SECOND EDITION

MAKING PLAY JUST RIGHT

Unleashing the Power of Play in Occupational Therapy

HEATHER KUHANECK, PhD, OTR/L, FAOTA
Sacred Heart University
Fairfield, CT

SUSAN L. SPITZER, PhD, OTR/L
Private Practice
Pasadena, CA

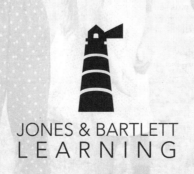

JONES & BARTLETT
LEARNING

World Headquarters
Jones & Bartlett Learning
25 Mall Road
Burlington, MA 01803
978-443-5000
info@jblearning.com
www.jblearning.com

Jones & Bartlett Learning books and products are available through most bookstores and online booksellers. To contact Jones & Bartlett Learning directly, call 800-832-0034, fax 978-443-8000, or visit our website, www.jblearning.com.

32131-9

Production Credits
Vice President, Product Management: Marisa R. Urbano
Vice President, Content Strategy and Implementation: Christine Emerton
Director, Product Management: Matthew Kane
Product Manager: Whitney Fekete
Manager, Content Strategy: Carolyn Pershouse
Content Strategist: Carol Brewer Guerrero
Content Coordinator: Sam Gillespie
Director, Project Management and Content Services: Karen Scott
Manager, Project Management: Kristen Rogers
Project Manager: Dan Stone
Senior Digital Project Specialist: Angela Dooley
Director, Marketing: Andrea DeFronzo
Marketing Manager: Mark Adamiak

Content Services Manager: Colleen Lamy
Vice President, Manufacturing and Inventory Control: Therese Connell
Composition: Straive
Project Management: Straive
Cover Design: Briana Yates
Text Design: Kristin E. Parker
Senior Media Development Editor: Troy Liston
Rights & Permissions Manager: John Rusk
Rights Specialist: Benjamin Roy
Cover Image (Title Page, Part Opener, Chapter Opener):
    © Rawpixel.com/Shutterstock
Printing and Binding: McNaughton & Gunn

Library of Congress Cataloging-in-Publication Data
Names: Kuhaneck, Heather, author. | Spitzer, Susan L., author.
Title: Making play just right : unleashing the power of play in
    occupational therapy / Heather Kuhaneck, Susan Spitzer.
Other titles: Activity analysis, creativity, and playfulness in pediatric
    occupational therapy
Description: Second edition. | Burlington, Massachusetts : Jones & Bartlett
    Learning, [2023] | Preceded by: Activity analysis, creativity, and
    playfulness in pediatric occupational therapy : making play just right /
    Heather Miller Kuhaneck, Susan L. Spitzer, Elissa Miller. 2010. |
    Includes bibliographical references and index. | Summary: "At the heart
    of Making Play Just Right: Activity Analysis, Creativity, and
    Playfulness in Pediatric Occupational Therapy, Second Edition is the
    belief that occupational therapists must incorporate play into
    interventions with children in order to ensure that pediatric
    occupational therapy is maximally effective. This text provides the
    background, history, evidence, and general knowledge needed to use a
    playful approach to pediatric occupational therapy, as well as the
    specific examples and recommendations needed to help therapists adopt
    these strategies. The authors provide a number of case examples and
    companion videos to allow the reader to engage in learning activities to
    improve understanding of the content"– Provided by publisher.
Identifiers: LCCN 2021051304 | ISBN 9781284194654 (paperback)
Subjects: MESH: Play Therapy–methods | Occupational Therapy–methods |
    Disabled Children–rehabilitation | Developmental
    Disabilities–rehabilitation | Child
Classification: LCC RJ505.P6 | NLM WS 350.4 | DDC
    618.92/891653–dc23/eng/20220209
LC record available at https://lccn.loc.gov/2021051304

6048

Printed in the United States of America
25 24 23 22 21   10 9 8 7 6 5 4 3 2 1

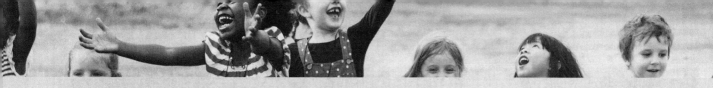

Brief Contents

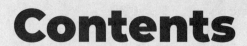

Contents

SECTION 1   The Knowledge You Need

SECTION 2 The Skills You Need

CHAPTER 3 Examining Play in Our Pediatric Clients: Formal Assessments 77

CHAPTER 4 Informal Play Assessment and Activity Analysis 109

APPENDIX 4.1 Safety and Accessibility Checklist. 133

APPENDIX 4.2 History of Activity Analysis. 139

APPENDIX 4.3 Training of Students in Activity Analysis. 140

SECTION 3 And How To Apply Them

CHAPTER 5 The Occupational Therapist as a Tour Guide to the Land of "PLAY" 141

CHAPTER 6 Being Playful: Therapeutic Use of Self in Pediatric Occupational Therapy 157

Chapter 12 **Play to Promote Mental Health in Children and Youth** 321

CHAPTER 13 **Creative Play and Leisure for Adolescents** **347**

CHAPTER 14 **Improving Social Play and Friendships Through Play in Groups** **375**

CHAPTER 15 **Perspectives on the Meaning of Play: International, Cultural, and Individual Contexts** . . . **399**

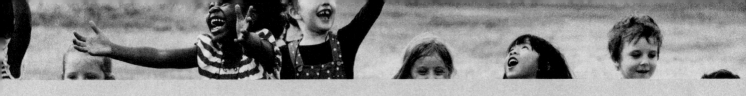

eBook Video Contents

The following videos are included within the *Navigate eBook*:

Chapter 4 Videos
Activity Analysis: Bike Riding
Activity Analysis: Building
Activity Analysis: Finger Painting (also in Chapter 7)

Chapter 6 Videos
Communicating in Play
Humor and Trash Cans (also in Chapter 16)
Lights Out: Adjusting to the Unexpected
Play and Therapeutic Relationship with a Parent and Child
Therapeutic Use of Self in Motor Play
Therapeutic Use of Self in Sensory Play

Chapter 7 Videos
Activity Analysis: Finger Painting (also in Chapter 4)

Chapter 8 Videos
Darts: Work and Play
Drawing and Writing as Playful Work
Drawing: Work and Play
Occupational Analysis and Modifying of Jacks in the Moment
Playful Work with Shoes
Snow and Grading Sensory Play
The Work and Play of Shoelaces
Trains as Work and Play

Chapter 16 Videos
Ghost in the Dark: Scary Play
Humor and Trash Cans (also in Chapter 6)
Play Interests, Structure, and Flexibility
Playful and Therapeutic Choice Cards
Pretending Something New

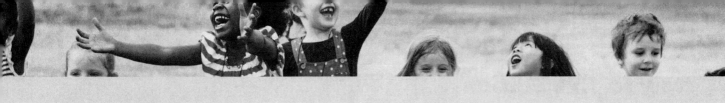

Preface

This book revolves around two core tenets. The first is that the meaning of the activities we engage in with our clients is the key to intervention effectiveness. The second is that play is fundamentally important for all children. For all pediatric clients, their primary meaningful occupation is play. Therefore, for pediatric occupational therapy to be maximally effective, we believe that it is our professional responsibility not only to incorporate play into our interventions with children but also to support play as an important outcome of therapy for children of all ages. We must unleash the power of play in both of these ways.

We have experienced and seen how elusive play can be at times. It is not uncommon for students and novice practitioners to have difficulty creating a fluid, playful atmosphere, balancing the competing priorities of obtaining new skills through therapeutic "work" while engaging in enjoyable meaningful occupation. When work is required to overcome barriers to participation, play for its own sake often becomes devalued. It is our hope that we may assist occupational therapy practitioners in more clearly practicing client-centered, occupation-focused playful and joyful pediatric therapy.

This text provides the background, history, evidence, and general knowledge needed to use a play approach as well as the specific examples and recommendations needed to help practitioners adopt these strategies. Additionally, we provide a number of case examples and companion videos to allow the reader to engage in learning activities to improve understanding of the content. We believe the videos to be especially important as we value the experiences we have had being mentored while we observed a master clinician treating. Although it is impossible to ensure every therapist gets that opportunity, by demonstrating key principles within videotaped intervention sessions, it is our hope that the skills and strategies will come alive and be more readily understood and adopted. Hopefully, this will be one facet of your learning, learning that will be applied in practice with a mentor.

For us, this book is very personal, like play. We are passionate about play and occupational therapy. Together, we have over 55 years of experience in pediatric practice using a play-based approach. We were both shaped by the work of A. Jean Ayres, as well as a wealth of incredible mentors and colleagues who are experts in practice. We have shared so many of our experiences to illustrate and expand on current research. We are so thankful for the way play has empowered our practice. Yet even with our knowledge and experience, we too have struggled with play at times. We *worked* on this book about *play* amid the global COVID-19 pandemic, a decidedly unplayful time, a time when the quest for play became increasingly important for ourselves, our clients, and our world. We found solace in the topic and endeavored onward because of our love for play-based occupational therapy. It is worth it if this book empowers other occupational therapy practitioners and, through them, children and adolescents.

This book, like many projects that span a long period of time, evolved and changed as it emerged into the form you read today. The initial focus of the book, using activity analysis in pediatric intervention, morphed and changed as our commitment to a playful approach to therapy took center stage. This second edition focuses extensively on the use of play in pediatric occupational therapy. Although pediatric activity analysis continues to be featured prominently, it is well overshadowed by the growth in play research and practice. Because of this incredible growth, we found it necessary to bring on a number of colleagues with added expertise to author additional chapters. We find it exciting to see that the power of play both in intervention and in daily life is being recognized increasingly.

In keeping with the content of the text, we have tried to maintain a playful, more personal, and somewhat informal writing style. Given the enormity of recent research, the tone in this edition is inevitably more formal as we struggled to balance play with scholarly work. Nonetheless, we hope that the style, content, and format allow you to enjoy your learning experience as you progress through this text. As you read and practice the strategies suggested here, we hope you have fun and unleash the power of play.

New to This Edition

Eight new chapters have been added to this edition to include comprehensive coverage of new areas of focus in pediatric occupational therapy, such as school-based therapy, mental health, and cultural perspectives:

- Chapter 9: Playful Play Spaces
- Chapter 10: Play in School-Based Occupational Therapy
- Chapter 11: Parent–Child Play and Attachment: Promoting Play Within Families
- Chapter 12: Play to Promote Mental Health in Children and Youth
- Chapter 13: Creative Play and Leisure for Adolescents
- Chapter 14: Improving Social Play and Friendships Through Play in Groups
- Chapter 15: Perspectives on the Meaning of Play: International, Cultural, and Individual Contexts
- Chapter 16: Creatively Negotiating Play Dilemmas

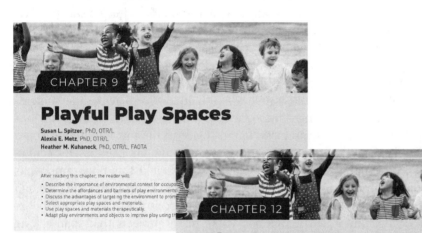

CHAPTER 9

Playful Play Spaces

Susan L. Spitzer, PhD, OTR/L
Alexia E. Metz, PhD, OTR/L
Heather M. Kuhaneck, PhD, OTR/L, FAOTA

After reading this chapter, the reader will:

- Describe the importance of environmental context for occupa...
- Determine the affordances and barriers of play environments...
- Discuss the advantages of targeting the environment to prom...
- Select appropriate play spaces and materials.
- Use play spaces and materials therapeutically.
- Adapt play environments and objects to improve play using t...

Good play environments have magical qualities that transcend the here and now, the humdrum and the typical. They have flow qualities—qualities that take the child to other places and other times. They are permeated with awe and wonder, both in rarity and in imaginative qualities.

—Joe Frost

Alongside other professional fields and with a wealth of well-established research, occupational therapy has adopted a transactional model of performance that recognizes that the environment is inseparable from human function (American Occupational Therapy Association [AOTA], 2020; Law et al., 1996). For children's play spaces, occupational therapy practitioners seek to create a person–environment fit for play by attending to the affordances offered by play environments and objects (Aziz & Said, 2015). Children's preferred play spaces provide an array of affordances for play, while balancing familiarity and novelty to promote exploration (Robinson, 1977). They are safe and accessible, allowing independent mobility and

© Rawpixel.com/Shutterstock

CHAPTER 12

Play to Promote Mental Health in Children and Youth

Lola Halperin, EdD, OTR/L
Sharon M. McCloskey, EdD, MBA, OTR

After reading this chapter, the reader will:

- Identify the benefits of play in relation to m...
- Describe the effects of adversity and men...
- Make play "just right" for children with men...
- Manage barriers to implementing play-ba...

When we treat children's play as seriously as...
we are helping them feel the joy that is to be...
creative spirit. It's the things we play with an...
who help us play that make a great differenc...

Play contributes to the social emotional he... dren (Ginsburg, 2007). Play is primarily a... experience that often results in positive emo... in turn, helps build a child's resilience a... well-being (Donaldson et al., 2011; Fredri... Seligman & Csikszentmihalyi, 2000). In co... tal illness can disrupt occupations (Krupa... including the essential occupation of play. M... conditions may become a barrier to play... negative effect on participation in other... (Keyes, 2007; Passmore, 2003; Singh & A... Zawadzki et al., 2015). The benefit of pla...

© Rawpixel.com/Shutterstock

CHAPTER 15

Perspectives on the Meaning of Play: International, Cultural, and Individual Contexts

Helen Lynch, PhD, MSc, Dip COT, Dip Montessori

After reading this chapter, the reader will:

- Describe play occupation from contrasting sociocultural contexts and from child and adult perspectives.
- Compare and contrast play as a universal concept versus play as a cultural concept.
- Identify reasons for protecting a child's right to play.
- Describe the core international documents that address a child's right to play.
- Explain challenges in occupational therapy for enabling play in international contexts.
- Apply play-centered occupational therapy that reflects local sociocultural and policy contexts.
- Formulate ways to enable play, informed by international examples of good practice.

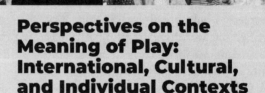

A fundamental problem with universal claims about play is that they basically ignore the contrasting realities of childhood experiences and the cultural forces that may help shape caregiver's ideas about play and early learning, and children's role in their own play.

—Roopnarine

Play is a phenomenon evident in cultural communities across all continents of the world (Lancy, 2007; Roopnarine, 2011). Although play is a universal behavior recognized in humans (Burghardt, 2014), play develops as a synthesis of nature *and* nurture. Indeed, the United Nations Committee on the Rights of the Child (CRC) General Comment 17, has contextualized play as a cultural expression whereby "children reproduce, transform, create and transmit culture through, for example, their imaginative play, songs, dance, animation, stories, painting, games, street theatre, puppetry, festivals, etc." (CRC, 2013, p. 5). Consequently, we need to ask: Does this mean that play is not universal after all? And how does play differ across cultures?

Occupational therapy practitioners who are committed to enhancing play for the children they serve, must understand how the form, function, and meaning of play can differ in different cultures. Occupational therapists need to understand play as a cultural phenomenon and not just a developmental one in order to build capacity to design interventions that have a goodness of fit for the child and family (Pierce, 2003). To strengthen their therapeutic power, therapists need

© Rawpixel.com/Shutterstock

Practice Examples feature specific cases, written by the authors.

PRACTICE EXAMPLE 9.2 Leyla's Play with Unsafe Objects

Leyla was a 9-year-old who sustained a head injury when hit by a car last year. As part of a home evaluation, an occupational therapist observed Leyla playing while holding an unused scented dryer sheet, which she repeatedly smelled. The therapist asked the father if this was common, and he explained that since the accident, the dryer sheets had become a favorite play item. Althou_____ therapist was concerned about the chemicals _____ because Leyla was exposing herself to chemic_____

PRACTICE EXAMPLE 3.2 Philip's Evaluation

Philip was a 7-year-old child who came with his mother for a_____ difficulties with social interaction and struggling at school w_____ that he was isolated socially and was failing in story comprel_____ the occupational therapist determined that it was important_____ pretend play especially due to its links to social ability, narrat_____ addressed by the ChIPPA 2 for this age.

Philip was chatty when I met him and was curious about_____ and started to explore the toys. He moved the toys around an_____ to balance all of them vertically. He was also interested wher_____ did experiments with them. He did not sequence play actions_____ and was not interested in imitating any modeled play actions_____ derivative was of $2x^3$. He was shocked I didn't know! Philip w_____

The ChIPPA 2 play assessment showed Philip's strengths_____ play, and also how difficult he found it to create play scenes_____ come again, and he did engage in play activities (with numbe_____ within spontaneous pretend play.

PRACTICE EXAMPLE 9.5 Mateo: Getting in the Game

Mateo was a third grader with cerebral palsy who used an AAC program on a tablet computer to communicate. Although his learning disabilities resulted in delayed academic skills, Mateo was included in a regular education classroom with an assistant. His parents had repeatedly stated that their top goal for Mateo was to be part of the class so that he could have friends and learn to be with other people for a full and meaningful life. And Mateo himself showed a strong interest in his peers.

The teacher requested the occupational therapist come during math games. Math games were used several times a week so that the children could help each other learn and practice new math skills. The teacher said that they did not know what to do with Mateo because he was behind in math and could not keep up with the other students in the games. The occupational therapist observed the class playing two math games, one using dice and the other using tile pieces. Each group of students pushed into a rough circle, with Mateo behind the circle with his assistant. All the students were very focused on the math concepts and seemed to be enjoying the games except Mateo, whose affect was flat. Mateo's only action was to enter what his assistant said into his tablet. The occupational therapist noted that Mateo was physically separate from the other students as well as uninvolved in their interactive play. The occupational therapist determined that the "games" for Mateo had been focused on the labor-intensive process of getting his work done. He had no control, choice, or opportunities to engage in the play.

The occupational therapist then suggested several modifications designed to promote play opportunities for Mateo:

- The addition of a plastic cup in the dice game so that Mateo could take an equal turn in rolling the dice
- Offering Mateo opportunities to hand out materials such as math tiles to give him a role in the group
- Use of screen shots of answers in his AAC program to be used as his work so that he could use his AAC program for communication
- Tape on the floor to mark a large enough space for Mateo to fit into the same space as his peers (with his assistant behind/outside the circle)
- Assistant's role to be assisting with screen shots and encouraging him to initiate and respond to the comments of other students about the math games
- Consider establishing a role of student scribe, who rotates in recording math problems and answers.

After a few weeks, the occupational therapist observed Mateo physically, verbally, and emotionally engaged in the math games.

Practice Opportunities provide case-study-type content focused on case study situations intended to broaden perspectives around race, gender identity, and other issues related to practice.

Practice Opportunity 5.1 Children as the Experts on Inclusivity

Ariana Brazier, PhD, and Julia Brazier
ATL Parent Like A Boss, Inc.

While working with the multigrade combo group in the summer camp, I noticed that most of the group

prompting or coaching was necessary for them to be inclusive. In addition to the immense value of learning in mixed-age groups, the children of various ages were learning how to accommodate differences—

...ntly, in this specific instance, the other ... were appreciative of his differences as they ... reason for the new game.

... time the group engaged in his game, they ... to view him through an asset- or strengths- ...s. As an adult in their company, we should ... habit of revisiting these teachable moments ...nal dialogue. Revisiting the game through ... allows us the opportunity to challenge ... to recreate this kind of cooperative play and ... with available resources. In turn, we can ... and remind each of them of their existing ... community-building skills.

...ver, instead of leaning into our inclination ...bleism that would have us challenge or ... is child to perform according to someone ...nate in a game structured

...nceptualization of able- ...cting our students to ... of deprivation might ... our personal ignorance, ...curity with regard to ability, ... forth. Intentional or not, ...individualized attention. ...le to facilitate this play ...ering it, and I could ...o perform at his capacity. ...ultimately necessitated that ..., *be within* the group, *not*

Practice Opportunity 1.1 José, Josie, Role-Playing, and Gender Identity

Amers Goff, MA, OTR/L

José is a 16-year-old who attends a special day class. He has a huge personality, always has something to say, and often comes into the OT room at his school already talking about his favorite movies or characters. He passionately loves My Little Ponies and Disney movies, and he imagines fusion movies, where his favorite characters meet each other. José has a dual diagnosis of autism spectrum disorder and Down syndrome. For José, this means that he is very passionate about the things that interest... difficult for him to focu... become "stuck" on a s... his speech is sometim... program on his tablet...

José comes from... family. He is the only... Maria speaks about a... younger than he actu... love of Disney and My... encourage him towar... "masculine," such as... little interest in these...

José's school occupational therapy goals address increasing frustration tolerance to reduce emotional outbursts in class and improving time spent on-task. José works with several boys his own age in a group focused on building self-regulation and problem-solving skills. In this group, each student selects a character of a knight or a prince to role-play frustrating or challenging situations in which they get to problem solve, practice appropriate responses to social scenarios, and "save the day." José consistently

---

Practice Opportunity 15.1 Exploring Play in Cultural Contexts

When you read reports from children about their play, you can see inside their play worlds and begin to notice their cultural contexts. Here is an example from a group of children, ages 4 to 5 years, in San Juan, Puerto Rico, playing together in school:

J. knocks on the door to a playhouse on the playground in which L., R., N., M., J., A1., & E. are hiding. A2. stands next to him at the door. "We're visiting," J. says. "Open up the door for visitors." Children inside the house scream and hold the door closed. "No, they're witches!" one child inside the house cries. "Witches!" several other children shout, laughing and screaming. "Open the door. We won't eat you," A2. says. "We aren't even hungry." He laughs. The children inside the house scream and laugh and hold the door closed. "It is witches!" one unidentified child shouts. "Hold the door!" (Trawick-Smith, 2010, p. 552).

Their play is focused on a common play event where children try to frighten each other, and in this case, it involves witches. Witches are a feature of many diverse cultures, have a historical and sometimes religious relevance, and, in children's fairy tales, often represent evil. In some cultures, witches are primarily regarded as being part of festivals such as Halloween. These children are reproducing their cultural contexts through their play and using a shared notion of what is scary to enhance the risk and excitement in their play.

Student and Instructor Resources

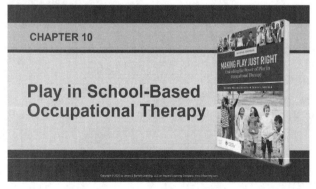

CHAPTER 10

Play in School-Based Occupational Therapy

Each new purchase of this textbook includes an access code to an enhanced *Navigate eBook*, which includes the following resources:

- Engaging video cases, illustrating the analysis of play and treatment applications
- Knowledge check questions, allowing students to test their knowledge along the way
- Chapter quizzes, allowing instructors to gauge each student's chapter learning
- Forms and worksheets to apply material to practice

The following **instructor resources** are available to qualified instructors:

- Slides in PowerPoint format
- Instructor Manual
- Test Bank available in LMS-compatible formats
- Image bank

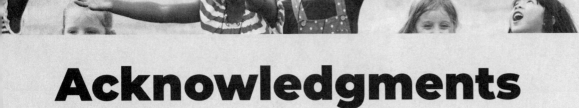

Acknowledgments

Completing any body of work requires the collaborative efforts of many individuals, and this text is no exception. We are grateful to the following people for their contributions and assistance: Carol Guerrero for her patience and assistance with our endless questions and queries; the numerous friends, family, and clients who agreed to be photographed and videotaped; Heather's former students, who provided photos and videos of their children playing; our clients throughout the years, as each one has taught and inspired us, and that cumulative experience is reflected and embedded in these pages; and our colleagues, who contributed their expertise directly to author-expanded material to complete this text. Finally, we each need to acknowledge the sacrifice of our families, who allowed us the time to devote to this creative enterprise and labor of love.

There is nothing that screams "PLAY" to me more than watching my two dogs, Ellie and Oliver, totally in the moment romping through the woods on our hikes, and their playful nature energizes mine. So, I must recognize their sacrifice, as over the years they often had to cheerfully wait for me to finish my work before we could go out to play. Well, maybe they weren't so cheerful about it, but they learned to wait if not to understand. More importantly, to my husband, Shayne, my enduring love and gratitude. Your playful, silly side helps keep me sane when I become too serious, and your steady support and encouragement allows me to grow.

—*HMK*

To my friends and family, I am so grateful for your understanding, patience, and humor. Together we have forgone so much as I put lots of play on hold to work on this book. Most of all, to my husband, David Morales, my love, gratitude, and admiration for you are only deepened by your enduring sacrifices and support. You have given up the most on a daily basis and yet have remained my greatest supporter, always believing in me even when I doubt myself. The moments of playfulness and silliness on which you insist are a welcome respite from work and the reminder I needed of the value of play. Thank you.

—*SLS*

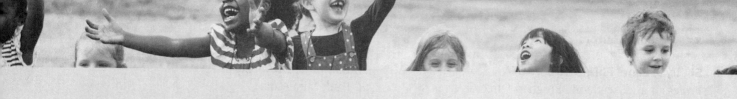

Contributors

Susan Bazyk, PhD, OTR/L, FAOTA
Professor Emerita, Occupational Therapy Program
Cleveland State University, and
Project Director, Every Moment Counts, LLC
Cleveland, Ohio

Amy Y. Burton, OTD, OTR/L
Assistant Professor of Occupational Therapy
Western New England University
Springfield, Massachusetts

Elissa Cunningham, OTD, OTR/L
Team District Leader/Occupational Therapist
Constellation School Based Therapy
Norwalk, Connecticut

Sarah E. Fabrizi, PhD, OTR/L
Associate Professor
Florida Gulf Coast University
Fort Myers, Florida

Lola Halperin, EdD, OTR/L
Assistant Professor in the Graduate Occupational
   Therapy Program
Sacred Heart University
Fairfield, Connecticut

Helen Lynch, PhD, MSc, Dip Montessori
Senior Lecturer
Department of Occupational Science and
   Occupational Therapy
University College Cork (UCC)
Cork, Ireland

Sharon M. McCloskey, EdD, MBA, OTR/L, DipCOT
Department Chair and Program Director
Graduate Program in Occupational Therapy
Sacred Heart University
Fairfield, Connecticut

Alexia E. Metz, PhD, OTR/L
Associate Professor & Program Director
Occupational Therapy Doctorate Program
University of Toledo
Toledo, Ohio

Kyle H. O'Brien, PhD, DHSc, MSW, MSOT, LCSW, OTR/L
Director of Health Science | Department of Health
   and Movement Sciences
Associate Professor | Department of Social Work
Southern Connecticut State University
New Haven, Connecticut

Karen E. Stagnitti, PhD, BOccThy, GCHE
Emeritus Professor
Deakin University
Geelong, Victoria
Australia

Amiya Waldman-Levi, PhD, OTR/L
Clinical Associate Professor of Occupational Therapy
Katz School of Science and Health
Yeshiva University
New York, New York

Practice Opportunity Contributors

Ariana Brazier, PhD
Founder & CEO
ATL Parent Like A Boss, Inc.
Atlanta, Georgia

Julia Brazier
Chairwoman of the Board of Directors
ATL Parent Like A Boss, Inc.
Atlanta, Georgia

Amers Goff, MA, OTR/L
Glendale Unified School District
Glendale, California

Reviewers

Nancy Gabres, MS, OTR/L
Assistant Professor
College of St. Scholastica
Duluth, Minnesota

Shelly J. Lane, PhD, OTR/L, FAOTA
Professor and Academic Program Director
Occupational Therapy, Colorado State University
Fort Collins, Colorado

Paula Rabaey, PhD, OTR/L
Associate Professor of Graduate Occupational
   Therapy Department
St. Catherine University
St. Paul, Minnesota

Joylynne D. Wills, MGA, OTR/L
Clinical Assistant Professor
Department of Occupational Therapy
Howard University
Washington, District of Columbia

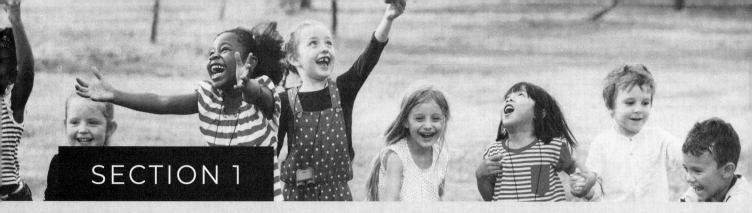

SECTION 1

The Knowledge You Need

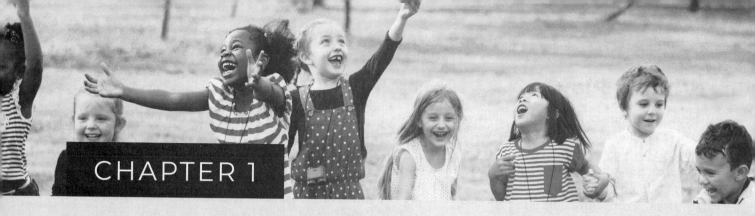

CHAPTER 1

Answering the Big Questions About Play

Heather M. Kuhaneck, PhD, OTR/L, FAOTA
Kyle O'Brien, PhD, DHSc, MSOT, MSW, OTR/L, LCSW

After reading this chapter, the reader will:

- Define play and describe its characteristics.
- Summarize theories of why children play.
- Compare and contrast play and playfulness.
- Recognize the universality and diversity of play.
- Identify the typical patterns of development of play and play preferences in humans.
- Apply this knowledge to practice.

Play is a uniquely adaptive act, not subordinate to some other adaptive act, but with a special function of its own in human experience.

—Johan Huizinga

Occupational therapy practitioners who wish to support and advocate for children's play must be armed with an array of important knowledge derived from both theory and evidence. Play theory has developed over more than 100 years, but interest in play and the ensuing research about play has grown exponentially since the prior edition of this text. As play research can be considered in its infancy compared to other areas of inquiry, there are many unanswered questions about play. However, this chapter will attempt to answer the BIG questions about play for therapists to promote play as an essential occupation in daily life.

Information gained from research increasingly is answering the big questions about play. Expanding ideas about play garnered through the study of children at play in natural environments, examination of species other than humans, and via advancing technology for imaging the brain increasingly justify the importance of play. Occupational therapists, in our conceptualization of play as an occupation, must use this information both to consider the myriad consequences for our clients of an inability to play as they prefer and to identify the appropriate methods for assessing and intervening. This knowledge base is crucial to support evidence-based practice in occupational therapy through thoughtful therapeutic reasoning to promote play in our practice with intentional interventions. So, let us begin with the most fundamental question.

What Is Play?

The word *play* is used in multiple fashions and has many connotations. People use the word *play* as a noun, as in theater productions on stage. People also use the word *play* to discuss sensory experiences, as in observing the "play" of light on the surface of the ocean. One could also play dead, play the radio, play with food, play it safe, or make a play for something. The task of defining play has been noted by many to be difficult. For example, Reilly (1974) likened the task of defining play to "defining a cobweb" and stated, "only the naïve could believe from reviewing the evidence of the literature that play is a behavior having an identifiable nature. While common sense may confidently assert that there is such a thing as play, the literature assumes a rather weak position about what this phenomenon is" (p. 113). Burghart (2005) similarly suggested that the problems with defining play are "legendary" (p. 49). For almost 100 years authors have tried to define the word *play*. Some examples of the many definitions are included in **Table 1.1**. In reviewing these attempts, one notes many similarities. However, one of the primary problems in defining play is the variety of play that exists. None of these definitions have gained the consensus to become "the" definition of play. However, across time, as will be seen in this chapter, progress has been made in this endeavor through greater interest by scientists and new avenues of research.

Knowing Play When You See It

Despite the difficulty of defining play, most readers, parents, teachers, and children know what play is. Play may be easier to recognize than define. The assertion that you can, in fact, "know play when you see it" has been studied and found to be true to a

Table 1.1 Notable Conceptions of Play throughout the Years

Year	Author	Definition or Description
1935	Buhler	Activity with or without materials, where bodily movement is an end in itself.
1950	Huizinga	Activity occurring for its own sake. Fully absorbing, providing elements of uncertainty, illusion, or exaggeration. Disconnected from material interest, or profit, proceeding according to rules.
1984	Fagan	Active behavioral interactions, player adjusts to/creates environment.
1990	Garvey	Voluntary, intrinsically motivated, associated with recreational pleasure/enjoyment.
1997	Sutton-Smith	Novel adaptation similar to the evolutionary struggle for survival.
2005	Scarlett et al.	Almost anything that would be considered enjoyable.
2014	Burghart	Seemingly nonfunctional and repeated behavior, initiated in a relaxed, low-stress setting.
2014	Eberle	Pleasurable, voluntary, emergent process, deepens positive emotions, instructs in social skills, enables a state that leaves us ready to play more.
2015	Van Vleet & Feeney	Carried out for amusement and fun, enthusiastic, in-the-moment attitude, highly interactive.
2017	LEGO Foundation	Activities to promote agency, supported vs. directed, experienced as joyful, meaningful, active, engaged, social, iterative thinking.
2018	Wright	Exists within a safe, bounded reality, absence of coercion, an imaginative method for engaging the real, one of the ways to learn boundaries between fantasy and reality. Connected to purposeful and nonpurposeful accomplishments, but never meaningless.
n.d.	National Institute for Play	Gateway to vitality, intrinsically rewarding, generates optimism and novelty, fun, leads to mastery and empathy, boosts the immune system, promotes belonging/community.

degree (Smith & Voldstedt, 1985). However, certain characteristics appear more important than others in making the determination, and observers may need to have at least two or more of the criteria present to be able to do so. The characteristic of nonliterality, or pretend, may be the most important characteristic in judging an episode as play, and the three criteria that best identify play are nonliterality, positive affect, and flexibility.

Characteristics of Play

With the difficulty of defining play, authors have instead created lists of characteristics that combine to make an activity play (see **Box 1.1**). The commonly agreed-upon characteristics for humans include that play is self-chosen or self-directed, is intrinsically motivated, is imaginative, and occurs in a relatively stress-free but active state of mind. Other characteristics include that play is pleasurable, is meaningful, and occurs with an attitude of playfulness (Bundy, 1993, Eberle, 2014; Gray, 2009, 2013; Lego Foundation, 2018c; Parham, 1996). In relation to animal play, Burghardt (2005) developed five criteria to denote play that include: the behavior should not be completely functional in the context in which it occurs, it should be voluntary, it should be modified in some way when compared to the typical occurrence in the functional activity, it should occur repeatedly (but not necessarily invariantly), and it should appear in animals when they are healthy and unstressed.

Occupational therapy practitioners are cautioned not to idealize play, however. Although the list of characteristics describing play sounds wonderful, not all play is wonderful. Some play may be scary

for some children. Play can be dangerous and risky (**Figure 1.1**). Some play is cruel. Play can be about struggles for power and dominance. Sometimes children must defer to more powerful or dominant children. Some play is highly sexualized. Play is not always completely free, and opportunities may not be accessible or available for all. And not all play is flexible; some play is highly rule bound and structured.

The Play vs. Nonplay Dichotomy

Sometimes it is easiest to define or describe something by comparing it to its opposite. A recently developed play-coding scheme attempted to identify play versus nonplay episodes using criteria across three dimensions, social-emotional, sensorimotor, and cognitive (Neale et al., 2018). These researchers coded what they called play congruent or nonplay congruent episodes based on these three dimensions simultaneously. In play congruent episodes, toys were available, and mothers were instructed to play with their infants. The coding scheme was effective in identifying the play congruent episodes in a small sample of mother–infant interactions. Play congruent episodes were found to result in higher scores on the social–emotional and sensorimotor dimensions. However, the cognitive dimension did not differ between play and nonplay episodes (Neale et al., 2018).

The Play-Work Dichotomy

In trying to define play, it has often been considered to be the opposite of work. Play was considered different from work because of its voluntary nature and lack of coercion (Wright, 2018). These ideas about this dichotomy originally grew out of economic concerns and the push for humans, and even children, to be oriented toward production. However, others rejected these notions and asserted the importance of play. The dispute over the relative importance of play vs. work for children also arose in part because of adult perceptions regarding the nature of children. Some advocated for childhood freedom (and play) because of their beliefs in the innate goodness of children, whereas others believed children left to their own devices would get into trouble, and therefore supported greater control over childhood activities and the provision of more work and more discipline (Goodman, 1994).

This artificially created division of two different constructs—work and play, often considered to be mutually exclusive—has fostered research supporting the dichotomy and ignoring the idea that one

Box 1.1 Characteristics of Activities Typically Defined as Play

- Flexible
- Spontaneous
- Intrinsically motivated
- Nonliteral or symbolic
- Voluntary
- Freely chosen
- Fun/enjoyable/joyful
- Meaningful
- Nonfunctional
- Resembling real behaviors but without the real consequences
- Active, engaged
- Iterative
- Social

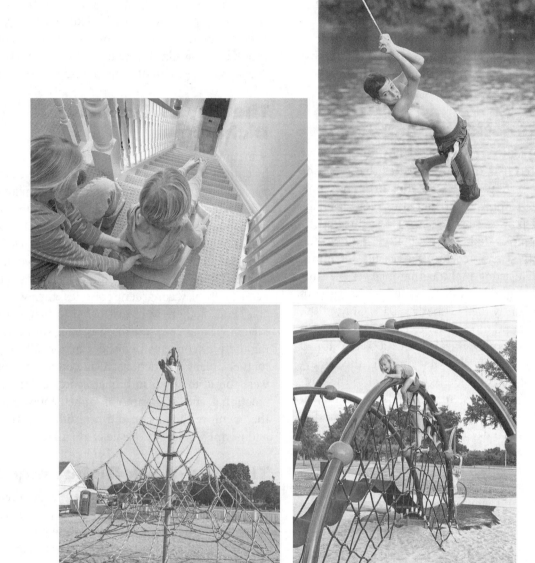

Figure 1.1 Some play is risky, dangerous, or just a little scary

Top left: © sturti/E+/Getty Images; top right: © Solid photos/Shutterstock. Bottom left: Courtesy of Leah Maniscalco Pirro. Bottom right: Courtesy of Kylene Wenzl Carroll.

could play while working or that one could take one's play very seriously and approach it almost like work (Holmes, 1999). There is likely a continuum between work and play rather than separate categories. Children asked to classify activities as either work or play label some things as "in between" (Wing, 1995), and this idea of a continuum has been noted in other similar studies (Holmes, 1999). Children do recognize these differences between play and work (Wiltz & Fein, 2015). They can differentiate between things they do at school that are and are not play but their understanding of what is play and work changes during the preschool and kindergarten years. Over time, the issues of choice and the voluntary nature of the activity becomes a defining factor. Play is considered to be fun, whereas work is not. While 5-year-olds consider the terms mutually exclusive, college students do not, suggesting that an understanding of the continuum may require a certain cognitive ability or level of experience (Holmes, 1999).

This dichotomy is not universal cross-culturally either. In many non-Western cultures, children work when they are able to produce something of economic value and play when they cannot (Chick, 2010). The age when the ratio of children's time at play and time at work shifts varies by culture and may relate to the primary way in which the culture supports itself (Ember & Cunnar, 2015). In at least some hunter-gatherer societies, there may be a type of "work-play" that is in between (Crittenden, 2016).

In current times and in Western societies, with child labor laws, educational requirements, and advanced technology, many of the early ideas about the dichotomy of work and play require further examination. These societal changes may warrant a continuum approach to considering what play is, or entirely new models and ideas that can accommodate new modes of play such as computer gaming that appear to blur the lines between work and play (Wright, 2018; Yee, 2006). In the middle areas of the continuum, where play and work overlap, children initiate purposeful activity (worklike) that they find enjoyable (playlike) (Goodman, 1994).

Some have proposed that play *is* the "work" of children (Stetsenko, & Ho, 2015), allowing them to develop into unique human individuals within a sea of social connection, while also learning to embody the culture of which they are a part (Rettig, 1995). In education, there is much discussion about play-based learning, and classrooms vary in their attempts to be more playlike or worklike (Goodhall & Atkinson, 2017; Pyle & Danniels, 2017). These issues and concerns exist in occupational therapy as well, as therapists must decide how playlike to be in their therapeutic sessions.

Defining Play as a Continuum

One way to manage the dichotomy is to consider play as a continuum or a spectrum based on the level of freedom and child-directedness present (Zosh et al., 2018; **Figure 1.2**). At one end is free play, considered the "gold standard" for play. Free play, and pretend play in particular, is the type of play on which many of the definitions and list of characteristics are based.

Along the play continuum, however, as a child is provided with more structure from an adult, there are additional forms of guided play and games that are still child directed, but have increasingly greater therapeutic goals. Then, the other end of the continuum is adult facilitated play and direct instruction through play. This sort of continuum might address some of the time when play seemingly does not match the full list of characteristics ascribed to it, yet still could be considered play. As will be seen in later chapters, occupational therapists have adopted the idea of a play continuum as well, as they try to navigate the amount of direction provided during sessions with children.

Play as an Attitude: Playfulness

The idea that play may be more of an *attitude* than a *thing* encourages a different type of definition. Ferland (2005) defined play as a subjective attitude in which pleasure, interest, and spontaneity are combined and that is expressed through freely chosen behavior where no specific performance is expected. Definitions of play as an attitude consider criteria such as the source of motivation, the level of goal orientation, and the degree of stimuli domination, as well as flexibility, affect, rule boundaries, and active involvement of the person observed. Each aspect occurs in degrees, and, as the relative combination of them increases, an activity is more likely to be described as playful or play (Rogers et al., 1998). The Lego Foundation (2018c) has suggested that playful experiences are joyful; help children find meaning; are active, engaging, and social; and foster learning. Bundy (1997) theorized that the combination of three elements, intrinsic motivation, internal control, and the ability to suspend reality, together make play playful. Playfulness as an attitude or a disposition appears easier to define and measure, and many authors have worked at both defining playfulness and creating measures of it (Barnett, 1990, 1991; Lieberman, 1965,

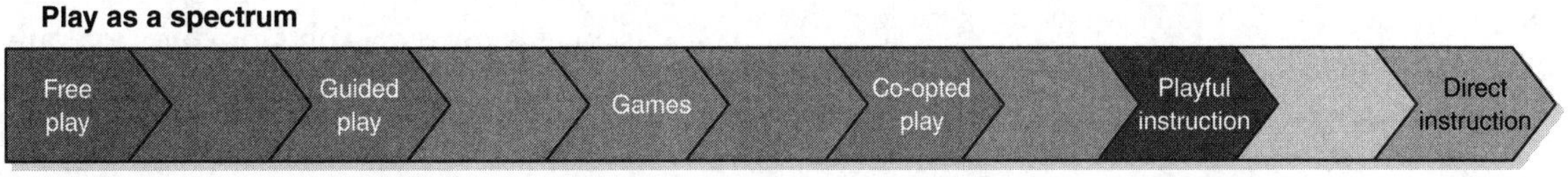

Play as a spectrum

	Free play	Guided play	Games	Co-opted play	Playful instruction	Direct instruction
Initiated by:	Child	Adult	Adult	Child	Adult	Adult
Directed by:	Child	Child	Child	Adult	Adult	Adult
Explicit learning goal:	No	Yes	Yes*	Yes	Yes	Yes

*Here, we refer to "serious games" as outlined in Hassinger-Das et all., 2017 in which the game has a learning goal.

Figure 1.2 Play as a continuum

Reproduced from Zosh, J. M., Hirsh-Pasek, K., Hopkins, E. J., Jensen, H., Liu, C., Neale, D., Solis, S. L., & Whitebread, D. (2018). Accessing the inaccessible: Redefining play as a spectrum. *Frontiers in Psychology, 9*, 1124. doi:10.3389/fpsyg.2018.01124

1966; Skard & Bundy, 2008). Occupational therapists may apply this information to invoke a playful attitude even while completing the work of therapy.

Play as Experience

Another way to consider play is as an experience (Henricks, 2015). As an experience, play can be an individual behavior, an action. Or play can be interaction, something that occurs between two or more people or between a person and object(s). Play can be an activity, situated in a culture, a behavior situated within a context, or a disposition/attitude. Each of these ways of considering play, though, differ in their consideration of the essential subjective experience, the affective experience of play. There is a way to examine "what are the many possibilities for action presented by the situation at hand and what are the personal implications of these?" (Henricks, 2015, p. 42). Therefore, play fosters self- awareness and allows cultivation of curiosity, fun, exhilaration, and gratification. During play, there is the potential for satisfying feelings, happiness, and confidence. Occupational therapists must consider the meaningfulness of the play activity in which a child is engaged and promote the development of mastery, confidence, and self-esteem through play-based therapeutic interventions.

Play as a Process

Perhaps defining play is difficult because most attempts do not account for the process that occurs during play, with change and variability. In one newer conception, play is an emergent system that self-organizes (Eberle, 2014). The six interconnected elements of anticipation, surprise, pleasure, understanding, strength, and poise emerge sequentially. These elements also occur in differing levels of intensity or "expression" in play, growing over time as one plays. For those interested in more information about this conceptualization of play, you can view a chart online (The Strong, n.d.).

The Definition for This Text

Here we offer a definition of play to provide a shared understanding for this book. For our purposes, we define play as *any activity freely entered into that is fun or enjoyable and that is appropriately matched to one's skill to represent an attainable challenge* (Kuhaneck, Spitzer, & Miller, 2010). Our definition is both similar to others in the literature and different as well. We have included each portion of this definition for specific reasons.

The inclusion of fun and enjoyment is intended to give voice to the importance and meaning of play as

described by children themselves. If play is defined as children define play, play is fun (Heah, Case, McGuire, & Law, 2007; Miller & Kuhaneck, 2008; Scarlett et al., 2005; Wiltz & Fein, 2006). Using "fun" in our definition of play, however, provides us with yet another dilemma. "If we could come up with a workable definition of fun and measure it objectively, we would still be left with the begging question 'why is this particular behavior fun?'" (Heinrich & Smolker, 1998, p. 28).

Fun often means that the game, toy, or activity provides an appropriate level of challenge (Csikszentmihalyi, 1990; Vygotsky, 1978). Therefore, our definition captures the importance of the *just right challenge* (Ayres, 1972; Burke, 1977; Michelman, 1974). The concept of the *just right challenge* suggests that a task must not be too hard but also not too easy. This concept originated from the University of Southern California faculty and students in their development of sensory integration and occupational behavior (Ayres, 1972; Burke, 1977; J. Burke and F. Clark, personal communication, November 10, 2021; Michelman, 1974, Robinson, 1977). It has been discussed by occupational therapists in relation to play and sensory integration for children (Ayres, 1972; Gaylard, 1966; Lindquist, Mack & Parham, 1982; Michelman, 1974; Robinson, 1977), the flow state (Jacobs, 1994; Rebeiro, & Polgar, 1999) and good occupational therapy practice (Burke, 1977; Christie, 1999; Hinojosa, 1994; Rogers, 1982; Yerxa, 1994).

Finally, the idea of play as voluntary and freely entered into is included because of the literature on the importance of intrinsic motivation for fun and play. Thus, someone else may suggest the idea for play, but the child is motivated and willing to participate. This definition is purposefully broad to allow us to encompass the continuum of play, the range of play of children with disabilities and particularly those with autism, as well as the sport and leisure of teenagers, and even some of the playful work of adults.

Who Plays?

Now let us turn to the next big question. Who plays? Is play a universal phenomenon or only engaged in by those with a certain level of evolutionary development? We can start with humans, as we know that most humans play.

Children Play

Play appears to be a universal aspect of child development. There is evidence indicating that children have played throughout history since the ancient Greeks,

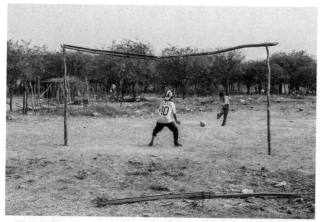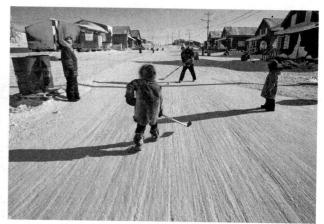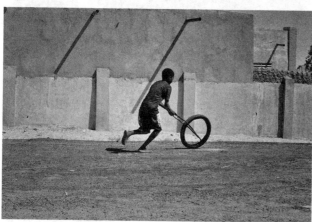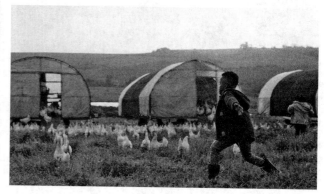

Figure 1.3 Children across the globe play

Top left: © Gonzalo Bell/Shutterstock; top right: © Ton Koene photography/Moment Open/Getty Images; bottom left: © yoh4nn/E+/Getty Images; bottom right: © PeopleImages/E+/Getty Images.

Sumerians, and Egyptians (Barnes, 2006). Children in both modern societies and hunter-gatherer societies play, and children across the globe in diverse cultures play (Gaskins, Haight, & Lancy, 2007; Hewlett, 2017; Konner, 2016; Roopnarine & Davidson, 2015) (**Figure 1.3**). Children with disabilities also play, but they may play somewhat differently than those without disabilities for a variety of reasons such as limited access; motor difficulties; cognitive, social, or language difficulties; or attitudes of adults (Chiarello et al., 2019; Lee et al., 2016; Pfeifer, Pacciulio, Santos, Santos, & Stagnitti, 2011; Sterman, Naughton, Bundy, Froude, & Villeneuve, 2020).

Adults Play

Although play is often considered something that only children do, adults play as well (Van Vleet & Feeney, 2015). Adults are certainly capable of play, and some adults are in fact quite playful (Barnett, 2007; Proyer & Jehle, 2013). For adults, play may be an expression of intimacy, acceptance, and trust and may be a method of stress reduction (Van Vleet & Feeney, 2015). Playfulness, a dispositional tendency to engage in play may also be related to life satisfaction

for adults (Proyer, 2013; Van Vleet & Feeney, 2015). Some adults embrace and engage in their play in large public groups through fandom, character dress up, zombie walks, renaissance festivals, and the like (Austin, 2015; Brownie, 2015; Gunnels, 2009; Maier, 2019; Shipley, 2010) (**Figure 1.4**). Others may characterize their play differently and engage more privately, such as through collecting toys or completing private hobbies (Heljakka, 2018; Heljakka, Harviainen, & Suominen, 2018).

Not all adults play or like to play, however. Adults may not actively seek to engage in play with children or may not feel they know how. Some adults dislike play or at least certain types of play. A quick internet search finds multiple blog posts by parents describing their lack of desire to play and also their guilt over not wanting to play with their children.

The Play of Nonhumans: Both Juveniles and Adults

In addition to humans of all ages, many nonhuman species play too. Play has been documented in 5 of the 30 different phyla of nonhuman species (Burghardt, 2005, 2014, 2015; Pellis, Pellis, & Himmler 2014).

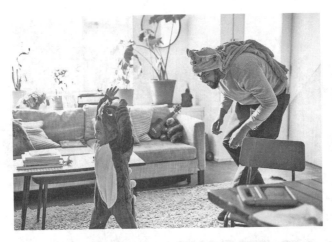

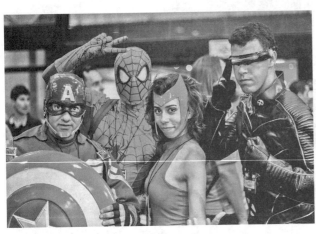

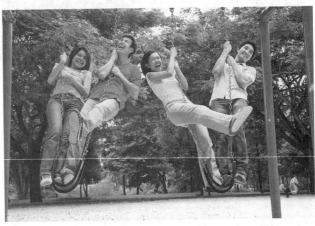

Figure 1.4 Adults play too

Top: © 10'000 Hours/DigitalVision/Getty Images; bottom left: © Andre Luiz Moreira/Shutterstock; bottom right: © Asia Images Group/Shutterstock.

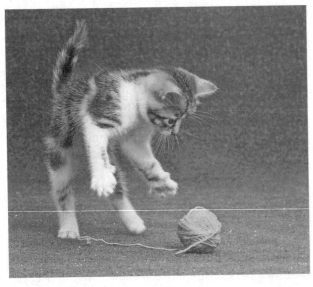

Figure 1.5 Cats play

© DenisNata/Shutterstock.

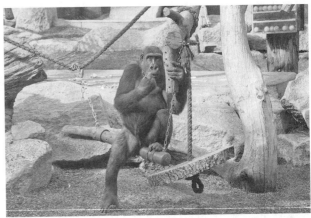

Figure 1.6 Primates play

© Artem Dulub/Shutterstock.

Dogs play, cats play, and rodents play, and elaborate play has been observed in both ravens and primates (**Figures 1.5**, **1.6**, and **1.7**). Play has been observed in dolphins, turtles, lizards, and fish as well as octopuses, spiders, and wasps (Burghardt, 2014, 2015; Ikeda et al., 2018; Kuba et al., 2006). Animals have been observed to engage in locomotor play, object play, and social play (Burghardt, 2010). Similar to humans, play is primarily observed in juvenile animals, and often juveniles are each other's preferred play partners. However, adults play as well (Burghardt, 2014; Hill, Dietrich, & Cappiello, 2017). Some believe that human play is different because humans pretend. However, primates have been seen to pretend (Matsuzawa, 2020). In particular, pretense has been observed in both chimps and gorillas who have been trained to use language (Gomes & Martin-Andrade, 2005; Lyn,

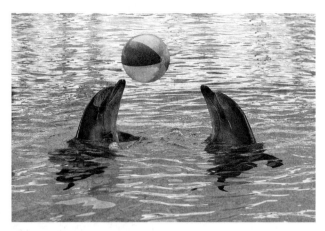

Figure 1.7 Even dolphins play
© ForGaby/Shutterstock.

Greenfield, & Savage-Rumbaugh, 2006). The study of play in animals has been informative for researchers who investigate why humans play (Burghardt, 2010).

Why Do We Play?

The comparative study of play across other species illuminates the evolution and function of human play (Smaldino, Palagi, Burghardt, & Pellis, 2019). According to evolutionary theory, there must be an advantage to this behavior for it to continue. If one completed a cost–benefit analysis in many species, one could see play had the potential to be quite costly. There is an expenditure of energy and the opportunity to be noticed and attacked by predators. Play can in fact be quite dangerous for animals (Caro, 1995; Harcourt, 1991; Kuehl et al., 2008). So, what advantage could play provide for a species? Why has it continued throughout evolution? Why do we play? For years, this was a difficult question to answer with any certainty.

Perhaps some of the difficulty in understanding the function of play was the combined consideration of play's primary purpose along with its beneficial consequences. The initial *cause* of play and the *function* of play that developed over time could be quite different (Burghardt, 2014, 2015; Smaldino et al., 2019). One can separately speculate about the primary processes that may have led to play evolving in ancient animals and the secondary processes that evolved over time as play conferred benefits to animals that engaged in it. Play perhaps emerged initially out of exploration to escape boredom in animals where food was plentiful, where predators were limited, and where parental care provided for most needs. Then, after a period, play evolved to facilitate rapid behavioral and mental development through natural selection. Through mechanisms of evolution, play continued because of

a host of secondary and tertiary benefits. See **Box 1.2** for a depiction of this model of the various potential causes and benefits of play (Burghardt, 2014). This model suggests that we likely play for many reasons, not just one.

A hundred years of theories about why we play can be broadly grouped based on the time period in which they were developed. Earlier "classical" theories about the function of play were developed often via opinion or observation of children. Most of these theories suggest some future benefit in relation to survival. One difficulty with many of them is that until quite recently there was very little evidence to support them (Burghardt, 2014; Sharpe, 2011). However, studies are now beginning to document that play in juvenile animals does actually confer future benefits to them (Blumstein, Chung, & Smith, 2013; Fagen & Fagen, 2009; Heintz, Murray, Markham, Pusey, & Lonsdorf, 2017; Nunes, 2014). For example, baby squirrels who play are more coordinated later on and become better mothers if female; and brown bears who play more are more likely to survive. The evidence is not wholly

---

Box 1.2 Hierarchy of Evolutionary Processes Leading to Animal Play

Primary Processes

- High activity levels or the need for stimulation to elicit typical behavior systems and optimal arousal
- Intention
- Excess metabolic energy
- Animals buffered from severe stress and food shortages
- Complex behaviors in varying conditions

Secondary Processes

- Provides neurological benefits
- Produces behavioral flexibility
- Fosters perceptual motor coordination
- Maintains physical fitness

Tertiary Processes

- Improved social status and reproductive success
- Novel behavior and creativity
- Ability for mental play
- Aids neurobehavioral development
- Reorganized and more complex behavioral systems

Modified from Burghardt, G. M. (1984). On the origins of play. In P. K. Smith (Ed.), *Play in animals and humans* (pp. 5–41). New York: Basil Blackwell; Burghardt, G. M. (2005). *The genesis of animal play: Testing the limits.* Cambridge, MA: MIT Press; and Burghardt, G. M. (2014). A brief glimpse at the long evolutionary history of play. *Animal Behavior and Cognition,* 1(2), 90–98.

supportive, however. The incredible variation in play complexity across species that do play as well as the number of creatures in the animal kingdom that do not play indicates to scientists that the function of play likely developed in different animals for different reasons, and not all species that play gain the same benefits from it. Perhaps play has arisen independently in different animals many times (Pellis et al., 2014). A description and discussion of the theories are provided in **Table 1.2**.

Animal research now suggests that perhaps one important reason for play is that it is a mechanism whereby an individual learns to modify behavior creatively and flexibly in the face of changes in conditions (Burghardt, 2014; Hill et al., 2017; Marks, Vizconde, Gibson, Rodriguez, & Nunes, 2017; Pellis et al., 2014). Play may provide stress regulation and enhanced ability to handle future stresses (Burghardt, 2014). In some species, play both creates and also promotes the transmission of novel behaviors to other young and adults of the species (Hill et al., 2017). This transmission strengthens the species' ability to adapt to environmental changes. There would be an evolutionary advantage for creatures that played and that were able to respond more adaptively to novel situations and had a broader mental repertoire that allowed greater success in adult life. During play, random actions are common. Play creates the unexpected and allows animals to learn to deal with novelty. Play may enhance creativity and the facilitation of

Table 1.2 Theories Regarding the Function of Play

Proponents and Theorists	Proposed Play Function	Explanation	Discussion
Schiller (1875) Spencer (1873)	Play to burn off or restore energy	Play emerged in individuals and animals that had more energy than they needed for basic survival and, therefore, played to "blow off steam."	Children do play when they are at the brink of exhaustion. Some play actually seems to refresh, rejuvenate, or restore the individual. Particularly with sedentary life, people need to use their muscles and engage in activities in more natural outdoor environments. However, these theories cannot explain play that is more cognitive in nature, such as puzzle play. They cannot account for play that is scary, stressful, or highly competitive and not at all relaxing (Saracho & Spodek, 1998).
Hall (1882)	Play as legacy from the past (recapitulation theory)	Each generation repeats the work of prior generations in a developmental sequence. First is survival then the experiences of early nomadic peoples, and then agricultural and tribal stages.	Children may act out activities in play that would have been from our ancient past, such as hunting, for example. However, there are many forms of play that hold little relationship to any past human history (e.g., hang gliding or video games).
Groos (1901)	Play as preparation	Play prepares children for the skills and abilities they would need in adult life.	Children do appear to practice certain adult forms of behavior through play, but they still learn even when they do not have opportunities to play.
Erickson (1950) Freud (1955)	Play to develop emotional well-being	Play allows children to make sense of feelings, gain a sense of control, work through loss or grief, and deal with anger in an acceptable fashion.	This theory ignores the play of much younger children and animals that lack the wide range of emotions experienced by humans. This perspective cannot explain a wide variety of recreational activities such as collecting and hiking.

Proponents and Theorists	Proposed Play Function	Explanation	Discussion
Piaget (1952, 1975) Vygotsky (1976) Bruner (1982)	Play to develop cognition	Play allows children to develop and integrate new skills. Play expresses or reflects children's learning.	Although play may assist development, children will still develop without it (for example, in societies where it is not encouraged or promoted).
Berlyne (1960) White (1959) Zuckerman (1971)	Play to be engaged	Play arises to seek arousal when one is not adequately stimulated by the environment. Children gain competence and satisfaction through play. Children gain pleasure from the ability to do something.	Cannot account for the entire range of motivation to play, nor for the continuum of playful work and "workful" play. Children may still play or want to play even when they are overstimulated.
Byers (1998) Thompson (1998)	Testing motor competence and exercise	Play is a mechanism of managing development so as to provide feedback on one's current level of ability. Play provides exercise for motor skills.	Evidence contradicts the motor exercise aspect of this theory. During play, the motions used are often too short in duration to provide any real muscular benefit. Also, if play is for muscular exercise, why does it not begin right at birth and continue throughout life? Muscular development declines rapidly if exercise is not continued. Additionally, this type of "play at the brink of capability" could lead to injury.
Hol, Van den Berg, Van Ree, & Spruijt (1999) Van den Berg et al. (1999) Panksepp & Burgdorf, (2003) Panksepp, Burgdorf, Turner, & Gordon (2003) Lewis (2005)	Building social competence	Animal play is for learning the local environment, the members of the social group, and the local culture; it allows animals to learn fairness and social morality.	There is some evidence for social theories of play in animals.
Bekoff (2002) Bateson (2005) Fry (2005)	Preparing for adulthood	Play in juvenile animals prepares the animal for adulthood. (Also see Groos above.)	Evidence often contradicts this idea. The movements used in juvenile animal play are often different from those used in adulthood. During play fighting, one animal will back down or ease off to allow play to continue, but this does not occur in real violent contests. Some aspects of play fighting are actually counterproductive to learning real fighting such as play partners going out of their way to make partners feel safe.

Data from Saracho, O. N. (2017). Theoretical framework of developmental theories. In T. Waller, E. Ärlemalm-Hagsér, E. B. H. Sandseter, L. Lee-Hammond, K. Lekies, & S. Wyver (Eds.), *The SAGE handbook of outdoor play and learning* (pp. 25–29). London: Sage; Kuhaneck, H., Spitzer, S., & Miller, E. (2010). *Activity analysis, creativity and playfulness in pediatric occupational therapy: Making play just right.* Burlington, MA: Jones & Bartlett Learning; Saracho, O. N., & Spodek, B. (2003). Understanding play and its theories. In O. N. Saracho & B. Spodek (Eds.), *Contemporary perspectives on play in early childhood education* (1–19). Greenwich, CT: Information Age; Mellou, E. (1994). Play theories: A contemporary review. *Early Child Development and Care*, 102(1), 91–100; and Takhvar, M. (1988). Play and theories of play: A review of the literature. *Early Child Development and Care*, 39(1), 221–244.

innovation and problem solving. The ability to investigate the brain's structures and functions through technological advances in imaging now support these hypotheses (Pellis et al., 2014).

What Do Children Play?

Often, because of the difficulty defining and explaining play as one large construct, play has been divided into different categories or types. Some authors have divided play simply into two categories, play and exploration, whereas others have created elaborate lists of multiple forms of play behaviors. Often, the categories of play behaviors follow developmental sequences, and thus intermingle play forms with developmental achievements.

Two commonly used typologies are Piaget's cognitive categories of play (1962) and Parten's social categories of play (1932). Parten suggested that children move from solitary play, to parallel play, side by side with another child, to associative play where materials are shared but cooperation is rare (**Figure 1.8**). The final stage in this hierarchy is cooperative play, where children may have a shared goal and shared leadership of the activity (**Figure 1.9**). Piaget described the growth in cognition through play, from early functional play, which is sensorimotor in nature, to constructive play, symbolic play, and then games with rules.

Two more recent lists of categories exist as well. One recent categorization scheme from the National Institute for Play (n.d.) suggests seven types or patterns of play, including object play, social play, attunement play, body and movement play, imaginative/pretend play, story-telling/narrative play, and creative play **(Figure 1.10**). The Lego Foundation proposed the categories of physical play, symbolic play, pretend play, play with objects, and games with rules (Lego Foundation, 2018). These lists of categories of play may be helpful to occupational therapists in their explanation of the types of play children engage in during assessment and intervention. See **Table 1.3** for descriptions of the types of play in the literature.

The Influence of Financial Means on What Children Play

There are multiple ways that financial assets can influence the play of children (Edwards, 2005; Miller, 2015; Pew, n.d.; Shapiro, 2014; Ziviani et al., 2008). Money often provides access, for example, in the situation of commercial play spaces. Money

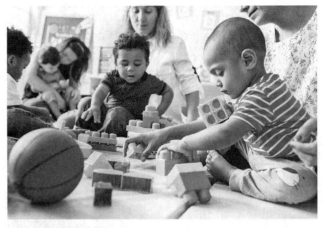

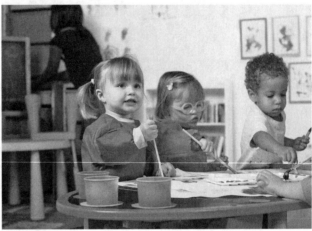

Figure 1.8 Young children engage in parallel play

Top: © Rawpixel.com/Shutterstock; bottom: © lostinbids/E+/Getty Images.

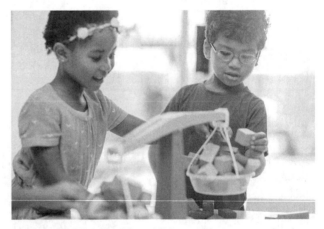

Figure 1.9 Slightly older children will cooperate in play to achieve a goal

© Westend61/Getty Images.

allows for purchasing of toys, media equipment, and equipment needed for sports and craft activities. Money influences the neighborhood one lives in. Children in lower socioeconomic status (SES) areas may not easily be able to get to a local park or playground, and those parks and playgrounds may have poor maintenance (to remove hazards), limited materials or equipment for play activities, and

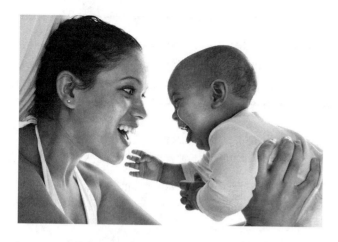

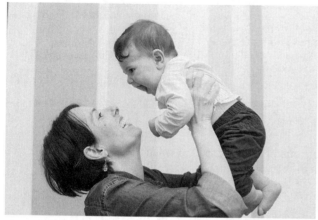

Figure 1.10 Adult–infant attunement play with positive emotion

Top: © Flashon Studio/Shutterstock; bottom: © Guaraciaba Seckler/Shutterstock.

SES may also be more likely to have parents who are working long hours or multiple jobs. Parents in low-income urban areas have reported that their work impacts their amount of time and engagement in play with their child, and this may in turn lead to more media usage for those children (Shah, Gustafson, & Atkins, 2019).

Affluence can also impact play spaces. Affluent children may have more access to toys; digital, virtual, and online play; and a variety of structured "play" activities as well as outdoor parks, playgrounds, and neighborhoods that allow outdoor play (Ginsburg et al., 2007; Kafai & Fields, 2013; Miller, 2015; Rigby & Rodger, 2006; Scarlett et al., 2005). Affluence may also allow for the ownership of specific brands of toys, thus allowing greater access into specific forms of peer culture (Hémar-Nicolas & Rodhain, 2017). Affluence may allow for a greater number of toys in the home. More affluent families are better able, and perhaps more likely to, purchase and provide toys or at least certain types of toys (Freitas et al., 2013; Le-Phuong Nguyen, Harman, & Cappellini, 2017).

However, children without commercial toys can create toys from whatever materials are available (Edwards, 2005) (**Figure 1.11**). Adult "trash" and household materials often can be used to fashion toys, and very elaborate and imaginative games can be made from buttons, bottle caps, paper, scraps of cloth, cans, and so on (Edwards, 2005). Although they have few commercially manufactured toys, children living in hunter-gatherer societies use materials available to them to create a variety of outdoor games and playful activities (Gosso et al., 2005) (**Figure 1.12**).

minimal security, (e.g., lighting and oversight) to allow for safe use. Children from homes with lower SES may have less access to toys and materials for creating playthings. Children in homes with lower

Table 1.3 Types or Categories of Play Described in the Literature

Type of Play	Description	Author(s)
Unoccupied play	Children exploring and manipulating.	Parten (1932)
Solitary play	Children play alone.	
Onlooker play	Children sit back and observe other children but do not join in.	
Parallel	Children play near each other doing similar things but with minimal interaction.	
Associative	Children interact in an activity but not with a shared goal, for example, children playing in a play kitchen pretending different scenarios.	
Cooperative	Children work together toward shared play goals.	

(continues)

Table 1.3 Types or Categories of Play Described in the Literature   *(continued)*

Type of Play	Description	Author(s)
Sensory-motor play/body play/exploratory play	Play with movement for the enjoyment that the movement/sensation provides, exploration of the body and the environment.	Piaget (1962) National Institute for Play (n.d.)
Object play/manipulative play	Play with toys or other materials with exploration using hands, fingers, mouth.	Belsky & Most (1981) Pellegrini & Bjorklund, (2004) National Institute for Play (n.d.) Whitebread et al. (2017)
Functional play	Appropriate use of objects (for example, spoon-feeding a doll).	Smilansky (1968) Ungerer & Sigman (1981)
Constructive play	Building with materials, combining items to create	Smilansky (1968) Christie & Johnsen (1987)
Story-telling or narrative play	Telling or acting out stories	National Institute for Play (n.d.)
Imaginative/socio-dramatic/pretend play/symbolic play/fantasy play	Representational and symbolic skills are used to pretend and/or role-play. May include object substitution, imagining absent objects, using objects functionally but with pretend, imitation.	Piaget (1962) Smilansky (1968) Ungerer & Sigman (1981) Pellegrini & Bjorklund, (2004) National Institute for Play (n.d.) Barton (2010) Whitebread et al. (2017)
Games with rules	Table games and physical games with peers that have logic and order, beginning and end, and penalties.	Piaget (1962) Smilansky (1968) Whitebread et al. (2017)
Rough-and-tumble/physical play	Vigorous play "fighting" with positive affect and gross motor activity.	Pellegrini (1988, 2006) Whitebread et al. (2017)
Language and musical play	Joke telling, chants, rhymes.	Whitebread et al. (2017) Eckert, Winkler, & Cartmill (2020).
Risky play	Play that provides exhilaration and positive emotions but exposes children to activities they fear.	Sandseter, 2009
Attunement play	Adult–infant play with eye contact and emotion	National Institute for Play (n.d.)

The Influence of Adults on What Children Play

The individuals in a child's social environment can include family members, teachers, day care workers, playground supervisors, and many others. Each of these individuals can support or hinder a child's play. The ways in which play can be supported socially, in relation to play spaces and materials, are primarily through engagement, access, and availability. Other people may provide access to toys, play spaces, and play opportunities through their physical presence and responsive engagement with a child, their provision of time for play, their provision of access to peers for play if siblings are not available, and through their monetary support for toys and play areas. Other

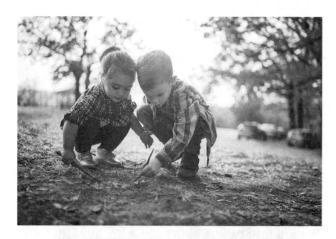

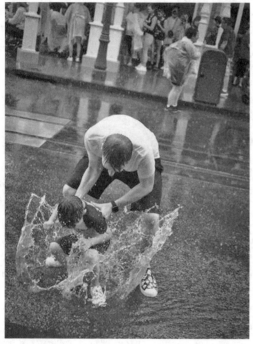

Figure 1.11 Nature provides opportunities for play without the need for commercial toys

Top: © Lucky Business/Shutterstock; bottom: Courtesy of Kyle O'Brien.

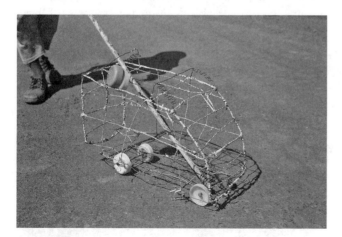

Figure 1.12 Children will play with whatever they have available, even building toys from adult trash

© Grigory Kubatyan/Shuuterstock.

adult individuals can have positive or negative attitudes toward play and either value or devalue play as a way to spend time in the home and/or classroom (Bulotsky-Shearer et al., 2017a, 2017b).

Adult influence is specifically noted in child access to outdoor and commercial play spaces. Parents may select outdoor play spaces for features important for adults such as shade and availability of toilets and drinking water (Sallis, McKenzie, Elder, Broyles & Nader, 1997), rather than the types of play opportunities available. Research has suggested that commercial play spaces, though in theory built for and designed for children, are actually more sought after by parents. Children appear to have less of an influence on visitation, with a large majority of visits being initiated or directed by the parent rather than the child (McKendrick, Bradford, & Fielder, 2000). Parents reported that their decisions to visit these play spaces often had to do with reducing the active play of children in the home.

Similarly, teacher attitudes can be important environmental supports. Teachers often take one of two stances (Pyle & Danniels, 2017). Teachers may believe that free play is important and that the teacher should not interfere unless necessary for safety. Others view play as an opportunity for academic growth and use it to structure learning around specific concepts. Teachers who believe that play supports learning are more likely to actively work to incorporate a range of play in the classroom (Pyle & Danniels 2016; Tsai, 2015).

What Do Children Like to Play?

Research throughout the past hundred or more years has carefully described the activities children like to play. The large body of literature allows us to make some generalizations regarding children's play preferences. First, children's play preferences change with age and the development of new physical, cognitive, and social skills. Second, children's play preferences vary by sex and gender and appear to be a function of both innate and social forces (Davis & Hines, 2020; Todd et al., 2018). Finally, children's preferences are influenced by the physical and sociocultural environment in which they live and play. Although the *content* of preferred play may have changed over time, development and sex/gender appear to be consistent factors influencing play preferences. Children also appear to prefer some level of risk.

Preferences and Context in Time

The toys children play with and the play activities children enjoy have changed over time. Evidence of early playthings suggests ancient and early people played with dolls, balls, rattles, drums, hobby horses, toy "men" or soldiers, games with rules, puzzles, and construction toys (Barnes, 2006). Although many of these toys and games remain, the advent of a variety of commercially available, technologically sophisticated toys has allowed new forms of play to emerge.

Preferences Related to Age and Development

As children grow and learn, they progress through stages and exhibit different play behaviors (Garner & Bergen, 2006; Johnson, 2015). Many authors have written about specific sequences in play development; one of the most familiar may be Piaget's cognitive levels in regard to play (Piaget, 1952, 1962). Piaget's stages are the sensorimotor stage, the preoperational stage, the stage of concrete operations, and the stage of formal operations. In the sensorimotor stage, the infant's reflexive behaviors eventually grow into independent interaction with the environment. The infant's sensorimotor behaviors become more intentional and more refined. Through processes of assimilation and accommodation, the infant learns about the world and begins to solve simple problems. By 2 years of age the toddler begins to use mental representation and begins more social interactions. Language skills grow during this period, and the child can use sensorimotor behaviors to solve problems. The child over time begins to have moral reasoning and eventually becomes focused on rules. From ages 7 to 11 years, the child is developing logical thought and can solve most concrete problems. During the next stage, the child's ability to think abstractly grows and emerges, and the child can use logic for an argument or to solve hypothetical problems. When considering Piaget's stages of cognitive development, one views the development of play as intertwined with cognitive development (Piaget, 1952/1975, 1962). As occupational therapists, however, the relationship between physical development and play must also be considered.

In infancy, play begins to emerge and differentiate from early body exploration (Garner & Bergen, 2006). Actions that occur by chance begin to be repeated purposely (Piaget, 1952, 1962). In play, the infant learns what he or she can do with objects and body parts that provide enjoyment. In this infant stage, the enjoyment received is typically sensory in nature, although enjoyment can occur from social interactions as well. Because infants cannot tell people when they are playing or not playing, adults infer this from their cues. Infant cues for play include smiles, giggles, positive affect, and the desire for repetition of a motion or action. As infants grow and develop, imitative abilities begin to figure prominently in play, and simple turn-taking emerges. Infants learn from adults to read play from nonplay and over time learn to invent their own games and provide cues to others to signal that what they are doing is also play. These skills of reading play cues begin early in infancy with games like "peekaboo," and by the second year of life, children are creating their own games with their own play cues (Garner & Bergen, 2006) (**Figure 1.13**).

Object play and sensorimotor play predominates at young ages (Garner & Bergen, 2006; Whitebread et al., 2017). Noticeable preferences for specific objects may be observed as early as 3 months of age, although a favorite toy is indicated by less than 50% of infants that young (Furby & Wilke, 1982). Closer to 90% of infants have one favored object by 1 year of age (Furby & Wilke, 1982). Many favorite objects of infants through preschool-age children are soft and can be held close to the body, perhaps as a mechanism of self-soothing (Jonsson, Reimbladh-Taube, & Sjöswärd, 1993). As early as 3 years of age, children prefer their own unique toy possessions to a matched new one (Gelman, & Davidson, 2016).

Object play has primarily been studied in children under the age of 7 (Whitebread et al., 2017). Object play progresses from single-object use to combined object play (Gowen, Johnson-Martin, Goldman, & Hussey, 1992). Single-object play is seen in infancy and decreases from 7 to 18 months of age as the child begins to combine objects in greater frequency. Object

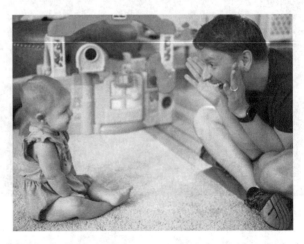

Figure 1.13 Early social games with infants often include "peekaboo"-type interactions
Courtesy of Kyle O'Brien.

play also progresses from use of an object indiscriminately to the use of an object in a way that demonstrates understanding of its unique features (Gowen et al., 1992). Children about 1 year of age investigate and explore new objects, but by 15 months, discriminative play is more common (Garner & Bergen, 2006). Later object play involves using objects as they are intended.

Early object play is also sensorimotor in nature, with mouthing, banging, and waving (**Figure 1.14**). The differential use of mouthing and fingering/manipulation of objects supports varied types of play with mouthing common with simpler play and greater manipulation occurring with more advanced forms of object play (Orr, 2019). As manipulation skills improve, object play becomes more advanced (**Figure 1.15**).

The second year of life is important as symbolic play begins to take hold (Garner & Bergen, 2006). Pretend play expands from simple pretense, such as talking into a play phone, to more complex pretense, such as feeding a baby doll. As the child matures, symbolic play and more complex pretense and role-play emerge. Role-play often is accompanied by the use of props and/or costumes (**Figure 1.16**). Initially, a child requires the props for pretense, and early props

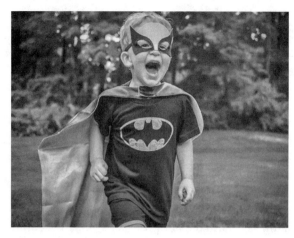

Figure 1.16 Pretending and role-play often occur with props or costumes
Courtesy of Kyle O'Brien.

must look quite real. Over time, the need for these replicas diminishes, and objects can be substituted for other objects. Eventually, props are not needed as a child imagines their existence while playing.

The preschool period brings greater language abilities and a significant emphasis on pretend play. Children of this age often pretend with toys of a variety of media, for example, creating pretend games while completing a puzzle or building with Legos. Pretend play can occur while drawing or painting or while climbing on a structure in a playground. Pretend play is often strongly connected with emotions and feelings. Children act out experiences they have had and desires that they cannot actually experience outside of play. Pretend play is also more and more social as children age.

With the increase in the social aspects of pretense, the ability to read and send cues is crucial because pretend actions often can look identical to the real action. How do people know a child is pretending? They must infer from the behaviors; they see facial expressions, smiles, different eye gaze, and positive affect. Contextual cues may help as well, such as a child pretending to be asleep in a location where he or she would not normally be sleeping. Generally, a child who is pretending may wish to take turns in the "game" with another. These contextual cues assist adults in determining that the child is playing (Garner & Bergen, 2006).

Preschool also brings a greater level of activity (Pellegrini & Smith, 1998a, 1998b, 2003) and a variety of gross motor and playground play that appears sensory seeking in nature. Preschool-age children love to swing, spin, run, climb, hang, jump, and be upside down (Chew, 1985; Sandseter, 2007). Why is movement so important for young children? While the vestibular apparatus is fully formed at birth, functionally it continues to develop for many years as children move, explore, and play (Cherng, Chen, & Su, 2001;

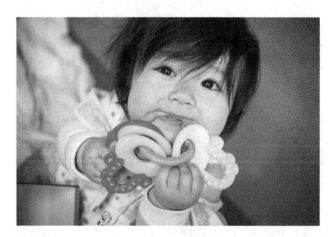

Figure 1.14 Infant play typically includes mouthing and sensory motor exploration
© bradleyhebdon/E+/Getty Images.

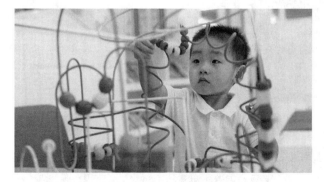

Figure 1.15 As infants mature, they engage in more manipulative and object play
© baona/E+/Getty Images.

Lai & Chan, 2002). These sensory-rich activities that children engage in during preschool and early school age correspond with significant new motor skills as children learn to balance on one foot, hop, skip, gallop, and challenge gravity. See **Figure 1.17** for an example of active play against gravity.

Elementary school-age children play somewhat differently (Johnson, 2015). In school, pretend play diminishes as peer play increasingly occurs outside the classroom on the playground. This peer play is made up of more physical or social games, such as rough-and-tumble play, jump-rope, and rhyming games. Pretending still may occur in the home or after school. Pretend play during this period is quite complex and often more tied to reality than it was in preschool. For example, children may pretend to be famous singers. The amount of preparation that goes into play during this stage is substantial.

Younger children just want to play, whereas older children want to properly set the stage (Johnson, 2015).

Outside school, board games and video games become very popular. During this time, children often play with peers with collections of items and trading games. Large amounts of negotiation can occur in the attempt for children to grow their collections. These games with rules can require elaborate planning and preparation as the children establish what the rules are. Competition and collaboration can become more emphasized in both genders as children engage in more games with rules and team competitive sports (Johnson, 2015; Piaget, 1962).

Aggressive-themed play and true aggression in play also can emerge during this time period (Blurton Jones, 1978). Wrestling, soldiers, space warriors, pirates, and superheroes are common themes where

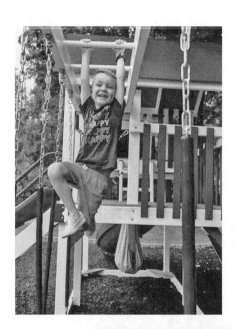

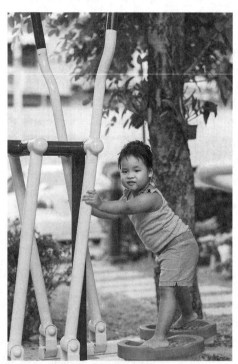

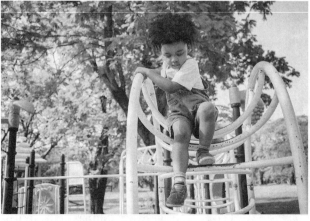

Figure 1.17 Preschool and young school-age children enjoy challenging gravity

Top left: Courtesy of Kyle O'Brien; top right: © Mr.Moo/Shutterstock; bottom: © Blue Titan/Shutterstock.

a form of aggression arises. This form of play appears to be universal but is influenced by cultural norms. In cultures where aggression is less tolerated, the play fighting includes more chase and flee games and less aggressive rough-and-tumble play (Fry, 2005). These culturally defined judgments about aggressive play are not yet supported by research to determine the benefits or detriments of such play. Power (2000) suggested that rough-and-tumble play may have positive functions for children in general but may be detrimental for overly aggressive or rejected children. Play fighting is only correlated with real aggression for children who are rejected by their peers but not for children in general (Pellegrini, 1988, 1994). Various adaptive functions have been proposed for this form of play, such as the development of aggression prevention and control, social relationships, and flexibility in handling social problems (Blurton Jones, 1978; Glassner, 1976; Goldstein, 1995; Pellegrini, 1995; Power, 2000). Play fighting may provide an acceptable excuse for physical contact and opportunities to care for each other (e.g., helping someone get up and checking if that person is okay) (Reed, 2005). It may also provide a sense of excitement as long as there is confidence that the players are in a safe environment (Apter, 1991). Play fighting may be beneficial at younger ages but may morph into something dangerous if it continues into adolescent bullying. Some teens do use rough-and-tumble play as a way to exert their dominance (Pellegrini, 2006).

In adolescence, play changes in other ways as well, and teens tend to spend much of their time socializing with peers (Cummings & Vandewater, 2007; Gordon & Caltabiano, 1996; Pawelko & Magafas, 1997; Zill, Winquist Nord, & Loomis, 1995). Common teen forms of play or leisure include formal and informal sports, video game play, watching videos with friends, and texting. However, often the leisure time of teens is spent in risky, unproductive, or sedentary behaviors. Given the potential link between adolescent leisure patterns and the leisure patterns of adults and the possible impact of playful adult leisure and psychological health, the importance of a well-balanced and active play leisure profile in adolescence seems clear (Hektner & Csikszentmihalyi, 1996; Scott & Willits, 1998; Staempfli, 2007). See Chapter 13 for more information about adolescence and leisure.

The changes in play seen with children's cognitive, social-emotional, and physical development are clear. Does play drive development or merely reflect it? We believe that development and play together grow in a spiraling process whereby play both reflects *and* contributes to the development of the child in all areas. **Table 1.4** summarizes the typical development of play. However, additional factors influence the expression of play across all ages, especially gender and context.

Table 1.4 Summary of the Typical Development of Play in Children*

Age	Object Play	Motor Play	Pretend Play	Social Play
Infancy	Mostly single-object use, combining of objects begins to emerge by the end of the first year. Uses objects in sensorimotor ways.	Reflexive or random actions repeated as the infant gets older and has more motor control. Early motor play includes manipulating, banging, and throwing.	Begins to emerge about age 1 year.	Visual attention and focus develop, leading to joint attention; social referencing emerges. Infant is initially more interested in objects than peers, but interest in peers increases by the end of the first year.
Toddlerhood	Increasingly combines objects and uses objects appropriately. Trial and error and invention occurs.	Exploration of greater distances and learning to walk, run, climb, and jump.	Beginning simple pretense (wave bye-bye, talk into pretend phone); most pretense is about self, and often pretense is imitative.	Social referencing increases. Increased interest in peers occurs. Toddlers do have friends, and friendship is generated by imitation. Onlooker play at age 1 becomes parallel.

(continues)

Table 1.4 Summary of the Typical Development of Play in Children* *(continued)*

Age	Object Play	Motor Play	Pretend Play	Social Play
Preschool	Uses a variety of objects and enjoys combining objects. Constructive play is quite common.	Exercise play or practice play occurs. Intense gross motor activities and physical challenges often sought after.	Combines scenes into simple narratives. Pretend extends to objects and others; becomes more inventive, creative, and supported by language. By age 5 creates complex scenes. Begins to use language to inform others ("Pretend that...").	Has definite friends and enjoys play with others. Associative play begins and moves into cooperative play before kindergarten.
Elementary/ middle childhood	Constructs elaborate creations with a variety of materials. Leisure crafts may begin.	Engages in rough-and-tumble play and games with rules.	Simple pretend play declines. Engages in complex fantasy games and may begin to play specific games with pretend elements such as Dungeons and Dragons and video games.	Seeks companions for play and processes more complex play activities with others.
Adolescence	May continue with leisure crafts/hobbies.	Greater participation in recreation and sports.	Engagement in theater, fantasy games, and video games with entire worlds online.	Teamwork and cooperation develop; begins to "hang out" with friends.

*As described in Westernized countries

Preferences Related to Sex and Gender

Differences in children's play and toy preferences based on sex and gender have been studied for decades by multiple experimental and observational methodologies and in a range of social contexts (Davis & Hines, 2020; Todd et al., 2018). For an overview of the findings of this body of research, please see **Box 1.3**. However, to understand sex and gender differences in play preferences among children, it's important to first understand the differences between biological sex alone and gender itself as a social construct. At birth, the sex of babies is assigned as male or female based on biological and physical characteristics, while gender identity, the experience of identifying as a boy, a girl, or nonbinary (gender identities that are not exclusively masculine or feminine) is an internal sense people have based on the interaction of biological traits, developmental influences, one's environment (Rafferty, 2018), and a continuum of complex psychosocial self-perceptions, attitudes, and expectations that society has about members of both sexes (Tseng, 2008). Those whose gender and biological sex are the same (male and boy/man or female girl/woman) are *cisgender*, and those whose gender and biological sex are not the same are *transgender*. People who are

---

Box 1.3 Toy Preferences for Girls and Boys Suggested by Years of Research

Toys typically preferred by girls according to research

- Dolls and doll-related activities
- House toys, such as a tea set
- Dramatic play/dress-up
- Crayons and painting
- Musical instruments
- Cooperative play often in dyads or smaller groups
- Crafts

Toys typically preferred by boys according to research

- Transportation toys (trucks/cars)
- Construction toys (blocks)
- Physical play/rough-and-tumble play
- Ball play
- Competitive play and risky play
- Superhero play/aggressive play (army/war/ pretend weapons)
- Video games

Data from Benenson (1993), Benjamin (1932), Connor and Serbin (1977), Fein (1981), Goldstein (1995), Hartup (1983), Humphreys and Smith (1987), Kafai (1998), Lyytinen et al. (1999), Pellegrini (1988, 1992, 1995), Pellegrini and Bjorklund (2004), Power (2000), Salonius-Pasternak and Gelfond (2005), Saracho (1990), Saunders et al. (1999), Servin et al. (1999), Todd et al. (2018), Von Klitzing et al. (2000), and Wall et al. (1989).

nonbinary may be gender-fluid (a sense of being both masculine and feminine at the same time), bigender (having two genders that may fluctuate), or agender (not identifying with any gender).

Being a boy or girl is something that feels natural for most children (Rafferty, 2018). Differences in play preferences may originate from biological predispositions and are then strengthened by socialization or may be solely attributed to social factors. Studies have suggested that biological predispositions among boys, which may impact their choice in toys, may include their gross motor skills, propulsive movement, higher activity levels, and lower impulse control (Todd et al., 2018). Having an early advantage in mental rotation of figures and event-mapping may contribute to the interest in construction and mechanical movement among boys. Girls have a typical advantage in fine motor control, processing facial expression, and attention to social stimuli, which may account for toy preferences such as dolls and beads (Todd et al. 2018).

Biological predispositions for toy preferences may be attributed to pre- and peri-natal exposure to sex hormones. Boys, for example, are typically exposed to greater levels of androgens than girls, and some evidence has found that level of androgen exposure may influence visual preferences in infants between the ages of 3 and 8 months, as boys made more visual fixations on trucks than dolls, and girls made more fixations on dolls than trucks (Todd et al., 2018). Studies have also found that girls with congenital adrenal hyperplasia (CAH) who are exposed to higher levels of androgens show great levels of interest in "male-typed" toys compared to "female-typed" toys (Hines, 2004; Meyer-Bahlberg et al., 2004) and a greater interest in "male-typed" toys compared to girls less affected by CAH (van de Beek et al., 2009). In addition to studies on people, evidence that suggests biological predispositions to toy preference has been found in vervet monkeys, where females have been observed to make more contact with a doll and cooking pots compared to males, who spent more time playing with a car and ball (Alexander & Hines, 2002), and male rhesus monkeys were found to prefer plush toys that had wheels over those without wheels (Hassett, Siebert, & Wallen, 2008). Taken together, a number of studies do provide findings that predict biological object preferences for boys and girls, at least during the stages of late infancy and early childhood (Todd et al., 2018).

While biological predispositions of being more male or female may initially influence play preferences, the effect of gender socialization must also be considered. Gender-normative stereotypes, including attitude and behavioral differences between boys and girls,

dominate children's media and popular culture with portrayals of boys in masculine gender roles, girls in feminine gender roles, and boys and girls engaging with stereotypically masculine and feminine play and toys, respectively (Spinner, Cameron, & Calogero, 2018).

As early as 12.5 months of age, preferences for gender-typed toys begins to emerge, and as early as the age of 2, children develop an interest in same-gender playmates (Boe & Woods, 2018; Caldera et al., 1989; Maccoby and Jacklin, 1987; Serbin et al., 1994; Wood et al., 2002). Between the ages of 3 and 6, a child's awareness of gender stereotypes has been found to increase rapidly (Aubry et al., 1999) and as a consequence, gender-typed play increases in rigidity between the ages of 3 and 5 (Halim et al., 2013). Once gender-related knowledge is established, gender flexibility, which is the open-minded attitude around gender roles, peaks and plateaus as children approach the age of 7, when their acceptance of gender stereotypes as "correct or fixed" begins to decline (Huston, 1983; Miller et al., 2006; Signorella et al., 1993; Trautner, 1992). A recent study tested the effect of exposing children to stereotypic and counterstereotypic displays of toy play in magazines on children's gender flexibility in toy and playmate preferences (Spinner et al., 2018). Results found that children who were shown counterstereotypic pictures (i.e., boys who played with My Little Pony and girls who played with cars), were more flexible with their answers when asked who should play with toys such as a baby doll, a jet fighter, a tool set, and a tea set and were also less rigid when asked which children from the pictures they wanted to play with compared to children who were only shown images that promoted stereotypical gender-based toys. Children who were shown counterstereotypic pictures were equally unlikely to make counterstereotypic choices themselves, but were more open to the idea that boys and girls could play with a variety of toys (Spinner et al., 2018).

Research on children who are transgender has found that these children show a consistent pattern of gender development associated with their identified gender and not their biological sex assigned at birth. This includes patterns of play behavior, toy preference, and gravitating toward friends that matched their gender rather than sex. Surprisingly, findings suggest that how, and for how long, a child who is transgender was treated and parented as the gender associated with their assigned sex does not appear to affect their actual gender identity and expression and that children who are transgender show almost no difference in how and the extent to which they identify with and express their gender compared to their cisgender peers (Gülgöz et al., 2019).

These findings suggest, when it comes to play in occupational therapy, practitioners should support the natural interests of the children we engage with by promoting self-directed play or using the toys that most interest them, without defaulting to assumed play preferences based on gender stereotypes. Incorporating a child's gender can be a tool to engage children in play. Conversely, if a child's gender is in conflict with their sociocultural context, an occupational therapist can provide support by analyzing and identifying the strengths and barriers a child may face toward self-expression in play (Kimelstein, 2019). See **Practice Opportunity 1.1** for an example of how one occupational therapist navigated gender issues with a client.

Occupational therapists should be mindful about the gender divide in toy preferences given that different types of toys facilitate different types of play and, taken together, can yield different developmental trajectories for social and cognitive skills in children. Toys such as cars, tracks, and video games that are typically targeted for boys promote the visual-spatial skill development and an agentic orientation to self and others (De Lisi & Wolford, 2002; Jirout & Newcombe, 2015), while toys targeted for girls such as dolls and Disney princesses promote the development of nurturing and empathy skills and a more communal orientation toward self and others (Coyne et al., 2016; Dittmar et al., 2006; Li & Wong, 2016).

Gender stereotypes at an early and formative stage of development have implications for children's identities, aspirations, and achievements (Cimpian et al., 2012). Therefore, actively achieving gender desegregation in children may address the perpetuation of gender-related social exclusion or bullying (Killen & Stangor, 2001), and may have an impact on career cognition and future career options as adults (Sherman & Zurbriggen, 2014) related to skill acquisition associated with varied toys. As occupational therapy practitioners, the toy choices made during therapeutic sessions can either reinforce or broaden specific toy related skills as well as notions of "appropriate" toys, and practitioners must make these choices carefully.

Parents and caregivers are often the primary purchasers of children's toys. Given that gender socialization influences children at early ages, toys provided by their parents deliver some of the earliest gender-based messages by encouraging children to play with gender-typed toys such as dolls for girls and trucks for boys (Boe & Woods, 2018). In a study of parents' influence on infants' gender-typed toy preferences, researchers found that even with brief encouragement by a parent to play with toys from each gender category, gender-typical toy preferences at 12.5 months were not altered. Instead, the most influential predictor of toy preferences was a child's exposure to types of toys in their own homes. These findings suggest

Practice Opportunity 1.1 José, Josie, Role-Playing, and Gender Identity

Amers Goff, MA, OTR/L

José is a 16-year-old who attends a special day class. He has a huge personality, always has something to say, and often comes into the OT room at his school already talking about his favorite movies or characters. He passionately loves My Little Ponies and Disney movies, and he imagines fusion movies, where his favorite characters meet each other. José has a dual diagnosis of autism spectrum disorder and Down syndrome. For José, this means that he is very passionate about the things that interest him, to the point that it can be difficult for him to focus on anything else. He can also become "stuck" on a specific topic or concern. Because his speech is sometimes unintelligible, José uses an AAC program on his tablet to clarify his spoken messages.

José comes from a very religious Guatemalan family. He is the only child of a single mother, Maria. Maria speaks about and to José as if he were much younger than he actually is. She is indulgent of his love of Disney and My Little Pony, but she tries to encourage him toward activities typically perceived as "masculine," such as sports or cars. José expresses little interest in these things.

José's school occupational therapy goals address increasing frustration tolerance to reduce emotional outbursts in class and improving time spent on-task. José works with several boys his own age in a group focused on building self-regulation and problem-solving skills. In this group, each student selects a character of a knight or a prince to role-play frustrating or challenging situations in which they get to problem solve, practice appropriate responses to social scenarios, and "save the day." José consistently requests to be a princess or a queen instead of a prince, and his occupational therapist agrees in order to promote a true self-directed play experience. José relishes wearing a dress and crown and swishing around the room. When dressed this way, he engages in deeper self-reflection and more complex problem solving. In order to support José's choice making and avoid any stigma (AOTA, 2020b), the occupational therapist changes to a gender-neutral structure and instead of asking what knight or prince each boy wants to be, she asks what character each wants to be.

José begins talking about gender identity and other LGBTQ themes in OT sessions. He asks to

(continues)

Practice Opportunity 1.1 José, Josie, Role-Playing, and Gender Identity   *(continued)*

wear a dress beyond the role-playing activities, describes himself as bisexual, asks questions about queer terms, and comments on a photo he sees in the OT's office that depicts her with her wife. It seems that play and the therapist's approach allowed José to feel accepted and comfortable discussing topics that he was not discussing with others. Because of the sensitive nature of sexuality, the OT consults regularly with her supervisor and the school psychologist to be sure her responses to José's questions are appropriate and professional.

José repeatedly expresses fear about what would happen if his mother ever found out about his orientation and asks his OT to keep his secret. He states that his mom doesn't believe being gay is real. This creates an ethical dilemma for the OT that she discusses with her supervisor and the school psychologist. Together, they review the AOTA (2020a) Occupational Therapy Code of Ethics and discuss their ethical obligations to both José and to Maria. They feel an obligation to Maria to truthfully share the details of her child's intervention. However, they fear that harm could come to José if they disclosed his queer identity because of her beliefs. They then consider the harm to José of his search for information, which could put him at risk if he ends up exploring these topics outside the safety of school. They conclude that José has a right to self-determination and confidentiality under the ethical principle of autonomy, and that asking these questions in the safety of OT does not pose any danger to him, whereas disclosure of his gender identity could potentially cause harm. Considering the principle of nonmaleficence, they decide to refrain from sharing José's gender identify and specific questions about LGBTQ themes with his mother. Because some of the terminology he uses is sex related, the IEP team reaches out to Maria about providing José with developmentally appropriate sexual education. They cite the fact that individuals with developmental disabilities are at higher risk of sexual and physical abuse. Maria responds negatively to this conversation. She states that her son is too young to be thinking about sexuality. Because of her religious beliefs, she does not want José learning about sex in school. The school psychologist mentions that José has been asking some general questions about sexuality. Maria denies that there could be any truth in this and asks to change the subject. The IEP team informs Maria that they are required by law to provide students with developmentally appropriate education about sexual and physical abuse. They share an example of the curriculum with Maria, and she agrees to allow José to participate in this curriculum, but not in a more comprehensive sexual education curriculum.

Following the meeting, the IEP team discusses how to manage the fact that Maria's wishes conflict with José's. They weigh the importance of culturally sensitive, family-centered care with the need to avoid discrimination of José's expressed sexual identity (AOTA 2020b). They decide to take a client-led approach and answer José's questions simply and honestly, but to honor Maria's beliefs, they do not volunteer information outside of a direct question from José.

Soon after this meeting, José asks the occupational therapist to "call me Josie not José." When asked why, Josie states "I feel like a girl inside and want to use a girl name." The occupational therapist simultaneously considers the importance of embedding play for mental health and motivation, the importance of developing teen self-advocacy, and the importance of not stigmatizing Josie's gender identity, and she agrees to Josie's request. The occupational therapist continues to feel conflicted, but when she discusses these concerns with her supervisor and the school psychologist, they agree that creating a safe and supportive environment in which Josie can learn and explore must be the highest priority as long as Josie is not in danger.

Over time, Josie becomes more settled in her identity. She asks to use female pronouns and starts using the name Josie with her close friends. She expresses that although she doesn't want her mom to know she is trans, she likes that her friends know who she really is and can use the right name and pronouns to describe her. Josie's teacher reports that over the past year, since Josie started using her girl name and pronouns, her emotional outbursts and destructive behaviors in class have decreased substantially. Several school staff comment that Josie seems happier and calmer than she did before.

The occupational therapist reflects on how play created opportunities for Josie to problem-solve and express what was most important to her in ways that could not have been anticipated. She is grateful to her school team for collaborative professional reasoning and respectfully supporting Josie's self-determination. She hopes that it will be possible someday for Josie and her mother also to come together similarly.

References

American Occupational Therapy Association (AOTA). (2020a). AOTA 2020 occupational therapy code of ethics. *American Journal of Occupational Therapy*, 74(Suppl. 3), 7413410005. https://doi.org/10.5014/ajot.2020.74S3006

AOTA. (2020b). Guide to acknowledging the impact of discrimination, stigma, and implicit bias on provision of services. https://www.aota.org/-/media/Corporate/Files/Practice/Guide-Acknowledging-Impact-Discrimination-Stigma-Implicit-Bias.pdf

that socialization processes may play a role in "the formation of early gender-typical toy preferences and highlight the importance of equal toy exposure during infancy to ensure optimal development" (Boe & Woods, 2018, p. 1). As such, findings indicate that parent encouragement alone, may not influence toy preference; however, the toys parents purchase for their children early on in life may. In another study, the predictors of gender-typed toy purchases by prospective parents were examined, and participants who reported playing with gender-typed toys more than cross-gender toys when they were children planned to purchase gender-typed toys for their own children (Weisgram & Bruun, 2018). Participants endorsed more stereotypes for feminine toys than for masculine toys and indicated that they believe gender differences in children's interest are mostly influenced by the environment. Women who reported having nontraditional interests as a child were more likely to purchase nontraditional toys for their own children (Weisgram & Bruun, 2018). Toy choices of preschool-age boys were most stereotypical if they perceived that their fathers would not approve of them playing with cross-gendered typed toys such as dishes (Raag & Rackliff, 1998). Findings from these select studies appear to echo a broad area of research on the examination of gender socialization and parent influence. Taken together, findings indicate that parents have the power to influence toy preferences in their children by exposing children to not only gender-typed toys but also cross-gender toys or gender-neutral toys. Occupational therapists can use this knowledge to advocate for access to a variety of toys.

Preferences Related to Risk

Risky play occurs at great heights, at high speeds, with potentially harmful tools, or near danger such as a fire. Rough-and-tumble play is considered risky play, as is play where children might get lost (Sandseter, 2007). This form of play is quite common, children appear to have a propensity for it, and it appears to be important to their development (Brussoni, Olsen, Pike, & Sleet, 2012; Little & Stapleton, 2021; Sandseter, Kleppe, & Sando, 2021). Children have varied preference levels for risky play, however, depending on the type of play, for example, preferring higher risk with high speeds but lower risk with dangerous objects or elements (Yurt & Keleş, 2019). Even very young children seek out play with elements that they perceived to be risky, although they might offer little objective risk for older children (Kleppe, 2018). Young children in centers that

provided greater opportunities for risky play with more categories of risky play demonstrated more varied risky play (Kleppe, 2018). They were more likely to find a challenging and risky play experience that "fit" their developmental abilities. This is likely essential for children during an age range with large variation in development and varied tolerance for risk. Therefore, play spaces that allow for risky play should provide versatility, flexibility, and complexity (Kleppe, 2018) to ensure that children have access to a wide range of experiences, with equipment and environments that can be manipulated by the children themselves, allowing for activities that accommodate a range of developmental abilities and tolerance for risk.

What Do Children Play With?

Any objects that children can play with can be called toys. This can range from natural items such as small rocks and sticks, to fancy human made items such as battery-powered small cars that children can actually steer and drive. Toy products are tangible items "designed to function primarily for play with the intention of being manufactured" (Kudrowitz & Wallace, 2010, p. 3).

There is archeological evidence of human-made toys for children's play dating back centuries before the common era and from around the world (Mann, 1975). In some cases, items were included in burial sites suggesting they were prized possessions and. They reflected elements of children's environments and were likely used for sensorimotor and pretend play: animals, human forms, miniaturized furniture and tools, and wheeled vehicles. The idea of commercial manufacture of specific objects created as toys to amuse and educate children is a relatively modern invention (Crawford, 2009; Cross, 1999; Ogata, 2004). Major toymakers began to mass-produce toys during the time period between the two world wars, initially for schools and then later for homes (Ogata, 2004). Early toys for this purpose were often made of wood and meant to provide for motor or cognitive skill development. Although the onset of World War II curtailed their development, postwar toy making resumed and expanded, with the concomitant development of toy marketing to parents and later to children (Ogata, 2004). The impetus for parental purchasing of toys shifted as well. After the war, parents were encouraged to select toys that fostered creativity, and with that change came a change in toy design and characteristics. Postwar toy materials also changed with the greater availability of tin and plastic.

Over time, varied forms of toys began to be associated with specific forms of play (Rubin, & Howe, 1985). Currently, according to the Toy Industry, there are 11 categories or types of toys, including action figures and accessories, arts and crafts, building sets, dolls, explorative, games and puzzles, infant/toddler/preschool, outdoor and sports, plush, vehicles, and electronics (Toy Industry, 2020). Within and across categories, the types of toys available to children have changed significantly over time (Cross, 9For example, in the past many toys imitated or were situated within real-life tasks such as adult homemaking activities and construction. However, over time, toys more frequently created or supported imaginary or fantasy environments such as magical places and supernatural abilities, as well as out-of-this-world spaces such as outer space.

Characteristics of Toys

A large variety of features of objects could influence their use, usefulness, and/or desirability as toys. These include availability, materials and type, realism, novelty, control, and complexity.

Availability

There currently is little descriptive information about toy availability in homes in the United States, but the Toy Association (2020) estimates that the current U.S. market for toys is approximately 27 billion dollars. In the United States, many studies that have described toy availability were completed to examine sex differences and gendered play. For example, one older study suggested significant gender differences in the toys available in children's rooms, with boys having access to more military and vehicle toys, sports equipment, animal toys, educational toys, and machines, whereas girls had significantly more dolls, dollhouses, and other forms of domestic type items (Rheingold & Cook 1975). In a weeklong observational study, the types of toys available in the homes of preschool-age children enrolled in a university campus summer program were coded as either vehicles, dolls, pretending toys with domestic role functions or dress-up, educational or art-related items, games, and spatiotemporal (puzzles/shape sorting) toys. Children in this study also played with natural materials, kitchen items, furniture, tools, and manufactured items such as boxes or paper clips (Giddings & Halverson, 1981). Boys and girls differed in the amount of time they played with some items but not

others. No recent studies on toy availability have been completed in the United States. In homes, parents/caregivers are primarily responsible for the availability of toys for children's play. In interviews with Pierce (1999), mothers reported intentional management of toy collections and explained that most toys in their homes were the result of targeted purchases, often selected because of their perceived ability to promote development or educational value. Their children also frequently received toys as gifts.

What is the "correct" number of toys for a child to have? There are currently debate and controversy. Advocates are beginning to suggest that fewer toys in the home are better (Becker, 2019; Harms, 2018). Given that toy availability is associated with motor and cognitive development (Freitas et al., 2013; Kavousipor, Golipour, & Hekmatnia, 2016; Malhi, Menon, Bharti, & Sidhu, 2018; Saccani et al., 2013), this is an important aspect of the environment to examine, although not the only important feature related to child development. Variety may be more important, for example (Wachs, 1985). However, this has not been well studied.

One aspect of availability is a toy's perceived desirability, as parents report that they purchase toys that are educational or their child expresses interest in (Christensen & Stockdale, 1991; Fallon & Harris, 1989; Giddings & Halverson, 1981; Al Kurdi, 2017; Parsons & Ballantine, 2008; Le-Phuong Nguyen, Harman, & Cappellini, 2017; Field Agent, 2018; Ummanel, 2017). This knowledge has increasingly led to intense marketing of toys to children and their parents, with ads that focus on educational value as well as generating toy desirability more generally (Common Sense, 2014; Gardner, Golinkoff, Hirsh-Pasek, & Heiney-Gonzalez, 2012; Healey & Mendelsohn, 2019; Ogata, 2004; Seiter, 1992).

Toy availability may also be related to cultural ideals and views on parenting and child development (Le-Phuong Nguyen et al., 2017; Ogata, 2004; Ummanel, 2017). Recent studies have investigated toy availability in India (Venkatesan & Yashodharakumar, 2017b). For children with disabilities in India, boys had an average of 11 toys and girls 8 (Venkatesan, 2014). In a study of toddlers, less than a third of those toddlers included had the following types of toys in their homes: coloring books, chalkboards, clay, toy letters and numbers, nesting toys, blocks, beads, or puzzles, and only half had crayons (Malhi, Menon, Bharti, & Sidhu, 2018). There are likely many factors that play into toy availability in different countries, at different SES levels, and with different types of families and children.

Toy Materials and Type

The different materials, methods of manufacture, types of toy designs, and their functions may influence the play that occurs, although little is known to date about the exact mechanisms of influence. It is clear that certain types of toys such as blocks appear to lead to more social play, whereas others, such as puzzles, lead to more independent play (Ivory & McCollum, 1999; Rubin & Howe, 1985; Stoneman, Cantrell, & Hoover-Dempsey, 1983). Certain toys and playthings are most often used or most preferred. For example, in one classroom playdough and art materials; pretending toys such as house, fireman, and so on; sand and water play; and blocks and puzzles were the most preferred (Rubin, 1977). These materials most often led to nonsocial, functional, and constructive play. Social play occurred most often with the pretending toys. Some toys are objects for the child to act upon, while others are tools for the child's imagination, something to talk to and interact with (Smirnova, 2011). Different categories of toys seem to generate more or less interest or preference as measured by time in contact (Bjorkland & Bjorkland, 1979). For example, toddlers appeared to spend most time with organizational toys.

Studies of toy design are just beginning to more clearly describe the ways children respond to varied aspects of toys. For example, toy designers have investigated how interactive and digital toys impact pretend play, finding that these toys were used to pretend in a variety of ways but also that the shape of the toy mattered, as well as the method of manipulation (Hong & Lee, 2019). More abstract shapes led to more diverse types of play. Another examined how preschool-age children responded to varied toys and similarly found that open-ended toys that allowed the most "doing" were most preferred (Balzan, Farrugia, Casha, & Wodehouse, 2018). Another study of a new toy presented in two ways demonstrated that with the toy, small groups of children ages 8 to 12 were able to create on average 6 to 7 new games in 30 minutes, but the types of games varied by the toy's affordances in the two conditions (Bekker, Hopma, & Sturm, 2010).

Realism

Children prefer real activities to pretend (Lillard & Taggart, 2019; Taggart, Heise, & Lillard, 2018). However, when using toys as opposed to real activities with real materials, the realism of the toy is important as well. Realistic looking toys as opposed to those that are more abstract influence the amount and type of pretend play (Trawick-Smith, 1990). Although younger children benefit from realistic props for pretense, props that are more realistic looking may reduce the varied forms of play that occur with the materials, restricting play to the theme that was intended by the realistic prop, particularly with older children (Dodge & Frost, 1986; Howe & Hogan, 2001).

Novelty

One aspect of play objects that has been extensively studied is novelty (Cahill-Solis & Witryol, 1994; Henderson & Moore, 1980; Hunter, Ross, & Ames, 1982; McLoyd & Ratner, 1983; Rabinowitz, Moely, Finkel, & McClinton, 1975; Trawick-Smith et al., 2015). Novel play objects are most attractive to children, and promote higher-quality play and greater levels of exploration. However, a child's response to novel toys may be influenced by who the child is playing with (Henderson, 1981; Rabinowitz et al., 1975).

Control

Certain forms of toys, called dynamic toys (Abdulaeva & Smirnova, 2011) allow a child to control the motion of the toy and experience, learn about, and play with physical laws such as gravity. Examples of these types of toys include tops, push cars, characters or animals that can be made to walk or hop or fly, and rolling toys such as balls or marble mazes. These toys require the control of the child to create the motion and often lead to child imitation of the movement in question. Although the desire for independence and autonomy in toddlers is legendary, few studies have examined the impact of level of control allowed by a toy or activity, a child's preference for it, or the play performance that ensues. In one example, for infant boys in particular, having control over when a toy activated reduced their fear of the toy and for girls, appeared to increase their enjoyment (Gunnar-Vongnechten, 1978).

Complexity

Toys vary from the very simple to the extremely complex. Complexity may be considered based on a variety of toy characteristics such as the size, shape, and number of parts; the way the parts relate to each other; the motor skills required to use the toy; the level of cause and effect needed; the materials the toy is made from; the color and contrast and other sensory elements; the level of realism; and level of robotic, digital, or smart features (Richards, Putnick, Suwalsky, & Bornstein, 2020). The past two decades have seen large jumps in complexity with the addition of game versions on laptops, tablets, phones, and other mobile devices, and toys with increasingly complex digital features such as speech, motor actions, and sensory stimulation (lights/sounds, etc.) (Healey & Mendelsohn, 2019).

Smart toys, such as robots and talking dolls, have very different affordances for play than simpler toys (Berriman & Mascheroni, 2019). These new toys have been described as providing "phygital play." *Phygital* is a marketing term denoting a blend of physical and digital. Smart toys are both toys and media objects and as media or digital objects offer affordances of "liveliness, affective stickiness, and mobility" (Berriman & Mascheroni, 2019, p. 798). Liveliness means that the toy appears to act autonomously. The animatronic toys can be activated a variety of ways and appear to "live." Many of these toys require or even demand children to care for them, and they only "live" in response to the child. Therefore, the affordances of these types of toys are corealized. The child animates the toy, but the ability of the toy to be animated encourages the child to engage. The toy "provokes" the child to enliven it. This is the aspect of these types of toys that is new and different. Older dolls and teddy bears could be animated by a child, but they didn't not demand it. *Affective stickiness* is the aspect of the toys whereby children form emotional attachments to them. Again, this attribute was present in of older toys, but in different ways, as older toys did not demand attention. The "personalities" of these newer toys have been designed to trigger care and emotional responses. Affective stickiness also refers to the nature of these new technologies as binding oneself to a device, much as adults are now "tethered" to their mobile phones. Mobility or portability is an affordance of many of the newer toys that allow them to easily be carried out of the home, to be played with in social groups with friends, and to create shared peer culture and materiality.

While all of these novel forms of toys provide new affordances, many experts are concerned with the changes in play they create. Often simple toys allow more varied uses and engender higher-quality play and better play interactions with parents (Miller, Lossia, Suarez-Rivera, & Gros-Louis, 2017; Trawick-Smith, Wolff, Koschel, & Vallarelli, 2014). While children are best able to utilize toys that are within their developmental capacity (Richards et al., 2020), within that range they may prefer toys with more detail as opposed to less (Robinson & Jackson, 1987) and appear to sustain greater attention to more complex toys that generate feedback such as sounds and lights (Miller et al., 2017). Parents and teachers, therefore, may need to ensure that children have toys with a range of complexity levels and also ensure that toy play occurs with appropriate adult scaffolding (Healey & Mendelsohn, 2019) (**Figure 1.18**).

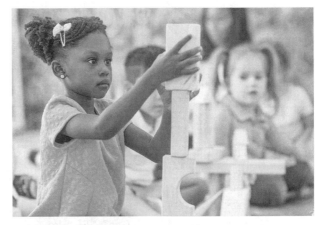

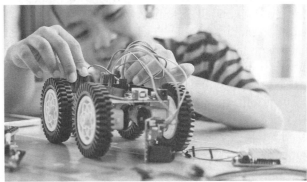

Figure 1.18 Toys can range from the very simple, such as blocks, to those that are quite complex

Top: © FatCamera/E+/Getty Images; bottom: © Cavan Images/Cavan/Getty Images.

Social Norms

Children at times will report that they prefer or want a toy because of their peers, or the knowledge that a friend would like to play with them with that toy (Mertala, Karikoski, Tähtinen, & Sarenius, 2016). Even young children may select a toy based on the selections of others (Gerson, Bekkering, & Hunnius, 2017). Lately, children may have been prompted to choose a toy based on an internet persona such as Ryan from Ryan's World (see https://www.youtube.com/c/RyanToysReview/videos).

Over many years, toy fads have spread like wildfire. Yo-yos were an early toy fad in the 1920s followed by Slinky, Mr. Potato Head, and eventually the Rubik's Cube. This idea of "everyone has one/it" is not a new invention, but in the digital age, this phenomenon can become global. Toy "fads" that came seemingly out of nowhere within the last decade or so include fidget spinners and Shopkins. Before that there were Pokémon, Webkinz, Furbies, Pogs, Silly Bandz, and Bratz. Toy trends commonly have an element of collecting as a form of play, where children gather, trade, build, and compare libraries of toys in a theme.

Preferences for Virtual Environments

Most children today will undoubtedly be exposed to the digital realm at some point during their childhood. Digital natives are growing up somewhat differently than the generations that have come before them (UNICEF, 2017). These differences can be seen in their play in multiple ways (Bryant, 2011), such as a greater likelihood for children to cocreate and to blur the lines of "ownership," particularly in the digital realm. This can readily be noted through generation of content on sites such as Scratch (see https://scratch.mit.edu/) (Resnick & Robinson, 2017). Children are eager to modify, change, hack, recycle, and engineer for themselves. They move easily between the real physical word and the virtual world.

New forms of more complex and connected digital toys offer new avenues for social connectedness (Kafai & Fields, 2013) and media mix (Ito, 2005). Media mix suggests an ecology that integrates home media such as television and home gaming with external media such as movies and other portable and collectible media such as trading cards or handheld games. Overall there is also a greater blending of the virtual worlds and real ones, for example, with games such as Pokémon Go. These new forms of virtual play spaces have led to expanded opportunities for play for many, including those with disabilities.

How Do Children with Disabilities Play?

As occupational therapists, we must be informed not only about the play of typically developing children but also about the play of children with disabilities. We know that although children with disabilities do play and may have similar playful attitudes to peers without disabilities, they play differently (Angelin, Sposito, & Pfeifer, 2018; Barton, 2015; Wolfberg, 2015). A thorough review of the play of children with varied disabilities is available freely online (Besio, Bulgarelli, & Stancheva-Popkostadinova, 2016). These authors report that children with disabilities may progress through similar stages of play development as children without disabilities but at delayed ages and reduced rates, depending on the type and severity of disability present. Children with physical limitations are more greatly challenged by barriers to access play. They may need greater assistance to play, demonstrate less active involvement with objects, spend more time with adults rather than peers, and may spend more time in passive activities such as television watching

rather than active and varied play. The difficulties with play experienced by children with autism spectrum disorder are well documented and include lack of symbolic play, less motivation to play socially, limited imitation of others in play, and repetitive play with objects. Because the development of play is closely tied to cognitive and motor development, the development of play in children with disabilities may be less affected by changes in chronological age than by developmental level. For children with severe disabilities, play skills may improve slowly.

Playfulness has also been studied in children with various disabilities with varying results, which may be related to the specific disability or to the environment in which the study was completed (Pinchover, Shulman, & Bundy, 2016). At times, children with physical disabilities and difficulties with specific play skills will demonstrate adequate playfulness, whereas children with cognitive disabilities may be more impaired in characteristics of playfulness (Benson, Nicka, & Stern, 2006; Bulgarelli, Bianquin, Besio, & Molina, 2018; Bundy, 1989; Harkness & Bundy, 2001; Leipold & Bundy, 2000; Muys, Rodger, & Bundy, 2006; Okimoto, Bundy, & Hanzlik, 2000; Reed, Dunbar, & Bundy, 2000; Skaines, Rodger, & Bundy, 2006).

Differences in play skills or the ability to access play do not necessarily equate to differences in play preferences. Although one can readily observe actual play *behaviors*, examining the play *preferences* of children with disabilities is more difficult because physical limitations may hinder access to preferred activities, and limited communication may hinder discussion. However, there are ways to assess the preferences of children even with severe disabilities (Reid, DiCarlo, Schepis, Hawkins, & Stricklin, 2003; Virués-Ortega et al., 2014), and research on the play preferences of children with disabilities suggests they can and do indicate specific play preferences. For example, children with an autism spectrum disorder have been found to demonstrate clear preferences for play activities and objects with sensorimotor properties, favored characters, and predictable situations (Desha, Ziviani, & Rodger, 2003; Ferrara & Hill, 1980). Children with developmental delays are reported by their parents to exhibit a preference for rough-and-tumble play and gross motor play above more sedentary play such as watching television, drawing, or coloring (Case-Smith & Miller Kuhaneck, 2008). Children with physical disabilities who were asked about their play choices and the technical aids they needed for play indicated they enjoyed play and thought play was fun, and many played typical games for their age and gender. However, many reported barriers to outdoor play because of poor physical access to play environments (Skar,

2002). Therefore, many of these children reported they preferred indoor play and passive activities, which is different from preferred activities reported by typically developing children.

So do children with disabilities have different preferences from typically developing children? One study found that children with mild motor disabilities hold preferences similar to children without disabilities (Clifford & Bundy, 1989), whereas another study (Case-Smith & Miller Kuhaneck, 2008) found differences in preferences. In a survey of parents of children with and without disabilities, the play preferences of children ages 3 to 7 were examined and compared (Case-Smith & Miller Kuhaneck, 2008). From a sample of 83 children with developmental delay and a total sample of 166 children, the authors found the preferences of children who were typical and developmentally delayed were somewhat different. Children with developmental delays preferred rough-and-tumble play more than typically developing children, while typically developing children preferred quiet tabletop activities, and peer-play more than the children with delays. Preferences may be shaped by physical or cognitive limitations that restrict access to certain play opportunities.

Technology and virtual reality have opened new doors for children with disabilities to play (Adams et al., 2017; Garzotto, Gelsomini, Occhiuto, Matarazzo, & Messina, 2017). These new options may lead to entirely new avenues for assessing and determining their play preferences and abilities as access improves. However, much of the research to date has focused on the effectiveness of technology-related play for improving motor skills (see, for example, Wu, Loprinzi, & Ren, 2019).

Where Does Play Occur?

Play happens all over the world and has been observed in many cultures and within many forms of societal structure (Barnes, 2015; Ramsey, 2015). Western industrialized cultures have increasingly afforded more importance to play. Children in these cultures are therefore often provided with specific places for play such as playgrounds, playrooms, and commercial play areas. Some of these can be quite elaborate. However, access is important and also uneven. Transportation services may or may not allow access to play spaces. Neighborhood geographies, safety, traffic, sidewalks, lighting, and so on may support or limit children's ability to play near their own home as well. Accessibility issues may specifically hinder access for children with disabilities (Ripat & Becker, 2012). These types of issues are best influenced through broad policy changes (Whitebread, 2012).

There is significant variation across the globe, as well, in the places where play occurs. Elaborate playgrounds, woods with trees to climb, or streams and rivers in which to swim are not evenly distributed. In very rural locations across the globe, play, by necessity, occurs in fields, in the dirt or grassy spaces between homes, in the local woods, or in the home.

Environmental features, the "where" of play, likely impact play behaviors. One study comparing the games of Nigerian children and American children found that the overall participation in categories of play was similar. However, the terrain where the children's games were played was different, thus somewhat altering the specific games available to the children (Nwokah & Ikekeonwu, 1998).

Another issue to consider in terms of where play occurs is whether it happens near adults or away from adults. In certain cultures, play is more likely to occur with or without adults nearby (Edwards, 2005; Lancy, 1996; Nwokah & Ikekeonwu, 1998). For example, in many hunter-gatherer societies, children under age 7 are encouraged to play together, away from adults, to allow adults to work (Gosso et al., 2005). In many farming and industrial societies, boys in middle childhood in particular roam away from home in gender-segregated groups to play (Edwards, 2005). In other cultures, children are encouraged to stay near adults, observe adults, and participate in the "work" of the community. As a result, play happens near the adults during or in between work chores (Bazyk, Stalnaker, Llerena, Ekelman, & Bazyk, 2003; Lancy, 1996).

Development of Westernized Play Spaces and Playgrounds

In Western societies, spaces began to be developed specifically for play more than 100 years ago. Public parks and fields were developed in earnest as Americans began to embrace outdoor and organized sports and recreation (Dulles, 1940). Social reformers and settlement workers of the time sought to "move" children's play from the streets to public areas where it could be supervised and where children could be "molded" (Cavallo, 1981). Therefore, the development of playgrounds for children grew out of the settlement movement. These ideas were especially prevalent in urban areas; thus, early playgrounds were in the cities. For example, Boston's first sand gardens, beginning in 1886, were established in poorer areas, near settlement houses (Frost, 2010). Settlement workers, such as Lillian Wald, were instrumental in establishing the Society for Parks and Playgrounds, the Outdoor Recreation League, and New York City's first playgrounds in the late 1800s (Cavallo, 1981; New York City Department of Parks and Recreation, n.d.).). The league developed nine playgrounds with swings, slides, and seesaws. The first municipal park with play equipment was created in 1903. Similar growth was occurring in Chicago as well. Jane Adams, a settlement worker, had built a playground at the Hull House in Chicago by the late 1800s. By 1903, she had successfully lobbied the city of Chicago for public playgrounds, the first of which was the one at Hull House, that the city took over (Ibrahim, 1989).

By 1906, the Playground Association of America was established (Cavallo, 1981; Ibrahim, 1989; Playworld, 2019). Between 1906, when the organization began, and 1924, the number of playgrounds in the United States grew to over 5,000. This movement was well funded, as municipal governments spent more than 100 million dollars for building and staffing public playgrounds between 1880 and 1920 (Cavallo, 1981). Lee, a social worker in Massachusetts, was also influential in the development of playgrounds across the country. Boston was one of the first cities to have public parks and outdoor areas for sports such as baseball; however, Lee quickly realized that children needed more than just flat open space. By 1900 Lee was instrumental in establishing the first playground in Boston that included many of the typical pieces of play equipment we would recognize today: swings, slides, teeters, and sandboxes (Sapora, 1989).

During this same time period, state legislation began to create playground commissions and recreation legislation, while colleges that educated teachers began instructing teachers in playground equipment usage. For example, the University of Virginia developed a playground, with homemade inexpensive equipment that included typical playthings of the time: sand, seesaw, slide, swings, and flying dutchman.

Playgrounds as Spaces for Play

Playgrounds can be loosely defined as outdoor play spaces that allow opportunities for children to play. Certain structures and playthings have come to be associated with the word *playground*, such as sandboxes, swings, slides, and climbing structures. Children consider a playground as a place where they can be social and where there are enough items that allow for "fun" (Jansson, 2008).

The typical choices of playground structures have evolved over time. Playgrounds of the 1950s and 1960s were often created with metal and cement climbing structures. By the 1980s a national survey of playgrounds identified the most common playground fixtures as swings and slides (Bowers, 1990). "Traditional" playgrounds are those that typically include jungle gyms, seesaws, slides, swings, and merry-go-rounds with the purpose primarily of gross-motor play (Frost, 1978). Ideally, playgrounds should offer a variety of opportunities for dramatic, construction, and social play (Beckwith, 1998) in addition to movement, climbing, and ball play (Olsen & Smith, 2017; The Trust for Public Land, 2017).

Playgrounds can often be found at local public or private schools or in public park spaces that are open to the community. However, current statistics suggest that only one in five children live within walking distance of a playground, and there are great disparities in access between communities and neighborhoods of differing socioeconomics (McKenzie, Moody, Carlson, Lopez, & Elder, 2013; National Recreation and Park Association, n.d.; The Trust for Public Land, 2019).

A criticism of traditional playgrounds was that they were quite dangerous (Frost, 1978), leading to changes to the types of structures as well as the ground surfaces under the structures. The first safety standards were published in 1981 by the U.S. Consumer Product Safety Commission, and they now keep data on injuries and deaths that occur at playgrounds. The majority of child injuries on playgrounds occur with falls, and with equipment such as seesaws/teeter-totters, swings, slides, and composite play structures (Hanway & Motabar, 2016). Playground safety varies from site to site, with a majority of public playgrounds surveyed demonstrating signs of wear, rust, or rot, and with about one-quarter having potential hazards (Olsen & Kennedy, 2018). However, when children are asked about the removal of specific items from playgrounds for safety, they may have strong reactions to the removal. They may be dissatisfied with what has been left behind and miss the items that are gone (Jansson, 2008).

Although many changes have occurred in the types of playgrounds available, in response to their earlier lack of safety, the new guidelines meant that for many schools and communities, playgrounds needed to be updated or removed (Playworld, 2019). Many states now have their own guidelines, and playgrounds are much safer; however, injuries do still occur, and playground safety remains a concern. Please see **Appendix 1.1** for more information about the history of playgrounds.

Modern playgrounds, while somewhat safer than traditional ones, have also been criticized for their poor design and their poor site selection with limited accessibility and variety (Czalczynska-Podolska, 2014; Veitch, Salmon, & Ball, 2007). They have been called boring and cookie cutter (Beckwith, 1998) and have been found to primarily promote functional play as opposed to other play forms (Czalczynska-Podolska,

2014; Hart & Sheehan, 1986). Many U.S. playgrounds limit the types of motor activities available, compared to playgrounds in other countries (Talarowski et al., 2019). For example, U.S. playgrounds appeared to be less likely to offer rocking, seesawing, or spinning. The most common features in U.S. playgrounds appear to be slides, ladders, and swings (Cohen et al., 2020). Playgrounds may also be standardized in their construction, for example, with items and objects spaced with equal distances between them or with equal heights or differences in heights (Jongeneel, Withagen, & Zaal, 2015). These types of configurations are not what children build for themselves when given the chance. Children appear to prefer variety and create play areas that match but can challenge their perceived abilities (Jongeneel, Withagen, & Zaal, 2015). Children note that playgrounds often were more fun when they were younger, as many of the activities available no longer pose a challenge for the older children (Jansson, 2008).

Different playgrounds afford varied forms of play (Adams, Veitch, & Barnett, 2018; Czalczynska-Podolska, 2014; Dyment & O'Connell, 2013; Mahony, Hyndman, Nutton, Smith, & Te Ava, 2017). Playgrounds that have more options and opportunities, more flexible options, and thus varied affordances for different children, provide the best play opportunities for children ; Talarowski, Cohen, Williamson, & Han, 2019). Playgrounds with more affordances for play allow all children to play together, regardless of their physical competence and motor skill (Barbour, 1999; Herrington & Brussoni, 2015). They also provide opportunities for practice and motor learning (Prieske et al., 2015). They allow children to create novel ways to use objects that were unintended (Castonguay & Jutras, 2009;). Playgrounds that provide the greatest opportunities for preferred movement may be most sought after by children. Often, the more variety of structures on a playground the better (**Figure 1.19**).

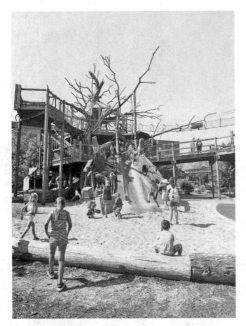

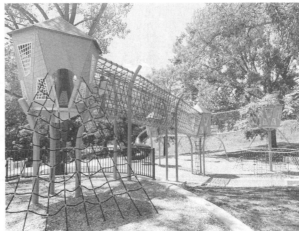

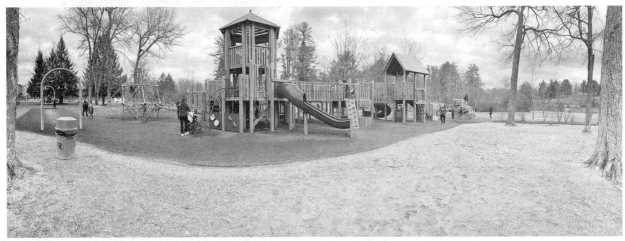

Figure 1.19 Different playgrounds afford very different forms of play

Top left and top right: Courtesy of Kylene Wenzl Carroll. Bottom: Courtesy of Kyle O'Brien.

Natural playscapes have traditional playground equipment but also have a variety of naturally landscaped features such as water, sand, stones, or wood, as well as natural loose parts such as pinecones and sticks. These spaces attempt to combine the best of natural areas with positive playground features. In spaces with both manufactured and natural areas children may prefer the mixed and manufactured areas, over the purely natural ones, although the natural environments lend themselves to greater dramatic play and provide props and materials for use in play in the manufactured areas (Zamani, 2016) (**Figure 1.20**).

With the current state of U.S. playgrounds, some authors have actually distinguished the term *playgrounds* from *play grounds* (Aziz & Said, 2015). Playgrounds are constructed of equipment often meant for specific uses and typically designed by adults. Play grounds, in contrast, are spaces that children find themselves, with space and materials to feed their curiosity and exploration, without the control of adults. In play grounds, children are free to do what they choose.

Adventure Playgrounds. Adventure playgrounds are a specific type of play space where children are free to build, create, destroy, and rebuild using a variety of scrap materials (Staemfli, 2009). Adventure playgrounds often look like a junkyard. There may also be a garden area to grow food and an area where children can climb and swing. One main purpose of an adventure playground is for children to encounter and learn to manage risk. There are typically one or two adults present to facilitate play and remove barriers, and they are there to ensure no children are hurt.

Originally available in Denmark in 1943 and Great Britain in 1946 (Matthews, 1985), these types of playgrounds spread across Europe. Although there are some adventure playgrounds available in the United States, in our country, the focus on child safety and the minimization of the threat of lawsuit has hindered their development here (Danzig, 2012; Staemfli, 2009). This may be to the detriment of our population in the United States, as these playgrounds have created lasting memories for many who frequented them as children (please see https://www.youtube.com/watch?reload=9&v=sQVWRb4SSdc). A reason children may prefer adventure playgrounds is the perception of freedom and choice (Brown, 2007; Frost, 2007; Jenkins, 2006).

Themed and Inclusive Playgrounds. According to the National Park and Recreation Association (Munsell, 2018), the current playground

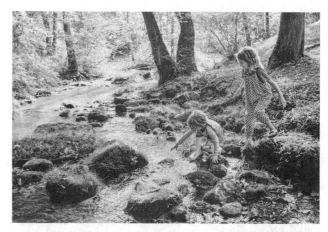

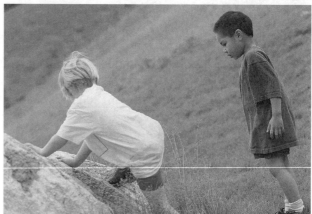

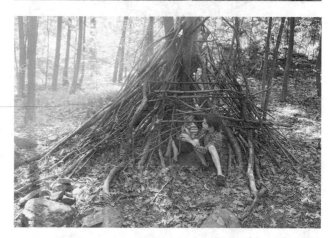

Figure 1.20 Natural play spaces may be the best playgrounds of all

Top: © Lisa5201/E+/Getty Images; middle: © Stockbyte/Stockbyte/Getty Images; bottom: © EvgeniiAnd/Shutterstock.

trend is for themed and inclusive playgrounds. Themed playgrounds have playground structures built around a particular idea, such as a farm (Pinon-iemi, 2003), or to look like a particular object, such as a firetruck, train, castle, or pirate ship. Themed playgrounds are believed to promote pretend play (Oke & Middle, 2016), whereas inclusive playgrounds are meant to promote social participation and full inclusion for children with disabilities. Fully inclusive playgrounds are desired by parents of children with disabilities (Stanton-Chapman & Schmidt,

2017). The best of these playgrounds would have the following features: accessible surfacing and enough space for maneuvering, equal amounts of ground-level and elevated play areas with ramps or other methods of accessing the elevated areas, multiniche areas to promote interactive play, cozy places and spaces, loose parts and props for imaginative play, equipment that allows for varied levels of challenge and risk, opportunities for sensory play such as tactile, auditory, and visual equipment, and they have multiple places to "jump in" to play (Fernelius & Christensen, 2017). Although not every community has access to inclusive playgrounds, organizations are attempting to create comprehensive lists of where they currently exist to provide greater access (see https://www.accessibleplayground.net/playground-directory/).

Interactive Playgrounds. A relatively new invention, interactive playgrounds use digital and electronic media in a play space to promote a variety of social and motor play activities (Bekker, Hopma, & Sturm, 2010; Poppe, van Delden, Moreno, & Reidsma, 2014). Interactive playgrounds often use lights, cameras, speakers, sensors, and large projection screens to immerse children in a virtual environment in which they can play. The sensors allow the interactive playground to adapt to the child's ability level, and novel elements can be introduced to maintain engagement and attention. Interactive playgrounds may be room sized, or in hallways, and this size allows for social interaction and also physical activity play. These play spaces are "activated" by the movements of the child as opposed to some handheld controller. In this way, they can promote active play. For example, one interactive playground encouraged physically active play by having children compete to "catch" shapes displayed on the floor via a projector from above. When a child neared a shape it would attach itself to the child but the shape could be stolen away if another child stepped on the same shape (Poppe, van Delden, Moreno, & Reidsma, 2014). Sensors also can measure the skill level of the child and actually be used to diagnose developmental difficulties in some cases. When these types of play spaces are designed specifically to be open ended, they are believed to promote creativity (Bekker, Hopma, & Sturm, 2010).

Natural Environments for Play

Natural environments for play include outdoor spaces such as fields, woods, or beaches that invite exploration and activity. Parks also provide natural play spaces. Recent surveys suggest that parks are available nearby

for the majority (75%) of Americans (National Recreation and Parks Association, 2018). The availability of other types of natural spaces, such as beaches, forests, and mountains, of course, varies based on geography.

Natural play environments are believed to promote development and well-being in a way that other play spaces cannot (Kemple, Oh, Kenney, & Smith-Bonahue, 2016). When allowed to play in a natural play environment, early elementary or kindergarten-aged children engage in different forms of play in different topographies and in areas with different vegetation (Fjørtoft, 2004). Children engage in climbing, sliding, running, building, and symbolic play in natural spaces, using the trees, rocks, and slopes. In these types of environments, functional play may predominate. However, construction play can occur with the materials available in nature such as sticks and pinecones (Fjørtoft, 2004). Symbolic play such as "house" and pirates also may occur with large rocks and trees as special spaces.

Natural play spaces are often preferred as well. A majority of adults surveyed about their childhoods and their perceptions of current play spaces for children report that they preferred natural environments for play (Brunelle, Herrington, Coghlan, & Brussoni, 2016). Children, too, often prefer natural play spaces (Castonguay & Jutras, 2009; Cloward Drown, 2014; Dowdell, Gray, & Malone, 2011; Luchs & Fikus, 2013). Within those spaces, children often specifically prefer features such as trees, plants, and water features over human-made environments (Mahidin & Maulan, 2012). However, natural environments provide aspects children may find either positive or negative. For example, positive aspects of a natural environment might include the natural colors, trees and shade, leaves and grass, woods, varied terrain level with places to climb or hide or challenge motor abilities, and animals and wildlife to observe and investigate. Negative elements of a natural play space could include pollution, trash, or litter; broken objects; unnatural colors, animals, or vegetation; bodies of water; wildlife that could be dangerous, unpleasant, or scary; lack of elements that provide shade; and places that are "boring" or too "open" with nowhere to hide (Tapsell, 1997; Tunstall, Tapsell, & House, 2004). Safety is a common concern related to disliked spaces (Castonguay & Jutras, 2009).

Community and Neighborhood Play Spaces

Young children may play outdoors in their neighborhoods, in the street, in parking lots, or alleys. The amount of time and the frequency of this type of play has changed, perhaps due to barriers put in place by parents because of fears for safety (Ferguson, 2019; Karsten, 2005; Tandy, 1999; Tranter & Doyle, 1996), societal expectations of how children should be supervised, and increased time spent using in screen-based devices time (Anderson, Economos, & Must, 2008). Currently, play in neighborhood areas not expressly meant for play (streets as opposed to parks, for example) occurs less often than play in areas "designed" for that purpose such as playgrounds (Cunningham & Jones, 1999; Veitch, Bagley, Ball, & Salmon, 2006). This form of outdoor play may be most likely to occur in neighborhoods that are socially cohesive (Aarts, Wendel-Vos, van Oers, Van de Goor, & Schuit, 2010). Children are more likely to play outside near their homes when there are other neighborhood children to play with, and when the physical aspects of the neighborhood such as sidewalks and traffic patterns support their ability to do so (Lambert, Vlaar, Herrington, & Brussoni, 2019). For example, street play may be more likely when there are cul-de-sacs nearby (Brockman, Jago, & Fox, 2011).

In some studies, only a small percentage of children report they prefer to play in the street (Tandy, 1999). Streets and alleys were favorite spaces for 20%, liked by 20%, and disliked by 19% of middle school children asked about space preferences in one study (Castonguay & Jutras, 2009). Adults, however, recall fondly their experiences of freely roaming their environments in childhood, whether by bus in the city, or by bicycle or foot in more rural areas (Cunningham & Jones, 1999).

There have been recent attempts by adults to reverse the trend of declining neighborhood and street play. To improve access to neighborhood play where parks and playgrounds are not available, researchers have placed mobile playgrounds built within old buses in local parking areas and have closed streets to allow play to occur safely without traffic (Espinoza, McMahan, Naffzinger, & Wiersma, 2012; Murray & Devecchi, 2016; Zieff, Chaudhuri, & Musselman, 2016). Children made use of these opportunities, and parents appreciated them. These types of altered community play spaces are not yet the norm, however.

Indoor Home and Classroom Environments

Although children prefer outdoor play to indoors (Burke, 2005; Glenn, Knight, Holt, & Spence, 2013; Miller & Kuhaneck, 2008) and are more active in their play outdoors (Kneeshaw-Price et al., 2013), having indoor play spaces allows for play when the weather is poor, when it is dark outside, or for younger children when parents are unable to supervise their outdoor play. Indoor play spaces in the home vary in as many ways as there are different types of homes. Play spaces may differ in size, location in the home, level of safety, warmth, or comfort (i.e., carpeted or concrete floor, heated or unheated, finished or unfinished). Differences are often due to home location, as well as socioeconomic status (Bradley, Corwyn, McAdoo, & García Coll, 2001; Freitas, Gabbard, Caçola, Montebelo, & Santos, 2013). Home environments vary in many factors, but the child's home environment may influence multiple aspects of child development, including play (Kavousipor, 2019).

Children are able to articulate their preferences for indoor play spaces. They appear to prefer closed and private spaces (Burke, 2005). Although children playing in the home may more frequently play in a family room or den than their own bedroom (Giddings & Halverson, 1981), their own bedroom is their preferred home space for most activities (Schiavo, 1987). In a study of 59 middle-class public-school children ages 8 to 18, when asked to draw their current home and their ideal home, 21% reported they currently had a playroom, and 29% of children who did not have a playroom, added one to their drawing of the ideal home (Schiavo, 1990).

Classroom spaces for play can be considered through the lens of a number of environmental variables, such as space available and arrangement of the physical layout (Rettig, 1998). Studies of indoor classroom spaces in relation to play and social behaviors suggest that indoor classroom play areas need to have sufficient space. Larger spaces may encourage more gross motor and individual play, and smaller spaces may promote interaction, but spaces that are too small may lead to disruptive behavior between children and poorer performance, particularly for girls (Brown, Fox, & Brady, 1987; Maxwell, 2003; Smith & Connelly, 1980). In smaller classrooms, or in areas of the classroom where child density is too high, children may become stressed (Legendre, 2003; Maxwell, 2003; 1996) and may be less likely to play when stressed in this way (Kantrowitz & Evans, 2004). Authors have noted that young children often prefer to have an area that is private or enclosed, sometimes called a "womb space" (Rettig, 1998; Richter & Oetter, 1990).

Well-defined classroom spaces appear to encourage cooperative play and socialization (Abbas & Othman, 2010; Moore, 1986; Moore & Sugiyama, 2007; Zimmons, 1997). However, visual barriers in classrooms, by removing children from the adult line of sight, can hinder play and socialization for young children

(Legendre & Fontaine, 1991). The physical layout of the furniture can impact the quantity and quality of socialization and joint play as well, in particular for children with weaker social connections (Legendre, 1999).

Classroom spaces can be considered in terms of their number and variety of toys and materials as well (Getz & Bernt, 1982; Rettig, 1998). Teachers are broadly given ideas about what ideal classrooms should be like and look like (Gordon Biddle et al., 2014). Some studies have indicated that the amount of play materials available can influence the amount of conflict in a classroom (Getz & Bernt, 1982). Many teachers want an inviting space with many toys, while others believe children today have too many toys. In a program begun over 25 years ago in Germany, which has spread to other countries as well, participating kindergarten classrooms remove *all* toys to promote greater imaginative and creative play and attempt to prevent addiction (Schubert & Strick, 1996; Zaske, 2017). Other recent examples of changing toy availability in a classroom setting include the toy-free week (Kiliańska-Przybyłoa & Górkiewiczb, 2017). During this toy-free week, children are guided to make their own playthings from provided materials, but all manufactured toys are removed. The children, with support of their parents, contributed to development of play materials from household supplies, such as recyclable packaging. The teachers noted creativity, cleverness, and humor in their creations.

Commercial Play Areas

Commercial play spaces generally are indoors and often are "branded" in some way. They typically provide a viewing area for parents or caregivers, who are responsible for supervising their child but are only allowed limited access to the actual play space (McKendrick, Bradford, & Fielder, 2000a, 2000b). Although there are multiple reasons for their growth, commercial playgrounds have arisen in part because of the recognition that children constitute a market that can generate profit. These play areas also provide access to physically active play in an environment that parents may consider safer than other play spaces (Jones, 2017; McKendrick, Bradford, & Fielder, 2000b).

There are different "types" of commercialized play spaces. There are a variety of for-profit franchises specializing in indoor play for children using trampolines, laser tag, or even indoor skydiving (e.g., Little Gym, Gymboree Play and Music, Sky Zone) (Bailey, 2016; McKendrick, Bradford, & Fielder, 2000a, 2000b). These types of play spaces all charge a fee for

their use; therefore, access is not equally distributed. The second type includes businesses such as malls or fast-food restaurants that may entice adult customers to their venues with their free indoor play spaces for the children to enjoy. These free play environments provide access to commercial play spaces for families within the full range of financial means.

The Relationship of Climate to Where and How Children Play

Although clearly not something humans have any control of, both the daily weather and seasonal patterns of weather do impact play, particularly in outdoor play spaces. Although most studies have examined weather-related changes in physical activity, as opposed to play per se, poor weather, related to temperature and precipitation often leads to lesser physical activity and more time indoors (Brockman, Jago, & Fox, 2011; Ergler, Kearns, & Witten, 2013; Harrison et al., 2011; Hyndman, Chancellor, & Lester, 2015; Pagels et al., 2014; Remmers et al., 2017). However, these changes in activity are not universal. For the majority of countries, extreme temperature (both hot and cold), windy, and wet, poorer weather conditions mean less physical activity outdoors, but that does not appear to be the case for countries such as Australia, Denmark, and Estonia, for example (Harrison et al., 2017). In some areas, outdoor physical activity remains high even in poor weather. The reasons for these differences require further investigation. One recent examination of outdoor play suggested that weather-related changes in outdoor affordances for play led to markedly different play activities (Fjørtoft, 2004). For example, deep snow allowed children to reach and climb new areas of trees and to slide down hills. In some areas, what might be considered "poor weather" may allow for "good play," particularly for children of certain ages. Rising temperatures associated with climate change, however, may jeopardize children's health and decrease their tolerance for vigorous physical play or result in higher use of indoor spaces with artificial climate controls (Committee on Environmental Health, 2007).

Play Can Occur Almost Anywhere

An infinite number of human-caused events could theoretically impact where children play. Important ones include war, refugeeism, and terrorism. Even in the worst of conditions, children may find places to play in and items to play with. This has been documented over and over again. For example, children have been captured in photographs playing on the overturned remains of bombed cars, swimming in water in the craters left by bombs, and playing ball in the dust of refugee camps (Hu, 2015). Play is believed to be healing for children after exposure to trauma (Cohen & Gadassi, 2018). Children need a place of relative safety and some basic materials, and they will find a way to make a play space. But when adults help, there are even better outcomes for children in these areas. For example, UNICEF has both helped create places to play and documented with photos the places that children play in war zones and as refugees (Suriyaarachchi, 2017). The U.S. border patrol similarly is building a playground for the migrant children it is detaining (Rohrlich, 2020).

Specific Evidence Regarding the Influence of *Where* Play Occurs

As occupational therapists, we understand the importance of context and know that contextual features can impact occupational performance. In the realm of play, these ideas are being supported by science. For example, research on playgrounds has indicated that the structures available and the location and layout of the structures does influence how children use the spaces and the type of play that they engage in (Cohen et al., 2020; Czalczynska-Podolska, 2014). Adventure playgrounds promote greater use of equipment and materials, whereas traditional playgrounds may promote more motor skills and movement (Adams, Veitch, & Barnett, 2018). Adventure playgrounds promote more social play than traditional playgrounds, and playgrounds with greater variety and more flexible objects promote creativity. Children are more likely to converse with other children on adventure playgrounds (Frost, 2006), but adventure playgrounds may be less supportive of physically active play than traditional playgrounds (Adams, Barnett, & Veitch, 2018). In a national study of playgrounds, Cohen et al. (2020) reported that each additional element on the playground increases the number of users and the amount of vigorous play that occurs.

Natural environments such as fields and forests allow for more complex and creative play (Herrington & Brussoni, 2015; Luchs & Fikus, 2013) and longer play episodes (Luchs & Fikus, 2013), in part because natural environments provide more affordances for play (Refshauge et al., 2013). Natural outdoor play seems to encourage peer socialization (Shim, Herwig,

& Shelley, 2009). Animal studies also support the influence of contextual features on play, suggesting that changes in habitat and environment can lead to marked changes in play (Ernst et al., 2018; Nogueira, Soledade, Pompéia, & Nogueira-Filho, 2011; Sharpe et al., 2002; Vanderschuren et al., 1995).

When Does Play Occur?

Play can occur almost anytime. One prerequisite for play to occur, however, is a feeling of safety and security. In both humans and nonhuman species, play occurs when basic survival needs are met and there is at least a minimum level of safety. Play is often the first activity to be lost, however, when things are not going well for an animal (Bateson, 2005).

Whenever a child is not otherwise occupied, for example, with school or chores, the child can play. In addition, children can approach those work tasks with a playful attitude (Glynn, 1994) and play while they are working (Bazyk et al., 2003; Lancy, 1996; Nwokah & Ikekeonwu, 1998).

One other distinction needs to be made in terms of the "when" of play. Some researchers divide play into two types: exploration and true play. These authors suggest that for play to occur, the play object must be fully explored. The child must know the characteristics of the object to know what the object can do (Hutt, 1966). We disagree with this. For our purposes, exploration is often an aspect of play, and we believe an appropriate level of novelty and exploration is necessary for play to continue. Simple objects can become rapidly boring if they are unable to be used in multiple ways. Children stop playing, as do some animals, when the play object lacks novelty. In a study of cats, habituation to a cat toy led to the stoppage of play, whereas reintroduction of novelty led to the return of play (Hall, 1998). Novelty was important to the maintenance of play behavior over time. As therapists, we have all seen the child who becomes bored with a game or object without any flexibility. Therefore, exploration is not a prerequisite for when play occurs, but rather exploration can also occur during play.

In relation to *when* children play, the amount of time a child has available in order to play also can impact play behaviors. Seasonal variations in play also have largely to do with changes in free time based on whether or not children are in school. Seasonal variations also impact the amount of daylight available for outdoor activities (Harrison et al., 2017). School calendars affect free time. The length of time per play session can also be important in play. Studies suggest that longer play periods lead to higher levels of play or more complex play (Christie, Johnsen, & Peckover, 1988; Christie & Wardle, 1992; Rettig, 1998; Tegano & Burdette, 1991).

Is Play a Privilege or Right?

In addition to considering where, when, and who children play with, it is also important to consider the difference between play considered as a privilege or a right, as each position can influence which children play and which do not. The United States remains one of the only countries that has not ratified the United Nations Rights of the Child, in which Article 31 declares play as a right of all children not a privilege. If framed as a privilege, play is granted to children of a dominant group, while others are denied the right to play because children and parents are blamed for opportunity gaps (Souto-Manning, 2017). The right to play is highly racialized, for example, in a society that denies African American children the right to play without fear of being rejected (i.e., when cultural norms differ) or fear of being criminalized to the point that play may cost their lives for example if an authority mistakes a water gun as an actual gun (Souto-Manning, 2017). See **Practice Opportunity 1.2**, and see the learning activities for ways to reflect on these ideas for application to occupational therapy practice.

Practice Opportunity 1.2 Responding to "Tiger Jail": Addressing Our Discomfort with "Cops and Robbers"

Ariana Brazier, PhD and Julia Brazier
ATL Parent Like a Boss, Inc.

During an ordinary summer camp afternoon, a small group of joyful Black second-grade girls lightly shoved a male classmate from behind before fleeing the scene—running and screaming through the open grassy hill outside the school. As they ran toward the wall behind me, panting and laughing, I asked what they were playing. One eagerly responded, "Sisters Adventure."

Judging by their responses, shared in spurts of energy between heavy breathing, it became apparent that this was an impromptu game that followed their imaginative impulses. I asked the rules of their game anyway. Excitedly speaking at once, the group of four or five girls shared the following parameters (these parameters are transcribed as shared without edit or correction; my personal observations of the discussion are in the brackets):

> First you gotta find a tiger, then you got to touch it while it's sleeping and you got to wake it up then run around the playground screaming "AHHHHH!!!!"

> Another student is a tiger, and the wall is the base [she trailed off as if to ponder what will be next before quickly circling back with a few more rules.]

> You gotta find another tiger … [Wait. I guess there's two tigers now...] another person holds the tiger back until the tiger is released and they chase the "sisters."

> Tigers are trying to get them and take them to tiger jail.

Clearly this fantastical narrative-based game was provoking incredible amounts of joy for the children involved. However, I was troubled by the final rule that effectively framed their play as a variation of the popular "Cops and Robbers" game that countless generations of children have grown accustomed to engaging without question or critique.

The summer camp program was located in a predominantly Black neighborhood within a majority Black city in the southeast United States. Their community is publicly defined by concentrated poverty, housing insecurity, systemic and interpersonal violence, and political negligence. Many children have witnessed police remove family members from their communities, and/or themselves have been subjected to emotional and physical violence by hired security companies and city police officers alike. Even with their neighborhoods being located within a 5-mile (or less) radius of a federal penitentiary, the police show up when they are least wanted, but are never present when they are supposedly most needed.

As one teacher intimated to me that summer, "[They don't play regular tag.] They play 'Go to Jail' [and they really pretend handcuffing them]." Growing up in a police state, these Black and Brown children are playing, and in some cases experiencing, a reality-informed version of "Cops and Robbers" in which there is no chase—there is no possibility of escape; the end result is always jail.

Nevertheless, in acknowledging this sociocultural context, we must also acknowledge the noteworthy strengths and benefits evident in their play such as cooperative rule development, as well as how their play invites belonging and shifts possibilities. Without explicit discussion, rather through practice,

(continues)

Practice Opportunity 1.2 Responding to "Tiger Jail": Addressing Our Discomfort with "Cops and Robbers" *(continued)*

the children were identifying common experiences and building relationships as they processed difficult experiences with joy at the center.

Children tend to react to and reenact experiences that happen in their lives through play and pretend situations. Their play is akin to the ways adults might process traumatic situations through dialogue, but because children do not have the language, they are processing as they play. Children need play as an outlet. Play is a way for children to share their stories and inform outside observers of the systems and injustices to which their communities have been exposed.

Accordingly, as adults it is not our place to interrupt or shut down their play even as we navigate our own triggers and discomforts around policing. While observing, we should be careful not to involve ourselves as anything more than passive guests. If we act as observers of their play, we can become a necessary sounding board. We can ask critical questions using nonjudgmental tones and phrases such as "I noticed that…," "I wonder about…," and/or "… how did you?" In the process, we may become privy to their perceptions, interpretations, and experiences. Once informed of their knowledge and opinions, their play and dialogue can be received as an opportunity to facilitate methods for the children to reimagine and extend the game.

Children should have the freedom to independently create and lead their own play experiences. We can provide safe spaces and allow adequate time for this to happen. Our expressions of disapproval based on value systems, expectations, or experiences not explicitly shared or fully processed by the children and their families may cause them to think they [the children themselves] are "bad" or doing something wrong. This could foreclose the possibility of discussing what is actually the problem—hyperpolicing of Black people and their communities.

In addition to racial inequities in play, social class must also be considered as some children are not afforded the opportunity to regularly play if they are from low-income communities. According to the U.S. Census, poverty rates have fluctuated greatly since 1970; however, sustained, long-term progress in lowering poverty has been difficult to achieve (Edwards, 2018). For those living in low-income communities, there may not be appropriate areas for play (i.e., open green spaces, large yards, parks, or playgrounds). Additionally, parents may be less available to provide children with play opportunities (i.e., going outside, going to parks, setting up playdates) if parents are working long hours or multiple jobs just to sustain basic needs such as shelter and food.

Play allows children to build the skills needed to ask questions, develop community, and stand up for fairness to enact change. By advocating for play as a right for all children, we unleash "their infinite potential and capacity—to learn, to grow, to get along, and to strive for fairness and justice" (Souto-Manning, 2017, p. 787). As professionals working with families, occupational therapists should reject the notion that play is a privilege and embrace a responsibility to all children and families by advocating for their right to play by identifying and addressing barriers to play they may face.

Conclusion

Play is one of the most powerful tools wielded by children for learning and growing. Through play, children learn about diversities, engage with familiar and unfamiliar materials, share their own experiences and perspectives and consider those of others, collaborate, make discoveries, create new narratives, take risks, and engage in resistance. In this chapter, we provided an overview of the important concepts relevant to play that readers need to know before continuing to the following chapters on application to intervention. Knowledge about play provides a foundation for assessing and incorporating play in occupational therapy as well as supporting advocacy outside of our profession. With this introduction to the many facets of play examined by researchers in animal biology, evolutionary science, education, psychology, and child development, we next turn to the way play is viewed and used in occupational therapy.

**NOTE: To protect confidentiality, all names and identifying information used throughout this book have been changed, except when specifically requested to use the real name.

References

Abbas, M. Y., & Othman, M. (2010). Social behavior of preschool children in relation to physical spatial definition. *Procedia-Social and Behavioral Sciences*, 5, 935–941. https://doi.org/10.1016/j.sbspro.2010.07.213

Abdulaeva, E. A., & Smirnova, E. O. (2011). The role of dynamic toys in child's development. *Psychological Science & Education*, *2011*(2), 30–38. https://doi.org/10.17759/pse

Adams, K. D., Rios Rincon, A. M., Becerra Puyo, L. M., Castellanos Cruz, J. L., Gómez Medina, M. F., Cook, A. M., & Encarnação, P. (2017). An exploratory study of children's pretend play when using a switch-controlled assistive robot to manipulate toys. *British Journal of Occupational Therapy*, *80*(4), 216–224. https://doi.org/10.1177/0308022616680363

Adams, J., Veitch, J., & Barnett, L. (2018a). Physical activity and fundamental motor skill performance of 5–10 year old children in three different playgrounds. *International Journal of Environmental Research and Public Health*, *15*(9), 1896. https://doi.org/10.3390/ijerph15091896

Adams, J., Barnett, L., & Veitch, J. (2018b). What sort of playground design facilitates physical activity and encourages children to use diverse motor skills?. *Journal of Science and Medicine in Sport*, *21*, S12.

Alexander, G. M., & Hines, M. (2002). Sex differences in response to children´s toys in nonhuman primates (Cercopithecus aethiops sabaeus). *Evolution and Human Behavior*, *23*, 467–479. https://doi.org/10.1016/S1090-5138(02)00107-1

Al Kurdi, B. (2017). *Investigating the factors influencing parent toy purchase decisions: Reasoning and consequences*. International Business Research, *10*(4), 104–116. https://doi.org/10.5539/ibr.v10n4p104

Anderson, S.E., Economos, C.D., & Must, A. (2008). Active play and screen time in US children aged 4 to 11 years in relation to sociodemographic and weight status characteristics: A nationally representative cross-sectional analysis. *BMC Public Health*, *8*, 366. https://doi.org/10.1186/1471-2458-8-366

Angelin, A. C., Sposito, A. M., & Pfeifer, L. I. (2018). Influence of functional mobility and manual function on play in preschool children with cerebral palsy. *Hong Kong Journal of Occupational Therapy*, *31*(1), 46–53. https://doi.org/10.1177/1569186118783889

Apter, M. J. (1991). A structural-phenomenology of play. In J. H. Kerr & M. J. Apter (Eds.), *Adult play: A reversal theory approach* (pp. 13–29). Amsterdam: Swets & Zeitlinger.

Aarts, M. J., Wendel-Vos, W., van Oers, H. A., Van de Goor, I. A., & Schuit, A. J. (2010). Environmental determinants of outdoor play in children: A large-scale cross-sectional study. *American Journal of Preventive Medicine*, *39*(3), 212–219. https://doi.org/10.1016/j.amepre.2010.05.008

Aarts, M. J., de Vries, S. I., Van Oers, H. A., & Schuit, A. J. (2012). Outdoor play among children in relation to neighborhood characteristics: A cross-sectional neighborhood observation study. *International Journal of Behavioral Nutrition and Physical Activity*, *9*(1), 98. https://doi.org/10.1186/1479-5868-9-98

Aubry, S., Ruble, D. N., & Silverman, L. B. (1999). The role of gender knowledge in children's gender-typed preferences. In L. Balter & C. S. Tamis-LeMonda (Eds.), *Child psychology: A handbook of contemporary issues* (pp. 363–390). New York: Psychology Press.

Austin, E. (2015). Zombie culture: Dissent, celebration and the carnivalesque in social spaces. In *The zombie renaissance in popular culture* (pp. 174–190). London: Palgrave Macmillan.

Ayres, A. J. (1972). *Sensory integration and learning disorders*. Los Angeles: Western Psychological Services.

Ayres, A. J. (1979). *Sensory integration and the child*. Los Angeles: Western Psychological Services.

Ayres, A. J. (2005). *Sensory integration and the child: 25th anniversary edition*. Los Angeles: Western Psychological Services.

Aziz, N. F., & Said, I. (2015). Outdoor environments as children's play spaces: Playground affordances. *In Play, Recreation, Health, and Well Being*, 1–22. https://doi.org/10.1007/978-981-4585-96-5

Bailey, R. (2016). Child-Related Franchise Report 2016. Retrieved June 12, 2018 from: https://www.franchisedirect.com/information/childrelatedfranchisereport2016/.

Balzan, E., Farrugia, P., Casha, O., & Wodehouse, A. (2018). Evaluating the impact of design affordances in preschool children's toy preferences. *Proceedings of International Design Conference, DESIGN*, *5*, 2165–2176. https://doi.org/10.21278/idc.2018.0155

Barbour, A.C. (1999). The impact of playground design on the play behaviors of children with differing levels of physical competence. *Early Child Res Quarterly*, *14*, 75–98. https://doi.org/10.1080/14733285.2013.812272

Barnes, D. R. (2006). Play in historical and cross-cultural contexts. In D. P. Fromberg & D. Bergen (Eds.), *Play from birth to twelve* (pp. 243–260). New York: Routledge.

Barnes, D. R. (2015). Play in historical and cross cultural contexts. In D. P. Fromberg & D. Bergen (Eds.), *Play from birth to twelve* (pp. 257–270). New York: Routledge.

Barnett, L. A. (1990). Playfulness: Definition, design, and measurement. *Play and culture*, *3*, 319–336.

Barnett, L. A. (1991). Characterizing playfulness: Correlates with individual attributes and personality traits. *Play & Culture*, *4*, 371–393.

Barnett, L. A. (2007). The nature of playfulness in young adults. *Personality and Individual Differences*, *43*(4), 949–958.

Barton, E. E. (2010). Development of a taxonomy of pretend play for children with disabilities. *Infants & Young Children*, *23*(4), 247–261.

Barton EE. (2015). Teaching Generalized Pretend Play and Related Behaviors to Young Children With Disabilities. *Exceptional Children*. ;*81*(4):489–506. https://doi.org/10.1177/0014402914563694

Bateson, P. (2005). The role of play in the evolution of great apes and humans. In A. D. Pellegrini & P. K. Smith (Eds.), *The nature of play: Great apes and humans* (pp. 13–24). New York: Guilford Press.

Bazyk, S., Stalnaker, D., Llerena, M., Ekelman, B., & Bazyk, J. (2003). Play in Mayan children. *American Journal of Occupational Therapy*, *57*, 273–283.

Becker, J. (2019). *Why fewer toys will benefit your kids*. https://www.becomingminimalist.com/why-fewer-toys-will-actually-benefit-your-kids/.

Beckwith, J. (1998). *No more cookie cutter parks*. Viewpoint. Berkeley, CA: Berkeley Partners for Parks. http://bpfp.org/PlaygroundDesign/NoMoreCookieCutter.php

Bekker, T., Hopma, E., & Sturm, J. (2010). Creating opportunities for play: The influence of multimodal feedback on open-ended play. *International Journal of Arts and Technology*, 3(4), 325–340. https://doi.org/10.1504/IJART.2010.035825

Bekoff, M. (2002). *Minding animals*. London: Oxford University Press.

Belsky, J., & Most, R. K. (1981). From exploration to play: A cross-sectional study of infant free play behavior. *Developmental Psychology*, 17(5), 630–639. https://doi.org/10.1037/0012-1649.17.5.630

Benenson, J. F. (1993). Greater preference among females than males for dyadic interaction in early childhood. *Child Development*, 64, 544–555.

Benjamin, H. (1932). Age and sex differences in toy preferences of young children. *Journal of Genetic Psychology*, 41, 417–429.

Benson, J. D., Nicka, M. N., & Stern, P. (2006). How does a child with sensory processing problems play? *Internet Journal of Allied Health Sciences and Practice*, 4. Retrieved July 28, 2008, from http://ijahsp.nova.edu/articles/vol4num4/benson.pdf

Berlyne, D. E. (1960). *Conflict, arousal, and curiosity*. New York: McGraw-Hill.

Berriman, L., & Mascheroni, G. (2019). Exploring the affordances of smart toys and connected play in practice. *News Media & Society. Sage*. 21(4), 798. https://doi.org/10.1177/1461444818807119

Besio, S., Bulgarelli, D., & Stancheva-Popkostadinova, V. (2016). *Play development in children with disabilities*. Berlin: Walter de Gruyter.

Bjorklund, G., & Bjorklund, R. (1979). An exploratory study of toddlers' satisfaction with their toy environments. *NA - Advances in Consumer Research*, 6, 400–406.

Blumstein, D. T., Chung, L. K., & Smith, J. E. (2013). Early play may predict later dominance relationships in yellow-bellied marmots (Marmota flaviventris). *Proceedings of the Royal Society B: Biological Sciences*, 280(1759), 20130485.

Blurton Jones, N. G. (1978). An ethological study of some aspects of social behavior of children in nursery school. In D. Muller-Schwarze (Ed.), *Evolution of play behavior* (pp. 349–366). Stroudsburg, PA: Dowden, Hutchinson & Ross.

Boe, J. L., & Woods, R. J. (2018). Parents' influence on infants' gender-typed toy preferences. *Sex Roles*, 79, 358–373. https://doi.org/10.1007/s11199-017-0858-4

Bowers, L. (1990). Results of the survey. In S.C. Wortham & J. Frost (eds). Playgrounds for young children: National survey and perspectives. *American Alliance for Health, Recreation, & Dance*. Reston, VA. https://files.eric.ed.gov/fulltext/ED326492.pdf

Bradley, R. H., Corwyn, R. F., McAdoo, H. P., & García Coll, C. (2001). The home environments of children in the United States part I: Variations by age, ethnicity, and poverty status. *Child Development*, 72(6), 1844–1867. https://doi.org10.1111/1467-8624.t01-1-00382

Brockman, R., Jago, R., & Fox, K. R. (2011). Children's active play: Self-reported motivators, barriers and facilitators. *BMC Public Health*, 11(1), 461. https://doi.org/10.1186/1471-2458-11-461

Brown, F. (2007). Services for children: The Venture - A case study of an adventure playground. Pearson Publishing

Brown, W. H., Fox, J. J., & Brady, M. P. (1987). Effects of spatial density on 3-and 4-year-old children's socially directed behavior during freeplay: An investigation of a setting factor. *Education and Treatment of Children*, 10(3), 247–258.

Brownie, B. (2015). The masculinization of dressing-up. *Clothing Cultures*, 2(2), 145–155.

Bruner, J. S. (1982). The organization of action and the nature of adult–infant transaction. In M. Cranach & R. Harre (Eds.), *The analysis of action* (pp. 313–327). New York: Cambridge University Press.

Brunelle, S., Herrington, S., Coghlan, R., & Brussoni, M. (2016). Play worth remembering: Are playgrounds too safe?. *Children, Youth and Environments*, 26(1), 17–36. https://doi.org/10.7721/chilyoutenvi.26.1.0017

Brussoni, M., Olsen, L. L., Pike, I., & Sleet, D. A. (2012). Risky play and children's safety: Balancing priorities for optimal child development. *International Journal of Environmental Research and Public Health*, 9(9), 3134–3148.

Buhler, C. (1935). *From birth to maturity*. London: Kegan Paul, Trench, Trubner & Co., Ltd.

Bryant, M. (2011). What today's digital native children can teach the rest of us about technology. https://thenextweb.com/insider/2011/09/10/what-todays-digital-native-children-can-teach-the-rest-of-us-about-technology/

Bulgarelli, D., Bianquin, N., Besio, S., & Molina, P. (2018). Children with cerebral palsy playing with mainstream robotic toys: Playfulness and environmental supportiveness. *Frontiers in Psychology*, 9, 1814.

Bulotsky-Shearer, R. J., Manz, P. H., Mendez, J. L., McWayne, C. M., Sekino, Y., & Fantuzzo, J. W. (2012). Peer play interactions and readiness to learn: A protective influence for African American preschool children from low-income households. *Child Development Perspectives*, 6(3), 225–231. https://doi.org/10.1111/j.1750-8606.2011.00221.x

Bundy, A. C. (1989). A comparison of the play skills of normal boys and boys with sensory integrative dysfunction. *Occupational Therapy Journal of Research*, 9, 84–100.

Bundy, A. C. (1993). Assessment of play and leisure: Delineation of the problem. *American Journal of Occupational Therapy*, 47, 217–222.

Bundy, A. C. (1997). Play and playfulness: What to look for. In L. D. Parham & L. S. Fazio (Eds.), *Play in occupational therapy for children* (pp. 52–66). St. Louis, MO: Mosby.

Burghardt, G. M. (1984). On the origins of play. In P. K. Smith (Ed.), *Play in animals and humans* (pp. 5–41). New York: Basil Blackwell.

Burghardt, G. M. (2005). *The genesis of animal play: Testing the limits*. Cambridge, MA: MIT Press.

Burghardt, G. M. (2010). The comparative reach of play and brain: Perspective, evidence, and implications. *American Journal of Play*, 2(3), 338–356.

Burghardt, G. M. (2014). A brief glimpse at the long evolutionary history of play. *Animal Behavior and Cognition*, 1(2), 90–98.

Burghardt, G. M. (2015). Play in fishes, frogs and reptiles. *Current Biology*, 25(1), R9–R10.

Burke, C. (2005). "Play in focus": Children researching their own spaces and places for play. *Children, Youth, and Environments*, 15(1), 27–53. http://doi.org/10.7721/chilyoutenvi.15.1.0027.

Burke, J. P. (1977). A clinical perspective on motivation: pawn versus origin. *American Journal of Occupational Therapy*, 31(4), 254–258.

Byers, J. A. (1998). Biological effects of locomotor play: Getting into shape, or something more specific? In M. Bekoff & J. A. Byers (Eds.), *Animal play: Evolutionary, comparative, and ecological perspectives* (pp. 205–220). Cambridge University Press. https://doi.org/10.1017/CBO9780511608575.011

Cahill-Solis, T. L., & Witryol, S. L. (1994). Children's exploratory play preferences for four levels of novelty in toy constructions. *Genetic, Social, and General Psychology Monographs. 120*(4), 393–408.

Caldera, Y. M., Huston, A. C., & O'Brien, M. (1989). Social interactions and play patterns of parents and toddlers with feminine, masculine, and neutral toys. *Child Development, 60*(1), 70–76.

Caro, T. M. (1995). Short-term costs and correlates of play in cheetahs. *Animal Behaviour, 49*(2), 333–345.

Case-Smith, J., & Miller Kuhaneck, H. (2008). Play preferences of typically developing children and children with developmental delays between the ages of 3 and 7 years. *OTJR: Occupation, Participation and Health, 28,* 19–29.

Castonguay, G., & Jutras, S. (2009). Children's appreciation of outdoor places in a poor neighborhood. *Journal of Environmental Psychology, 29*(1), 101–109 https://doi.org/10.1016/j.jenvp.2008.05.002

Cavallo, D (1981). *Muscles and morals: organized playgrounds and urban reform, 1880–1920.* Philadelphia: University of Pennsylvania Press

Cherng, R. J., Chen, J. J., & Su, F. C. (2001). Vestibular system in performance of standing balance of children and young adults under altered sensory conditions. *Perceptual Motor Skills, 92,* 1167–1179.

Chew, T. (1985). The developmental progression of vestibular based playground play of preschool children. Unpublished master's thesis, University of Southern California, Los Angeles.

Chiarello, L. A., Bartlett, D. J., Palisano, R. J., McCoy, S. W., Jeffries, L., Fiss, A. L., & Wilk, P. (2019). Determinants of playfulness of young children with cerebral palsy. *Developmental Neurorehabilitation, 22*(4), 240–249.

Chick, G. (2010). Work, play, and learning. In D. F. Lancy, J. Bock, & S. Gaskins (Eds.), *The anthropology of learning in childhood* (p. 119–143). Lanham, MD: AltaMira Press.

Christensen, K. E., & Stockdale, D. F. (1991). Predictors of toy selection criteria of preschool children's parents. *Children's Environments Quarterly, 8*(1), 25–36.

Christie, A. (1999). A meaningful occupation: The just right challenge. *Australian Occupational Therapy Journal, 46*(2), 52–68.

Christie, J. F., & Johnsen, E. P. (1987). Reconceptualizing constructive play: A review of the empirical literature. *Merrill-Palmer Quarterly (1982–),* 439–452.

Christie, J. F., Johnsen, E. P., & Peckover, R. B. (1988). The effects of play period duration on children's play patterns. *Journal of Research in Childhood Education, 3*(2), 123–131.

Christie, J. F., & Wardle, F. (1992). How Much Time Is Needed for Play?. *Young Children, 47*(3), 28–33.

Cimpian, A., Mu, Y., & Erickson, L. C. (2012). Who is good at this game? Linking an activity to a social category undermines children's achievement. *Psychological Science, 23*(5), 533–541. https://doi. org/10.1177/0956797611429803.

Clifford, J. M., & Bundy, A. (1989). Play preference and play performance in normal boys and boys with sensory integrative dysfunction. *Occupational Therapy Journal of Research, 9,* 202–217.

Cloward Drown, K. (2014). Dramatic play affordances of natural and manufactured elements in outdoor settings for preschool-aged children. Graduate Research Symposium. Paper 19. https://digitalcommons.usu.edu/grs/19.

Cohen, E., & Gadassi, R. (2018). The function of play for coping and therapy with children exposed to disasters and political violence. *Current psychiatry reports, 20*(5), 1–7.

Cohen, D. A., Han, B., Williamson, S., Nagel, C., McKenzie, T. L., Evenson, K. R., & Harnik, P. (2020). Playground features and physical activity in US neighborhood parks. *Preventive Medicine, 131,* 105945.

Committee on Environmental Health. (2007). Global climate change and children's health. *Pediatrics, 120,* 1149–1152, https://doi.org/10.1542/peds.2007-2645

Common Sense Media (2014). Advertising to Children and Teens: Current Practices. San Francisco, CA: https://www.commonsensemedia.org/research/advertising-to-children-and-teens-current-practices.

Connor, J. M., & Serbin, L. A. (1977). Behaviorally based masculine and feminine activity preferences scales for preschoolers: Correlates with other classroom behaviors and cognitive tests. *Child Development, 48,* 1411–1416.

Coyne, S. M., Linder, J. R., Rasmussen, E. E., Nelson, D. A., & Birkbeck, V. (2016). Pretty as a princess: Longitudinal effects of engagement with Disney princesses on gender stereotypes, body esteem, and prosocial behavior in children. *Child Development, 87*(6), 1909–1925. https://doi.org/10.1111/cdev.12569

Crawford, S. (2009) The archaeology of play things: Theorising a toy stage in the "biography" of objects. *Childhood in the Past, 2*(1), 55–70. https://doi.org/10.1179/cip.2009.2.1.55

Crittenden, A. N. (2016). Children's foraging and play among the Hadza. *Origins and Implications of the Evolution of Childhood,* 155–172.

Cross, G. S. (1999). *Kids' stuff: Toys and the changing world of American childhood.* Harvard University Press.

Csikszentmihalyi, M. (1990). *Flow: The psychology of optimal experience.* New York: Harper & Row.

Cummings, H. M., & Vandewater, E. A. (2007). Relation of adolescent video game play to time spent in other activities. *Archives of Pediatric and Adolescent Medicine, 161,* 684–689.

Cunningham, C. J., & Jones, M. A. (1999). The playground: a confession of failure?. *Built Environment (1978-),* 11–17.

Czalczynska-Podolska, M. (2014). The impact of playground spatial features on children's play and activity forms: An evaluation of contemporary playgrounds' play and social value. *Journal of Environmental Psychology, 38,* 132–142. https://doi.org/10.1016/j.jenvp.2014.01.006

Danzig, C. (2012, July 17). Infographic of the day: American litigiousness statistics that will make you angry. Retrieved June 13, 2018, from https://abovethelaw.com/2012/07/infographic-of-the-day-american-litigiousness-statistics-that-will-make-you-angry/.

Davis, J. T., & Hines, M. (2020). How large are gender differences in toy preferences? A systematic review and meta-analysis of toy preference research. *Archives of Sexual Behavior, 49*(2), 373–394.

De Lisi, R., & Wolford, J. L. (2002). Improving children's mental rotation accuracy with computer game playing. *The Journal of Genetic Psychology, 163*(3), 272–282. https://doi.org/10.1080/00221320209598683

Desha, L., Ziviani, J., & Rodger, S. (2003). Play preferences and behavior of preschool children with autistic spectrum disorder in the clinical environment. *Physical and Occupational Therapy in Pediatrics, 23*(1), 21–42.

Dittmar, H., Halliwell, E., & Ive, S. (2006). Does Barbie make girls want to be thin? The effect of experimental exposure to images of dolls on the body image of 5- to 8-year-old girls. *Developmental Psychology*, 42(2), 283–292. https://doi.org/10.1037/0012-1649.42.2.283

Dodge, M. K., & Frost, J. L. (1986). Children's dramatic play: Influence of thematic and nonthematic settings. *Childhood Education*, 62(3), 166–170. https://doi.org/10.1080/00094056.1986.10520728

Dowdell, K., Gray, T., & Malone, K. (2011). Nature and its influence on children's outdoor play. *Journal of Outdoor and Environmental Education*, 15(2), 24. https://doi.org/10.1007/BF03400925

Dulles, F. R., & Dulles, F. R. (1965). history of recreation; America learns to play. https://archive.org/details/americalearnstop007872mbp

Dyment, J., & O'Connell, T. S. (2013). The impact of playground design on play choices and behaviors of pre-school children. *Children's Geographies*, 11(3), 263–280. https://doi.org/10.1080/14733285.2013.812272

Eberle, S. G. (2014). The elements of play: Toward a philosophy and a definition of play. *American Journal of Play*, 6(2), 214.

Eckert, J., Winkler, S. L., & Cartmill, E. A. (2020). Just kidding: The evolutionary roots of playful teasing. *Biology Letters*, 16(9), 20200370.

Edwards, A. (2018). Poverty rate drops for third consecutive year in 2017. Retrieved January 28, 2021, from https://www.census.gov/library/stories/2018/09/poverty-rate-drops-third-consecutive-year-2017

Edwards, C. P. (2005).Children's play in cross cultural perspective: A new look at the six culture study. In F. F. McMahon, D. E. Lytle, & B. Sutton-Smith (Eds.), *Play & culture studies: Volume 6. Play: An interdisciplinary synthesis* (Vol. 6, pp. 81–96). Lanham, MD: University Press of America.

Ember, C. R., & Cunnar, C. M. (2015). Children's play and work: The relevance of cross-cultural ethnographic research for archaeologists. *Childhood in the Past*, 8(2), 87–103.

Ergler, C. R., Kearns, R. A., & Witten, K. (2013). Seasonal and locational variations in children's play: Implications for wellbeing. *Social Science & Medicine*, 91, 178–185. https://doi.org/10.1016/j.socscimed.2012.11.034

Ernst, K., Ekkelboom, M., Kerssen, N., Smeets, S., Sun, Y., & Yin, X. (2018). Play behavior and environmental enrichment in pigs. *WUR*, 1–59. https://edepot.wur.nl/507108

Erikson, E. H. (1950). *Childhood and society*. New York: W. W. Norton & Co.

Espinoza, A., McMahan, S., Naffzinger, T., & Wiersma, L. D. (2012). Creating Playgrounds, Where Playgrounds Do Not Exist. *Californian Journal of Health Promotion*, 10(SI-Obesity), 13–19. https://doi.org/10.32398/cjhp.v10iSI-Obesity.1466

Fagan, R. (1984). Play and behavioral flexibility. In P. K. Smith (Ed.), *Play in animals and humans* (pp. 159–174). New York: Basil Blackwell.

Fagen, R., & Fagen, J. (2009). Play behaviour and multi-year juvenile survival in free-ranging brown bears, *Ursus arctos*. *Evolutionary Ecology Research*, 11(7), 1053–1067.

Fallon, M. A., & Harris, M. B. (1989). Factors influencing the selection of toys for handicapped and normally developing preschool children. *The Journal of Genetic Psychology*, 150(2), 125–134. https://doi.org/10.1080/00221325.1989.9914584

Fein, G. G. (1981). Pretend play in childhood and integrative review. *Child Development*, 52, 1095–1118.

Ferguson, A. (2019). Playing out: A grassroots street play revolution. *Cities & Health*, 3(1-2), 20–28. https://doi.org/10.1080/23748834.2018.1550850

Ferland, F. (2005). *The Ludic model: Play, children with physical disabilities and occupational therapy* (2nd ed.). Ottawa, Ontario: Canadian Association of Occupational Therapists.

Fernelius, C. L., & Christensen, K. M. (2017). Systematic review of evidence-based practices for inclusive playground design. *Children, Youth and Environments*, 27(3), 78–102. https://doi.org/10.7721/chilyoutenvi.27.3.0078

Ferrara, C., & Hill, S. D. (1980). The responsiveness of autistic children to the predictability of social and nonsocial toys. *Journal of Autism and Developmental Disorders*, 10, 51–57.

Field Agent. (2018). All things toys. https://info.fieldagent.net/all-things-toys-download

Fjørtoft, I. (2004). Landscape as playscape: The effects of natural environments on children's play and motor development. *Children Youth and Environments*, 14(2), 21–44. http://www.colorado.edu/journals/cye/.

Freud, S. (1955). *The interpretation of dreams*. New York: Perseus Books. https://www.researchgate.net/file.PostFileLoader.html?id=5624b63c614325ab3f8b4595&assetKey=AS:286198816886793@1445246523980

Freitas, T. C., Gabbard, C., Caçola, P., Montebelo, M. I., & Santos, D. C. (2013). Family socioeconomic status and the provision of motor affordances in the home. *Brazilian journal of physical therapy*, 17, 319–327.

Frost, J. L. (2010). *A history of children's play and play environments: Toward a contemporary child-saving movement*. Routledge.

Frost, J. L. (2007). Special feature: The changing culture of childhood: A perfect storm. *Childhood Education*, 83(4), 225–230.

Frost, J. (2006). The dissolution of children's outdoor play: Causes and consequences. Glenn, Knight, Holt, & Spence.

Frost, J. L. (1978). The american playground movement. *Childhood Education*, 54(4), 176–182. https://doi.org/10.1080/00094056.1978.10729698

Fry, D. (2005). Rough and tumble social play in humans. In A. D. Pellegrini & P. K. Smith (Eds.), *The nature of play: Great apes and humans* (pp. 54–85). New York: Guilford Press.

Furby, L., & Wilke, M. (1982). Some characteristics of infants preferred toys. *Journal of Genetic Psychology*, 140(2d Half), 207–210.

Gardner, M. P., Golinkoff, R. M., Hirsh-Pasek, K., & Heiney-Gonzalez, D. (2012). Marketing toys without playing around. *Young Consumers Insight and Ideas for Responsible Marketers*, 13(4), https://doi.org/10.1108/17473611211282626

Garner, B. P., & Bergen, D. (2006). Play development from birth to age four. In D. P. Fromberg & D. Bergen (Eds.), *Play from birth to twelve: Contexts, perspectives and meanings* (2nd ed., pp. 3–12). New York: Routledge.

Garvey, C. (1990). *Play*. Cambridge, MA: Harvard University Press.

Garzotto, F., Gelsomini, M., Occhiuto, D., Matarazzo, V., & Messina, N. (2017, June). Wearable immersive virtual reality for children with disability: A case study. In *Proceedings of the 2017 Conference on Interaction Design and Children* (pp. 478–483). New York: Association for Computing Machinery.

Gaskins, S., Haight, W., & Lancy, D. F. (2007). The cultural construction of play. *Play and Development: Evolutionary, Sociocultural, and Functional Perspectives*, 179202.

Gaylard A. (1966). Treatment of Children with Perceptual Problems: An Introduction to the Role of the Occupational Therapist. *Canadian Journal of Occupational Therapy.* ;33(2):53–61. https://doi.org/10.1177/000841746603300202

Gelman, S. A., & Davidson, N. S. (2016). Young children's preference for unique owned objects. *Cognition, 155,* 146–154.

Gerson, S. A., Meyer, M., Hunnius, S., & Bekkering, H. (2017). Unravelling the contributions of motor experience and conceptual knowledge in action perception: A training study. *Scientific reports, 7*(1), 1–10.

Getz, S. K., & Berndt, E. G. (1982). A test of a method for quantifying amount, complexity, and arrangement of play resources in the preschool classroom. *Journal of Applied Developmental Psychology, 3*(4), 295–305.

Giddings, M., & Halverson, C. F. (1981). Young children's use of toys in home environments. *Family Relations, 30*(1), 69–74. https://doi.org/10.2307/584238

Ginsburg, K. R. American Academy of Pediatrics Committee on Communications; American Academy of Pediatrics Committee on Psychosocial Aspects of Child and Family Health. (2007). The importance of play in promoting healthy child development and maintaining strong parent-child bonds. *Pediatrics, 119*(1), 182–191. https://doi.org/10.1542/peds.2006-2697.

Glassner, B. (1976). Kid society. *Urban Education, 11*(1), 5–22.

Glenn, N. M., Knight, C. J., Holt, N. L., & Spence, J. C. (2013). Meanings of play among children. *Childhood, 20*(2), 185–199.

Glynn, M. A. (1994). Effects of work task cues and play task cues on information processing, judgment, and motivation. *Journal of Applied Psychology, 79,* 34–45.

Goldstein, J. (1995). Aggressive toy play. In A. D. Pellegrini (Ed.), *The future of play theory* (pp. 127–147). Albany: State University of New York Press.

Gomes, J., & Martin-Andrade, B. (2005). Fantasy play in apes. In A. D. Pellegrini & P. K. Smith (Eds.), *The nature of play: Great apes and humans* (pp. 139–172). New York: Guilford Press.

Goodhall, N., & Atkinson, C. (2017). How do children distinguish between "play" and "work"? Conclusions from the literature. *Early Child Development and Care, 189*(10), 1695–1708.

Goodman, J. F. (1994). "Work" versus "play" and early childhood care. *In Child and Youth Care Forum, 23*(3), 177–196.

Gordon, W. R., & Caltabiano, M. L. (1996). Urban–rural differences in adolescent self-esteem, leisure boredom, and sensation-seeking as predictors of leisure-time usage and satisfaction. *Adolescence.* Retrieved July 21, 2008, from http://findarticles.com/p/articles/mi_m2248/is_n124_v31/ai_19226145

Gosso, Y., Otta, E., DeLima, M., Morais, S. E., Ribeiro, F. J. L., & Bussab, V. S. R. (2005). Play in hunter-gatherer society. In A. D. Pellegrini & P. K. Smith (Eds.), *The nature of play: Great apes and humans* (pp. 213–253). New York: Guilford Press.

Gowen, J. W., Johnson-Martin, N., Goldman, B. D., & Hussey, B. (1992). Object play and exploration in children with and without disabilities: A longitudinal study. *American Journal on Mental Retardation, 97,* 21–38.

Gray, P. (2013). *Free to learn: Why unleashing the instinct to play will make our children happier, more self-reliant, and better students for life.* Basic Books/Hachette Book Group.

Gray, P. (2009). Play as the foundation for hunter-gatherer social existence. *American Journal of Play, 1*(4), 476–522.

Groos, K. (1901). *The play of man.* New York: Appleton.

Gülgöz, S., Glazier, J. J., Enright, E. A., Alonso, D. J., Durwood, L. J., Fast, A. A., Lowe, R., Ji, C., Heer, J., Martin, C. M., & Olson, K. R. (2019). Similarity in transgender and cisgender children's gender development. *PNAS, 115*(49), 24480–24485. https://doi.org/10.1073/pnas.1909367116; https://depts.washington.edu/scdlab/all-publications/publications-by-year/

Gunnar-Vongnechten, M. R. (1978). Changing a frightening toy into a pleasant toy by allowing the infant to control its actions. *Developmental Psychology, 14*(2), 157.

Gunnels, J. (2009). "A Jedi like my father before me": Social identity and the New York Comic Con. *Transformative Works and Cultures, 3*(3).

Halim, M. L., Ruble, D., Tamis-LeMonda, C., & Shrout, P. E. (2013). Rigidity in gender-typed behaviors in early childhood: A longitudinal study of ethnic minority children. *Child Development, 84*(4), 1269–1284. https://doi.org/10.1111/cdev.12057.

Hall, G. S. (1882). Moral and religious training of children. *Princeton Review, 9,* 26–48.

Hall, S. I. (1998). Object play by adult animals. In M. Bekoff & J. A. Byers (Eds.), *Animal play: Evolutionary, comparative, and ecological perspectives* (pp. 45–60). New York: Cambridge University Press.

Hanway, S., & Motabar, L. (2016). Injuries and investigated deaths associated with playground equipment 2009–2014. Consumer Product Safety Commission Report. https://www.cpsc.gov/Research-Statistics/sports-recreation/playgrounds

Harcourt, R. (1991). Survivorship costs of play in the South American fur seal. *Animal Behaviour, 42*(3), 509–511.

Harkness, L., & Bundy, A. C. (2001). Playfulness and children with physical disabilities. *Occupational Therapy Journal of Research, 21,* 73–89.

Harms, C. (2018). How many toys do kids really need? https://www.todaysparent.com/family/parenting/how-many-toys-do-kids-really-need/

Harrison, F., Goodman, A., van Sluijs, E. M., Andersen, L. B., Cardon, G., Davey, R., ... & Pate, R. (2017). Weather and children's physical activity; How and why do relationships vary between countries?. *International Journal of Behavioral Nutrition and Physical Activity, 14*(1), 74. https://doi.org/10.1186/s12966-017-0526-7

Harrison, F., Jones, A. P., Bentham, G., van Sluijs, E. M., Cassidy, A., & Griffin, S. J. (2011). The impact of rainfall and school break time policies on physical activity in 9-10 year old British children: A repeated measures study. *International Journal of Behavioral Nutrition and Physical Activity, 8*(1), 47. https://doi.org/10.1186/1479-5868-8-47

Hart, C. H., & Sheehan, R. (1986). Preschoolers' play behavior in outdoor environments: Effects of traditional and contemporary playgrounds. *American Educational Research Journal, 23*(4), 668–678. https://doi.org/10.2307/1163097

Hartup, W. W. (1983). Peer relations. In P. H. Mussen (Ed.), *Handbook of child psychology* (4th ed., pp. 103–196). New York: Wiley.

Hassett, J. M., Siebert, E. R., & Wallen, K. (2008). Sex differences in rhesus monkey toy preferences parallel those of children. *Hormones and Behavior, 54,* 359–364

Heah, T., Case, T., McGuire, B., & Law, M. (2007). Successful participation: The lived experience among children with disabilities. *Canadian Journal of Occupational Therapy, 74*(1), 38–47.

Healey, A., & Mendelsohn, A. (2019). Selecting appropriate toys for young children in the digital era. *Pediatrics, 143*(1), 1–10. https://doi.org/10.1542/peds.2018-3348

Heinrich, B., & Smolker, R. (1998). Play in common ravens. In M. Bekoff & J. A. Byers (Eds.), *Animal play: Evolutionary, comparative, and ecological perspectives* (pp. 27–44). New York: Cambridge University Press.

Heintz, M. R., Murray, C. M., Markham, A. C., Pusey, A. E., & Lonsdorf, E. V. (2017). The relationship between social play and developmental milestones in wild chimpanzees (Pantroglodytes schweinfurthii). *American Journal of Primatology, 79*(12), e22716.

Hektner, J. M., & Csikszentmihalyi, M. (1996, April). A longitudinal exploration of flow and intrinsic motivation in adolescents. Paper presented at the annual meeting of the American Educational Research Association, New York, NY. Retrieved July 21, 2008, from http://eric.ed.gov/ERICDocs/data/ericdocs2sql/content_storage_01/0000019b/80/14/84/e3.pdf

Heljakka, K. I. (2018). More than collectors: Exploring theorists', hobbyists' and everyday players' rhetoric in adult play with character toys. *Games and Culture, 13*(3), 240–259.

Heljakka, K., Harviainen, J. T., & Suominen, J. (2018). Stigma avoidance through visual contextualization: Adult toy play on photo-sharing social media. *New Media & Society, 20*(8), 2781–2799.

Hémar-Nicolas, V., & Rodhain, A. (2017). Brands as cultural resources in children's peer culture, *Consumption Markets & Culture, 20*(3), 193– 214, https://doi.org/10.1080/10253866.2016.1205494

Henderson, B. B. (1981). Exploration by preschool children: Peer interaction and individual differences. *Merrill-Palmer Quarterly of Behavior and Development*, 241–255.

Henderson, B., & Moore, S. G. (1980). Children's responses to objects differing in novelty in relation to level of curiosity and adult behavior. *Child Development, 51*(2), 457–465. https://doi.org/10.2307/1129279

Henricks, T. S. (2015). Play as experience. *American Journal of Play, 8*(1), 18–49.

Herrington, S., & Brussoni, M. (2015). Beyond physical activity: The importance of play and nature-based play spaces for children's health and development. *Current Obesity Reports, 4*(4), 477–483. https://doi.org/10.1007/s13679-015-0179-2

Hewlett, B. S. (2017). *Hunter-gatherer childhoods: Evolutionary, developmental, and cultural perspectives*. New York: Routledge.

Hill, H. M., Dietrich, S., & Cappiello, B. (2017). Learning to play: A review and theoretical investigation of the developmental mechanisms and functions of cetacean play. *Learning & Behavior, 45*(4), 335–354.

Hines, M. (2004). *Brain gender*. London: Oxford University Press.

Hinojosa, J. (1994). The Just Right Challenge. *Work, 4*(4), 253–258.

Hol, T., Van den Berg, C. L., Van Ree, J. M., & Spruijt, B. M. (1999). Isolation during the play period in infancy decreases adult social interactions in rats. *Behavioral Brain Research, 100*, 91–97.

Holmes, R. M. (1999). Kindergarten and college students' views of play and work at home and school. In S. Reifel (Ed.), *Play & culture studies: Volume 2. Play contexts revisited* (pp. 59–72). Stamford, CT: Ablex. https://www.legofoundation.com/en/why-play/

Hong, J., & Lee, W. (2019). The use of interactive toys in children's pretend play: An experience prototyping approach. *Archives of Design Research, 32*(3), 35–47. https://doi.org/10.15187/adr.2019.08.32.3.35

Howe, N., & Hogan, C. (2001). Do props matter in the dramatic play center? The effects of prop realism on children's play. *The Canadian Journal of Infancy and Early Childhood, 8*(4), 51.

Hu, C. (2015). Photos: The games children play in war zones. https://qz.com/385446/photos-the-games-children-play-in-war-zones/

Huizinga, J. (1950). *Homo ludens*. Boston: Beacon Press.

Humphreys, A., & Smith, P. K. (1987). Rough and tumble play, friendship and dominance in school children: Evidence for continuity and change with age. *Child Development, 58*, 201–212.

Hunter, M. A., Ross, H. S., & Ames, E. W. (1982). Preferences for familiar or novel toys: Effect of familiarization time in 1-year-olds. *Developmental Psychology, 18*(4), 519. https://doi.org/10.1037/0012-1649.18.4.519

Huston, A. C. (1983). Sex-typing. In E. M. Hetherington (Ed.), *Handbook of child psychology: Socialization, personality, and social development* (Vol. 4, pp. 388–467). New York: Wiley.

Hutt, C. (1966). Exploration and play in children. In P. A. Jewell & C. Loizos (Eds.), *Play, exploration and territory in mammals* (pp. 61–80). New York: Academic Press.

Hyndman, B. P., Chancellor, B., & Lester, L. (2015). Exploring the seasonal influences on elementary schoolchildren's enjoyment of physical activity during school breaks. *Health Behavior and Policy Review, 2*(3), 182–193.

Ibrahim, H. (1989). *Pioneers in Leisure and Recreation*. AAHPERD Publications, Inc., PO Box 704, Waldorf, MD 20604. https://files.eric.ed.gov/fulltext/ED308157.pdf

Ikeda, H., Komaba, M., Komaba, K., Matsuya, A., Kawakubo, A., & Nakahara, F. (2018). Social objects play between captive bottlenose and Risso's dolphins. *PLoS One, 13*(5), e0196658.

Ihmeideh, F. (2019). Getting parents involved in children's play: Qatari parents' perceptions of and engagement with their children's play. *Education 3-13, 47*(1), 47–63.

Ito, M. (2005). Technologies of the childhood imagination: Yu-Gi-Oh, media mixes, and everyday cultural production. In J. Karaganis and N. Jeremijenko (Eds.), *Network/netplay: Structures of participation in digital culture*. Durham, NC: Duke University Press. http://www.itofisher.com/mito/archives/technoimagination.pdf

Ivory, J. J., & McCollum, J. A. (1999). Effects of social and isolate toys on social play in an inclusive setting. *Journal of Special Education, 32*, 238–243. https://doi.org/10.1177/002246699903200404

Jacobs, K. (1994). Flow and the occupational therapy practitioner. *American Journal of Occupational Therapy, 48*(11), 989–996.

Jansson, M. (2008). Children's Perspectives on Public Playgrounds in Two Swedish Communities. *Children Youth and Environments, 18*(2), 88–109.

Jenkins, N. (2006). 'You can't wrap them up in cotton wool!' Constructing risk in young people's access to outdoor play. *Health, Risk & Society, 8*(4), 379–393. https://doi.org/10.1080/13698570601008289

Jenvey, V. (2013). Play and disability. *Encyclopedia on Early Childhood Development*.

Jirout, J. J., & Newcombe, N. S. (2015). Building blocks for developing spatial skills: Evidence from a large, representative U.S. sample. *Psychological Science, 26*(3), 302–310. https://doi.org/10.1177/0956797614563338

Jongeneel, D., Withagen, R., & Zaal, F. T. J. M. (2015). Do children create standardized playgrounds? A study on the gap-crossing affordances of jumping stones. *Journal of Environmental Psychology*, *44*, 45–52. https://doi.org/10.1016/j.jenvp.2015.09.003

Johnson, J.E. (2015). Play Development from Ages Four to Eight Years. In *Play from birth to twelve*, 21–29.

Jones, M. A. (2017). Effect of sex and body mass index on children's physical activity intensity during free play at an indoor soft play center: An exploratory study. *International Journal of Environmental Research and Public Health*, *14*(9), 1052. https://doi.org/10.3390/ijerph14091052

Jonsson, C. O., Reimbladh-Taube, G., & Sjöswärd, E. (1993). Forms, uses and functions of children's favourite objects. *Scandinavian Journal of Psychology*, *34*(1), 86–93.

Kafai, Y. B. (1998). Video game designs by girls and boys: Variability and consistency of gender differences. In J. Cassell & H. Jenkins (Eds.), *From Barbie to Mortal Kombat: Gender and computer games* (pp. 90–114). Cambridge, MA: MIT Press.

Kafai, Y. B., & Fields, D. (2013). *Connected Play: Tweens in a Virtual World*. MIT Press.

Kantrowitz, E. J., & Evans, G. W. (2004). The relation between the ratio of children per activity area and off-task behavior and type of play in day care centers. *Environment and Behavior*, *36*(4), 541–557. https://doi.org/10.1177/0013916503255613

Karsten, L. (2005). It all used to be better? Different generations on continuity and change in urban children's daily use of space. *Children's Geographies*, *3*(3), 275–290. https://doi.org/10.1080/14733280500352912

Kavousipor, S. (2019). Which aspects of child development are related to the home environment?: A narrative review. *Journal of Rehabilitation Sciences & Research*, *6*(1), 1–5. https://doi.org/10.30476/jrsr.2019.44716

Kavousipor, S., Golipour, F., & Hekmatnia, M. (2016). Relationship between a child's cognitive skills and the inclusion of age appropriate toys in the home environment. *Journal of Rehabilitation Sciences & Research*, *3*(4), 103–108. https://doi.org/10.30476/jrsr.2016.41108

Kemple, K. M., Oh, J., Kenney, E., & Smith-Bonahue, T. (2016). The power of outdoor play and play in natural environments. *Childhood Education*, *92*(6), 446–454. https://doi.org/10.1080/00094056.2016.1251793

Kiliańska-Przybyłoa, G., & Górkiewiczb, B. (2017). No toy, no joy?–Some reflections on the potential of toy-free week to promote children's creativity and active learning. *Journal of Early Childhood Education Research*, *6*(1), 136–147.

Killen, M., & Stangor, C. (2001). Children's social reasoning about inclusion and exclusion in gender and race peer group contexts. *Child Development*, *72*(1), 174–186. https://doi.org/10.1111/1467-8624. 00272

Kimelstein, J. (2019), Gender as an occupation: The role of OT in the transgender community. *Ithaca College Theses*, 424.

Kleppe R. (2018). Affordances for 1- to 3-year-olds' risky play in Early Childhood Education and Care. *Journal of Early Childhood Research*. 16(3):258–275. https://doi.org/10.1177/1476718X18762237

Kneeshaw-Price, S., Saelens, B. E., Sallis J. F., et al. (2013). Children's objective physical activity by location: Why the neighborhood matters. *Pediatric Exercise Science*, *25*(3), 468–86. https://doi.org/10.1123/pes.25.3.468

Konner, M. (2016). Hunter-gatherer infancy and childhood in the context of human evolution. In C. L. Meehan & A. N. Crittenden (Eds.), *Childhood: Origins, evolution, and implications* (pp. 123–154). Santa Fe, NM: School for Advanced Research Press.

Kuba, M. J., Byrne, R. A., Meisel, D. V., & Mather, J. A. (2006). When do octopuses play? Effects of repeated testing, object type, age, and food deprivation on object play in Octopus vulgaris. *Journal of Comparative Psychology*, *120*(3), 184–190.

Kudrowitz, B. M., & Wallace, D. R. (2010). The play pyramid: A play classification and ideation tool for toy design. *International Journal of Arts and Technology (IJART)*, *3*(1).

Kuehl, H. S., Elzner, C., Moebius, Y., Boesch, C., & Walsh, P. D. (2008). The price of play: Self-organized infant mortality cycles in chimpanzees. *PLoS One*, *3*(6), e2440.

Kuhaneck, H., Spitzer, S., & Miller, E. (2010). *Activity analysis, creativity and playfulness in pediatric occupational therapy: Making play just right*. Burlington, MA: Jones & Bartlett Learning.

Lai, C. H., & Chan, Y. S. (2002). Development of the vestibular system. *Neuroembryology*, *1*, 61–71.

LaForett, D. R., & Mendez, J. L. (2017). Play beliefs and responsive parenting among low-income mothers of preschoolers in the United States. *Early Child Development and Care*, *187*(8), 1359–1371. https://doi.org/10.1080/03004430.2016.1169180

Lambert, A., Vlaar, J., Herrington, S., & Brussoni, M. (2019). What is the relationship between the neighbourhood built environment and time spent in outdoor play? A systematic review. *International Journal of Environmental Research and Public Health*, *16*(20). https://doi.org/10.3390/ijerph16203840

Lancy, D. F. (1996). *Playing on the mother-ground: Cultural routines for children's development*. New York: Guilford Press.

Le-Phuong Nguyen, K., Harman, V., & Cappellini, B. (2017). Playing with class: Middle-class intensive mothering and the consumption of children's toys in Vietnam. *International Journal of Consumer Studies*, *41*(5), 449–456.

Lee, Y. C., Chan, P. C., Lin, S. K., Chen, C. T., Huang, C. Y., & Chen, K. L. (2016). Correlation patterns between pretend play and playfulness in children with autism spectrum disorder, developmental delay, and typical development. *Research in Autism Spectrum Disorders*, *24*, 29–38.

Legendre, A. (2003). Environmental features influencing toddlers' bioemotional reactions in day care centers. *Environment and Behavior*, *35*(4), 523–549. https://doi.org/10.1177/0013916503035004005

Legendre, A. (1999). Interindividual relationships in groups of young children and susceptibility to an environmental constraint. *Environment and Behavior*, *31*(4), 463–486.

Legendre, A., & Fontaine, A. M. (1991). The effects of visual boundaries in two-year-olds' playrooms. *Children's Environments Quarterly*, 2–16.

LEGO Foundation. (2017). *What we mean by learning through play*. https://www.legofoundation.com/media/1062/learningthroughplay_leaflet_june2017.pdf

Lego Foundation. (2018a). *Types of play*. Retrieved August 17, 2020, from https://www.legofoundation.com/en/learn-how/types-of-play/

Lego Foundation. (2018b). *Why play*. Retrieved March 28, 2020, from https://www.legofoundation.com/en/why-play/

Lego Foundation. (2018c). Characteristics of playful experiences. Retrieved October 30, 2021 from https://www.legofoundation .com/en/why-play/characteristics-of-playful-experiences/

Leipold, E., & Bundy, A. C. (2000). Playfulness and children with ADHD. *Occupational Therapy Journal of Research, 20,* 61–79.

Lewis, K. P. (2005). Social play in the great apes. In A. D. Pellegrini & P. K. Smith (Eds.), *The nature of play: Great apes and humans* (pp. 27–53). New York: Guilford Press.

Li, R. H., & Wong, W. I. (2016). Gender-typed play and social abilities in boys and girls: Are they related? *Sex Roles, 74*(9–10), 399–410. https://doi.org/10.1007/s11199-016 -0580-7

Lieberman, J. N. (1965). Playfulness and divergent thinking: Investigation of their relationship at the kindergarten level. *Journal of Genetic Psychology, 107,* 219–224.

Lieberman, J. N. (1966). Playfulness: An attempt to conceptualize a quality of play and of the player. *Psychological Reports, 19,* 1278.

Lillard, A. S., & Taggart, J. (2019). Pretend play and fantasy: What if Montessori was right?. *Child Development Perspectives, 13*(2), 85–90.

Lindquist, J. E., Mack, W., & Parham, L. D. (1982). A synthesis of occupational behavior and sensory integration concepts in theory and practice, Part 2: Clinical applications. *American Journal of Occupational Therapy, 36*(7), 433–437.

Little, H., & Stapleton, M. (2021). Exploring toddlers' rituals of "belonging" through risky play in the outdoor environment. *Contemporary Issues in Early Childhood,* 1463949120987656.

Luchs, A., & Fikus, M. (2013). A comparative study of active play on differently designed playgrounds. *J Adv Educ Outdoor Learn 13*(3), 206–222. https://doi.org/10.1080/14729679.2013.778784

Lyn, H., Greenfield, P., & Savage-Rumbaugh, S. (2006). The development of representational play in chimpanzees and bonobos: Evolutionary implications, pretense, and the role of interspecies communication. *Cognitive Development, 21*(3), 199–213. https://doi.org/10.1016/j.cogdev.2006.03.005

Lyytinen, P., Laakso, M. L., Poikkeus, A. M., & Rita, N. (1999). The development and predictive relations of play and language across the second year. *Scandinavian Journal of Psychology, 40,* 177–186.

Maccoby, E. E., & Jacklin, C. N. (1987). Gender segregation in childhood. *Advances in Child Development and Behavior, 20,* 239–287. https://doi.org/10.1016/S0065-2407(08)60404-8.

Mahidin, A. M. M., & Maulan, S. (2012). Understanding children preferences of natural environment as a start for environmental sustainability. *Procedia-Social and Behavioral Sciences, 38,* 324–333. 10.1016/j.sbspro.2012.03.354

Mahony, L., Hyndman, B., Nutton, G., Smith, S., & Te Ava, A. (2017). Monkey bars, noodles and hay bales: a comparative analysis of social interaction in two school ground contexts. *International Journal of Play, 6*(2), 166–176. https://doi.org/10 .1080/21594937.2017.1348319

Maier, K. (2019). Kids at heart? Exploring the material cultures of adult fans of all-ages animated shows. *The Journal of Popular Television, 7*(2), 235–254.

Malhi, P., Menon, J., Bharti, B., & Sidhu, M. (2018). Cognitive development of toddlers: Does parental stimulation matter?. *The Indian Journal of Pediatrics, 85*(7), 498–503. https://doi .org/10.1007/s12098-018-2613-4

Mann, T. (1975). The child at play. *Proceedings of the Royal Society of Medicine, 68,* 39–42. https://journals.sagepub.com/doi/abs /10.1177/003591577506800120

Marks, K. A., Vizconde, D. L., Gibson, E. S., Rodriguez, J. R., & Nunes, S. (2017). Play behavior and responses to novel situations in juvenile ground squirrels. *Journal of Mammalogy, 98*(4), 1202–1210.

Matsuzawa, T. (2020). Pretense in chimpanzees. *Primates, 61,* 543–555.

Matthews, S. (1985). Adventure Playgrounds vs Traditional Playgrounds. https://digitalcommons.unf.edu/etd/55/

Maxwell, L. E. (2003). Home and school density effects on elementary school children: The role of spatial density. *Environment and Behavior, 35*(4), 566–578. https://doi.org /10.1177/0013916503035004007

Maxwell, L. E. (1996). Multiple effects of home and day care crowding. *Environment and Behavior, 28*(4), 494–511. https://doi .org/10.1177/0013916596284004

McKendrick, J. H., Bradford, M. G., & Fielder, A. V. (2000a). Kid customer? Commercialization of playspace and the commodification of childhood. *Childhood, 7*(3), 295–314. https://doi.org/10.1177/0907568200007003004

McKendrick, J. H., Bradford, M. G., & Fielder, A. V. (2000b). Making sense of the commercialization of leisure space for children. *Children's Geographies: Playing, Living, Learning, 8,* 86. http://www.tandfebooks.com/isbn/9780203017524

McKenzie, T. L., Moody, J. S., Carlson, J. A., Lopez, N. V., & Elder, J. P. (2013). Neighborhood income matters: Disparities in community recreation facilities, amenities, and programs. *Journal of park and recreation administration, 31*(4), 12.

McLoyd, V. C., & Ratner, H. H. (1983). The effects of sex and toy characteristics on exploration in preschool children. *The Journal of Genetic Psychology, 142*(2), 213–224.

Mellou, E. (1994). Play theories: A contemporary review. *Early child development and care, 102*(1), 91–100.

Mertala, P., Karikoski, H., Tähtinen, L., & Sarenius, V. M. (2016). The value of toys: 6–8-year-old children's toy preferences and the functional analysis of popular toys. *International Journal of Play, 5*(1), 11–27.

Meyer-Bahlburg, H. F. L., Dolezal, C., Baker, S. W., Carlson, A. D., Obeid, J. S., & New, M. I. (2004). Prenatal androgenization affects gender-related behavior but not gender identity in 5–12-year-old girls with congenital adrenal hyperplasia. *Archives of Sexual Behavior, 33*(2), 97–104. https://doi .org/10.1023/B:ASEB.0000014324.25718.51

Michelman, S. S. (1974). Play and the deficit child. In M. Reilly (Ed.), *Play as exploratory learning: Studies of curiosity behaviour* (pp. 157–207). Beverly Hills, CA: Sage Publications.

Miller, C. C. (2015). Class differences in child-rearing are on the rise. *The New York Times.* https://www.nytimes .com/2015/12/18/upshot/rich-children-and-poor-ones-are -raised-very-differently.html

Miller, J. L., Lossia, A., Suarez-Rivera, C., & Gros-Louis, J. (2017). Toys that squeak: Toy type impacts quality and quantity of parent–child interactions. *First Language, 37*(6), 630–647. https://doi.org/10.1177/0142723717714947

Miller, C. F., Trautner, H. M., & Ruble, D. N. (2006). The role of gender stereotypes in children's preferences and behavior. In L. Balter & C. S. Tamis-LeMonda (Eds.), *Child psychology:*

A handbook of contemporary issues (pp. 293–323). New York: Psychology Press.

Miller, E., & Kuhaneck, H. (2008). Children's perceptions of play experiences and play preferences: A qualitative study. *American Journal of Occupational Therapy*, 62, 407–415.

Moore, G.T. (1986). "Effects of the Spatial Definition of Behavior Settings on Children's Behavior: A Quasi-Experimental Field Study." *Journal of Environmental Psychology*, 6, 205–231.

Moore, G. T., & Sugiyama, T. (2007). The children's physical environment rating scale (CP ERS): Reliability and validity for assessing the physical environment of early childhood educational facilities. *Children Youth and Environments*, 17(4), 24–53.

Munsell, F. (2018). Some Innovative Playground Design Trends and Fundraising Resources. https://www.nrpa.org/parks-recreation -magazine/2018/february/some-innovative-playground-design -trends-and-fundraising-resources/

Murray, J., & Devecchi, C. (2016). The Hantown street play project. *International Journal of Play*, 5(2), 196–211. https://doi .org/10.1080/21594937.2016.1203662

Muys, V., Rodger, S., & Bundy, A. C. (2006). Assessment of playfulness in children with autistic disorder: A comparison of the Children's Playfulness Scale and the Test of Playfulness. *OTJR: Occupation, Participation, & Health*, 26, 159–170.

National Institute for Play. (n.d.). Patterns of play. http://www .nifplay.org/science/pattern-play/

National Recreation and Parks Association. (n.d.). Parks and recreation in underserved areas: A public health perspective. https://www.nrpa.org/uploadedFiles/nrpa.org/Publications _and_Research/Research/Papers/Parks-Rec-Underserved -Areas.pdf

National Recreation and Parks Association. (2018). Americans engagement with parks report. https://www.nrpa.org/global assets/engagement-survey-report-2018.pdf

Neale, D., Clackson, K., Georgieva, S., Dedetas, H., Scarpate, M., Wass, S., & Leong, V. (2018). Toward a neuroscientific understanding of play: A dimensional coding framework for analyzing infant–adult play patterns. *Frontiers in Psychology*, 9, 273.

New York City Department of Parks & Recreation. (n.d.) History of Playgrounds in Parks. https://www.nycgovparks.org/about/history /playgrounds

Nogueira, S. S. C., Soledade, J. P., Pompéia, S., & Nogueira-Filho, S. L. G. (2011). The effect of environmental enrichment on play behaviour in white-lipped peccaries (Tayassu pecari). *Animal Welfare: The UFAW Journal*, 20(4), 505.

Nunes, S. (2014). Juvenile social play and yearling behavior and reproductive success in female Belding's ground squirrels. *Journal of Ethology*, 32(3), 145–153.

Nwokah, E. E., & Ikekeonwu, C. (1998). A sociocultural comparison of Nigerian and American children's games. In M. C. Duncan, G. Chick, & A. Aycock (Eds.), *Play & culture studies: Volume 1:. Diversions and divergences in fields of play* (pp. 59–76). Greenwich, CT: Ablex. Octopus vulgaris. *Journal of Comparative Psychology*, 120(3), 184–190. https://doi .org/10.1037/0735-7036.120.3.184.

Ogata, A. F. (2004). Creative playthings: Educational toys and postwar American culture. *Winterthur Portfolio*, 39(2/3), 129–156. https://doi.org/10.1086/433197

Oke, A., & Middle, G. J. (2016). Planning playgrounds to facilitate children's pretend play: A case study of new suburbs in Perth, Western Australia. *Planning Practice &*

Research, 31(1), 99–117. https://doi.org/10.1080/0269745 9.2015.1081336

Okimoto, A. M., Bundy, A., & Hanzlik, J. (2000). Playfulness in children with and without disability: Measurement and intervention. *American Journal of Occupational Therapy*, 54, 73–82.

Olsen, H., & Kennedy, (2018). Final report National Program for Playground Safety. https://playgroundsafety.org/sites/default /files/inline-files/NPPS_CPSC__Final_Report_0.pdf

Olsen, H., & Smith, B. (2017). Sandboxes, loose parts, and playground equipment: A descriptive exploration of outdoor play environments. *Early Child Development and Care*, 187(5–6), 1055–1068. https://doi.org/10.1080/0300 4430.2017.1282928.

Orr, E. (2019). Mouthing and fingering affect the achievement of play milestones. *Early Child Development and Care*, 1–10.

Pagels, P., Raustorp, A., De Leon, A. P., Martensson, F., Kylin, M., & Boldemann, C. (2014). A repeated measurement study investigating the impact of school outdoor environment upon physical activity across ages and seasons in Swedish second, fifth and eighth graders. *BMC Public Health*, 14(1), 803. https:// doi.org/10.1186/1471-2458-14-803

Panksepp, J., & Burgdorf, J. (2003). "Laughing" rats and the evolutionary antecedents of human joy?. *Physiology & behavior*, 79(3), 533–547.

Panksepp, J., Burgdorf, J., Turner, C., & Gordon, N. (2003). Modeling ADHD-type arousal with unilateral frontal cortex damage in rats and beneficial effects of play therapy. *Brain & Cognition*, 52, 97–105.

Parham, L. D. (1996). Perspectives on play. In R. Zemke & F. Clark (Eds.), *Occupational science: The evolving discipline* (pp. 71–88). Philadelphia, PA: F. A. Davis.

Parsons, A. G., & Ballantine, P. W. (2008). The gifts we buy for children. *Young Consumers*, 9(4), 308–15. https://doi .org/10.1108/17473610810920515

Parten, M. B. (1932). Social participation among preschool children. *Journal of Abnormal Psychology*, 27, 243–69.

Pawelko, K. A., & Magafas, A. H. (1997, July). Leisure well being among adolescent groups: Time choices and self determination. *Parks & Recreation*. Retrieved July 21, 2008, from http://findarticles.com/p/articles/mi_m1145/is_n7_v32 /ai_19649715/pg_1?tag=artBody;col1

Pellegrini, A. D. (1988). Elementary-school children's rough-and-tumble play and social competence. *Developmental Psychology*, 24, 802–806.

Pellegrini, A. D. (1992). Preference for outdoor play during early adolescence. *Journal of Adolescence*, 15, 241–254.

Pellegrini, A. D. (1994). The rough play of adolescent boys of differing sociometric status. *International Journal of Behavioral Development*, 17, 525–540.

Pellegrini, A. D. (1995). Boys' rough-and-tumble play and social competence. In A. D. Pellegrini (Ed.), *The future of play theory* (pp. 107–126). Albany: State University of New York Press.

Pellegrini, A. D. (2006). Rough and tumble play from childhood to adolescence. In D. P. Fromberg & D. Bergen (Eds.), *Play from birth to twelve: Contexts, perspectives and meanings* (2nd ed., pp. 111–118). New York: Routledge.

Pellegrini, A. D., & Bjorklund, D. E. (2004). The ontogeny and phylogeny of children's object and fantasy play. *Human Nature*, 15, 23–42.

Pellegrini, A. D., & Smith, P. K. (1998a). Physical activity play: The nature and function of a neglected aspect of play. *Child Development*, 69, 577–598.

Pellegrini, A. D., & Smith, P. K. (1998b). The development of play during childhood: Forms and possible function. *Child Psychology & Psychiatry Review, 3*(2), 51–57.

Pellegrini, A. D., & Smith, P. (2003). Development of play. *Handbook of developmental psychology*, 276–291.

Pellis, S. M., Pellis, V. C., & Himmler, B. T. (2014). How play makes for a more adaptable brain: A comparative and neural perspective. *American Journal of Play, 7*(1), 73–98.

Pew Research Center (2015). Parenting in America. https://www.pewresearch.org/social-trends/2015/12/17/parenting-in-america/

Pfeifer, L. I., Pacciulio, A. M., Santos, C. A. D., Santos, J. L. D., & Stagnitti, K. E. (2011). Pretend play of children with cerebral palsy. *Physical & Occupational Therapy in Pediatrics, 31*(4), 390–402.

Piaget, J. (1952). *The origins of intelligence in children* (M. Cook, Trans.). New York: W. W. Norton & Co. https://doi.org/10.1037/11494-000

Piaget, J. (1962). *Play, dreams and imitation in childhood.* New York: W. W. Norton.

Piaget, J. (1975). *The origins of intelligence in children.* New York: International Universities Press. (Original work published 1952)

Pierce, D. (2000). Maternal management of the home as a developmental play space for infants and toddlers. *American Journal of Occupational Therapy, 54*(3), 290–299.

Pinchover, S., Shulman, C., & Bundy, A. (2016). A comparison of playfulness of young children with and without autism spectrum disorder in interactions with their mothers and teachers. *Early Child Development and Care, 186*(12), 1893–1906.

Pinoniemi, L. (2003). Theme parks: Creating memorable playgrounds by building on a theme. *Parks & Recreation, 38*(11), 48–51.

Playworld (2019). The Evolution of Public Playgrounds in the United States. https://playworld.com/blog/evolution-public-playgrounds-united-states/

Poppe R., van Delden R., Moreno A., & Reidsma D. (2014). Interactive playgrounds for children. In A. Nijholt (Ed.), *Playful user interfaces. Gaming media and social effects.* Singapore: Springer. https://doi.org/10.1007/978-981-4560-96-2_5

Power, T. G. (2000). *Play and exploration in children and animals.* Mahwah, NJ: Erlbaum.

Prieske, B., Withagen, R., Smith, J., & Zaal, F. T. J. M. (2015). Affordances in a simple playscape: Are children attracted to challenging affordances? *Journal of Environmental Psychology, 41*, 101–111. https://doi.org/10.1016/j.jenvp.2014.11.011

Proyer, R. T. (2013). The well-being of playful adults: Adult playfulness, subjective well-being, physical well-being, and the pursuit of enjoyable activities. *The European Journal of Humour Research, 1*(1), 84–98.

Proyer, R. T., & Jehle, N. (2013). The basic components of adult playfulness and their relation with personality: The hierarchical factor structure of seventeen instruments. *Personality and Individual Differences, 55*(7), 811–816.

Pyle, A., & Danniels, E. (2017). A continuum of play-based learning: The role of the teacher in play-based pedagogy and the fear of hijacking play. *Early Education and Development, 28*(3), 274–289.

Raag, T., & Rackliff, C. L. (1998). Preschoolers' awareness of social expectations of gender: relationships to toy choices. *Sex Roles, 38*, 685–700. https://doi.org/10.1023/A:1018890728636

Rabinowitz, F. M., Moely, B. E., Finkel, N., & McClinton, S. (1975). The effects of toy novelty and social interaction on the exploratory behavior of preschool children. *Child Development,* 286–289.

Rafferty, J. (2018). Gender identity development in children. *American Academy of Pediatrics.* Retrieved from https://www.healthychildren.org/English/ages-stages/gradeschool/Pages/Gender-Identity-and-Gender-Confusion-In-Children.aspx

Ramsey, P. G. (2015). Influences of race, culture, social class, and gender: Diversity and play. In *Play from birth to 12* (3rd ed., pp. 271–282). New York: Routledge.

Reed, C. N., Dunbar, S. B., & Bundy, A. C. (2000). The effects of an inclusive preschool experience on the playfulness of children with and without autism. *Physical and Occupational Therapy in Pediatrics, 19*, 73–89.

Reed, T. L. (2005). A qualitative approach to boys' rough and tumble play: There is more than meets the eye. In F. F. McMahon, D. E. Lytle, & B. Sutton-Smith (Eds.), *Play & culture studies: Volume 6. Play: An interdisciplinary synthesis* (pp. 53–71). Lanham, MD: University Press of America.

Rebeiro, K. L., & Polgar, J. M. (1999). Enabling occupational performance: Optimal experiences in therapy. *Canadian Journal of Occupational Therapy, 66*(1), 14–22.

Refshauge, A. D., Stigsdotter, U. K., Lamm, B., et al. (2013). Evidence-based playground design: Lessons learned from theory to practice. *Landsc Res Routledge, 40*, 226–46. https://doi.org/10.1080/01426397.2013.824073

Reid, D. H., DiCarlo, C. F., Schepis, M. M., Hawkins, J., & Stricklin, S. B. (2003). Observational assessment of toy preferences among young children with disabilities in inclusive settings: Efficiency analysis and comparison with staff opinion. *Behavior Modification, 27*(2), 233–250.

Reilly, M. (1974). Defining a cobweb. In M. Reilly (Ed.), *Play as exploratory learning: Studies of curiosity behavior* (pp. 57–116). London: Sage.

Remmers, T., Thijs, C., Timperio, A., Salmon, J. O., Veitch, J., Kremers, S. P., & Ridgers, N. D. (2017). Daily weather and children's physical activity patterns. *Medicine and Science in Sports and Exercise, 49*(5), 922–929. https://doi.org/10.1249/MSS.0000000000001181

Resnick, M., & Robinson, K. (2017). *Lifelong kindergarten: Cultivating creativity through projects, passion, peers, and play.* MIT press.

Rettig, M. (1995). Play and cultural diversity. *The Journal of Educational Issue of Language Minority Students, 15*(4), 1–9.

Rettig, M. (1998). Environmental Influences on the Play of Young Children with Disabilities. *Education and Training in Mental Retardation and Developmental Disabilities, 33*(2), 189–194. http://www.jstor.org/stable/23879166

Rettig, M. (1998). Environmental influences on the play of young children with disabilities. *Education and Training in Mental Retardation and Developmental Disabilities,* 189–194.

Rheingold, H. L., & Cook, K. V. (1975). The contents of boys' and girls' rooms as an index of parents' behavior. *Child development,* 459–463.

Richards, M. N., Putnick, D. L., Suwalsky, J. T., & Bornstein, M. H. (2020). AGE DETERMINATION GUIDELINES: Relating Consumer Product Characteristics to the Skills, Play Behaviors, and Interests of Children. https://cpsc.gov/s3fs-public/pdfs/blk_media_adg.pdf

Richter, E., & Oetter, P. (1990). Environmental matrices for sensory integrative treatment. *Environment implications for*

Occupational Therapy practice. Rockville, MD, USA: The American Occupational Therapy Association

Rigby, P., & Rodger, S. A. (2006). *Developing as a player. Occupational therapy with children: Understanding children's occupations and enabling participation*. Edited by S. Rodger and J. Ziviani. Oxford: Blackwell. 177–199.

Ripat, J., & Becker, P. (2012). Playground usability: what do playground users say?. *Occupational therapy international*, 19(3), 144–153.

Robinson, A. L. (1977). Play: The arena for acquisition of rules for competent behavior. *American Journal of Occupational Therapy*, 31(4), 248–253.

Robinson, C. C., & Jackson, R. (1987). The effects of varying toy detail within a prototypical play object on the solitary pretend play of preschool children. *Journal of Applied Developmental Psychology*, 8(2), 209–220.

Rogers, J. C. (1982). The spirit of independence: The evolution of a philosophy. *American Journal of Occupational Therapy*, 36(11), 709–715.

Rogers, C. S., Impara, J. C., Frary, R. B., Harris, T., Meeks, A., Semanic-Lauth, S.,& Reynolds, M. R. (1998). Measuring playfulness: Development of the Child Behaviors Inventory of Playfulness. In M. C. Duncan, G. Chick, & A. Aycock (Eds.), *Play & culture studies: Volume 1*. Diversions and divergences in fields of play (pp. 121–136). Greenwich, CT: Ablex.

Rohrlich, J. (2020). The US Border Patrol is building a caged playground for migrant children. https://qz.com/1845181/border-patrol-is-building-a-caged-playground-for-migrant-children/

Roopnarine, J. L., & Davidson, K. L. (2015). Parent–child play across cultures: Advancing play research. *American Journal of Play*, 7(2), 228–252.

Rubin, K. H. (1977). The social and cognitive value of preschool toys and activities. *Canadian Journal of Behavioural Science/ Revue canadienne des sciences du comportement*, 9(4), 382.

Rubin KH, Howe N. (1985). Toys and Play Behaviors: An Overview. *Topics in Early Childhood Special Education*. 5(3):1–9. https://doi.org/10.1177/027112148500500302

Saccani, R., Valentini, N. C., Pereira, K. R., Müller, A. B., & Gabbard, C. (2013). Associations of biological factors and affordances in the home with infant motor development. *Pediatrics International*, 55(2), 197–203. https://doi.org/10.1111/ped.12042

Sallis, J. F., McKenzie, T. L., Elder, J. P., Broyles, S. L., & Nader, P. R. (1997). Factors parents use in selecting play spaces for young children. *Arch Pediatr Adolesc Med.*, 151(4), 414–417. https://doi.org/10.1001/archpedi.1997.02170410088012.

Salonius-Pasternak, D., & Gelfond, H. (2005). The next level of research on electronic play: Potential benefits and contextual influences for children and adolescents. *Human Technology*, 1(1), 5–22.

Sandseter, E. B. (2007). Risky play among four- and five-year-olds in preschool. *Vision into Practice CECDE International Conference*. Retrieved February 15, 2007, from http://www.cecde.ie/english/conference_2007.php

Sandseter, E. B. H. (2009). Characteristics of risky play. *Journal of Adventure Education & Outdoor Learning*, 9(1), 3–21.

Sandseter, E. B. H., Kleppe, R., & Sando, O. J. (2021). The prevalence of risky play in young children's indoor and outdoor free play. *Early Childhood Education Journal*, 49(2), 303–312.

Sapora A (1989) In Ibrahim, H. (Ed). *Pioneers in Leisure and Recreation*. AAHPERD Publications, Inc., Waldorf, MD 65–78 https://files.eric.ed.gov/fulltext/ED308157.pdf

Saracho, O. N. (1990). Preschool children's cognitive styles and their social orientations. *Perceptual and Motor Skills*, 70(3 Pt. 1), 915–921.

Saracho, O. N. (2017). Theoretical framework of developmental theories. In T. Waller, E. Ärlemalm-Hagsér, E. B. H. Sandseter, L. Lee-Hammond, K. Lekies, & S. Wyver (Eds.), *The SAGE handbook of outdoor play and learning* (pp. 25–29). London: Sage Publishing.

Saracho, O. N., & Spodek, B. (1998). A historical overview of theories of play. *Multiple perspectives on play in early childhood education*, 1–10.

Saracho, O. N., & Spodek, B. (2003). Understanding play and its theories. In O. N. Saracho & B. Spodek (Eds.), *Contemporary perspectives on play in early childhood education*, 1–19. Greenwich, CT: Information Age Publishing.

Saunders, I., Sayer, M., & Goodale, A. (1999). The relationship between playfulness and coping in preschool children: A pilot study. *American Journal of Occupational Therapy*, 53, 221–226.

Scarlett, W. G., Naudeau, S., Salonius-Pasternak, D., & Ponte, I. (2005). *Children's play*. London: Sage.

Schiavo, R. S. (1990). Children's and adolescents' designs of ideal homes. *Children's Environments Quarterly*, 7(4), 37–46.

Schiavo, R. S. (1987). Home use and evaluation by suburban youth: Gender differences. *Children's Environments Quarterly*, 4(4), 8–12.

Schiller, F. (1875). *Essays, Aesthetical and philosophical*. London: Bell and Sons.

Scott, D., & Willits, F. K. (1998). Adolescent and adult leisure patterns: A reassessment. *Journal of Leisure Research*. Retrieved July 22, 2008, from http://findarticles.com/p/articles/mi_qa3702/is_199807/ai_n8784241

Seiter, E. (1992). Toys are us: Marketing to children and parents. *Cultural Studies*, 6(2), 232–247. https://doi.org/10.1080/09502389200490121

Serbin, L. A., Moller, L. C., Gulko, J., Powlishta, K. K., & Colboume, K. A. (1994). The emergence of gender segregation in toddler playgroups. In C. Leaper (Ed.), *Childhood gender segregation: Causes and consequences* (pp. 7–18). San Francisco: Jossey-Bass.

Servin, A., Bohlin, G., & Berlin, L. (1999). Sex differences in 1-, 3-, and 5-year-olds' toy-choice in a structured play-session. *Scandinavian Journal of Psychology*, 40, 43–48.

Schubert, E., & Strick, R. (1996). Toy-free Kindergarten. *A Proyect to Prevent Addiction for Children and with Children*. München: München Aktion Jugendschutz, Landesarbeitsstelle Bayern eV. http://wildthingtoys.com/wp-content/uploads/2017/04/englisch.pdf

Shah, R., Gustafson, E., & Atkins, M. (2019). Parental attitudes and beliefs surrounding play among predominantly low-income urban families: A qualitative study. *Journal of Developmental and Behavioral Pediatrics*, 40(8), 606–612. https://doi.org/10.1097/DBP.0000000000000708

Shapiro, J. (2014). 3 ways to close the "play gap" between rich and poor kids. https://www.forbes.com/sites/jordanshapiro/2014/10/24/3-ways-to-close-the-play-gap-between-rich-and-poor-kids/?sh=667df0211233

Sharpe, L. (2011). So you think you know why animals play…. *Scientific American* https://blogs.scientificamerican.com/guest-blog/so-you-think-you-know-why-animals-play/

Sharpe, L. L., Clutton-Brock, T. H., Brotherton, P. N., Cameron, E. Z., & Cherry, M. I. (2002). Experimental provisioning increases play in free-ranging meerkats. *Animal Behaviour*, *64*(1), 113–121. https://doi.org/10.1006/anbe.2002.3031

Sherman, A. M., & Zurbriggen, E. L. (2014). Boys can be anything: Effect of Barbie play on girls' career cognitions. *Sex Roles, 70*(5–6), 195–208. https://doi.org/10.1007/s11199-014-0347-y

Shim, S., Herwig, J. E., & Shelley, M. (2009). Preschoolers' play behaviors with peers in classroom and playground settings. *Journal of Research in Childhood Education, 15*(2), 149–163. https://doi.org/10.1080/02568540109594956

Shipley, M. (2010). Dressing the part: How Twilight fans self-identify through dress at an Official Twilight Convention. *Communication Honors Theses, 3*.

Signorella, M. L., Bigler, R. S., & Liben, L. S. (1993). Developmental differences in children's gender schemata about others: A meta-analytic review. *Developmental Review, 13*(2), 147–183. https://doi.org/10.1006/drev.1993.1007

Skaines, N., Rodger, S., & Bundy, A. (2006). Playfulness in children with autistic disorder and their typically developing peers. *British Journal of Occupational Therapy, 69*, 505–512.

Skar, L. (2002). Disabled children's perceptions of technical aids, assistance and peers in play situations. *Scandinavian Journal of Caring Sciences, 16*(1), 27–33.

Skard, G., & Bundy, A. C. (2008). Test of playfulness. In L. D. Parham & L. S. Fazio (Eds.), *Play in occupational therapy for children* (2nd ed., pp. 71–93). St. Louis, MO: Mosby Elsevier.

Smaldino, P. E., Palagi, E., Burghardt, G. M., & Pellis, S. M. (2019). The evolution of two types of play. *Behavioral Ecology, 30*(5), 1388–1397.

Smilansky, S. (1968). *The effects of sociodramatic play on disadvantaged preschool children*. New York: Wiley.

Smirnova, E. O. (2011). Character toys as psychological tools. *International Journal of Early Years Education, 19*(1), 35–43.

Smith P., & Connolly K (1980). *The ecology of preschool behavior*. Cambridge, England: Cambridge University Press.

Smith, P. K., & Vollstedt, R. (1985). On defining play: An empirical study of the relationship between play and various play criteria. *Child Development*, 1042–1050.

Souto-Manning, M. (2017). Is play a privilege or a right? And what's our responsibility? On the role of play for equity in early childhood education. *Early Child Development and Care, 187*(5-6), 785–787. https://doi.org/10.1080/03004430.2016.1266588

Spencer, H. (1873). *The principles of psychology*. New York: D. Appleton and Co.

Spinner, L., Cameron, L., & Calogero, R. (2018). Peer toy play as a gateway to children's gender flexibility: The effect of (counter) stereotypic portrayals of peers in children's magazines. *Sex Roles, 79*, 314–328. https://doi.org/10.1007/s11199-017-

Staempfli, M. B. (2007). Adolescent playfulness, stress perception, coping and well being. *Journal of Leisure Research*. Retrieved July 20, 2008, from http://findarticles.com/p/articles/mi_qa3702/is_200707/ai_n21185992?tag=rel.res4

Staempfli MB. Reintroducing Adventure Into Children's Outdoor Play Environments. *Environment and Behavior*. 2009;41(2):268–280. https://doi.org/10.1177/0013916508315000

Stanton-Chapman, T. L., & Schmidt, E. L. (2017). Caregiver perceptions of inclusive playgrounds targeting toddlers and preschoolers with disabilities: Has recent international and national policy improved overall satisfaction?. *Journal of Research in Special Educational Needs, 17*(4), 237–246. https://doi.org/10.1111/1471-3802.12381

Sterman, J. J., Naughton, G. A., Bundy, A. C., Froude, E., & Villeneuve, M. A. (2020). Is play a choice? Application of the capabilities approach to children with disabilities on the school playground. *International Journal of Inclusive Education, 24*(6), 579–596.

Stetsenko, A., & Ho, P. C. G. (2015). The serious joy and the joyful work of play: Children becoming agentive actors in co-authoring themselves and their world through play. *International Journal of Early Childhood, 47*(2), 221–234.

Stoneman, Z., Cantrell, M. L., & Hoover-Dempsey, K. (1983). The association between play materials and social behavior in a mainstreamed preschool: A naturalistic investigation. *Journal of Applied Developmental Psychology, 4*(2), 163–174.

Suriyaarachchi, R. (2017). Where do children play in a war zone? https://www.unicef.org.au/blog/stories/december-2017/where-children-play-war-zone-conflict

Sutton-Smith, B. (1997). *The ambiguity of play*. Cambridge, MA: Harvard University Press.

Taggart, J., Heise, M. J., & Lillard, A. S. (2018). The real thing: Preschoolers prefer actual activities to pretend one. *Developmental Science, 21*, e12582. https://doi.org/10.1111/desc.12582

Takhvar, M. (1988). Play and theories of play: A review of the literature. *Early Child Development and Care, 39*(1), 221–244.

Talarowski, M., Cohen, D. A., Williamson, S., & Han, B. (2019). Innovative playgrounds: Use, physical activity, and implications for health. *Public health, 174*, 102–109. https://doi.org/10.1016/j.puhe.2019.06.002

Tandy, C. A. (1999). Children's diminishing play space: A study of inter-generational change in children's use of their neighbourhoods. *Australian Geographical Studies, 37*(2), 154–164. https://doi.org/10.1111/1467-8470.00076

Tapsell, S. M. (1997). Rivers and river restoration: A child's-eye view. *Landscape Research, 22*(1), 45–65. https://doi.org/10.1080/01426399708706500

Tegano, D. W., & Burdette, M. P. (1991). Length of activity periods and play behaviors of preschool children. *Journal of Research in Childhood Education, 5*(2), 93–99.

The Strong. (n.d.). Reading the play elements chart. https://www.museumofplay.org/sites/default/files/uploads/Elements%20of%20Play050114.pdf

Thompson, K. V. (1998). Self assessment in juvenile play. In M. Bekoff & J. A. Byers (Eds.), *Animal play: Evolutionary, comparative, and ecological perspectives* (pp. 183–204). New York: Cambridge University Press.

Todd, B. K., Fischer, R. A., Di Costa, S., Roestorf, A., Harbour, K., Hardiman P., & Barry, J. A. (2018). Sex differences in children's toy preferences: A systematic review, meta-regression, and meta-analysis. *Infant and Child Development, 27*(2), e2064. https://doi.org/10.1002/icd.2064

Toy Industry (2020). U.S. Sales data. https://www.toyassociation.org/ta/research/data/u-s-sales-data/toys/research-and-data/data/us-sales-data.aspx

Tranter, P., & Doyle, J. (1996). Reclaiming the residential street as play space. *International Play Journal, 4*(91–97).

Trautner, H. M. (1992). The development of sex-typing in children: A longitudinal analysis. *German Journal of Psychology, 16*(3), 183–199.

Trawick-Smith, J. (1990). Effects of realistic vs. non-realistic play materials on young children's symbolic transformation of objects. *Journal of Research in Childhood Education, 5*, 27–36. https://doi.org/10.1080/02568549009594800

Trawick-Smith, J., Wolff, J., Koschel, M., & Vallarelli, J. (2015). Effects of toys on the play quality of preschool children: Influence of gender, ethnicity, and socioeconomic status. *Early Childhood Education Journal*, 43(4), 249–256. https://doi.org/10.1007/s10643-014-0644-7

Trawick-Smith, J., Wolff, J., Koschel, M., & Vallarelli, J. (2014). Preschool: Which toys promote high-quality play? Reflections on the five-year anniversary of the TIMPANI study. *YC Young Children*, 69(2), 40–46.

The Trust for Public Land. (2017). *2017 City park facts*. San Francisco: Playscore. https://www.tpl.org/parkscore

The Trust for Public Land. (2019). Annual report. https://www.tpl.org/2019-annual-report

Tsai, C. Y. (2015). Am I Interfering? Preschool Teacher Participation in Children Play. *Universal Journal of Educational Research*, 3(12), 1028–1033.

Tseng, J. (2008). Sex, gender, and why the differences matter. *Virtual Mentor*, 10(7), 427–428.

Tunstall, S., Tapsell, S., & House, M. (2004). Children's perceptions of river landscapes and play: What children's photographs reveal. *Landscape Research*, 29(2), 181–204. https://doi.org/10.1080/01426390410001690365

Ummanel, A. (2017). A comparative analysis of children's, mothers' and teachers' views about play and toys. *International Journal of Humanities and Education*, 3(2), 222–241.

Ungerer, J. A., & Sigman, M. (1981). Symbolic play and language comprehension in autistic children. *Journal of the American Academy of Child Psychiatry*, 20(2), 318–337.

UNICEF. (2017). *Children in a digital world*. https://www.unicef.org/uzbekistan/media/711/file/SOWC:%20Children%20in%20a%20Digital%20World.pdf

Vanderschuren, L. J., Niesink, R. J., Spruijt, B. M., & Van Ree, J. M. (1995). Influence of environmental factors on social play behavior of juvenile rats. *Physiology & behavior*, 58(1), 119–123.

Van de Beek, C., van Goozen, S. H., Buitelaar, J. K., & Cohen-Kettenis, P. T. (2009). Prenatal sex hormones (maternal and amniotic fluid) and gender-related play behavior in 13-month-old infants. *Archives of Sexual Behavior*, 38(1), 6–15.

Van den Berg, C. L., Hol, T., Van Ree, J. M., Spruijt, B. M., Everts, H., & Koolhaas, J. M. (1999). Play is indispensable for an adequate development of coping with social challenges in the rat. *Developmental Psychobiology: The Journal of the International Society for Developmental Psychobiology*, 34(2), 129–138.

Van Vleet, M., & Feeney, B. C. (2015). Play behavior and playfulness in adulthood. *Social and Personality Psychology Compass*, 9(11), 630–643.

Venkatesan, S. (2014). Availability of toys for children with developmental disabilities. *Journal of Disability Management and Special Education*. 4(1), 58–70.

Venkatesan, S., & Yashodharakumar, G. Y. (2017a). Parent opinions and attitudes on toys for children with or without developmental disabilities. *The International Journal of Indian Psychology*, 4(4), 6–20. https://doi.org/10.25215/0404.061

Venkatesan, S., & Yashodharakumar, G. Y. (2017b). Toy index of children with or without developmental disabilities. *Indian Journal of Clinical Psychology*, 44(1), 60–67.

Veitch, J., Bagley, S., Ball, K., & Salmon, J. (2006). Where do children usually play? A qualitative study of parents' perceptions of influences on children's active free-play. *Health & Place*, 12(4), 383–393. https://doi.org/10.1016/j.healthplace.2005.02.009.

Veitch, J., Salmon, J., & Ball, K. (2007). Children's active free play in local neighborhoods: A behavioral mapping study. *Health Education Research*, 23(5), 870–879. https://doi.org/10.1093/her/cym074

Virués-Ortega, J., Pritchard, K., Grant, R. L., North, S., Hurtado-Parrado, C., Lee, M. S., . . . Yu, C. T. (2014). Clinical decision making and preference assessment for individuals with intellectual and developmental disabilities. *American Journal on Intellectual and Developmental Disabilities*, 119(2), 151–170.

Von Klitzing, K., Kelsay, K., Emde, R. N., Robinson, J., & Schmitz, S. (2000). Gender-specific characteristics of 5-year-olds' play narratives and associations with behavior ratings. *Journal of the American Academy of Child and Adolescent Psychiatry*, 39, 1017–1023.

Vygotsky, L. (1976). Play and its role in the mental development of the child. In J. Bruner, A. Jolly, & K. Sylva (Eds.), *Play, its role in development and evolution*. Harmondsworth, Middlesex: Penguin, 537–54.

Vygotsky, L. S. (1978). *Mind in society: The development of higher psychological processes*. Cambridge, MA: Harvard University Press.

Wachs, T. D. (1985). Toys as an aspect of the physical environment: Constraints and nature of relationship to development. *Topics in Early Childhood Special Education*, 5(3), 31–46. https://doi.org/10.1177/027112148500500304

Wall, S. M., Pickert, S. M., & Gibson, W. B. (1989). Fantasy play in 5- and 6-year-old children. *Journal of Psychology*, 123, 245–256.

Weisgram, E. S., & Bruun, S. T. (2018). Predictors of gender-typed toy purchases by prospective parents and mothers: The roles of childhood experiences and gender attitudes. *Sex Roles*, 79, 342–357. https://doi.org/10.1007/s11199-018-0928-2

White, R. (1959). Motivation reconsidered: The concept of competence. *Psychological Review*, 66, 297–333.

Whitebread, D. (2012). The importance of play: A report on the value of children's play with a series of policy recommendations. https://www.csap.cam.ac.uk/media/uploads/files/1/david-whitebread---importance-of-play-report.pdf

Whitebread, D., Neale, D., Jensen, H., Liu, C., Solis, S. L., Hopkins, E., Hirsh-Pasek, K., & Zosh, J. M. (2017). *The role of play in children's development: A review of the evidence (research summary)*. The LEGO Foundation, DK.

Wiltz, N. W., & Fein, G. G. (2006). Play as children see it. In D. P. Fromberg & D. Bergen (Eds.), *Play from birth to twelve: Contexts, perspectives and meanings* (2nd ed., pp. 127–140). New York: Routledge.

Wiltz, N. W., & Fein, G. G. (2015). Play as children see it. In D. P. Fromberg & D. Bergen (Eds.), *Play from birth to twelve: Contexts, perspectives, and meanings* (pp. 43–53). New York: Routledge.

Wing, L. (1995). Play is not the work of the child: Young children's perceptions of work and play. *Early Childhood Research Quarterly*, 10, 223–247.

Wolfberg, P., DeWitt, M., Young, G. S. et al. (2015). Integrated play groups: Promoting symbolic play and social engagement with typical peers in children with ASD across settings. *J Autism Dev Disord 45*, 830–845. https://doi.org/10.1007/s10803-014-2245-0

Wood, E., Desmarais, S., & Gugula, S. (2002). The impact of parenting experience on gender stereotyped toy play of children. *Sex Roles*, 47(1–2), 39–49. https://doi.org/10.1023/A:1020679619728

Wright, J. T. (2018). Liberating human expression: Work and play or work versus play. *American Journal of Play*, *11*(1), 3–25. https://files.eric.ed.gov/fulltext/EJ1200909.pdf

Wu, J., Loprinzi, P. D., & Ren, Z. (2019). The rehabilitative effects of virtual reality games on balance performance among children with cerebral palsy: A meta-analysis of randomized controlled trials. *International Journal of Environmental Research and Public Health*, *16*(21), 4161.

Yee, N. (2006). The labor of fun: How video games blur the boundaries of work and play. *Games and Culture*, *1*(1), 68–71.

Yerxa, E. J. (1994). Dreams, dilemmas, and decisions for occupational therapy practice in a new millennium: An American perspective. *American Journal of Occupational Therapy*, *48*(7), 586–589

Yurt, Ö., & Keleş, S. (2019). How about a risky play? Investigation of risk levels desired by children and perceived mother monitoring. *Early Child Development and Care*, 1–11.

Zamani, Z. (2017). Young children's preferences: What stimulates children's cognitive play in outdoor preschools?. *Journal of Early Childhood Research*, *15*(3), 256–274. https://doi.org/10.1177/1476718X15616831

Zaske, S. (2017). Germany Is Taking Away Kindergarteners' Toys to Curb Future Addiction. https://www.theatlantic.com/education/archive/2017/03/the-toy-free-kindergarten/520905/

Zieff, S. G., Chaudhuri, A., & Musselman, E. (2016). Creating neighborhood recreational space for youth and children in the urban environment: Play (ing in the) streets in San Francisco. *Children and Youth Services Review*, *70*, 95–101. https://doi.org/10.1016/j.childyouth.2016.09.014

Zill, N., Winquist Nord, C., & Loomis, L. S. (1995). *Adolescent time use, risky behavior and outcomes: Executive summary*. Retrieved from http://aspe.hhs.gov/HSP/cyp/xstimuse.htm

Zimmons, J. K. (1997). *The effects of spatial definition on preschool prosocial interaction* (Doctoral dissertation, Texas Tech University).

Ziviani, J., Wadley, D., Ward, H., Macdonald, D., Jenkins, D., & Rodger, S. (2008). A place to play: socioeconomic and spatial factors in children's physical activity. *Australian occupational therapy journal*, *55*(1), 2–11.

Zosh, J. M., Hirsh-Pasek, K., Hopkins, E. J., Jensen, H., Liu, C., Neale, D., . . . Whitebread, D. (2018). Accessing the inaccessible: Redefining play as a spectrum. *Frontiers in Psychology*, *9*, 1124.

Zuckerman, M. (1971). Dimensions of sensation seeking. *Journal of Consulting and Clinical Psychology*, *36*, 45–52.

APPENDIX 1.1

For more information about the history of playgrounds, please see the following links.

How We Came to Play: The History of Playgrounds (Great photos of old playgrounds)

Playgrounds: A 150 Year Old Model (Download a chapter about the history and philosophy of playground design over time)

History of Playgrounds in NY (Extensive history of playground development in NY City and also very good old photographs of early playgrounds)

For interesting photos of playgrounds around the world and in other times:Ten Unusual Playgrounds from Around the World

- https://www.mentalfloss.com/article/22756/10-unusual-playgrounds-around-world
  Photos of very old playground equipment
- https://www.dailymail.co.uk/news/article-2321189/Is-worlds-playground-swing-Newly-discovered-photographs-children-fun-days-health-safety.html

APPENDIX 1.2 Internet Resources for and About Play

http://nifplay.org/
http://www.ipausa.org/
http://www.strongmuseum.org/
http://www.strongmuseum.org/about_play/play_journal.html
http://www.strongmuseum.org/about_play/recess_play.html
http://www.aap.org/pressroom/playFINAL.pdf

http://www.npr.org/templates/story/story.php?storyId=19212514
http://naecs.crc.uiuc.edu/position/recessplay.html

Rights of Children to Play

http://www.righttoplay.com/site/PageServer?pagename=aboutRTP

http://www.playireland.ie/
http://www.ipacanada.org/home_childs.htm
http://www.unicef.org.au/SchoolRoom-Subs
.asp?SchoolRoomID=1

Play in Refugee Camps

http://www.tornfromhome.com/
http://www.savethechildren.org/publications/technical
-resources/emergencies-protection/psychsocwellbeing2.pdf
http://www.refugeesinternational.org/who-we-are/our-issues

APPENDIX 1.3 Videos of Animals Playing

Primates
https://www.youtube.com/watch?v=E0ce8up7x6A
https://www.youtube.com/watch?v=luuX8oaC0w4
https://www.youtube.com/watch?v=Rad-sWnAiwI

Birds
https://www.youtube.com/watch?v=3dWw9GLcOeA
https://www.youtube.com/watch?v=Lw7L_3WCRfQ
https://www.youtube.com/watch?v=LpsDWFei9Z4

Turtles and lizards
https://www.youtube.com/watch?v=Rx2LnoPI_Dw
https://www.youtube.com/watch?v=tFWytrb2DUk
https://www.youtube.com/watch?v=fdE2Uuu8wHc

Dogs, Cats, and Goats
https://www.youtube.com/watch?v=uuph5-xXGH4
https://www.youtube.com/watch?v=Hly0vuXPG-M
https://www.youtube.com/watch?v=58-atNakMWw
https://www.youtube.com/watch?v=1CxK_jKKHHU

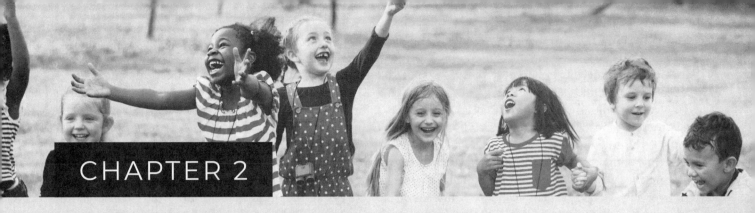

Contributions of the Profession of Occupational Therapy to the Understanding of the Phenomenon of Play as an Occupation

Heather M. Kuhaneck, PhD, OTR/L, FAOTA

After reading this chapter, the reader will:

- Describe the unique contribution of occupational therapy to the understanding of play as a phenomenon.
- Explain the profession's views on play both historically and currently.
- Differentiate play as an occupation from play as a tool.
- Demonstrate an understanding of the meaning of play for children.
- Situate occupational therapy's role within the changing societal context for play.
- Formulate a plan for collaboration with other "play ambassadors and champions" to improve the state of play.

Deep meaning lies often in childish play.

—Johann Friedrich von Schiller

Authors in various fields have studied play, trying to understand why play occurs in humans and other species. Each attempt has contributed to the total body of knowledge regarding play as a phenomenon. While it is important for occupational therapy practitioners to consume the play literature from professions such as psychology and education, it is equally important for us to understand our unique contributions and perspectives.

Occupational therapy practitioners use occupations to facilitate health and engagement and work to ensure that those we serve are able to participate in meaningful occupations as the primary outcome of our therapy. Occupational therapy practitioners are *experts in occupation* who promote health, well-being, and life satisfaction through enabling participation in occupation (AOTA, 2021; Wilding, 2009). We can and should be "play ambassadors," advocating and promoting the importance of play as one of the most important occupations of children, working alongside our colleagues from psychology, education, and child development.

Occupational therapists have been interested in, studied, and written about play for over 50 years. As a profession, ideas about play have shifted over time, and thus the writings reflect the times in which they were written. This chapter provides an overview of play as it has been understood, researched, and promoted within the profession of occupational therapy, highlights the particular contributions of occupational therapy to the study of play, and offers suggestions for the future.

Play at the Foundation of Occupational Therapy

The founders of occupational therapy clearly thought play and leisure were important, as their early writings emphasized the importance of play and the "play spirit" (Reed, 2019; Slagle, 1922). Adolph Meyer (1922), a proponent of occupational therapy and the founder of the first occupational therapy department, believed that mental illness arose from a lack of balance between work, rest, and play. Meyer was influenced by colleagues prominently involved with the mental hygiene movement such as Jane Addams and Julia Lathrop, who helped establish one of the first playgrounds in America at Hull House, a settlement house in Chicago (Dunton, 1954; Jane Addams-Hull House Museum, n.d.; Richmond, 1995). Meyer "acknowledged his debt to Jane Addams and other workers at Hull House, for in emphasizing that play … developed feelings of success and accomplishment, they showed concern for the physical and emotional health of old and young alike" (Dreyer, 1976, p. 996). Eleanor Clarke Slagle, a founding member of the organization that would become AOTA, took courses at Hull House and was similarly influenced to consider play important.

Although the primary recipients of occupational therapy services in the early years were adults, occupational therapy publications began to emerge that were specific to pediatrics in the middle of the 20th century. This was during a time of the creation of specialized fields of pediatrics in both medicine and psychology. The first published pediatric assessment in occupational therapy, in 1950, appears to have been a daily living skill checklist for children with cerebral palsy (Reed & Sanderson, 1999), rather than an assessment of play. However, by the second edition of Willard

and Spackman's *Principles of Occupational Therapy* in 1954 "children's play" was specifically identified as one of the activities assessed by occupational therapists (McNary, 1954, p. 16). Toys were considered to be important treatment tools. Gleave (1954) provided an early description of client-centered pediatric occupational therapy practice, specifically stressing the importance of the child's participation in choice making. She discussed the use of activities such as crafts, recreation (play), and music with children, stating, "the child should have an opportunity to contribute to the program" (p. 164), and "the development of play interests in the child must be considered" (p. 164). In addition, Gleave (1954) highlighted the usefulness of crafts, as they allowed the child "unlimited opportunities for self-expression and permit[ed] the child to pursue his natural interests" (p. 164).

In the 1960s and 1970s, Ayres's work in sensory integration, while not specifically about play, highlighted the importance of play in the way that the intervention is delivered (Ayres 1963, 1964, 1971, 1972). Child-directed play, with choice, is key to Ayres's Sensory Integration approach (Parham et al., 2011). Ayres's respect for children and the value she placed on play is clear in all of her work. Ayres believed that play both reflected learning and could be used to enhance learning, consistent with researchers and theorists from other disciplines of this time. As you may recall from Chapter 1, during this time period, she would have been exposed to the works of Piaget (1962) and others who considered play as reflective of and important for development. In addition, ideas about the importance of motivation for activity (White, 1959) were also influential in her thinking (Schaaf, Merrill, & Kinsella, 1987).

The emergence of play as a topic worthy of study in occupational therapy can be traced back to Mary Reilly (1974). The first occupational therapy text about play was edited by Reilly, and this instrumental work provided our profession with a base of knowledge specific to our field. Reilly proposed three hierarchical stages of play development—exploratory, competency, and achievement—and suggested that play allowed learning and mastery to occur for the child. Reilly's students contributed to this text and the profession in important ways (Florey, 1971; Knox, 1974; Takata, 1974). Florey identified the importance of play in natural environments and considered the power of the environment to either inhibit or facilitate play. Takata believed play and development were inextricably linked and that play therefore followed a predictable sequence of development. She created a taxonomy of play based on age and developmental level as well as the Takata Play History, an assessment that is still referred to today (Besio et al., 2018; Takata, 1974). Knox (1974) similarly believed in a developmental progression of play and believed in the idea that play reflected development in other areas. She developed an assessment called the Knox's Preschool Play Scale (PPS), which is still in use. For more on both of these tools, see Chapter 3.

During the 20 or so years following the publication of Reilly's book, there were few published studies on play, and as a group, these generally examined one aspect of play—the type, form, or category. Studies of this time period primarily examined play as a means to measure development in other areas (cognition, motor skills, etc.). The PPS was used to study play in varied populations such as children who were hospitalized (Kielhofner, Barris, Bauer, Shoestock, & Walker, 1983), abused (Howard, 1986), or diagnosed with autism (Restall & Magill-Evans, 1994). The PPS was also used to examine play behaviors of children of differing socioeconomic status (von Zuben, Crist, & Mayberry, 1991). The assessment of play was specifically targeted as a fruitful area for further development (Kielhofner & Barris, 1984). By 1993, Bundy stated, "it is telling that we who claim that play and leisure are a primary lifelong human occupation and who make it our business to assess occupation, have contributed so little to the existing theoretical and practical knowledge base of play" (p. 219).

Although some of the concepts of client-centered therapy existed in early pediatric occupational therapy practice, views on play were somewhat different from what they are now. Play was generally a diversion for a sick child, or it was primarily used as a method to assess or develop other skills. The idea that play itself is important and deserving of our time in intervention without an alternative agenda is a more modern perspective.

Play as an Occupation

During the 1990s, renewed interest in play resulted in the publication of the first comprehensive texts on play in occupational therapy since Reilly's work (Chandler, 1997; Parham & Fazio, 1996). During this time as well, ideas about play began to change,

influenced by new models of occupational therapy practice. With the growth and development of occupational science, writers promoted the idea that play and leisure should be an explicit goal of occupational therapy intervention and not merely a means to another developmental end (Bundy, 1993; Parham, 1996). Play began to be described as an integral part of the human experience (Parham, 1996), important for the quality of life of the child and for enhancing health. Occupational therapy literature throughout the 1990s stressed the importance of considering play *as an occupation* (Bundy, 1992, 1993; Couch, Deitz, & Kanny, 1998; Knox, 1997; Parham, 1996; Wood, 1996). But what exactly does this mean? Before we can focus on occupational therapy's unique perspective on play as an occupation, let us first define occupation.

Defining Occupation

In order to fully understand what play as an occupation means for our profession and our practice, first we must clarify our use of terminology and define "occupation." Our definitions matter (Pierce, 2001; Wilding, 2009). Good definitions allow for shared understanding, better teamwork and role delineation, and improved focus for education and research (Price et al., 2017; Wilding 2009). We must be able to articulate the contribution we can make to the health and well-being of those we serve (Wilding, 2009). However, studies have shown, and anecdotal evidence abounds, that occupational therapists have a hard time explaining what we do (Wilding, 2009; Wilding & Whiteford, 2006, 2007, 2008). Improper, unclear, or inarticulate definitions and explanations about what we do can lead to loss of service provision for those who need it.

Authors have suggested that a comprehensible definition of occupation is "simply ... chunks of culturally and personally meaningful activity in which humans engage that can be named in the lexicon of our culture" (Clark et al., 1991, p. 301). The World Federation of Occupational Therapists (2012) has suggested the definition of occupations as "the everyday activities that people do as individuals, in families and with communities to occupy time and bring meaning and purpose to life. Occupations include things people need to, want to and are expected to do."

Core Concepts of Occupation

The profession of occupational therapy has had almost as much difficulty defining occupation as scholars have had with defining play. Just as the list of characteristics of play described in Chapter 1 helps to create a common understanding of play, core concepts of "occupation" gathered from leaders within the profession are presented in **Box 2.1**. This list of concepts helps generate a shared interpretation of what is meant by occupation.

Occupation vs. Activity

There had been debate in the occupational therapy literature regarding the use of the words *occupation* and *activity* and changes in their usage across time (Bauerschmidt & Nelson, 2011; Hinojosa & Blount, 2004; Nelson, 1996, 1997; Pierce, 2001). The new edition of the OTPF (OTPF-4; AOTA, 2020) clearly differentiates these terms by stating that occupations are meaningful to a particular client, whereas activities are objective actions not specific to a client or a context.

Form, Function, and Meaning

Clark and colleagues (1991) suggested that occupations have *form, function*, and *meaning*. In terms of play, the form includes the specific types of play activities that are commonly accepted and named. As discussed in Chapter 1, the *function* of play may be to promote flexibility, creativity, problem solving, and adaptation to novel situations in the environment. However, as occupational therapy practitioners, we also believe in the power of play to make life joyful for a child and to enhance well-being for both children and adults.

Box 2.1 Core Concepts of Occupation

- Related to human health and life satisfaction
- Meaningful to the individual(s) participating in them
- Unique to the individual
- Reflect cultural or family values
- Provide satisfaction and fulfillment
- Goal directed and extended over time
- May involve multiple tasks
- Meet human needs (things people need to, want to, or are expected to do)
- Involve mental and/or physical skills and abilities but may or may not be observable (cooking vs. daydreaming or learning)
- Activities that can be named in the culture
- May be shared or done with others

The subjective meaning of play for an individual may be one of the most important considerations of play as an occupation (Hammell, 2004). There is no doubt that childhood play is meaningful. Ask any adult about their favored childhood playthings or experiences, and lengthy emotion-laden descriptions can ensue. Authors have suggested that occupational therapy practitioners should value engagement in occupation for the experience and how someone feels while it is occurring, rather than for its outcome (Hasselkus, 2002). In relation to play, our focus should be on the experience of play and how play impacts the child's quality of life, rather than only what play can be used to develop in a child (Hammell, 2004; Parham, 1996). There are many potential meanings of play for an individual, and likely these meanings will change over time with development. The meaning attributed to play may be as varied and unique as the individual players.

Occupations Occur in Natural Environments

Whereas much of the play research in the 1900s in other fields documented children's play in laboratory settings, occupational scientists proposed that occupations be examined as they occur in natural environments. Occupational therapy researchers, therefore, began to examine children's play in typical contexts. Knox (1997) studied children's play in the classroom, observing the play styles of children and the influence of environmental factors on their play style. Play style was conceptualized as including a child's preferences, attitudes, approach, and social reciprocity within a play situation or context. This qualitative study of six children documented a unique play style for each and also the effect of the context on the child's play. Primeau (1998) examined play as it occurred within the home during the typical day-to-day routines of 10 families with preschool-age children. Through extensive participant observation and interviewing, she found that parents used two strategies to play with their child: segregation and inclusion. Segregation strategies were used when parents removed themselves from their child's play or moved the child away from their housework. Inclusion occurred when the parent created some way of playing with the child while in the midst of completing household chores or work. Primeau suggested that these two different strategies lead to either play interspersed with work or play embedded in work. This scaffolded play allowed parents to involve their children in household tasks and assist their child in completing tasks as independently as possible. Nabors and Badawi (1997) observed preschool-age children on the playground repeatedly over 3 months, comparing typically developing children to those with disabilities. They reported differences in the level of social interaction during play between the groups as well as differences in types of play. Their field notes also suggested important roles for teachers as facilitators of play for students with disabilities on the playground. The physical and social contexts are well-recognized aspects of play today.

Current Focus: Emphasizing the Importance of Play

A variety of factors have coalesced to encourage occupational therapists to enhance our focus on play only not as a vehicle to improve other skills, but also as important for children for its own sake, critical for their health and wellness, and worthy of our time and attention. These factors include

- Multiple changes in American society limiting play
- Concerns about the decline of play related to creativity and problem solving
- An international push to support the rights of children
- Increased number of children with autism, corresponding to more study of their play challenges
- Greater numbers of children with mental health concerns

Societal Changes

One historical influence on play has to do with the amount of free time and freedom children have for play as well as access to toys, games, and activities (Chudacoff, 2007; Sandberg & Vuorinen, 2008). A variety of recent and long-term societal changes in the United States have negatively impacted play. Four primary changes will be discussed here.

First, there has been a decline in free-play for children, while structured activities have doubled (Doherty, 2004). When competing for time, academics have taken precedence over play and leisure activity during the school day. Similarly, engagement in structured sports and other extracurricular activities leaves children with minimal time left to their own devices to choose how they wish to play.

Second, fears of unintentional injury associated with play have also restricted play opportunities for children. Newer playground regulations have substantially altered the types of play equipment available on playgrounds, as well as the surfaces underneath them (Spiegal, Gill, Harbottle, & Ball, 2014), often on the basis of very few reported injuries. The reduction of access to risky play is a major change in the nature of free play for children in the United States as the culture has become increasingly concerned with safety (Staemfli, 2009). These concerns are reflected in the laws passed as well as the reaction to injuries; the fear of litigation has curtailed childhood access to risky play (Kleppe, 2018; Staemfli, 2009). This has consequences for children. In schools with reduced rules and greater opportunities for risks, children are more likely to report being happy and are more likely to play with other children on the playground (Farmer et al., 2017).

Third, play in our current culture is significantly more under adult supervision than in generations past. Overprotective parenting now often restricts children's activities or encourages supervised play (Little, 2015; McFarland & Laird, 2018). Children of this generation have been called the "bubblewrap" generation (Malone, 2007). There has also been a reduction in independent mobility of children within their own neighborhoods, often due to fears of traffic or "stranger danger" (Foster et al., 2014; Little, 2015).

Finally, the adoption of many sedentary, digital forms of activities in addition to television has changed the form of play substantially (Loprinzi & Davis, 2016; O'Keeffe & Clarke-Pearson, 2011), with some reports suggesting children spend more than 6 hours a day in front of screens and on a variety of social media platforms (Connected Kids, 2015, 2018). The rise in childhood obesity has led to an examination of childhood activity levels, which has revealed the importance of outdoor, physically active play (Janssen, 2014; McCambridge et al., 2006).

All of these changes have led to a call for greater outdoor and risky play opportunities for children and the recognition of the importance of play for childhood (Brown & Vaughan, 2009; Elkind, 2007; Ginsberg, 2007; Hirsh-Pasek, Golinkoff, Berk, & Singer, 2009; Tremblay et al., 2015). These calls originated from authors and professionals in the fields of medicine, psychology, psychiatry, child development, and education and are being joined by occupational therapists. Similar ideas have begun to circulate in business as well.

Growing Play Concerns and Organizational Responses

Business leaders and others have noted a decline in worker creativity, and some have attributed this to the lack of play in childhood (Bronson & Merryman, 2014; Florida, 2004; Kim, 2011; Mercer 2014; Tsai, 2012; Zosh et al., 2017). With the growing fear in the United States that the lack of play for children could have serious long-term consequences, some businesses and organizations have taken the step of formally encouraging play through various mechanisms of support. For example, the LEGO Foundation supports the mission of engaging children in learning through play, by contributing resources to education and research. The Toy Association has created an online presence to help families play more through their Genius of Play campaign. Playcore, a company that creates indoor and outdoor play spaces, has partnered with a variety of individuals to create research supportive of play. Similarly, the International Play Equipment Manufacturing Association now promotes the benefits of play and playgrounds through its online presence. These and other companies have also contributed to a new focus in business on promoting worker creativity through play (**Table 2.1**).

International Support for the Right to Play

The United Nations (UN) Convention on the Rights of the Child, approved in 1989 by the UN, is an international treaty that has been ratified by almost every country in the world, but as of yet, not the United States. In relation to play, Article 31 of the treaty states, "every child has the right to rest and leisure, *to engage in play and recreational activities appropriate to the age of the child* and to participate freely in cultural life and the arts. That member governments shall respect and promote the right of the child to participate fully in cultural and artistic life and shall encourage the provision of appropriate and equal opportunities for cultural, artistic, recreational and leisure activity" (UN, 1989). Subsequently, research and policy from around the world has had a greater focus on the importance of play for children with and without disabilities (Casey, 2017; Mulder, Carter, & Graf, 2019) and those in crisis (Rintoul, 2018). A variety of international organizations, many now with chapters in the United States, have grown to support children in play (**Table 2.2**), such as the International Play Association, Play England, and Right to Play. Pop Up Adventure Play promotes small, specially designed adventure playgrounds and playworker training to support children's ability to play, experience freedom, and take risks. In

Table 2.1 Businesses and Organizations Promoting Worker and Child Play and Creativity

Organization	Purpose Related to Play	Web Information
The LEGO Company: LEGO Serious Play Model for Business	Promotes creativity in workers through a facilitated play-based approach to problem solving.	https://www.lego.com/en-us/seriousplay
The LEGO Company: LEGO Prescription for Play	A program for healthcare providers of young (18 mo–24 mo) children.	https://www.lego.com/en-us/campaigns /prescription-for-play
The Toy Association Genius of Play	Promotes play in families through information and education.	https://thegeniusofplay.org/
International Play Equipment Manufacturing Association— The Voice of Play	Promotes understanding of the importance and benefits of play as well as the science behind these claims.	https://voiceofplay.org/
Playcore	Promotes play and recreation through provision of resources related to inclusive play and active play among other areas.	https://www.playcore.com/programs
Life Is Good Playmakers	Helps children by using the power of joyful play for healing. They focus on optimism and relationship building.	https://www.lifeisgood.com/kidsfoundation /about-playmakers.html

Table 2.2 International Organizations Supporting Play

Name of Organization or Resource	Purpose	Web Link
Play England	Promotes nature play, street play, adventure playgrounds, and more.	https://www.playengland.org.uk/
Right to Play	Promotes play to assist children in crisis.	https://righttoplay.com/en/
Pop Up Adventure Play	Supports play through playwork.	https://www.popupadventureplay.org/
Global Recess Alliance	Newly formed in response to COVID-19 to ensure that when children return to school after COVID, they will have access to recess.	https://globalrecessalliance.org/recess-statement/
The Playwork Foundation	Promotes playwork and advocates for play.	https://playworkfoundation.org/about/
Playworks Foundation	Provides assistance to schools to improve recess.	https://www.playworks.org/about/

response to the 2020 COVID-19 pandemic, an international group of scholars and researchers formed The Global Recess Alliance to support a return to recess when students resume in-person school. The Playwork Foundation is another recently founded organization, supporting playworkers and devoted to the rights of children to play.

The Rise in Prevalence of Autism Spectrum Disorder

A notable increase in the number of children diagnosed with autism spectrum disorder (ASD) has been documented by multiple studies (Centers for Disease Control [CDC], 2020). The spike may have begun earlier, but the evidence for the changes strengthened as the millennium changed (CDC, 2020; Nevison, Blaxill, & Zahorodny, 2018). The dramatic increase in ASD led to an explosion of research into the condition (Dawson et al., 2013). As one of the common symptoms of ASD is difficulties with symbolism and pretend play, the number of studies that has been completed on play in ASD has also grown (Jarrold, 2003; Memari et al., 2015; Thiemann-Bourque, Johnson, & Brady, 2019). Overall curiosity about the impact of play has expanded to interest researchers in many fields, including occupational therapy.

Rise in Childhood Mental Health Concerns

Mental health disorders among children are those that impact a child's ability to learn, behave, regulate emotions, cause distress, or lead to difficulty with daily activities (CDC, 2020). In the United States alone, 9.4% (6.1 million) of children ages 2–17 have been diagnosed with ADHD. Of children ages 3–17, 7.4% (4.5 million) have a diagnosed behavior problem, 7.1% (4.4 million) have diagnosed anxiety, and 3.2% (1.9 million) have diagnosed depression.

The number of children and adolescents experiencing a psychiatric disorder appears to be on the rise (Hamovitch, Acri, & Bornheimer, 2018). The CDC (2020) reports that rates of anxiety and depression among children have increased over time; the National Comorbidity Survey Adolescent Supplement showed an increase in the prevalence of anxiety and mood disorders, behavior disorders, and substance abuse/dependence (Merikangas et al., 2010), and the National Survey of Children's Health found an upward trend in mental health disorders among children between 1994 and 2011 (Perou et al., 2013). Findings regarding child mental health tend to reflect only those who are diagnosed and does not reflect or include those whose lives are still impacted by symptoms of anxiety and depression who may not meet diagnostic criteria or who have not been diagnosed for other reasons (i.e., access to health care, stigma associated with mental health). As such, the number of children who receive mental health treatment is far lower than the estimated need; however, despite this, more children and adolescents are using mental health services based on analyses of insurance claims and the Medical Expenditure Panel Surveys (Hamovitch et al., 2018).

Certain authors have specifically related the mental health concerns of today to a decline in play in our country (Gray, 2011). There is support for play as important to mental health, parent–child interaction, attachment, and quality of life (Bowlby, 1988; Ginsberg, 2007; Gray, 2011). Anxiety and depression are often experienced by people who perceive that they are not in control of their own lives, and conversely, those who do feel in control of their own lives experience anxiety and depression less often. This relationship may be related to a societal shift that once emphasized learning and doing that was intrinsically motivated (i.e., interest, competence, affiliation, autonomy) to more extrinsic factors (i.e., grades, financial gain, status) (Twenge et al., 2010). The current emphasis on academic readiness has led to an increased focus on structured activities to promote academic skills as early as preschool with a concomitant decrease in time and opportunity for free play (Yogman, Garner, Hutchison, Hirsh-Pasek, & Golinkoff, 2018). If the current societal trend of devaluing play continues to deprive children of opportunities to feel a sense of control with less structured experiences, the rates of mental health disorders among children may not improve and in turn worsen. Given what is known about the biological, psychological, and social benefits of play, it is important to consider the consequences that will impact subsequent developmental life stages if play is not a priority among young children.

Occupational Therapy's Continued Contributions

As a result of these factors, occupational therapists have added their voices to those of educators, mental health providers, businesses, and organizations in raising an alarm about the lack of free play, outdoor and nature play, and risky play, and in general supporting the importance of play for children (Lynch & Moore, 2016; Ray-Kaeser & Lynch, 2017; Stagnitti & Unsworth, 2000; Tanta & Kuhaneck, 2020). Occupational therapists also increasingly have engaged in scholarship in the area of play. Although encouraging, research in the United States and abroad continues to document our limited focus on play in our clinical practices (Lynch, Prellwitz, Schulze, & Moore, 2018; Miller Kuhaneck, Tanta, Coombs, & Pannone, 2013; Moore & Lynch, 2018). It is intended that research will translate broadly into practice so that play becomes a common part of pediatric occupational therapy practice.

The growth in occupational therapy play-related scholarship in the last 20 years is impressive. With our focus on play as an occupation, studies have considered the meaning of play for children, the way in which play occurs in natural environments and the impact of context on play experiences, the influence of play partners, and cultural factors surrounding play engagement. Additionally, occupational therapists have contributed to the evidence regarding specific interventions to promote play and have increasingly considered the role of sensory processing in relation to play.

The Meaning of Play for Children

Occupational therapy researchers have asked children and adolescents about their perceptions regarding the meaning of play (Caiazzo, Sarra, Vechionne, Miller, & Miller Kuhaneck, 2008; Heah, Case, McGuire, & Law, 2007; Miller & Kuhaneck, 2008; Pollack et al., 1997; Skär, 2002; Tamm & Skär, 2000). Through interviews or surveys, children and adolescents generally responded that they choose to play what they found fun. Fun, in turn, had to do with the level of challenge, the level of motor activity, and the level of interaction provided by the play activity. Although children reported highly individualized choices of what might be considered favored play, they indicated a strong preference for active play, outdoor play, and play with a medium challenge level. They also preferred to play with peers. Adolescents report similar rationales for their choices and a greater preference for activities with friends. For future research, occupational therapists may want to consider new methods of examining the meaning of play for children such as via a self-report tool (McDonald & Vigen, 2012).

Children with disabilities report many of the same interests and concerns as typically developing children. Children with ADHD reported similar preferences for who they preferred to play with (peers), but they were found to have different preferences for where and what to play (Pfieffer et al., 2011). Children with disabilities report the importance of playground spaces for their play that provide the appropriate challenge, opportunities for sensory and pretend play, and equitable access (Ripat & Becker, 2012). Adults with disabilities have also documented the meaning of their earlier play by reminiscing (Sandberg, Björck-Åkesson, & Granlund, 2004), noting themes of participation and exclusion and the importance of challenge in play.

For those children who have challenges with communicating, a different approach is required to become informed regarding the meaning of play. Spitzer (2003a, 2003b, 2004) used the qualitative method of participant observation to understand the occupations of five children with autism ages 3 and 4 years. None of the children had sufficient language to adequately explain why they were engaging in their chosen activities, which often were unique, unusual, and not readily named. Spitzer was able to begin to infer the meaning of the play occupations with careful observation of the "what" and the "how" to attempt to understand the "why." To do so, Spitzer recommends that adults suspend adult judgments, assume that the child's actions are meant as communication, share in activities with the child to try to understand their meaning, follow what the child is doing, and engage in the activity themselves to examine the sensations the activity provides.

Another way to attempt to understand the meaning of play for children without language is to ask their parents as surrogates (Askins, Diasio, Szewerniak, & Cahill, 2013; Case-Smith & Miller Kuhaneck, 2008; Graham, Truman, & Holgate, 2015; Schneider & Rosenblum, 2014; Shikako-Thomas et al., 2012). Parents report that, in examining their child's play, they gain better awareness and insight, suggesting potential value when occupational therapists include parents in assessing play. Studies with parents have documented that children with disabilities do indicate preferences for play that may be similar to nondisabled peers, they seek to create an outcome or have an effect upon their environment through their play, demonstrate pleasure with mastery, and improve their well-being with participation in preferred leisure.

An Occupational Therapy Model of Playfulness

Bundy developed a model of playfulness and an assessment tool to measure playfulness. She considered playfulness a style of approaching activities that transcended the activity itself. Playfulness manifested joy, flexibility, and spontaneity. Bundy's Model of Playfulness (Skard & Bundy, 2008) proposed three primary elements that must be present for playfulness: intrinsic motivation, internal control, and freedom to suspend reality. These three characteristics can be present to a greater or lesser degree in any play situation. A playful child with intrinsic motivation is focused on the activity process, not the product, and that child chooses the activity because he or she wants to do it. A child with internal control decides whom to play with, what to play with, and how and when to play. A child who has the freedom to suspend reality is

able to pretend and take risks. The Test of Playfulness (Bundy, 2003) measures motivation, control, freedom from the constraints of reality, and the ability to interact with others using cues to frame an activity as play.

Consideration of Context and Culture

Occupational therapy practitioners have increasingly documented the importance of contextual features in children's play. Skard and Bundy (2008) created an assessment tool to examine the environmental supports for playfulness and the fit between the player and the play environment. Important environmental features supportive of playfulness include physical safety, space for play, time for play, availability of developmentally appropriate and preferred play materials, and appropriate social interaction with either peers or adults. In an examination of the playground as a natural environment, Miller and colleagues (2017) documented the ability of a playground to provide enhanced sensory features, promote positive affect, socialization, and novel motor skills. They also documented the specific types of play that might be most often observed on various types of playground equipment.

The impact of culture on play has been less well studied in occupational therapy. In one qualitative examination of the play of 20 Mayan children in five families, the researchers found that play was allowed if it did not interfere with adult work but was not encouraged by adults as play, as it often is in the United States (Bazyk, Stalnaker, Llerena, Ekelman, & Bazyk, 2003). However, the authors' findings did support play as a universal desire of children because these children somehow found ways to play within their daily activities.

Consideration of the Relationship between Sensory Integration and Play

Using occupational therapy assessments such as the SIPT or the Sensory Processing Measure or both, researchers have documented play deficits related to dyspraxia in children with ASD (Bodison, 2015; Kuhaneck & Britner, 2013). These difficulties in praxis may be at least part of the reason for documented difficulties in the ability to create or generate novel ideas for play activities in children with ASD (Lee et al., 2016). Ideational praxis in particular may be specifically important for the development of play (Serrada-Tejeda, Santos-del-Riego, May-Benson, & Pérez-de-Heredia-Torres, 2021).

Children with sensory processing concerns or probable developmental coordination disorder (DCD) have been found to have less-advanced play skills and to be less likely to engage in play than typically developing peers (Kennedy-Behr et al., 2013). Sensory issues do not necessarily predispose a child to choose different play than typically developing peers, although qualitative differences in how children play may be noted (Cosbey, Johnston, Dunn, & Bauman, 2012).

A systematic review examining the relationship with sensory processing and play found some support for the idea that sensory processing may impact play preferences and perhaps play performance (Watts, Stagnitti, & Brown, 2014). Specific studies examining the relationship between sensory processing and pretend play have suggested that social participation, proprioception, vestibular, and tactile processing scores are predictive of scores on a measure of pretend play (Roberts, Stagnitti, Brown, & Bhopti, 2018).

The idea that sensory processing patterns of children and parents are related and may influence parent–child play has not been fully supported (Welters-Davis & Mische Lawson, 2011). However, occupational therapists have examined the relationships between child sensory processing, parental playfulness, and parental self-efficacy (belief in one's own abilities), finding that sensory issues do impact parental self-efficacy, and parent playfulness is related to a parent's emotional self-efficacy (Román-Oyola et al., 2017). These results prompt a consideration of parental support for play in establishing emotional connections with their child with ASD. Parents of children with ASD do relate their ability to interact with their child during play and their experience of positive emotions with play to their feelings of self-efficacy although mothers and fathers report different perceptions regarding these relationships (Román-Oyola et al., 2018).

Expanded Examination of Play and Playfulness in Varied Populations

Difficulties in play and playfulness for those with disabilities had been reported in the past; however, recent occupational therapy scholarship has furthered knowledge in this area. Researchers examined the pretend play of children with cerebral palsy, one area of play that had not been studied extensively in this population, and found that 65% of the children with cerebral palsy studied had challenges with pretend play (Pfeiffer et al., 2011). In a group of subjects reared in Romanian orphanages, play behaviors were assessed with a naturalistic observation method, and results suggested that these children engaged in a variety of play behaviors. The relationship between their cognitive abilities and their play behaviors was strong, and it appeared that the children played at a level that better matched their mental age (Daunhauer et al., 2007).

Multiple studies of playfulness have been completed. Studies have examined the playfulness of children with ASD (Skaines, Rodger, & Bundy 2006) in both unstructured and structured conditions. Children with ASD demonstrate less playfulness than typically developing peers, although they are more playful in a facilitated, structured play condition. Occupational therapists have considered the theoretical relationships between theory of mind (the ability to attribute mental states to others), pretend play deficits, and playfulness in those with ASD (Chan, Chen, Feng, Lee, & Chen, 2016), suggesting that playfulness may be unrelated to theory of mind. Children with ADHD also were found to be less playful but demonstrated uneven performance on items related to social dimensions of playfulness (Cordier et al., 2010).

Studies of play and playfulness have now also begun to document the importance of the interaction between parent, child, and teacher in relation to playfulness (Porter & Bundy, 2001). Studies have suggested that supportive maternal play behavior may encourage object play (Roach, Barratt, Miller, & Leavitt, 1998), and there is research to support that parent *responsiveness* is important for child playfulness (Chiarello, Huntington, & Bundy, 2006). There is also some evidence that play is more developmentally competent when an adult caregiver is present (Daunhauer et al., 2007). Some authors therefore promote playful parenting (Cohen, 2001). The developmental of an assessment called the Parent/Caregiver's Support of Young Children's Playfulness Scale (Waldman-Levi & Bundy, 2014, 2016) has allowed the examination of the complex relationships between child playfulness and adult behaviors in play (Waldman-Levi, Grinion, & Olson, 2019). (Please see Chapter 11 for more on this topic). Parents can encourage their child's playfulness by supporting their exploration and decision making. One study of playfulness in teachers led to the unsurprising finding that teacher silliness and spontaneity were related to child playfulness (Pinchover, 2017). Attempts have been made to better understand adult playfulness as well (Guitard, Ferland, & Dutil, 2005). However, little research yet exists documenting the ability of occupational therapy to specifically increase *playfulness* in parents or the effects of increasing playfulness in parents on their children. Thus, it may be important to consider the playfulness of the adults in a child's life; but much more research in this area is needed.

Efficacy of Interventions to Promote Play and Playfulness

A variety of specific interventions used by occupational therapists have been shown to promote play and playfulness, such as robots (Ríos-Rincón et al., 2015), Floortime (Dionne & Martini, 2011), and community playgroups (Fabrizi & Hubbell, 2017). Occupational therapists have documented the efficacy of aquatic community playgroups for children with ASD to promote playfulness (Fabrizi, 2015). Community playgroups were also effective in promoting playfulness in an early intervention setting (Fabrizi, Ito, & Winston, 2016). Please see Chapter 14 for more on this topic.

Occupational therapists have also studied the impact of video modeling, peer-mediated intervention, and parent-delivered interventions for promoting play and playfulness in children (Cordier et al., 2009; Henning, Cordier, Wilkes-Gillan, & Falkmer, 2016; Kent, Cordier, Joosten, Wilkes-Gillan, & Bundy, 2019; Wilkes et al., 2011; Wilkes-Gillan et al., 2014a, 2014b; Wilkes-Gillan, Bundy, Cordier, Lincoln, & Chen, 2016). As a whole, this group of research has suggested that occupational therapy intervention including parents and peer-mediated approaches can improve playfulness, particularly in children with ADHD. Parents generally found the intervention to be appropriate and acceptable (Wilkes-Gillan, Bundy, Cordier, Lincoln, & Hancock, 2015). Similar intervention may also be worthwhile for children with ASD (Kent, Cordier, Joosten, Wilkes-Gillan, & Bundy, 2018; Kent et al., 2020; Kent, Cordier, Joosten, Wilkes-Gillan, & Bundy, 2019).

Occupational therapists have also demonstrated effectiveness of a specific child-led and play-based program called "Learn to Play" that is meant to promote self-initiated play and pretense (Stagnitti, 1998, 2009; O'Connor & Stagnitti, 2011; Stagnitti, O'Connor, & Sheppard, 2012). Learn to Play is based on developmental appropriateness, ensuring attention to the play task, modeling and talking about the play as it occurs, engaging with the child emotionally, and using imitation and repetition with variation. The therapist creates a play story and promotes the development of symbolism while focusing on specific play sequences, substitution of objects during play, creation of play scripts, and specific forms of pretend play.

Two reviews of interventions to promote play for children with ASD found that play can be altered by intervention (Kent et al., 2020; Kuhaneck, Spitzer, & Bodison, 2020). Strategies may be most effective if targeted to an individual child with ASD as opposed to a child in a group, or via providing the intervention to the parent or teacher. It is not yet clearly established which combinations, dosages, and methods are most effective. However, there is moderate to strong evidence for modeling interventions (video/peer) and imitating the child with ASD.

Examining Our Own Practices

Recently, occupational therapists have more carefully considered our own practices in relation to play. This has resulted in promotion of new practices (Kuhaneck, Spitzer, & Miller, 2010) and new models and ideas about the way in which we use play in therapy (Ray-Kaeser, & Lynch, 2017). Bundy (2011) considers five facets of play that have importance to occupational therapy: the child's skills and abilities to play, the attitude or approach to play (playfulness), the activities of play, the environmental support for play, and the motivation for play. A variety of surveys of occupational therapists working with children (Miller Kuhaneck et al., 2013; Lynch et al., 2018; Mitchell, Hale, Lawrence, Murillo, Newman, & Smith, 2018; Moore & Lynch, 2018) have documented that the profession has work to do to realize our full potential in the realm of play.

In occupational therapy intervention, play may be used in one of three ways, as a reward, as a tool, and as an occupation (Tanta & Kuhaneck, 2020). As a reward, play is used as positive reinforcement to gain compliance with an adult agenda. In such a fashion, it is no different than using ice cream to encourage a child to eat vegetables first. When occupational therapists use play as a tool, there is also an adult agenda, but a more playful approach to "getting the work done." In these sessions, the specific form of play is chosen through activity analysis because the play activity will allow "work" on other important skills of therapy. There are various levels of adult direction available when one uses play as a tool (Ray-Kaeser & Lynch, 2017). There is a continuum from work to play, considering the amount of intrinsic to extrinsic motivation and adult direction to child direction provided in an occupational therapy session. The therapy may vary from completely adult directed with the child working (no play) to completely child directed, chosen, and led (play). In the middle the therapist has a choice of how much control to share with a child

Table 2.3 Explanations and Examples of the Ways Play Is Used in Occupational Therapy

	Play as a Reward	Play as a Tool	Play as an Occupation
Emphasis	Work	Blend of Work and Play	Play
Purpose	Reinforce behavior to gain compliance with adult agenda	Improve skills in areas other than play	Improve play Improve access Improve playfulness Improve motivation
Examples	Johnny if you do XYZ that I am asking you to do first, then you can play _____. Let's make a list of the things we need to do, and when all of that is done, you can play on the iPad for 3 minutes.	Mary, let's get this doll dressed for the tea party, can you button her dress? (to work on buttoning) Let's stack up as many blocks as we can, and then we can throw these bean bags to knock the tower down (to work on accuracy of throwing).	How can we make it so that you can play XYZ with your friends? (adapt materials or environment) Here are some new games, which should we try to play? Which of these things would you like to play? Let's work with your mom and dad and your neighbors to create a play street in your neighborhood so you can play with your friends outside. Let's pretend to be (X favorite character). What would X do? How can we play X?
Primary Approach to Intervention (AOTA, 2020)	Establish, Restore	Establish, Restore, Modify	Establish, Restore, Maintain, Modify Create, Promote, Prevent

and how playful to be. The therapist may select and choose activities or the child may select and choose activities, while the therapist supports and scaffolds (Ray-Kaeser & Lynch, 2017). The amount of sharing of control makes the play more or less work-like or play-like. When play is used in an occupational therapy session as an occupation, the focus is on developing the child's agency, engagement in play, expanding preferred forms of play, and improving the child's overall well-being and quality of life through play. See **Table 2.3** for examples of each of these forms of play in occupational therapy intervention. Please also refer to Chapter 1 for further discussion and a depiction of play as a continuum.

One Possible Future for the Occupational Therapy Practitioner in Relation to Play

An ambassador is a representative of, and someone who promotes, a specific activity. A champion is someone who argues for a cause on behalf of someone else (Merriam-Webster, 2020; Oxford, 2020). Our profession has been repeatedly called to act as

play ambassadors and champions since the 1990s (Bundy 1993 ; Couch, Deitz, & Kanny, 1998; Parham, 1996). This call becomes more urgent with the societal changes described in this chapter. Occupational therapists are not alone in understanding the impact of these changes on children and now have powerful allies available in business, education, medicine, and psychology. As you will read in detail throughout the rest of this text, there are a variety of interventions that occupational therapists can provide directly to children, but in order to change societal contexts, often public awareness and policy change must occur. Both typically occur in response to strong advocacy, and advocacy can begin with each individual therapist.

Continuing Education

Occupational therapists have reported that one of the barriers to their consistent inclusion of play as a focus of their therapy was their lack of knowledge (Miller Kuhaneck et al., 2013). A multitude of excellent continuing education options are available for learning about play outside traditional sources. For example, there are a variety of opportunities for

Table 2.4 Continuing Education Opportunities Related to Play

Name of Organization or Resource	Type of Continuing Education	Internet Link
The U.S. Play Coalition	Annual play conference	https://usplaycoalition.org/
The International Council for Children's Play	Annual conferences on play with international audiences	https://www.iccp-play.org/conferences.html
International Play Association	International conferences every 3 years	http://ipaworld.org/conferences/
The LEGO Foundation	Annual conference	https://www.legoideaconference.com/en/about/highlights/
The Association for the Study of Play	Annual conferences on play, annual journal, and quarterly newsletter	http://www.tasplay.org/conference/past/
Fairydust Teaching	Annual Play Summit	https://fairydustteaching.com/

interdisciplinary conferences on play (**Table 2.4**). Gaining competence with specific play assessments will allow the therapist to use them comfortably (see Chapters 3 and 4). Learning how to write goals that can be achieved through play and that will be acceptable for various work settings may be an important first step. Understanding policy regarding recess and local play spaces may be critical information in particular locales, as well as the skills necessary to advocate for changes through lobbying, writing to legislators, providing public testimony, participating in school board meetings, and so on. Occupational therapists not only can provide the scientific evidence to support the promotion of play, but also have a platform to share the stories and be the voice on behalf of those we work with who are often unheard. Occupational therapists must also educate themselves regarding the growing evidence of two things. First, that play is important and, second, that play can be improved by therapy (see **Box 2.2** for self-study resources regarding the importance of play). For example, play is easily associated with specific cognitive tasks related to academic functions, making it more likely to be considered acceptable school-based practice. Therefore, therapists working in school systems should be familiar with the multitude of studies linking pretend play with executive functioning (Berk & Meyers, 2013; Carlson, White, & Davis-Unger, 2014; Kelly, Dissanayake, Ihsen, & Hammond, 2011).

For those occupational therapists less acquainted with the literature on family-centered care, it is also important to find ways to educate oneself about the importance of providing assistance and therapy to families and not only the pediatric client (see https://

www.ipfcc.org/index.html). Parents may feel, at least in some cases, that peer play and friendships are an important outcome of occupational therapy (Cohen, 2001). A limited relationship is often found between competence with specific skills and quality of life in individuals with disability (Gibson et al., 2009). Therefore, in providing family-centered care, the therapist may ascertain that play, happiness, and friendships are, in fact, more important goals for the family of a client than remediation of specific skills. A focus on skills rather than play, in some cases, may indicate a lack of consideration for family-centered care.

Educating Others

Armed with new knowledge gained by one's own continuing education, the occupational therapy practitioner is now in a position to share that knowledge with others. These others may include professional colleagues, team members, policy makers, and parents. Education of others may take many forms, including direct conversation, write-ups and newsletter articles, or blogs.

Some occupational therapists have reported that one of the barriers to their consistent inclusion of play as a focus of their therapy was the idea that play was not part of their role in their work setting (Miller Kuhaneck et al., 2013). Therapists felt that other team members, such as teachers, had taken on the area of play as their domain. They also felt that other team members did not necessarily want them to focus on play in occupational therapy, considering other areas, for example, fine motor skills, a greater priority. To reduce this barrier, therapists must be sure to discuss play during team meetings, explain why play is part of the role of occupational therapy, consistently document occupational therapy assessment of play, and highlight the relationship of play to a child's happiness, quality of life, and well-being, in addition to its importance for learning, problem solving, and creativity.

For parents, occupational therapists can explain the importance of play, ask parents about their concerns regarding their child's play, and create newsletters or brochures providing resources to help parents generate play ideas for the home. Therapists can help parents with selection of appropriate toys and activities and ways to improve their playfulness while engaging with their child.

Improving Reimbursement

Occupational therapists need to become emboldened to fight for play as part of our role and something that should be reimbursed as part of our intervention. Therapists reported reimbursement as another barrier to their use of play in practice (Miller Kuhaneck et al., 2013). True, there is no "code" to be reimbursed for play. There is no code for "handwriting," either. Yet even without a specific CPT code, fine-motor and handwriting skills are a both a frequent reason for referral and a common intervention focus (Barnes et al., 2003; Case-Smith, 1995; Oliver, 1990; Reisman, 1991; Wehrmann, Chiu, Reid, & Sinclair, 2006). There are CPT codes that could be used that would allow for a focus on play as long as therapists write functional goals that are appropriate reimbursable outcomes of therapy. See Chapter 5 for more information about goals for play.

Changing Environments

Occupational therapists can work with local parks, local schools, and local community organizations to improve the opportunities for play. This may include the provision of loose parts play (Bundy et al., 2008; Gibson, Cornell, & Gill, 2017) or in developing Play Streets (Cortinez-O'Ryan, Albagli, Sadarangani, & Aguilar-Farias, 2017; D'Haese, Van Dyck, De Bourdeaudhuij, Deforche, & Cardon, 2015; Espinoza, McMahan, Naffzinger, & Wiersma, 2012; Zieff, Chaudhuri, & Musselman, 2016). It could include volunteering to assess local playgrounds using appropriate assessment tools, in order to make recommendations for improvements (Moore & Lynch, 2015; Prellwitz & Skär, 2007; Stout, 1988; also see Chapters 9 and 10).

Changing environments can also occur in the home. Occupational therapists have a unique skill-set to facilitate supportive environments to promote mental health among children and, as a means of prevention, can promote the participation in meaningful activities, such as through play, to enhance emotional well-being, mental health, and social competence (AOTA, 2020). Social connection is critical to one's sense of self and mental health. As such, emotional regulation, problem solving, and understanding social etiquette are skills an occupational therapist can promote through meaningful play in an effort to help children establish and maintain friendships (AOTA, 2020). Such friendships could then serve as a protective factor for mental health disorders

Involvement

Occupational therapists can write letters to the editor, write letters to their government officials, and create blog posts that improve awareness of the importance of play and occupational therapists' unique focus in relation to play. Therapists can get involved with local or national "Hill Day" events. Therapists often have stories from real events and families that can push legislators to understand the real impact of their decisions. More occupational therapists can join organizations that are advocating for play such as the US Play Coalition, the Association for the Study of Play, or the American Association for the Child's Right to Play. Therapists can sign up to get involved with outreach and educating others or could organize a play day. Therapists can write posts such as for thegeniusofplay.org to document occupational therapists' ability to contribute in unique ways. Therapists might also get involved with local university research centers and faculty members who are researching play to help with data collection, and occupational therapy researchers could collaborate with some of the organizations now doing play research to include the occupational therapy perspective in these studies. See **Table 2.5** for resources to become a play ambassador.

Table 2.5 Other Resources for Becoming a Play Ambassador

Name of Organization or Resource	Purpose	Internet Link
Play Streets	By temporarily closing a street to traffic, a play street allows children with limited access to other play spaces to have a safe place to play with others.	https://uploads.strikinglycdn.com/files/2d72cca6-1b05-4fc9-ac33-098b324c300e/CoDesign%20Studio_Play%20Streets%20Toolkit.pdf
The US Play Coalition	Therapists can sign up to be play ambassadors with this organization.	https://usplaycoalition.org/communication/play-ambassadors
The American Association for the Child's Right to Play	Supports advocacy to promote play. Supports Play days.	http://www.ipausa.org/ http://www.ipausa.org/pdf/PlayDayBooklet.pdf
The Strong Museum of Play	Explores how play encourages learning, creativity, and discovery. The Museum has online archives, and the organization publishes the *American Journal of Play*.	https://www.museumofplay.org/
Right to Play	Promotes play to assist children in crisis.	https://www.righttoplayusa.org/en/
Let Grow Project	Believes that the overprotectiveness of current society is harmful for children and seeks to allow children more freedom and to promote resilience.	https://letgrow.org/ https://letgrow.org/history-of-let-grow/
PlayCore	Supports communities through play and recreation.	https://www.playcore.com/research
National Institute for Play	Promotes play through research.	http://www.nifplay.org/
USA–International Play Association	Works to protect and promote a child's right to play.	https://ipausa.org/

Conclusion

The original articles of incorporation of the National Society for the Promotion of Occupational Therapy suggested that the profession "advance occupation as therapeutic" and "study of the effects of occupation on humans" (Nelson, 1997). In regard to play, how well have occupational therapists advanced play as a therapeutic occupation and studied the impact of play on human beings? Recent efforts have been promising. Much has changed since the last edition of this book, and occupational therapists have increasingly been studying play and promoting play. This chapter has provided an overview of some of the many contributions occupational therapists have made through their writing and research. Though the profession's views on play have changed since its inception, there has been a resurgence of interest in occupational therapy research in the realm of play. New conceptions of both occupations in general and play specifically have challenged occupational therapists to alter our views and examine the meaning and importance of play for children. Occupational therapy's emphasis on client-centered care pushes us to consider the preferences of the children we serve and to incorporate play and playfulness into our evaluations and interventions on a consistent basis. There is a growing acceptance of the importance of play and playfulness for children and adults in diverse professions outside of occupational therapy, which suggests that now, more than ever, we must assert ourselves as a profession able and willing to help children to play.

In this day and age of accountability and focus on reimbursement, play can be mistakenly believed to be unimportant enough to warrant our time. Therapists may be pushed to focus solely on the development of other skills. However, the premise of this entire book is that for the occupational therapist working with a child with a disability, play should be evaluated and included as a *primary* goal of intervention. Work and play should not be segmented. We must express to those on our team and those who employ us that play *is* important and is worthy of our time. This book provides the information to make well-founded arguments in support of play in general and in therapy for our clients. The editors and authors of this book hope you will follow your reading of this content with a plan to become a play ambassador and champion!

References

American Occupational Therapy Association. (2021). Occupational therapy scope of practice. *American Journal of Occupational Therapy*, 75(Suppl. 3), 7513410030. https://doi.org/10.5014/ajot.2021.75S3005

AOTA (2020). Occupational therapy practice framework: Domain and process (4th ed.). *American Journal of Occupational Therapy* 74(Supplement_2), 7412410010p1–7412410010p87. https://doi.org/10.5014/ajot.2020.74S2001

Askins, L., Diasio, B., Szewerniak, D., & Cahill, S. M. (2013). Children with developmental disabilities and their motivation to play. *The Open Journal of Occupational Therapy*, 1(4), 4.

Ayres, A. J. (1963). The development of perceptual-motor abilities: A theoretical basis for treatment of dysfunction. *American Journal of Occupational Therapy*, 17, 221–225.

Ayres, A. J. (1964). Tactile functions: The relation to hyperactive and perceptual motor behavior. *Perceptual and Motor Skills*, 20, 288–292.

Ayres A. J. (1971). Characteristics of types of sensory integrative dysfunction. *American Journal of Occupational Therapy*, 25, 329–334.

Ayres, A. J. (1972). *Sensory integration and learning disorders*. Los Angeles: Western Psychological Services.

Barnes, K. J., Beck, A. J., Vogel, K. A., Grice, K. O., & Murphy, D. (2003). Perceptions regarding school-based occupational therapy for children with emotional disturbances. *American Journal of Occupational Therapy*, 57(3), 337–341.

Bauerschmidt, B., & Nelson, D. L. (2011). The terms occupation and activity over the history of official occupational therapy publications. *American Journal of Occupational Therapy*, 65(3), 338–345.

Bazyk, S., Stalnaker, D., Llerena, M., Ekelman, B., & Bazyk, J. (2003). Play in Mayan children. *American Journal of Occupational Therapy*, 57, 273–283.

Berk, L. E., & Meyers, A. B. (2013). The role of make-believe play in the development of executive function: status of research and future directions. *American Journal of Play*, 6(1), 98–110.

Besio, S., Bulgarelli, D., & Stancheva-Popkostadinova, V. (2018). *Evaluation of children's play. Tools and methods* (pp. 1–147). De Gruyter.

Bodison, S. C. (2015). Developmental dyspraxia and the play skills of children with autism. *American Journal of Occupational Therapy*, 69(5), 6905185060p1-6905185060p6.

Bowlby, J. (1988). Developmental psychiatry comes of age. *The American journal of psychiatry*.

Bronson, P., & Merryman, A. (2009). *NurtureShock: New thinking about children*.

Brown, S., & Vaughan, C. (Collaborator). (2009). *Play: How it shapes the brain, opens the imagination, and invigorates the soul.* Avery/Penguin Group USA.

Bundy, A. (1992). Play: The most important occupation of children. *American Occupational Therapy Association's Sensory Integration Special Interest Section Newsletter*, 15(2), 1–2.

Bundy, A. C. (1993). Assessment of play and leisure: delineation of the problem. *American Journal of Occupational Therapy*, 47, 217–222.

Bundy, A. C. (2003). *Test of playfulness (ToP), version 4*. Sydney, Australia: School of Occupation and Leisure Sciences, The University of Sydney.

Bundy, A. (2011). Children: Analysing the occupation of play. In L. Mackenzie & G. O'Toole (Eds.), *Occupation Analysis in Practice* (1st ed.) (pp. 133–146). Oxford, UK: Blackwell Publishing ltd.

Bundy, A. C., Luckett, T., Naughton, G. A., Tranter, P. J., Wyver, S. R., Ragen, J., … Spies, G. (2008). Playful interaction: Occupational therapy for all children on the school playground. *American Journal of Occupational Therapy*, 62(5), 522–527. https://doi.org/10.5014/ajot.62.5.522

Caiazzo, L., Sarra, A., Vechionne, M., Miller, E., & Miller Kuhaneck, H. (2008). A survey of children's play preferences: Further examination of the dynamic model for play choice. Unpublished master's thesis, Sacred Heart University, Fairfield, CT.

Carlson, S. M., White, R. E., & Davis-Unger, A. C. (2014). Evidence for a relation between executive function and pretense representation in preschool children. *Cognitive Development*, 29, 1–16. https://doi.org/10.1016/j.cogdev.2013.09.001

Case-Smith, J. (2005). School-based occupational therapy. *Occupational therapy for children*, 795–826.

Case-Smith, J., & Kuhaneck, H. M. (2008). Play preferences of typically developing children and children with developmental delays between ages 3 and 7 years. *Occupational Therapy Journal of Research*, 28(1), 19–29. https://doi.org/10.3928/15394492-20080101-01

Casey, T. (2017). Outdoor play and learning in the landscape of children's rights. *The SAGE Handbook of Outdoor Play and Learning*. London: SAGE, 362–377.1 https://doi.org/10.4135/9781526402028.n24

Centers for Disease Control and Prevention (CDC). (2020). Data & statistics on autism spectrum disorder. *Centers for Disease Control and Prevention*. https://www.cdc.gov/ncbddd/autism/data.html

Chan, P. C., Chen, C. T., Feng, H., Lee, Y. C., & Chen, K. L. (2016). Theory of mind deficit is associated with pretend play performance, but not playfulness, in children with autism spectrum disorder. *Hong Kong Journal of Occupational Therapy*, 28(1), 43–52. https://doi.org/10.1016/j.hkjot.2016.09.002

Chandler, B. (Ed.). (1997). *The essence of play: A child's occupation*. Bethesda, MD: American Occupational Therapy Association.

Chiarello, L. A., Huntington, A., & Bundy, A. (2006). A comparison of motor behaviors, interaction, and playfulness during mother–child and father–child play with children with motor delay: Implications for early intervention practice. *Occupational & Physical Therapy in Pediatrics*, 26(1/2), 129–151. https://doi.org/10.1080/J006v26n01_09

Chudacoff, H. P. (2007). *Children at play: An American history*. New York: New York University Press.

Clark F. A., Parham, D., Carlson, M.E., et al. (1991). Occupational science: Academic innovation in the service of occupational therapy's future. *American Journal of Occupational Therapy*. 45(4). 300–310. https://doi.org/10.5014/ajot.45.4.300

Cohen, L. J. (2001). *Playful parenting: A bold new way to nurture close connections, solve behavior problems, and encourage children's confidence*. New York: Ballantine Books.

Connected Kids. (2015). *Children's entertainment is booming globally*, IHS says. ENP Newswire.

Connected Kids. (2018). *Trend watch*. Childwise https://groupmp15170118135410.blob.core.windows.net/cmscontent/2018/09/Connected-Kids-Trends-Watch-2018.pdf

Cordier, R., Bundy, A., Hocking, C., & Einfeld, S. (2009). A model for play-based intervention for children with ADHD. *Australian Occupational Therapy Journal*, 56(5), 332–340. https://doi.org/10.1111/j.1440-1630.2009.00796.x

Cordier, R., Bundy, A., Hocking, C., & Einfeld, S. (2010). Empathy in the play of children with attention deficit hyperactivity disorder. *OTJR: Occupation, Participation and Health*, 30(3), 122–132. https://doi.org/10.3928/15394492-20090518-02

Cortinez-O'Ryan, A., Albagli, A., Sadarangani, K. P., & Aguilar-Farias, N. (2017). Reclaiming streets for outdoor play: A process and impact evaluation of "Juega en tu barrio" (play in your neighborhood), an intervention to increase physical activity and opportunities for play. *PloS One*, 12(7). https://doi.org/10.1371/journal.pone.0180172

Cosbey, J., Johnston, S. S., Dunn, M. L., & Bauman, M. (2012). Playground behaviors of children with and without sensory processing disorders. *OTJR: Occupation, Participation and Health*, 32(2), 39–47. https://doi.org/10.3928/15394492-20110930-01

Couch, K. J., Deitz, J. C., & Kanny, E. M. (1998). The role of play in pediatric occupational therapy. *American Journal of Occupational Therapy*, 52, 111–117. https://doi.org/10.5014/ajot.52.2.111

Daunhauer, L. A., Coster, W. J., Tickle-Degnen, L., & Cermak, S. A. (2007). Effects of caregiver–child interactions on play occupations among young children institutionalized in Eastern Europe. *American Journal of Occupational Therapy*, 61, 429–440. https://doi.org/10.5014/ajot.61.4.429

Dawson, G. (2013). Dramatic increase in autism prevalence parallels explosion of research into its biology and causes. *JAMA Psychiatry*, 70(1), 9–10. https://doi.org/10.1001/jamapsychiatry.2013.488

D'Haese, S., Van Dyck, D., De Bourdeaudhuij, I., Deforche, B., & Cardon, G. (2015). Organizing "Play Streets" during school vacations can increase physical activity and decrease sedentary time in children. *International Journal of Behavioral Nutrition and Physical Activity*, 12(1), 14. https://doi.org/10.1186/s12966-015-0171-y

Dionne, M., & Martini, R. (2011). Floor time play with a child with autism: A single-subject study. *Canadian Journal of Occupational Therapy*, 78(3), 196–203.

Doherty, J. (2004). Reward representations and reward-related learning in the human brain: Insights from neuroimaging. *Current Opinion in Neurobiology*, 14(6), 769–776. https://doi.org/10.1016/j.conb.2004.10.016

Dreyer, B. A. (1976). Adolf Meyer and mental hygiene: An ideal for public health. *American Journal of Public Health*, 66(10), 998–1003. https://doi.org/10.2105/ajph.66.10.998

Dunton, W. R. (1954). History and development of occupational therapy. In H. S. Willard & C. S. Spackman (Eds.), *Principles of occupational therapy* (2nd ed., pp. 1–10). Philadelphia: J. B. Lippincott.

Elkind, D. (2007). *The power of play: How spontaneous, imaginative activities lead to happier, healthier children*. Boston, MA: Da Capo Lifelong Books.

Espinoza, A., McMahan, S., Naffzinger, T., & Wiersma, L. D. (2012). Creating playgrounds, where playgrounds do not exist. *Californian Journal of Health Promotion*, 10(SI-Obesity), 13–19. https://doi.org/10.32398/cjhp.v10iSI-Obesity.1466

Fabrizi, S. E. (2015). Splashing our way to playfulness! An aquatic playgroup for young children with autism, a repeated measures design. *Journal of Occupational Therapy, Schools, & Early Intervention*, 8(4), 292–306. https://doi.org/10.1080/19411243.2015.1116963

Fabrizi, S., & Hubbell, K. (2017). The role of occupational therapy in promoting playfulness, parent competence, and social participation in early childhood playgroups: A pretest posttest design. *Journal of Occupational Therapy, Schools, & Early Intervention*, 10(4), 346–365. https://doi.org/10.1080/19411243.2017.1359133

Fabrizi, S., Ito, M., & Winston, K. (2016). Effect of occupational therapy–led playgroups in early intervention on child playfulness and caregiver responsiveness: A repeated-measures design. *American Journal of Occupational Therapy*, 70(2), 700220020. https://doi.org/10.5014/ajot.2016.017012

Farmer, V., Williams, S., Mann, J., Schofield, G., McPhee J., Taylor, R. (2017). The effect of increasing risk and challenge in the school playground on physical activity and weight in children: A cluster randomised controlled trial (PLAY). *International Journal of Obesity*, 41, 793–800. https://doi.org/10.1038/ijo.2017.41

Florey, L. (1971). An approach to play and play development. *The American Journal of Occupational Therapy*, 25, 275–280.

Florida, R. (2004). *America's looming creativity crisis*. https://hbr.org/2004/10/americas-looming-creativity-crisis

Foster, S., Villanueva, K., Wood, L., Christian, H., & Giles-Corti, B. (2014). The impact of parents' fear of strangers and perceptions of informal social control on children's independent mobility. *Health & Place*, 26, 60–68. https://doi.org/10.1016/j.healthplace.2013.11.006

Gibson, B. E., Darrah, J., Cameron, D., Hashemi, G., Kingsnorth, S., Lepage, C.,... & Menna-Dack, D. (2009). Revisiting therapy assumptions in children's rehabilitation: clinical and research implications. *Disability and Rehabilitation*, 31(17), 1446–1453.

Gibson, J. L., Cornell, M., & Gill, T. (2017). A systematic review of research into the impact of loose parts play on children's cognitive, social and emotional development. *School Mental Health*, 9(4), 295–309. https://doi.org/10.1007/s12310-017-9220-9

Ginsburg, K. R., American Academy of Pediatrics Committee on Communications, & American Academy of Pediatrics Committee on Psychosocial Aspects of Child and Family Health. (2007). The importance of play in promoting healthy child development and maintaining strong parent–child bonds. *Pediatrics*, 119, 182–191. https://doi.org/10.1542/peds.2006-2697

Gleave, G. M. (1954). Occupational therapy in children's hospitals and pediatric service. In H. S. Willard & C. S. Spackman (Eds.), *Principles of occupational therapy* (2nd ed., pp. 138–167). Philadelphia: J. B. Lippincott.

Graham, N. E., Truman, J., & Holgate, H. (2015). Parents' understanding of play for children with cerebral palsy. *American Journal of Occupational Therapy*, 69(3), 6903220050. https://dx.doi.org/10.5014/ajot.2015.015263

Gray, P. (2011). The decline of play and the rise of psychopathology in children and adolescents. *American Journal of Play*, 3(4), 443–463.

Guitard, P., Ferland, F., & Dutil, E. (2005). Toward a better understanding of playfulness in adults. *OTJR: Occupation, Participation and Health*, 25(1), 9–22. https://doi.org/10.1177/153944920502500103

Hammell, K. W. (2004). Dimensions of meaning in the occupations of daily life. *Canadian Journal of Occupational Therapy*, 71(5), 296–305. https://doi.org/10.1177/000841740407100509

Hamovitch, E., Acri, M., & Bornheimer, L. (2018). Who is accessing family mental health programs? Demographic differences before and after system reform. *Children and Youth Services Review*. https://doi.org/10.1016/j.childyouth.2017.12.027

Hasselkus, B. R. (2002). *The meaning of everyday occupation*. Thorofare, NJ: Slack.

Heah, T., Case, T., McGuire, B., & Law, M. (2007). Successful participation: The lived experience among children with disabilities. *Canadian Journal of Occupational Therapy*, 74(1), 38–47. https://doi.org/10.2182/cjot.06.10

Henning, B., Cordier, R., Wilkes-Gillan, S., & Falkmer, T. (2016). A pilot play-based intervention to improve the social play interactions of children with autism spectrum disorder and their typically developing playmates. *Australian Occupational Therapy Journal*, 63(4), 223–232. https://doi.org/10.1111/1440-1630.12285

Hinojosa, J., & Blount, M. (2004). Purposeful activities within the context of occupational therapy. In J. Hinojosa & M. Blount (Eds.), *Texture of life* (pp. 1–16). Bethesda, MD: AOTA Press.

Hirsh-Pasek, K., Golinkoff, R. M., Berk, L. E., & Singer, D. (2009). *A mandate for playful learning in preschool: Applying the scientific evidence*. New York: Oxford University Press.

Howard, A. C. (1986). Developmental play ages of physically abused and nonabused children. *American Journal of Occupational Therapy*, 40, 691–695. https://doi/org/10.5014/ajot.40.10.691

Jane Addams Hull-House Museum. (n.d.). *About Jane Addams*. https://www.hullhousemuseum.org/about-jane-addams

Janssen, I. (2014). Active play: An important physical activity strategy in the fight against childhood obesity. *Canadian Journal of Public Health*, 105(1), e22–e27. https://doi.org/10.17269/cjph.105.4154

Jarrold, C. (2003). A review of research into pretend play in Autism. *Autism*, 7(4), 379–390. https://doi.org/10.1177/1362361303007004004

Kelly, R., Dissanayake, C., Ihsen, E., & Hammond, S. (2011). The relationship between symbolic play and executive function in young children. *Australasian Journal of Early Childhood*, 36(2), 21–27. https://doi.org/10.1177/183693911103600204

Kennedy-Behr, A., Rodger, S., & Mickan, S. (2013). A comparison of the play skills of preschool children with and without developmental coordination disorder. *OTJR: Occupation, Participation and Health*, 33(4), 198–208. https://doi.org/10.3928/15394492-20130912-03

Kent, C., Cordier, R., Joosten, A., Wilkes-Gillan, S., & Bundy, A. (2018). Peer-mediated intervention to improve play skills in children with autism spectrum disorder: A feasibility study. *Australian Occupational Therapy Journal*, 65(3), 176–186. https://doi.org/10.1111/1440-1630.12459

Kent, C., Cordier, R., Joosten, A., Wilkes-Gillan, S., & Bundy, A. (2019). Can I join in? Multiple case study investigation of play performance generalisation for children with autism spectrum disorder from dyad to triad. *Australian Occupational Therapy Journal*, 67(3), 199–209. https://doi.org/10.1111/1440-1630.12635

Kent, C., Cordier, R., Joosten, A., Wilkes-Gillan, S., & Bundy, A. Can we play together? (2020). A close look at the peers of a peer-mediated intervention to improve play in children with autism spectrum disorder [published online ahead of print, 2020 Feb 10]. *Journal of Autism and Developmental Disorders*, 50(8), 2860–2873. https://doi.org/10.1007/s10803-020-04387-6

Kent, C., Cordier, R., Joosten, A., Wilkes-Gillan, S., Bundy, A., & Speyer, R. (2020). A systematic review and meta-analysis of interventions to improve play skills in children with autism spectrum disorder. *Review Journal of Autism and Developmental Disorders*, 1–28. https://doi.org/10.1371/journal.pone.0172242

Kielhofner, G., & Barris, R. (1984). Collecting data on play: A critique of available methods. *Occupational Therapy Journal of Research*, 4, 150–180. https://doi.org/10.1177/153944928400400302

Kielhofner, G., Barris, R., Bauer, D., Shoestock, B., & Walker, L. (1983). A comparison of play behavior in non-hospitalized and hospitalized children. *American Journal of Occupational Therapy*, 37, 305–312. https://doi.org/10.5014/ajot.37.5.305

Kim, K. H. (2011). The creativity crisis: The decrease in creative thinking scores on the Torrance Tests of Creative Thinking. *Creativity Research Journal*, 23(4), 285–295. https://doi.org/10.1080/10400419.2011.627805

Kleppe, R. (2018). Affordances for 1- to 3-year-olds' risky play in early childhood education and care. *Journal of Early Childhood Research*, 16(3), 258–275. https://doi.org/10.1177/1476718X18762237

Knox, S. (1974). A play scale. In M. Reilly (Ed.), *Play as exploratory learning* (pp. 247–266). Los Angeles: Sage.

Knox, S. H. (1997). *Play and play styles of preschool children.* Unpublished doctoral dissertation, University of Southern California, Los Angeles. http://digitallibrary.usc.edu/cdm/ref/collection/p15799coll17/id/266518

Kuhaneck, H. M., & Britner, P. A. (2013). A preliminary investigation of the relationship between sensory processing and social play in autism spectrum disorder. *OTJR: Occupation, Participation and Health*, 33(3), 159–167.

Kuhaneck, H., Spitzer, S. L., & Bodison, S. C. (2020). A systematic review of interventions to improve the occupation of play in children with Autism. *OTJR: Occupation, Participation and Health*, 40(2), 83–98. https://doi.org/10.1177/1539449219880531

Kuhaneck, H., Spitzer, S., & Miller, E. (2010). *Activity analysis, creativity and playfulness in pediatric occupational therapy: Making play just right.* Burlington, MA: Jones & Bartlett Learning.

Lee, Y. C., Chan, P. C., Lin, S. K., Chen, C. T., Huang, C. Y., & Chen, K. L. (2016). Correlation patterns between pretend play and playfulness in children with autism spectrum disorder, developmental delay, and typical development. *Research in Autism Spectrum Disorders*, 24, 29–38.

Little, H. (2015). Mothers' beliefs about risk and risk-taking in children's outdoor play. *Journal of Adventure Education & Outdoor Learning*, 15(1), 24–39. https://doi.org/10.1080/14729679.2013.842178

Loprinzi, P. D., & Davis, R. E. (2016). Secular trends in parent-reported television viewing among children in the United States, 2001–2012. *Child: Care, Health and Development*, 42(2), 288–291. https://doi.org/10.1111/cch.12304

Lynch, H., & Moore, A. (2016). Play as an occupation in occupational therapy. *British Journal of Occupational Therapy*, 79(9), 519–520. https://doi.org/10.1177/0308022616664540

Lynch, H., Prellwitz, M., Schulze, C., & Moore, A. H. (2018). The state of play in children's occupational therapy: A comparison between Ireland, Sweden and Switzerland. *British Journal of Occupational Therapy*, 81(1), 42–50. https://doi.org/10.1177/0308022617733256

Malone, K. (2007). The bubble-wrap generation: Children growing up in walled gardens. *Environmental Education Research*, 13(4), 513–527, https://doi.org/10.1080/13504620701581612

McCambridge, T. M., Bernhardt, D. T., Brenner, J. S., Congeni, J. A., Gomez, J. E., Gregory, A. J., … Small, E. W. (2006). Active healthy living: Prevention of childhood obesity through increased physical activity, *Pediatrics*, 117(5), 1834–1842. https://doi.org/10.1542/peds.2006-0472

McDonald, A. E., & Vigen, C. (2012). Reliability and validity of the McDonald Play Inventory. *American Journal of Occupational Therapy*, 66, e52–e60. https://dx.doi.org/10.5014/ajot.2012.002493

McFarland, L., & Laird, S. G. (2018). Parents' and early childhood educators' attitudes and practices in relation to children's outdoor risky play. *Early Childhood Education Journal*, 46(2), 159–168. https://doi.org/10.1007/s10643-017-0856-8

McNary, H. (1954). The scope of occupational therapy. In H. S. Willard & C. S. Spackman (Eds.), *Principles of occupational therapy* (2nd ed., pp. 11–23). Philadelphia: J. B. Lippincott.

Memari, A. H., Panahi, N., Ranjbar, E., Moshayedi, P., Shafiei, M., Kordi, R., & Ziaee, V. (2015). Children with autism spectrum disorder and patterns of participation in daily physical and play activities. *Neurology Research International*, 2015, 531906. https://doi.org/10.1155/2015/531906

Mercer, J. (2014). Russ, Sandra W.: Pretend play in childhood: Foundation of adult creativity. *CHOICE: Current Reviews for Academic Libraries*, 8, 1494.

Merikangas, K., He, J., Burstein, M., Swanson, S., Aveneoli, S., Cui, L., … Swendsen, J. (2010). Lifetime prevalence of mental disorders in U.S. adolescents: Results from the National Comorbidity Survey Replication–Adolescent Supplement (NCS-A). *Journal of the American Academy of Child & Adolescent Psychiatry*, 49(10), 980–989 https://doi.org/https://doi.org/10.1016/j.jaac.2010.05.017

Merriam-Webster. (2020). Ambassador. *Merriam-Webster* https://www.merriam-webster.com/dictionary/ambassador

Meyer, A. (1922). The philosophy of occupational therapy. *Archives of Occupational Therapy*, 1, 1–10. https://www.aotf.org/Portals/0/Meyers%20full%20article.pdf

Miller, E., & Kuhaneck, H. (2008). Children's perceptions of play experiences and play preferences: A qualitative study. *American Journal of Occupational Therapy*, 62, 407–415. https://doi.org/10.5014/ajot.62.4.407

Miller, L. J., Schoen, S., Camarata, S., McConkey, J., Kanics, I., Valdez, A., & Hampton, S. (2017). Play in natural environments: A pilot study quantifying the behavior of children on playground equipment. *Journal of Occupational Therapy, Schools, & Early Intervention*, 10(3). 213–231. https://doi.org/10.1080/19411243.2017.1325818

Miller Kuhaneck, H., Tanta, K. J., Coombs, A. K., & Pannone, H. (2013). A survey of pediatric occupational therapists' use of play. *Journal of Occupational Therapy, Schools, & Early Intervention*, 6(3), 213–227. https://doi.org/10.1080/19411243.2013.850940

Mitchell, A. W., Hale, J., Lawrence, M., Murillo, E., Newman, K., & Smith, H. (2018). Entry-level occupational therapy programs' emphasis on play: A survey. *Journal of Occupational Therapy Education*, 2(1), 1–18. https://doi.org/10.26681/jote.2018.020105

Moore, A., & Lynch, H. (2015). Accessibility and usability of playground environments for children under 12: A scoping review. *Scandinavian Journal of Occupational Therapy*, 22(5), 331–344. https://doi.org/10.3109/11038128.2015.1049549

Moore, A., & Lynch, H. (2018). Play and play occupation: A survey of paediatric occupational therapy practice in Ireland. *Irish Journal of Occupational Therapy*, 81(1), 42–50. https://doi.org/10.1177/0308022617733256

Mulder, J., Carter, S., & Graf, M. (2019). Right to play for children with disabilities. *Canadian Journal of Children's Rights/Revue*

Canadienne Des Droits des Enfants, 6(1), 197–212. https://doi
.org/10.22215/cjcr.v6i1.2189

Nabors, L., & Badawi, M. (1997). Playground interactions
for preschool-age children with special needs. *Physical &
Occupational Therapy in Pediatrics*, 17(3), 21–31. https://doi
.org/10.1080/J006v17n03_02

Nelson, D. L. (1996). Therapeutic occupation: A definition.
American Journal of Occupational Therapy, 50, 775–782.
https://doi.org/10.5014/ajot.50.10.775

Nelson, D. L. (1997). Why the profession of occupational therapy
will continue to flourish in the 21st century (Eleanor Clarke
Slagle Lecture). *American Journal of Occupational Therapy*, 51,
11–24. https://doi.org/10.5014/ajot.51.1.11

Nevison, C., Blaxill, M., & Zahorodny, W. (2018). California
autism prevalence trends from 1931 to 2014 and comparison
to national ASD data from IDEA and ADDM. *Journal of Autism
and Developmental Disorders*, 48(12), 4103–4117. https://doi
.org/10.1007/s10803-018-3670-2.

O'Connor, C., & Stagnitti, K. (2011). Play, behaviour, language
and social skills: The comparison of a play and a non-play
intervention within a specialist school setting. *Research in
Developmental Disabilities*, 32(3), 1205–1211. https://doi
.org/10.1016/j.ridd.2010.12.037

O'Keeffe, G. S., Clarke-Pearson, K., & Council on Communications
and Media. (2011). The impact of social media on children,
adolescents, and families. *Pediatrics*, 127(4), 800–804. https://
doi.org/10.1542/peds.2011-0054

Oliver, C. (1990). Determinants of interorganizational
relationships: Integration and future directions. *Academy of
Management Review*, 15(2), 241–265.

Oxford. (2020). Ambassador: Definition of Ambassador by
Lexico. *Lexico Dictionaries* | English. https://www.lexico.com
/en/definition/ambassador

Parham, L. D. (1996). Perspectives on play. In R. Zemke & F. Clark
(Eds.), *Occupational science: The evolving discipline* (pp. 71–88).
Philadelphia: F. A. Davis.

Parham, L. D., & Fazio, L. S. (1996). *Play in occupational therapy
for children*. St. Louis, MO: Mosby.

Parham, L. D., Roley, S. S., May-Benson, T. A., Koomar, J., Brett-Green,
B., Burke, J. P., … Schaaf, R. C. (2011). Development of a fidelity
measure for research on the effectiveness of the Ayres Sensory
Integration® intervention. *American Journal of Occupational Therapy*,
65(2), 133–142. https://doi.org/10.5014/ajot.2011.000745

Perou, R., Bitsko, R. H., Blumberg, S. J., Pastor, P., Ghandour, R.
M., Gfroerer, J. C., … Huang, L. N. (2013). Mental health
surveillance among children—United States, 2005–2011.
MMWR. Morbidity and Mortality Weekly Report, 62, 1–35.

Pfeifer, L. I., Pacciulio, A. M., Santos, C. A. D., Santos, J. L. D., &
Stagnitti, K. E. (2011). Pretend play of children with cerebral
palsy. *Physical & Occupational Therapy in Pediatrics*, 31(4),
390–402. https://doi.org/10.3109/01942638.2011.572149

Piaget, J. (1962). *Play, dreams and imitation in childhood*. New York:
Norton.

Pierce, D. (2001). Untangling occupation and activity. *American
Journal of Occupational Therapy*, 55(2),138–146. https://doi
.org/10.5014/ajot.55.2.138

Pinchover, S. (2017). The relation between teachers' and children's
playfulness: A pilot study. *Frontiers in Psychology*, 8, 2214.

Pollack, N., Stewart, D., Law, M., Sahagian-Whalen, S., Harvey, S.,
& Toal, C. (1997). The meaning of play for young people with
physical disabilities. *Canadian Journal of Occupational Therapy*,
64, 25–31. https://doi.org/10.1177/000841749706400105

Porter, C., & Bundy, A. C. (2001). Validity of three tests of
playfulness with African American children and their parents
and relationships among parental beliefs and values and
children's observed playfulness. In S. Reifel (Ed.), *Theory in
context and out* (pp. 315–334). Westport, CT: Ablex.

Prellwitz, M., & Skär, L. (2007). Usability of playgrounds
for children with different abilities. *Occupational Therapy
International*, 14(3), 144–155. https://doi.org/10.1002/oti.230

Price, P., Hooper, B., Krishnagiri, S., Taff, S. D., & Bilics, A. (2017).
A way of seeing: How occupation is portrayed to students
when taught as a concept beyond its use in therapy. *American
Journal of Occupational Therapy*, 71, 7104230010. https://doi
.org/10.5014/ajot.2017.024182

Primeau, L. A. (1998). Orchestration of work and play within
families. *American Journal of Occupational Therapy*, 52, 188–195.
https://doi.org/10.5014/ajot.52.3.188

Ray-Kaeser, S., & Lynch, H. (2017). Occupational therapy
perspective on play for the sake of play. In *Play Development
in Children with Disabilities* (pp. 155–165). Berlin: De Gruyter.
https://doi.org/10.1515/9783110522143-014

Reed, K. L. (2019). The beliefs of Eleanor Clarke Slagle: Are they
current or history? *Occupational Therapy in Health Care*, 33,
265–285, https://doi.org/10.1080/07380577.2019.1619215

Reed, K. L., & Sanderson, S. (1999). *Concepts of occupational
therapy*. Philadelphia, PA: Lippincott, Williams & Wilkins.

Reilly, M. (1974). Defining a cobweb. In M. Reilly (Ed.), *Play as
exploratory learning: Studies of curiosity behavior* (pp. 57–116).
London: Sage.

Reisman, J. M. (1991). *A history of clinical psychology*. New York:
Taylor & Francis.

Restall, G., & Magill-Evans, J. (1994). Play and preschool children
with autism. *American Journal of Occupational Therapy*, 48,
113–120. https://doi.org/10.5014/ajot.48.2.113

Richmond, J. B. (1995). The Hull House era: Vintage years for
children. *American Journal of Orthopsychiatry*, 65(1), 10–20.
http://dx.doi.org/10.1037/h0085065

Rintoul, M. A. (2018). Access to play for children in situations of
crisis play: Rights and practice—A tool kit for staff, managers
and policy makers. *Children, Youth and Environments*, 28(2),
187–190. https://doi.org/10.7721/chilyoutenvi.28.2.0187

Ríos-Rincón, A. M., Adams, K., Magill-Evans, J., & Cook, A.
(2015). Playfulness in children with limited motor abilities
when using a robot. *Physical & Occupational Therapy in
Pediatrics*, 36(3), 232–246. https://doi.org/10.3109/0194263
8.2015.1076559

Ripat, J., & Becker, P. (2012). Playground usability: What do
playground users say? *Occupational Therapy International*,
19(3), 144–153. https://doi.org/10.1002/oti.1331

Roach, M. A., Barratt, M. S., Miller, J. F., & Leavitt, L. A. (1998).
The structure of mother–child play: Young children with Down
syndrome and typically developing children. *Developmental
Psychology*, 34(1), 77–87. https://doi.org/10.1037/0012-
1649.34.1.77

Roberts, T., Stagnitti, K., Brown, T., & Bhopti, A. (2018).
Relationship between sensory processing and pretend play in
typically developing children. *American Journal of Occupational
Therapy*, 72, 7201195050. https://doi.org/10.5014/ajot.2018
.027623

Román-Oyola, R., Figueroa-Feliciano, V., Torres-Martínez, Y.,
Torres-Vélez, J., Encarnación-Pizarro, K., Fragoso-Pagán, S.,
& Torres-Colón, L. (2018). Play, playfulness, and self-efficacy:
Parental experiences with children on the autism spectrum.

Occupational Therapy International, 2018, 1–10. https://doi.org/10.1155/2018/4636780

Román-Oyola, R., Reynolds, S., Soto-Feliciano, I., Cabrera-Mercader, L., & Vega-Santana, J. (2017). Child's sensory profile and adult playfulness as predictors of parental self-efficacy. *American Journal of Occupational Therapy, 71,* 7102220010. https://doi.org/10.5014/ajot.2017.021097

Sandberg, A., Björck-Åkesson, E., & Granlund, M. (2004). Play in retrospection: Play experiences from childhood in adults with visual disability, motor disability and Asperger syndrome. *Scandinavian Journal of Disability Research, 6*(2), 111–130. https://doi.org/10.1080/15017410409512645

Sandberg, A., & Vuorinen, T. (2008). Preschool–home cooperation in change. *International Journal of Early Years Education, 16,* 151–161. 10.1080/09669760802025165

Schaaf, R. C., Merrill, S. C., & Kinsella, N. (1987). Sensory integration and play behavior: A case study of the effectiveness of occupational therapy using sensory integrative techniques. *Occupational Therapy in Health Care, 4*(2), 61–75. https://doi.org/10.1080/J003v04n02_07

Schneider, E., & Rosenblum, S. (2014). Development, reliability, and validity of the My Child's Play (MCP) questionnaire. *American Journal of Occupational Therapy, 68,* 277–285. https://dx.doi.org/10.5014/ajot.2014.009159

Serrada-Tejeda, S., Santos-del-Riego, S., May-Benson, T. A., & Pérez-de-Heredia-Torres, M. (2021). Influence of Ideational Praxis on the Development of Play and Adaptive Behavior of Children with Autism Spectrum Disorder: A Comparative Analysis. *International journal of environmental research and public health, 18*(11), 5704.

Shikako-Thomas, K., Dahan-Oliel, N., Shevell, M., Law, M., Birnbaum, R., Rosenbaum, P., … Majnemer, A. (2012). Play and be happy? Leisure participation and quality of life in school-aged children with cerebral palsy. *International Journal of Pediatrics, 2012,* 387280. https://doi.org/10.1155/2012/387280

Skaines, N., Rodger, S., & Bundy, A. (2006). Playfulness in children with autistic disorder and their typically developing peers. *British Journal of Occupational Therapy, 69,* 505–512.

Skär, L. (2002). Disabled children's perceptions of technical aids, assistance and peers in play situations. *Scandinavian Journal of Caring Sciences, 16*(1), 27–33. https://doi.org/10.1046/j.1471-6712.2002.00047.x

Skard, G., & Bundy, A. C. (2008). Test of playfulness. In L. D. Parham & L. S. Fazio (Eds.), *Play in occupational therapy for children* (2nd ed., pp. 71–93). St. Louis, MO: Mosby Elsevier.

Slagle, E. C. (1922),Training aides for mental patients. *Archives of Occupational Therapy, 1,* 11–17.

Spiegal, B., Gill, T. R., Harbottle, H., & Ball, D. J. (2014). Children's play space and safety management: Rethinking the role of play equipment standards. *SAGE Open.* https://doi.org/10.1177/2158244014522075

Spitzer, S. L. (2003a). Using participant observation to study the meaning of occupations of young children with autism and other developmental disabilities. *American Journal of Occupational Therapy, 57*(1), 66–76. https://doi.org/10.5014/ajot.57.1.66

Spitzer, S. L. (2003b). With and without words: Exploring occupation in relation to young children with autism. *Journal of Occupational Science, 10*(2), 67–79. https://doi.org/10.1080/14427591.2003.9686513

Spitzer, S. L. (2004). Common and uncommon daily activities in individuals with autism: Challenges and opportunities for supporting occupation. In H. Miller-Kuhaneck (Ed.), *Autism:*

A comprehensive occupational therapy approach (2nd ed., pp. 83–106). Bethesda, MD: AOTA Press.

Staempfli, M. B. (2009). Reintroducing adventure into children's outdoor play environments. *Environment and Behavior, 41*(2), 268–280. https://doi.org/10.1177/0013916508315000

Stagnitti, K. (1998). *Learn to play: A practical program to develop a child's imaginative play skills.* Melbourne, Australia: Co-ordinates Publications.

Stagnitti, K. (2009). *Play intervention: The Learn to Play program.* Play as Therapy: Assessment and Intervention, 176–186.

Stagnitti, K., O'Connor, C., & Sheppard, L. (2012). Impact of the learn to play program on play, social competence and language for children aged 5–8 years who attend a specialist school. *Australian Occupational Therapy Journal, 59*(4), 302–311. https://doi.org/10.1111/j.1440-1630.2012.01018.x

Stagnitti, K., & Unsworth, C. (2000). The importance of pretend play in child development: An occupational therapy perspective. *British Journal of Occupational Therapy, 63*(3), 121–127. https://doi.org/10.1177/030802260006300306

Stout, J. (1988). Planning playgrounds for children with disabilities. *American Journal of Occupational Therapy, 42*(10), 653–657. https://doi.org/10.5014/ajot.42.10.653

Takata, N. (1974). Play as a prescription. In M. Reilly (Ed.), *Play as exploratory learning* (pp. 209–246). Los Angeles: Sage.

Tamm & Skär, M. T. L. (2000). How I play: Roles and relations in the play situations of children with restricted mobility. *Scandinavian Journal of Occupational Therapy, 7*(4), 174–182. https://doi.org/10.1080/110381200300008715

Tanta, K. J., & Kuhaneck, H. (2020). Assessment and treatment of play. In J. C. O'Brien & H. Kuhaneck (Eds.), *Case-Smith's occupational therapy for children and adolescents* (8th ed. pp. 239-266). St. Louis, MO: Elsevier.

Thiemann-Bourque, K., Johnson, L. K., & Brady, N. C. (2019). Similarities in functional play and differences in symbolic play of children with autism spectrum disorder. *American Journal on Intellectual and Developmental Disabilities, 124*(1), 77–91. https://doi.org/10.1352/1944-7558-124.1.77

Tremblay, M. S., Gray, C., Babcock, S., Barnes, J., Bradstreet, C. C., Carr, D., … Herrington, S. (2015). Position statement on active outdoor play. *International Journal of Environmental Research and Public Health, 12*(6), 6475–6505. https://doi.org/10.3390/ijerph120606475

Tsai, K. C. (2012). Play, imagination, and creativity: A brief literature review. *Journal of Education and Learning, 1*(2), 15–20. https://doi.org/10.5539/jel.v1n2p15

Twenge, J., Gentile, B., DeWall, N., Ma, D., Lacefield, K., & Schurtz, D. (2010). Birth cohort increases in psychopathology among young Americans, 1938–2007: A cross-temporal meta-analysis of the MMPI. *Clinical Psychology Review.* https://doi.org/https://doi.org/10.1016/j.cpr.2009.10.005

UN General Assembly, Convention on the Rights of the Child. (1989, November 20). United Nations, Treaty Series, vol. 1577, p. 3, available at: https://www.refworld.org/docid/3ae6b38f0.html [accessed September 20, 2021]

von Zuben, M., Crist, P., & Mayberry, W. (1991). A pilot study of differences in play behavior between children of low and middle socio-economic status. *American Journal of Occupational Therapy, 45,* 113–118. https://doi.org/10.5014/ajot.45.2.113

Waldman-Levi, A., & Bundy, A. (2014). *Parent/caregiver's support of young children's playfulness scale (PSYCP).* Unpublished Manual.

Waldman-Levi, A., & Bundy, A. (2016). A glimpse into co-occupations: Parent/caregiver's support of young children's playfulness scale. *Occupational Therapy in Mental Health, 32*(3), 217–227. https://doi.org/10.1080/0164212X.2015.1116420

Waldman-Levi, A., Grinion, S., & Olson, L. (2019). Effects of maternal views and support on childhood development through joint play. *The Open Journal of Occupational Therapy, 7*(4), 1–21. https://doi.org/10.15453/2168-6408.1613

Watts, T., Stagnitti, K., & Brown, T. (2014). Relationship between play and sensory processing: A systematic review. *The American Journal of Occupational Therapy, 68*(2), e37–46. https://doi.org/10.5014/ajot.2014.009787

Wehrmann, S., Chiu, T., Reid, D., & Sinclair, G. (2006). Evaluation of occupational therapy school-based consultation service for students with fine motor difficulties. *Canadian Journal of Occupational Therapy, 73*(4), 225–235.

Welters-Davis, M., & Mische Lawson, L. (2011). The relationship between sensory processing and parent–child play preferences. *Journal of Occupational Therapy, Schools, & Early Intervention, 4*(2), 108–120. https://doi.org/10.1080/19411243.2011.595300

White, R. (1959). Motivation reconsidered: The concept of competence. *Psychological Review, 66*, 297–333. https://doi.org/10.1037/h0040934

Wilding, C. (2009). *Defining occupational therapy*. Occupational Therapy and Physical Dysfunction E-Book: Enabling Occupation, 3–13.

Wilding, C., & Whiteford, G. (2006). Occupation and occupational therapy: Knowledge paradigms and everyday practice. *Australian Occupational Therapy Journal, 54*(3), 185–193. https://doi.org/10.1111/ j.1440-1630.2006.00621.x

Wilding, C., & Whiteford, G. (2007). Occupation and occupational therapy: Knowledge paradigms and everyday practice. *Australian Occupational Therapy Journal, 54*(3), 185–193. https://doi.org/10.1111/j.1440-1630.2006.00621.x

Wilding, C., & Whiteford, G. (2008). Language, identity and representation: Occupation and occupational therapy in acute settings. *Australian Occupational Therapy Journal, 55*(3), 180–187. https://doi.org/0.1111/j.1440-1630.2007.00678.x

Wilkes, S., Cordier, R., Bundy, A., Docking, K., & Munro, N. (2011). A play-based intervention for children with ADHD: A pilot study. *Australian Occupational Therapy Journal, 58*(4), 231–240. https://doi.org/10.1111/j.1440-1630.2011.00928.x

Wilkes-Gillan, S., Bundy, A., Cordier, R., & Lincoln, M. (2014a). Eighteen month follow-up of a play-based intervention to improve the social play skills of children with attention deficit hyperactivity disorder. *Australian Occupational Therapy Journal, 61*(5), 299–307. https://doi.org/10.1111/1440-1630.12124 PMID: 24762264 21.

Wilkes-Gillan, S., Bundy, A., Cordier, R., & Lincoln, M. (2014b). Evaluating a pilot parent-delivered play-based intervention for children with ADHD. *American Occupational Therapy Journal, 68*(6), 700–709. https:doi.org/10.5014/ajot.2014.012450 PMID: 25397765

Wilkes-Gillan, S., Bundy, A., Cordier, R., Lincoln, M., & Chen, Y. W. (2016). A randomised controlled trial of a play-based intervention to improve the social play skills of children with attention deficit hyperactivity disorder (ADHD). *PloS One, 11*(8). https://doi.org/10.1371/journal.pone.0160558

Wilkes-Gillan, S., Bundy, A., Cordier, R., Lincoln, M., & Hancock, N. (2015). Parents' perspectives on the appropriateness of a parent-delivered intervention for improving the social play skills of children with ADHD. *British Journal of Occupational Therapy, 78*(10), 644–652. https://doi.org/10.1177/0308022615573453

Wood, W. (1996). The value of studying occupation: An example with primate play. *American Journal of Occupational Therapy, 50*(5), 327–337. https://doi.org/10.5014/ajot.50.5.327

World Federation of Occupational Therapists. (2012). *Definition of occupation* http://wwww.wfot.org/aboutus/aboutoccupationaltherapy/definitionofoccupationaltherapy.asx

Yogman, M., Garner, A., Hutchinson, J., Hirsh-Pasek, K., Golinkoff, R. M., & Committee on Psychosocial Aspects of Child and Family Health. (2018). The power of play: A pediatric role in enhancing development in young children. *Pediatrics, 142*(3).

Zieff, S. G., Chaudhuri, A., & Musselman, E. (2016). Creating neighborhood recreational space for youth and children in the urban environment: Play(ing in the) streets in San Francisco. *Children and Youth Services Review, 70*, 95–101. https://doi.org/10.1016/j.childyouth.2016.09.014

Zosh, J. M., Hirsh-Pasek, K., Golinkoff, R. M., & Dore, R. A. (2017). Where learning meets creativity: The promise of guided play. In *Creative Contradictions in Education* (pp. 165–180). Cham: Springer.

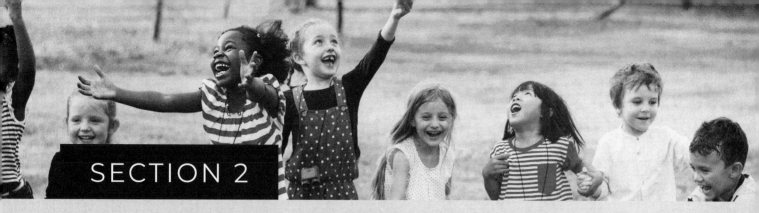

SECTION 2

The Skills You Need

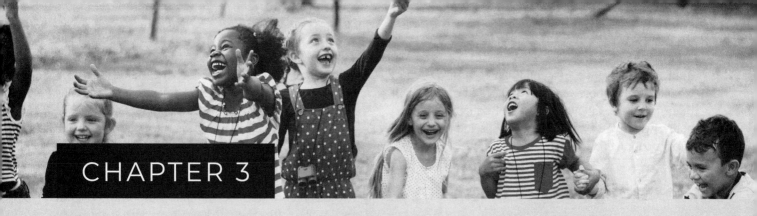

CHAPTER 3

Examining Play in Our Pediatric Clients: Formal Assessments

Karen E. Stagnitti, PhD, BOccThy, GCHE

After reading this chapter, the reader will:

- Explain the value of measuring play, and articulate the importance of formal assessment of play.
- Understand the relationship between formal assessments of play and play definitions.
- Describe the contradictions between formal assessment of play and play as a spontaneous action.
- Create the conditions for a formal assessment of play in occupational therapy.
- Discuss the essential elements for occupational therapists to consider when measuring play.
- Recognize the variety of formal assessment tools available for play assessment in occupational therapy.
- Apply the "when, where, why, and how" of formal assessment of play within occupational therapy practice.
- Appraise the value of different play assessments for use with different clients and in different settings.

You can discover more about a person in an hour of play than in a year of conversation.

—Plato

Occupational therapists view play as a primary and important occupation of childhood (Canadian Association of Occupational Therapists [CAOT], 1996; Moore & Lynch, 2018); therefore, the examination of a child's play ability should be a critical piece of any pediatric occupational therapy assessment. How a child plays provides insight into how a child functions within their social, cultural, and physical environment (Rodger & Ziviani, 2006; Spitzer, 2003), a child's enjoyment of play (Eberle, 2014), a child's ability to engage socially and emotionally with others (Whitebread & O'Sullivan, 2012), a child's language and narrative understanding (Nicolopoulou & Ilgaz, 2013; Quinn, Donnelly, & Kidd, 2018), and a child's

creativity and flexibility (Russ, Robins, & Christiano, 1999). Observations of a child playing can also highlight resources the child has to play with, the barriers they encounter such as space and time, and the safety of their environment (Rodger & Ziviani, 2006).

In Chapter 1, the big questions of play were discussed. This chapter further hones the questions in relation to formal play assessment. A formal assessment of play can offer answers to "what" "why," and "how" an individual child plays. Inference from a reliable and valid formal assessment may also provide insights into the when, who, and where of a child's play. To answer these questions for an individual, a variety of methods can be used, just as we use multiple tools and methods to evaluate activities of daily living or motor skills. This chapter provides information on the variety of formal play assessments for children. Assessments via parent/caregiver report and informal observation of a child's play are discussed in Chapter 4. For those reading this text, I hope you will be inspired to evaluate play more frequently and formally, just as you evaluate motor skills and other areas of occupational performance in children.

Formally Assessing Play

In formal assessments of play, play is measured. Measurement refers to determining quantitative differences by assigning numerals to objects, events, or people using a rule (Short-DeGraff & Fisher, 1993). When we measure something, a number or category is usually placed beside the activity we are measuring. In play measurement, we examine the differences between how varied children play, by assigning a number to what we are observing. To interpret the number or the child's score, we need to understand how play is conceptualized in the assessment.

Defining Play to Measure It

Play is conceptualized broadly and covers a wide range of abilities and skills. Chapter 1 provided background on the difficulty and discussion that has surrounded the defining of play. One of the biggest obstacles to the development of play assessments has been the lack of a single definition of play (Cooper, 2009; Kielhofner & Barris, 1984). For the purposes of this book, play is defined in Chapter 1 as: *any activity freely entered into that is fun or enjoyable and that is appropriately matched to one's skill to represent an attainable challenge.* This definition hones in on key elements of play, that is, play is self-initiated by the child (it is freely entered into), it is enjoyable, and children play at their skill level. Formal play assessment provides measures of different aspects of this information, which informs the occupational therapy practitioner as to where to start working with a child at the just right challenge in play (Ayres, 1975).

Our understanding or our definition of play informs which tool we select and what we observe when we assess a child's play. For example, if we understand play as being physically active, then we will observe whether a child is physically active and the child's motor and sensory skills, if a child can play with a ball, bat, and other objects that can be used in active play. Our understanding of play also informs how we interpret what we are observing. For example, does the child become physically active when given certain toys or objects, or in certain environmental spaces. If this understanding of play is a personal bias of the therapist, then the therapist's observations of

a child's play will miss the depth of additional rich observations that can come from using a formal play assessment with greater breadth or varied scope.

One of the benefits in measuring play is that the conceptualization of play becomes explicit, which in turn provides information on how the child is functioning. For over two decades in occupational therapy, play was theorized to be extremely important to child development (Stagnitti, 2004), a primary occupation (CAOT, 1996), and important in itself (Bundy, 1997; Parham & Fazio, 2008; Rodger & Ziviani, 1999). What, how, and why a child plays provides the occupational therapist with an insight and an understanding into which children require support to develop their play ability and where to begin to enable children "to engage in self-directed daily occupations in the areas of . . . play and leisure" (Rodger & Ziviani, 1999, p. 337).

Play assessment is based on different understandings of play. Play has been defined or conceptualized in five main ways. These are by characteristics (Smith & Vollstedt, 1985), by a process or attitude (Bundy, 1993; Cooper, 2009), by category (Pellegrini & Perlmutter, 1987), by type of play (Göncü & Perone, 2005; Russ, 2014), and by elements (Eberle, 2014).

The defining characteristics given to play have been the features of: more internally than externally motivated, transcending reality and reflecting reality, controlled by the player, attention to process, safe, fun, unpredictable, spontaneous, and nonobligatory active engagement (Parham & Primeau, 1997). Smith and Vollstedt (1985) recruited 70 people to rate video footage of children using criteria for play established in previous research. Smith and Vollstedt found that criteria for play, with high agreement by adults, was nonliterality, positive affect, and flexibility. When play is defined by an attitude or process, it is understood to be intrinsically motivated, internally controlled, and free of many of the constraints of objective reality (Bundy, 1997). Based on this definition of play, Bundy developed the Test of Playfulness (Bundy, 2005). Lautamo (2009) added to Bundy's definition of play and developed the Play in Group Settings with play conceptualized as spirit, skills, and environment.

Defining play by category typically divides into two broad areas, cognitive (functional, constructive, dramatic) and social (solitary, parallel, interactive) (Pellegrini & Perlmutter, 1987). The cognitive and social categories can then be combined into dramatic-constructive play, functional constructive play, and solitary play. This definition of play underpins the PLAY Behaviour Observation Scheme, which was designed to be used in early childhood educational settings (Farmer-Dougan & Kaszuba, 1999).

Assessments based on categories of play measure the amount, frequency, or level of cognitive or social play in which the child engages.

Type of play is another conceptualization of play reflected in assessment. Generally, the types of play are referred to as gross-motor play (large-muscle movement, physically active play), fine-motor play (activities involving hand movements such as threading), sensory-motor play (activities that involve sand, water, and movement of the body through obstacles), visual-perceptual play (play with puzzles, I spy), auditory play (such as memory games, listening games), and pretend play (imposing meaning on what is being played, use of object substitution, property attributions, and reference to absent objects). The Revised Knox Preschool Play Scale (Knox, 2008) is an example of a play assessment that reflects this view of play. Some authors combine types of play. For example, Perone and Göncü (2014) argued that pretend play can be social, and Whitebread and O'Sullivan (2012) argued that social pretend play is intellectually demanding for young children. Assessments based on types of play measure the amount, frequency, or level of specific types of the child's play.

Play has also been defined and measured by its elements. In 2014, Eberle argued that play has elements that are unique, and these elements are on a continuum. These elements are emotional and integrating of the body, for example, anticipation (looking forward positively), surprise (laughter, curiosity), pleasure (satisfaction, buoyancy), and poise (the body moves with ease and dignity in play). A play assessment that considers emotional engagement along with type of play is the Pretend Play Enjoyment Developmental Checklist (Stagnitti, 2017). Assessments that include a definition of play by its elements are assessments such as the Assessment of Ludic Behavior (Ferland, 1997, 2005), where the assessment includes observations of a ludic attitude such as curiosity, sense of humor, pleasure, and enjoyment of challenge.

To add to the complexity of understanding play, pretend play can be imposed on all other types of play. For example, in gross-motor play, an obstacle course may become an event in the Olympics, or in sensory-motor play, the sand becomes a beach, and the added water becomes the ocean. Pretend play has been argued to be the quintessence of play (Stagnitti, 2004) because pretend play involves nonliterality and the suspension of reality. Examples of assessments of pretend play are Symbolic Play Test (Lowe & Costello, 1988), Test of Pretend Play (Lewis & Boucher, 1997), Child-Initiated Pretend Play Assessment 2 (Stagnitti, 2019), and Affect in Play Scale (Russ, 2004).

What Is a Formal Assessment of Play?

Formal assessment of play, in this chapter, is conceptualized as a standardized assessment of play. A standardized assessment has procedures for administration and scoring detailed in a test manual, and therapists must use these same procedures each time they administer, score, and interpret the assessment (Richardson, 2001). That is, there is a set or standard way to administer and score an assessment of a child's play. Brown and McDonald (2009) noted that formal play assessments also have a test manual outlining administration and scoring criteria.

Formal play assessments are also different from other standardized assessments commonly used in occupational therapy. As Richardson (2001) argued, standardized assessments of motor skills and development do not measure functional skills but rather measure an aspect of a skill. For example, bilateral coordination on the Bruininks–Oseretsky Test of Motor Performance is measured by items that of themselves are not functional, such as tapping fingers and feet simultaneously (Richardson, 2001). Standardized assessments of play, in contrast, differ in that they measure play abilities that a child requires in order to play. In this respect, formal play assessments are functional assessments of how a child engages in play. For example, on the Child-Initiated Pretend Play Assessment 2 (Stagnitti, 2019), a child's scores provide information on whether a child can initiate a sequence of play actions (the play is organized, logical, coherent and planned), use symbols in play (indicating a child can impose meaning on an object, go beyond the literal), and if the child can self-initiate (that is, the child is not reliant on a model of how to play). The patterns in the scores provide deeper analysis on a child's play style and insight into how a child processes and understands play.

In summary, a formal play assessment typically has standardized procedures (administration and scoring) with an accompanying manual and measures functional play engagement and abilities. However, there are many formal play assessments that do not have a published manual, but rather, have the standardized procedures set out in a book or journal article.

Is Formal Assessment of Play an Oxymoron?

Given this description of formal play assessment and the definition of play in this book, is formal assessment of play an oxymoron? In the dictionary, *oxymoron* is defined as "a figure of speech in which apparently contradictory terms appear in conjunction" (Lexico, 2020). A formal play assessment, then, appears to be a contradiction in terms, as the definition of play—being a child's ability to self-initiate, have fun, and have skills to play—seems the opposite of "formal." The oxymoron is particularly acute when the majority of pediatric occupational therapy practitioners work from settings such as schools, hospitals, government organizations, or community-based practice (Miller Kuhaneck, Tanta, Coombs, & Pannone, 2013; Rodger, Brown, & Brown, 2005), often with high caseloads (Springfield, Rodger, & Maas, 1993), and have limited opportunity to observe children in their natural setting (Stagnitti, 2004). We must examine this oxymoron because as occupational therapists, "if we cannot think seriously about play, we cannot be serious about assessing, implementing or promoting it. If we cannot assess, implement and promote play, we do not take it seriously" (Bundy, 1993, p. 218). Formal assessments of play take play seriously.

Our perceptions of play within a formal assessment may challenge our explicit and implicit assumptions and understandings of play. We all have an implicit understanding of play. This was discussed in Chapter 1. An implicit understanding of play is when you recognize when a child is playing. It is intuitive. An explicit understanding of play is when you can articulate what you are observing and why and when it is play and when it is not play. A formal assessment of play requires an explicit understanding of play just as our practice does.

Formal assessments must have a clear definition of play and how to measure it. In my own work, developing a formal assessment of play challenged my assumptions about play. I had assumed that when typically developing children played with similar toys, they would play with them in wildly different ways from each other. I found this to be a false assumption, as typically developing children played with the same play materials in remarkably similar ways with only a minority using the play materials in different ways. The expected age range for play ability in the Child-Initiated Pretend Play Assessment 2 reflects this observation (Stagnitti, 2019). I also had assumed all children could play and enjoyed playing. After 28 years of developing the Child-Initiated Pretend Play Assessment and its revision, I came to realize that play is an ability, and not all children have the ability to play nor do all children enjoy play. I also came to understand that if a child did not have the ability to play, then that child's function within their social, cultural, and physical environment was impacted. Children who could not play

were observed to be socially isolated from peers. They missed cues in their environment and were often anxious. I realized that addressing such functional needs was clearly so important for these children.

A formal assessment of play and play itself can coexist because a formal assessment provides the occupational therapist with an explicit understanding of play and when to recognize when a child is playing and when they are having difficulties in play, by themselves or with others. A formal assessment of play can provide the therapist with detailed information about how a child is functioning in their environment because play as an occupation involves social interaction (Rodger & Ziviani, 2006), language (Quinn et al., 2018), problem solving (Wyver & Spence, 1999), and the integration of motor ability (Eberle, 2014). This is one of the many reasons occupational therapists should formally assess play.

Why Formally Assess Play?

The "why" of a formal play assessment is evidence-based practice, particularly if the play assessment has established reliability and validity. Formal play assessment provides critical information to guide intervention in efficient ways, increases understanding of what is important to individual children, is a nonthreatening way to gain accurate information, and identifies challenges of a child's function and enjoyment.

Efficient and Critical Information

A formal play assessment is time efficient, while providing a lot of information to the occupational therapist. For example, some formal play assessments provide information on a child's play ability, with many also providing information on a child's developmental level in play (such as Revised Knox Preschool Play Scale, Pretend Play Enjoyment Developmental Checklist, Westby Symbolic Play Scale, Children's Developmental Play Instrument, PIECES). Other assessments provide information on how a child plays and the quality of a child's play (such as Test of Playfulness, ChIPPA 2). How a child plays may provide the occupational therapist with insight into how a child participates in their everyday life with family, siblings, and peers. For example, participation with peers and siblings is often limited for children who cannot play. Children who do not understand play do not recognize play in others and often have few skills in how to participate socially with others. Formal assessment of the occupation of play is efficient because it can allow for concurrent assessment of co-occupation, necessary skills supporting play, and underlying client factors as well.

Play Is a Window into the Child's World

Play has been viewed over time as a window into a child's world and inner self (Fein, 1981). In play, children play out events from their own lives and gain a deeper emotional understanding of their own life story (Tessier, Normandin, Ensink, & Fonagy, 2016). From 2 to 3 years of age, children discover and explore representational aspects of thoughts and understand the intentionality of others in their play (Rakoczy, 2008; Tessier et al., 2016). Playing collaboratively with others in different pretend play scenarios contributes to the development of a child's autobiographical narrative (Tessier et al., 2016), the story of who they are, and their sense of self (Harter, 2012). Some formal play assessments gather information on the affective aspects of a child's play (for example, Children's Developmental Play Instrument, Affect in Play Scale, ChIPPA 2 through analysis of play themes, and a description of a child's emerging sense of self through play in the Pretend Play Enjoyment Developmental Checklist). This information about personal meaning is important to the occupational therapy evaluation (American Occupational therapy Association [AOTA], 2020).

Play Is Nonthreatening and Enjoyable

Play that is child-led activates opioids, oxytocin, and dopamine in the brain, which in turn reduces levels of stress chemicals (Sunderland, 2007). Opioids also have anti-aggressive properties and contribute to people having a feeling of contentment (Sunderland, 2007). Thus, children should respond to the idea of playing with toys without a sense of dread. Even for children who struggle with play ability, in a formal play assessment, the therapist sets up the environment with toys and an area to play with an invitation to play with the toys. The open-endedness of a formal play assessment creates a space where children should not perceive that they are under pressure to perform. I have observed children from the ages of 2 years to 15 years indicate their relief by a smile, a sigh, or nod of the head, that I am just inviting them to play with the toys or create a movie with props. I am not providing instructions that they need to adhere to and follow, as is the case in the majority of nonplay assessments.

To truly be able to play involves emotional enjoyment, with pleasure, joy, surprise, mastery, and integration of movement all being elements of true play (Eberle, 2014). Emotional engagement is a consideration in formal play assessments such as ChIPPA 2, Test of Playfulness, Pretend Play Enjoyment

Developmental Checklist, Children's Developmental Play Instrument, Assessment of Ludic Behaviors, Animated Movie Test, Play in Group Settings, and the Affect in Play Scale. Play is not a task or a rote learned skill. To truly be able to play, the child engages spontaneously with pleasure and anticipation with play materials, going beyond the literal meaning of the play objects and creating play scenes that reflect their interests, culture, and experiences.

Play Demonstrates and Creates Function and Ability

Sculpting of the brain occurs when children play (Brown & Vaughan, 2009; Sunderland, 2007), with the creation of new cognitive combinations and new connections when we imaginatively play (Brown & Vaughan, 2009). To pretend in play requires the ability to transform objects and then use them symbolically (for example, a box is used as a car); and it is more likely that many areas of the brain are activated in pretend play as it involves cognition (Bergen, 2002), language (Quinn et al., 2018), emotion (Tessier et al., 2016), problem solving, planning and negotiation (Bergen, 2002), social competence (Uren & Stagnitti, 2009), and coping (Fiorelli & Russ, 2012).

The implications of poor play ability for a child's function within their environment impact every aspect of their participation. To be able to play with others offers opportunities to socialize, to talk, to problem-solve, to learn about emotions, and to develop a sense of self (O'Connor & Stagnitti, 2011; Quinn et al., 2018; Tessier et al., 2016). Children who are referred to occupational therapists often come because they are not able to participate with others within their environment. Practitioners can provide more effective intervention when they understand the play ability of a child. An assessment of the play ability of children is an assessment of that child's function and ability to participate. With all of these reasons to do so, it would seem that formally assessing play would be common practice, yet that is not the case.

Current Frequency of Formal Play Assessment

Although many occupational therapists profess to value play as an occupation and believe play is important, few formally evaluate it (Couch, Deitz, & Kanny, 1998; Lynch, Prellwitz, Schulze, & Moore, 2018). In cross-cultural studies on the assessments used within pediatric occupational therapy, results consistently have shown that play assessments are used minimally by occupational therapists (Couch et al.,

1998; Lynch et al., 2018; Miller Kuhaneck et al., 2013; Rodger et al., 2005; Rodger, Brown, Brown, & Boever, 2006; Rodger, 1994). Instead, assessments for motor and sensory skills (body function) are reported as the most clinically used assessments (Miller Kuhaneck et al., 2013; Rodger et al., 2005). In Ireland, Moore and Lynch (2018) found that 34 out of 65 therapists surveyed did not use any formal assessments of play, and the most commonly used assessments did not assess play or assessed play by way of directive preference activities. In an Australian study in 1994, Rodger found that 25% of a sample of occupational therapists had access to the Knox Play Scale in their departments; however, no one reported using it in practice. By 2005, Rodger et al. reported that only 5 out of 330 therapists reported using the Revised Knox Preschool Play Scale. For more than 20 years, a mismatch has been shown between the value placed on play as an occupation and how it is used in practice. In fact, Miller Kuhaneck et al. (2013) found that in America there had been a decrease in the use of play in occupational therapy since 1998. This is alarming, as play is regarded as one of the most important occupations of childhood (CAOT, 1996: Rodger & Ziviani, 2006).

One of the recommendations of Lynch et al.'s (2018) study was to strengthen the education of occupational therapists about play assessment because two of the reported barriers to the use of play assessment in occupational therapy were a lack of availability and knowledge of play assessments and a lack of education about play (Miller-Kuhaneck et al., 2013). Other reported barriers included that other professionals also focused on play and that play was not reimbursed (Miller Kuhaneck et al., 2013). Miller Kuhaneck et al. counteracted this by arguing that the role of the occupational therapist differs from other professionals as occupational therapists work with children to improve their ability to play. This is a critical difference between occupational therapists and other professionals and requires an in-depth assessment of a child's play so clear play outcomes can be measured. As noted in Chapter 2, occupational therapists have been slow to include play in therapy goals for reimbursement. The reluctance to include play may be that play itself is misunderstood and undervalued by occupational therapists, as there are CPT® codes where play could be included in therapy (see Chapter 5). To establish the need for play as a personally meaningful occupation for a child, formal play assessments provide an objective measure of need as well as a measure of progress in occupational therapy (AOTA, 2020).

How to Formally Assess Play

To eliminate some of the barriers to the formal assessment of play, let us turn to the knowledge about how to formally assess play, how and when to select appropriate play assessments, and the availability of play assessments from which to choose. Please see **Box 3.1** for an example of the process of completing a formal play assessment.

Box 3.1 The Process of Administering the ChIPPA 2

The manual of the ChIPPA 2 (Stagnitti, 2019) explains the process of administration.

- If the child will be accompanied by their parent/carer, I will have spoken to the parent or carer before the session and explained that the assessment is child-initiated, therefore no instructions on what or how to play are given to the child.
- The toys and play space have been prepared, and the child and parent/carer enter the room.
- On the way to the room, I chat to the child to gain insight into whether the child is anxious, shy, or easy to engage.
- On entering the room, I invite the child to sit on the floor and show them the toys. I also let the child know the narrative of what will happen. That is, first I have these toys to play with, then I have some other toys, then I'll talk to [the parent/carer's name] and after I talk to [the parent/carer], then the child can go outside the room and go home with [the parent/carer]. For all children, it is important to tell them the narrative of what will happen. You cannot assume children will know what will happen next, so telling them the story of what will happen reduces the child's anxiety.
- In the process of the session, I am physically beside the child, not in front of the child and not physically close to the child. Anxious children relax more if the therapist is further away from them. Interestingly, the Latin origin of assessment means to sit beside (Renshaw & Parson, 2020). Sitting beside the child also provides a lot of space in front of the child, and the child does not feel hemmed in.
- I invite the child to play with the play materials, then I pause. To be fully present, the therapist is aware of the child's experience on a sensory and bodily level. That is, I note where the child is looking, the posture of the child, the facial expression of the child, and I give the child time to orient to the room. For some children, I may have sat on the floor before they sit on the floor.

- In a child directed assessment, the therapist is passive and calm. The therapist is authentic, or congruent with themselves (Geller & Greenberg, 2002). To be fully present, the therapist has warm facial expression, has open body posture, and is aware of vocal tone and intonation and rhythm of their vocalizations (Geller & Porges, 2014).
- In a play assessment, the therapist is totally focused on what is happening in the room and is attuned to the child. In a play assessment, where the child's ability to self-initiate play is a crucial observation, the therapist is not making demands of the child and not asking lots of questions. When children are anxious, no direct eye contact is made, but rather the therapist looks at the toys and glances at the child to ascertain when the child is starting to relax. Interactions are nonjudgmental and nondemanding.

The "Art" of the Therapist in Formally Assessing Play

Measuring play in a typical clinical setting such as a clinic, hospital, or school requires the occupational therapist to be artful in the administration of the assessment because a play assessment should measure a child's ability to self-initiate their own play (a key factor in any definition of play). This is in stark contrast to the majority of the assessments used by occupational therapists, which are therapist-directed assessments such as the Developmental Test of Visual Motor Integration or the Bruininks–Oseretsky Test of Motor Proficiency (Rodger et al., 2005). A formal play assessment necessitates therapeutic skills to ensure that the environment and interactions between the therapist and child allow the child to spontaneously engage with the play materials. The approach of the therapist in a formal play assessment is a different use of self, compared to how a therapist interacts with a child during a therapist-directed assessment, such as a motor assessment.

Formal play assessments with manuals have a section on how to interact with a child during the assessment. Many formal play assessments may also have a section of the assessment when the therapist comes in to play an action, for example, the ChIPPA 2, Pretend Play Enjoyment Developmental Checklist, Westby Symbolic Play Scale, and Revised Knox Preschool Play Scale. Other play assessments such as the Affect in Play Scale suggest verbal comments by the therapist but no modeling of play actions. The therapist's role in the administration of a formal play assessment is related to the purpose of the play assessment.

Creating a Safe Environment for Formal Play Assessment

For children who are referred for a play assessment, the creation of a sense of safety in the environment is paramount. The artful administration of a formal play assessment therefore requires the occupational therapist to create an atmosphere where the child feels safe and comfortable. The therapeutic skills, which become the art of the therapist in a play assessment, are presence, attunement, unconditional positive regard, congruence, and holding the child in the play as much as possible (Geller & Greenberg, 2002; Renshaw & Parson, 2020). If a child does not feel safe, that child will not freely engage with the play materials.

The feeling of being safe is based in our neurology (Allison & Rossouw, 2013; Geller & Porges, 2014). Polyvagal theory by Porges provides an explanation of why feeling safe is so important to human beings (Geller & Porges, 2014). The name of Polyvagal theory reflects that there are two vagal circuits (Geller & Porges, 2014). One circuit is ancient and is associated with defense when activated (for example, the freeze autonomic response) and the phylogenetically newer circuit, which is related to spontaneous social behavior (Geller & Porges, 2014, p. 181). Positive social engagement only occurs when the neurobiological defenses are inhibited or downregulated and we feel safe (Geller & Porges, 2014).

Many children referred to occupational therapy have autism spectrum disorder and experience chronic autonomic nervous system hyperarousal, which results in a perception of threat even when the child is in a safe context (Patriquin, Hartwig, Friedman, Porges, & Scarpa, 2019). Many other children also experience anxiety or just stress with being in a different setting or with an unfamiliar therapist. Therefore, the therapeutic skill of creating a safe environment for all the children who come for a play assessment is essential.

Creating a safe and comfortable environment requires the therapist to be fully present with the child (Geller & Porges, 2014). "Therapeutic presence involves therapists being fully in the moment on several concurrently occurring dimensions, including physical, emotional, cognitive, and relational" (Geller & Porges, 2014, p. 179). Therapeutic presence is what the therapist does when in the session with the child and parent/carer (Geller & Greenberg, 2002). To be fully present, an occupational therapist is grounded, centered, steady, open, and receptive to the child. For a therapist to be fully present in a formal play assessment, the chosen play assessment should be congruent with the therapist's understanding of play, otherwise the therapist cannot be authentic.

If a therapist is present, the client (child) has feelings of safety (Geller & Porges, 2014). If a child feels safe, they are more likely to demonstrate the play abilities they have and to settle and engage with the play materials freely. The spontaneous ability of a child to engage with the play materials is a key observation in a formal play assessment. A child's sense of safety with a therapist who is present, creates opportunities for the child to feel free to spontaneously engage with the play materials supplied for the assessment as seen in the case of a child called Jack (see **Practice Example 3.1**).

Working with Children During the Assessment

In a formal child-initiated play assessment, the occupational therapist must be open and accepting of the child and not prejudge what the child may do. When approaching a formal play assessment, the attitude of the therapist toward the child is an attitude of openness, interest, acceptance and nonjudgement (Axline, 1947/1974; Geller & Greenberg, 2002). The child may or may not show play skills. The child may show more skill than expected. When open to the child, the occupational therapist will be able to identify more of the child's abilities. See **Practice Example 3.2**.

PRACTICE EXAMPLE 3.1 Creating a Safe Environment for Jack

Background and Referral Information

Jack was 5 years old and referred for occupational therapy due to social as well as language difficulties. He had diagnoses of intellectual disability and autism spectrum disorder. I had spoken to Jack's mother before she brought Jack to the center. Jack's mother reported that he would push his peers in an attempt to engage them socially, and he did not contribute to the play of others, but rather was disruptive and destroyed other children's play scenes.

The Assessment

Given the way in which Jack's social and language abilities were impacting his play, a play assessment was indicated. His mother was informed that the assessment would be observational and child directed. When I met Jack, he did not speak to or otherwise acknowledge me. His mother and I chatted as we walked to the door of the playroom. On entering the room, Jack located the light switches and other switches on the walls. He stepped over the toys that had been placed on the floor and ignored the play space that had been set up. He was interested in the walls and the two-way mirror. I let Jack walk around the room and gave him time to orient. Jack appeared to "float" around the room and did not acknowledge me, his mother, or the toys. After a few minutes I made a noise with a toy on the floor to bring Jack's attention to the toy. He glanced at it but showed no curiosity or interest. He continued to walk around the room and showed interest in the walls and switches.

His mother stated that he liked doll's houses so I got my doll's house and placed it on the floor. Jack squatted down and lined up all the windows of the doll's house perfectly. This was the longest time he spent engaged with a toy (30 seconds). His behavior did not change when I brought out the unstructured objects.

As Jack showed no interest in toys and no self-initiated pretend play, I sat on the chair next to his mum and let him continue to wander around the room and become familiar with the space at his own pace. His mother told me that Jack had no interest in toys, screens, or objects, even though at home there were a variety of toys for him. He would wander around the house, staring into space. He would stare into space for long periods of time, so much so, that his mother had him checked for epilepsy. He was not epileptic. He had been expelled from several early childhood centers for pushing children and knocking them down and had no friends at school or in the neighborhood. Other children were afraid of him.

As we talked, his mother gasped and stopped. She said, "I've never seen him like this at a professional appointment." I looked at her, a little startled I must admit! She continued, "I've never seen him so calm. He is usually running around the room, hitting his head on the walls and trying to get out of the room." Jack had dismantled the play space, taken off his shoes and was sitting cross-legged on an adult chair staring contentedly at his reflection in the two-way mirror. I replied to his mum that this was a positive sign, as the therapy work would occur in this room, and it was important that Jack was relaxed and felt safe here as he would be more likely to want to return. (Jack did come back, and over time, he developed spontaneous ability to engage in pretend play and developed friendships.)

The specific actions the therapist took to create the safe space included allowing Jack to explore the new space on his own, without adult demands. The therapist kept a physical distance between herself and Jack, she used her upper facial expression (such as smiling, using her eyes), she spoke in soft tones and short sentences using a playful voice, she kept an open body posture, and she made no direct demands to Jack.

PRACTICE EXAMPLE 3.2 Philip's Evaluation

Philip was a 7-year-old child who came with his mother for an occupational therapy evaluation. The referral stated difficulties with social interaction and struggling at school with literacy. His mother and teachers were concerned that he was isolated socially and was failing in story comprehension and story writing. Based on these concerns, the occupational therapist determined that it was important to assess Philip's functional ability to engage in pretend play especially due to its links to social ability, narrative, and language in children, which is specifically addressed by the ChIPPA 2 for this age.

Philip was chatty when I met him and was curious about the toys I had in the room. He sat down immediately and started to explore the toys. He moved the toys around and did little experiments with the toys, such as trying to balance all of them vertically. He was also interested when I introduced the unstructured objects. Again, he did experiments with them. He did not sequence play actions into a story, he did not use any object substitutions and was not interested in imitating any modeled play actions. After the play assessment, he asked me what the derivative was of $2x^3$. He was shocked I didn't know! Philip was a natural born mathematician. He was exceptional.

The ChIPPA 2 play assessment showed Philip's strengths in how he processed information, his preferences in play, and also how difficult he found it to create play scenes and spontaneously play out a story. He was happy to come again, and he did engage in play activities (with numbers as a hook) to develop his ability to think narratively within spontaneous pretend play.

Play is a complex behavior, and coming into a play assessment, the occupational therapist needs to be aware of their own explicit understanding of play, so they are open to observing the child and understand what they are scoring. In a formal play assessment, the therapist is not instructing the child what to do. Rather, the child is introduced to the play materials and invited to play. It is open ended. The therapist is passive. However, how a therapist interacts with a child during a play assessment should be consistent with the administration instructions. For example, the Affect in Play Scale provides the responses that the therapist may use during this 5-minute assessment of the child playing with two puppets and blocks, such as reflecting what the child is doing in the play. In the Pretend Play Enjoyment Developmental Checklist and the Westby Symbolic Play Scale, after being passive and observing the child, the therapist may model a play action if the child is not responding to the play materials.

Selecting a Formal Play Assessment
Essential Elements

The essential elements to consider when choosing a formal play assessment are definition of play, theoretical underpinnings, purpose of the assessment, and the construction of the assessment. As described earlier, how play is defined and its underlying theory are essential elements of the play assessment because the definition of play and its underlying theory relate to the purpose of the assessment. From these elements flow the purpose and construction of the assessment.

The purpose of the assessment can dictate the setting of the play assessment. Examples of assessments constructed for use in early childhood settings are: PLAY Observation Scheme (Farmer-Dougan & Kaszuba, 1999), Play in Early Childhood Evaluation System (PIECES) (Kelly-Vance & Ryalls, 2005, 2020), and Play in Group Settings (Lautamo, 2009). Examples of assessments that were constructed for the purpose of assessing a child's play development in a therapy clinic or early childhood setting are Westby Symbolic Play Scale (Westby, 1991), Revised Knox Preschool Play Scale (Knox, 2008), and the Pretend Play Enjoyment Developmental Checklist (Stagnitti, 2017). Assessments designed to determine specific information about a child's play function to inform therapy interventions include Affect in Play Scale (Russ, 2004), Child-Initiated Pretend Play Assessment 2 (Stagnitti, 2019), Symbolic Play Test (Lowe & Costello, 1988), Test of Pretend Play (Lewis & Boucher, 1997), and the Animated Movie Test (Stagnitti, 2018).

After consideration of the definition of play, purpose, and underlying theoretical foundations of the play assessment, the therapist must consider the construction of a play assessment. Construction includes items of the assessment (that is, what is the focus of scoring), as well as how the assessment is administered, scored, and interpreted. Fewell and Glick (1993) noted that if the purpose of a play assessment was to gain knowledge about a child's preferences, learning styles, and function, then toy presentation and selection were often less structured. If comparison between children was a purpose of the assessment, then norms or developmental level with a specific scoring system was needed (Fewell & Glick, 1993). The therapist must provide thoughtful attention to the following questions:

- How do I interact with the child? (administration)
- Is this assessment child-initiated or adult-led? (administration)
- Do I set up a play situation or observe the child in their natural environment? (administration)
- Are toys or play materials required for the assessment, and if so, what are they? (materials and administration)
- How long (in time) is the assessment? (administration)
- What do I look for to score the child's play ability? (scoring)
- What scoring system is used in the assessment? (scoring)
- What do the scores mean? (interpretation)

Further considerations for play assessment are molar vs. molecular units of assessment (Gitlin-Weiner, Sandgrund, & Schaefer, 2000) and the reliability and validity of the assessment. Molar units are your general observations of the child during the assessment (Gitlin-Weiner et al., 2000). These observations provide a broader picture of the child's behavior, for example, the child needed time to process information during the assessment, the child was not curious about the play materials, the child was impulsive, the child was easily distracted, or the child talked constantly throughout the assessment. Molecular units are detailed information about specific aspects of play you are scoring, particular play behaviors, and the child's verbalizations during play (Gitlin-Weiner et al., 2000). Both types of observations may be helpful, but one may be more desirable in different cases. A reliable and valid play assessment is important if your play assessment is to be a true indication of the child's functioning. A formal play assessment should have documented reliability and validity. Please see **Box 3.2** for two examples illustrating the essential elements involved in selecting a formal play assessment.

Box 3.2 Two Play Assessments Illustrating the Essential Elements of Assessment Selection

Child-Initiated Pretend Play Assessment 2 (ChIPPA 2; Stagnitti, 2019)

- In the ChIPPA 2 (Stagnitti, 2019), play is *defined* as pretend play, comprising conventional-imaginative play and symbolic play. Conventional imaginative play is defined when a child plays with conventional toys in a conventional way (for example, a truck is pushed or a figurine is put in a bed) and imposes meaning on the play by attributing properties (for example, the animal is tired and needs to have a sleep), referring to absent objects (for example, the truck crashes into a rock, which is absent) and creating a story about what is being played. Symbolic play on the ChIPPA 2 is when the child uses symbols in play and creates play scenes using unstructured objects, for example, the box is a house and the stick is a person.
- The underlying theories are the cognitive developmental theories of play, particularly Vygotsky (1966/2016), who stated that pretend play is the mature form of play. Pretend play is related to social ability, language, narrative, problem solving, and creativity. The purpose of the ChIPPA 2 is to assess the quality of a child's ability to self-initiate their own pretend play for children ages 3 years to 7 years 11 months.
- The *construction* of the administration of the assessment was influenced by Axline's (1947/1974) interpretation of person-centered practice for children (a further *underlying theory*). In administration, the therapist is nondirective, passive, and responsive to the child. Hence, the child is not directed by the therapist because the *purpose* of the assessment is to measure a child's ability to initiate play. The *construction* and *materials* of the ChIPPA 2 reflect this definition of play, with the ChIPPA 2 having a Conventional-Imaginative Play Session and a Symbolic Play Session.
- As the *purpose* of the assessment is to measure a child's ability to self-initiate play, a play space is prepared with a sheet thrown over the back of two adult chairs (called a "cubby house") with the play materials set out on the floor in front of the play space. The therapist sits to the side and introduces the play materials to the child and invites the child to play. This position is less threatening or demanding to a child and allows the child more space to play. The items that are assessed are the elaborateness of the child's play (this reflects a child's ability to self-organize their play and engage in play for a period of time), the child's use of symbols in play, and if a child relies on the therapist's modeled actions (indicating the child struggles to initiate their own play ideas). A clinical observation form is used to collect further information on the quality of a child's play (both molar and molecular), for example, the child's play style, play themes, time played, and emotional enjoyment of the play.
- Reliability and validity are established across several countries (for example, Chiu et al., 2017; Pfeifer, Pacciulio, Abrão dos Santos, Licio dos Santos, & Stagnitti, 2011; Pfeifer, Queiroz Jair, dos Santos, & Stagnitti, 2011; Stagnitti & Unsworth, 2004; Uren & Stagnitti, 2009).

- The interpretation of this assessment provides detailed information on the child's ability to engage in the occupation of play and what this means for a child's function because pretend play ability is linked to social competence, understanding a social situation, language, narrative, creativity, flexibility, and self-regulation.
- A child who might benefit from a ChIPPA 2 assessment would be a child age 3 to 7 years who has been identified as having difficulties in social interaction, delays in language, and inability to engage in play with peers. The child may also present as anxious and rigid with little tolerance to changes in their routine or a child who wishes to engage with peers in play but is often observed watching others and not engaging until instructed what to play by others. Children may also be observed to have a short attention span, with play being manipulation of objects or moving toys around with no overall organization of their play.

Revised Knox Preschool Play Scale (RKPPS; Knox, 2008)

- The *purpose* of the Revised Knox Preschool Play Scale (RKPPS; Knox, 2008), originally called the Knox Play Scale and also known as the Preschool Play Scale (Bledsoe & Shepherd, 1982), is to provide a developmental description of play. *Theoretically* it is based on Developmental Theory (Schaefer, Gitlin, & Sandgrund, 1991). Knox was also influenced by Mary Reilly and the Arousal Modulation Theories of play (Stagnitti, 2004).
- Play is *defined* by 12 categories allocated across 4 dimensions (Pacciulio, Pfeifer, & Santos, 2010). The 4 dimensions with the 12 categories are space management (categories of gross motor and interest), material management (with categories of manipulation, construction, purpose, and attention), pretense/symbolic (with categories of imitation and dramatization), and participation (with categories of type, cooperation, humor, and language) (Jankovich, Mullen, Rinear, Tanta, & Deitz, 2008; Pacciulio et al., 2010).
- Hence, it was *constructed* to cover all areas of development (Jankovich et al., 2008) for children age 0 to 72 months. The *construction* of the assessment includes administration by observation of the child in free play in indoor and outdoor familiar environments. However, reliability and validity has been established for indoor settings only (see Bledsoe & Shepherd, 1982; Harrison & Kielhofner, 1986; Jankovich et al., 2008; Pacciulio et al., 2010; Shepherd, Brollier, & Dandrow, 1994). The examiner assigns a score within a category, based on their observations. The scores provide a developmental play age, 4 dimension ages, and 12 category ages (Jankovich et al., 2008).
- The instructions for scoring have been unclear, with Jankovich et al. (2008) and Pacciulio et al. (2010) devising refinements to the scoring. The Revised Knox Preschool Play Scale gives information about the skills involved that occur in play as well in other activities such as gross motor activities.
- The results of this assessment provide information on areas of delays in a child's development (Pacciulio et al., 2010). Thus, skills involved in play are assessed. Interestingly, Bundy pointed out that "researchers who . . . develop play assessments have failed to recognize that evaluation of the constituent skills used in play . . . does not constitute an evaluation of play" (Bundy, 1997, p. 53).
- Children who present with delays in their development would benefit from an assessment using the Revised Knox Preschool Play Scale because the assessment allows for observations over a range of developmental areas. For example, this assessment would be appropriate for a child of 2 years of age who was beginning to walk and showed no interest in toys, whose verbalizations were vocalizations with single words, whose interaction with toys was primarily manipulation with little imitation of others, and who showed a short attention span.

Types of Formal Play Assessments

There are two main types of formal play assessments, norm referenced and criterion referenced. These types serve different purposes and provide different information about a child's play. They also often have different methods of test development and varied protocols for administration. Both norm-referenced and criterion-referenced assessments have manuals and scoring booklets. The manual sets out the assessment's background, administration procedures, scoring guidelines, and interpretation of the scores (Brown & McDonald, 2009). The manual should also define play as measured by the assessment.

In a norm-referenced standardized assessment of play, the child's score can be compared to the scores of children in the normative sample (Richardson, 2001). A normative sample is usually comprised of hundreds of children from various geographical locations who are regarded as typically developing for their age. The obtained norms are only as good as the normative sample; therefore, these tools typically are developed with large, representative samples. In the United States, these are often based on the most recent U.S. census.

A norm-referenced standardized play assessment provides information about a child's play in comparison to a group of children of the child's age and, in some cases, gender. This allows the therapist to argue for services or funding, particularly if a child's scores are below that expected for age. A norm-referenced standardized play assessment also provides information as to the urgency of intervention and may be used to monitor progress of the child after intervention. The normative scores on a norm referenced assessment can comprise *z* scores, rescaled scores (that is, mean of 100 and standard deviation of 15), percentile ranks, T scores, or stanines (Brown & McDonald, 2009). For example, on the ChIPPA 2, a child's individual raw scores can be compared to same-age peers using *z* scores, rescaled scores, or percentile ranks.

A criterion-referenced play assessment provides information on a child's level of performance across a particular skill (Richardson, 2001). A child's performance is compared to a particular criterion, not other children (Richardson, 2001). Developmental checklists are examples of criterion-referenced assessment (Richardson, 2001).

Available Formal Play Assessments

There are many play assessments referred to in the literature (for example, see Bulgarelli, Bianquin,

Caprino, Molina, & Ray-Kaeser, 2018, and Gitlin-Weiner et al., 2000 for an overview of many play assessments). Play assessments are designed by health professionals (such as developmental psychologists, occupational therapists, speech pathologists) and educational professionals. **Table 3.1** provides an overview of norm-referenced and criterion-referenced play assessments that meet the formal play assessment criteria by Richardson (2001) and Brown and McDonald (2009) of having a test manual outlining administration and scoring criteria. **Table 3.2** includes standardized play assessments that do not meet Richardson's (2007) and Brown and McDonald's (2009) criteria of having a manual for a standardized formal play assessment; however, they do have administration and scoring procedures information published in books and journals.

Table 3.1 Formal Standardized Play Assessments with Manuals

Assessment and Author	Description	
	Norm-referenced standardized assessments	
Child-Initiated Pretend Play Assessment 2 (ChIPPA 2) Stagnitti (2019)	Purpose	Measure quality of a child's ability to spontaneously self-initiate pretend play.
	Theoretical orientation	Influenced by cognitive developmental theories of play particularly Vygotsky (1966/2016), client-centered approach (Axline, 1947/1974), and play as a meaningful and primary occupation of childhood.
	Age range	3 years to 7 years 11 months.
	Area/s assessed	Ability to sequence play actions (elaborateness of play, including attributing properties to objects and reference to absent objects), symbols in play (object substitution), reliance of a model (imitated actions) across conventional-imaginative play and symbolic play. Clinical observations include items such as: time played, scripts in play, enjoyment, talk during play, emotional engagement, specific behaviors during play, play style, play themes.
	Time to assess	18 minutes for 3-year-olds. 30 minutes for 4- to 7-year-olds.
	Setting	Quiet space in a clinic, school, community center, hospital, or home. The play space is physically framed by a "cubby house" (a sheet thrown over the backs of 2 adult chairs to make a playhouse, which is supplied in the kit).
	Play materials	Supplied in the kit. Play materials were trialed for gender neutrality and developmental appropriateness (Stagnitti, Rodger, & Clarke, 1997). Play materials vary according to research on cultural appropriateness.

Assessment and Author	Description	
	Reliability and validity	Interrater reliability was good to excellent via video rating kappa = 0.96–1.00 (Stagnitti, Unsworth, & Rodger, 2000) and in situ, kappa = 0.7 (Swindells & Stagnitti, 2006). Test-retest reliability was moderate to excellent being ICCs 0.73–0.57 (Stagnitti & Unsworth, 2004). Discriminative validity was strong for typically developing preschoolers and preschoolers with suspected preacademic skills ($p < 0.0001$) (Stagnitti et al., 2000). Social competence can be inferred from scores (Uren & Stagnitti, 2009). Scores are predictive of semantic organization and narrative retell (Stagnitti & Lewis, 2015) and theory of mind (Lin, Tsai, Li, Huang, & Chen, 2017). Used in research with children with autism (Chiu et al., 2017; Lin et al., 2017), acquired brain injury (Dooley, Stagnitti, & Galvin, 2019), and cerebral palsy (Pfeifer, Paccuilio, et al., 2011). Used as an outcome measure for children with additional needs (O'Connor & Stagnitti, 2011).
	Availability	https://www.learntoplayevents.com/shop/ Online training available through learntoplayevents.com.
	Comment	Normative sample comprises 693 children. Cross-cultural research has provided validity evidence for Australian Aboriginal children (Dender & Stagnitti, 2011), Brazilian children (Lucisano, Pfeifer, Santos, & Stagnitti, 2020; Pfeifer, Queiroz Jair, et al., 2011), and Iranian children (Dabiri Golchin, Mirzakhani, Stagnitti, Dabiri Golchin, & Rezaei, 2017). The ChIPPA 2 provides information on the quality of a child's play that informs the play intervention, Learn to Play Therapy (Stagnitti, 2021).
The Symbolic Play Test (SPT) Lowe and Costello (1988)	Purpose	Assess symbolic functioning independent of language, and predict future language competence (Power & Radcliffe, 1991).
	Theoretical orientation	Influenced by Piaget.
	Age range	12–36 months.
	Area/s assessed	Child is scored on how they relate the toys together.
	Time to assess	Child allowed all the time needed to complete the test. For the majority of children 20 minutes is the minimum time required for this assessment.
	Setting	Suitable for clinic or school setting.
	Play materials	Four sets of standardized toys: (1) large girl doll, saucer, spoon, cup, brush, comb. (2) Bed pillow, blanket, small girl doll. (3) Chair, table, tablecloth, fork, small boy doll, knife, plate. (4) Trailer, man doll, tractor, logs.

(continues)

Table 3.1 Formal Standardized Play Assessments with Manuals   *(continued)*

Assessment and Author	Description	
	Reliability and validity	Construct validity supported when SPT scores were found to identify a child's level of symbolic play and differentiate developmentally disordered children with and without significant social impairments (Power & Radcliffe, 1991; Whittaker, 1980). Power and Radcliffe (1991) found a significant positive relationship between the SPT and conventional measures of cognitive ability for a population of children referred to child developmental clinics. Udwin and Yule (1982) found a "reasonably significant relationship" between SPT and ratings of pretend play using Singer's Imaginativeness Scale, and the SPT differentiated between two groups of children.
	Availability	https://shop.acer.edu.au/symbolic-play-test
	Comment	Small normative sample of 241 assessments carried out on a group of 137 English children ranging in age from 12 to 36 months. Some children were assessed on five occasions. Despite its name, the SPT does not assess symbolic play. Lewis, Boucher, and Astell (1992) criticized the SPT for only assessing play using objects in a conventional or functional way (e.g., placing the doll on a chair). The play materials have been criticized for gender bias (Wilke, 1992). No new data were added for the second edition of the SPT in 1988. The scoring does not reflect the complexity of the child's play such as degree of organization or elaboration (Power & Radcliffe, 1991).

Criterion-Referenced Assessments

Assessment and Author	Description	
Animated Movie Test Stagnitti (2018)	Purpose	Assess a young person's ability in pretend play in an age-appropriate manner.
	Theoretical orientation	Cognitive developmental theories, particularly Vygotsky (1966/2016). Recognition that pretend play is a lifelong skill (Göncü & Perone, 2005) with pretend play ability in older children associated with social competence, understanding narrative, problem solving and creativity.
	Age range	8–15 years.
	Area/s assessed	Ability to plan and set up a scene, self-initiate ideas, sequence ideas, generate problems, emotional self-engagement, verbalization, understand character roles, use of symbols or symbolic representational thinking.
	Time to assess	Up to 30 minutes.
	Setting	Indoors standing or sitting at a table. Could be administered in a clinic, school, or home.

Assessment and Author		Description
	Play materials	Supplied by therapist, with consideration of the child's cultural background. Suggestions for play props are given in the manual.
	Reliability and validity	Interrater reliability good to excellent (ICC 0.8–0.99 (Stagnitti, Goldingay, & Pepin, 2017; Stagnitti, 2018). Total scores correlate positively, moderately and significantly ($r = 0.53$; $p < 0.01$) with narrative language and moderate positive significant relationship between generation of problems and Theory of Mind ($r = 0.47$; $p = 0.024$) (Stagnitti, 2018).
	Availability	https://www.learntoplayevents.com/shop/ Training is available (see Workshop in link above).
	Comment	The Animated Movie Test opens up new research for the importance of pretend play in older childhood and early adolescence. It has been used as an outcome measure for the Imagine, Create, Belong intervention program (Goldingay et al., 2020).
Play Assessment for Group Settings (PAGS) Lautamo and Laaksonen (2019)	Purpose	Measure children's social play skills and can be used as a checklist of children's performance in a social setting (Lautamo, 2009). Designed by an occupational therapist for early childhood education and rehabilitation professionals.
	Theoretical orientation	Play as a social occupation (Lautamo, 2009) is influenced by Wilcock's Occupational Perspective of Health (Wilcock, 1998), the cognitive developmental theorists of play (particularly Vygotsky) and playfulness work by Bundy. "Play performance was theoretically conceptualised by three elements influencing the dynamic process of playing: spirit, skills and environment" (Lautamo, 2009, p. 117). Spirit (that is inner drive, self-direction, attitude, self-actualization) and skill acquisition are internal features of play, and the social, physical, and cultural environments are the external features of where the playing occurs (Lautamo, 2009).
	Age range	2- to 6-year-old children.
	Area/s assessed	Scoring is a 4-point scale that is based on the frequency of certain behaviors that a child enacts in their social environment. Spirituality and skill acquisition items are scored on a continuum for expressing a playful attitude (that is, meaningful doing) and creating and engaging in play stories (that is, mindful doing).
	Time to assess	Observation time is variable.
	Setting	Children observed in groups in their early childhood setting such as a day-care setting.
	Play materials	Provided within the child's early childhood setting.

(continues)

Table 3.1 Formal Standardized Play Assessments with Manuals　　　　　　　　*(continued)*

Assessment and Author	Description	
	Reliability and validity	Construct validity established the items, which separated children into five different levels of play ability. The PAGS differentiated children who were at risk or disabled from children not at risk. Children with language-related problems were found to have significantly lower play ability than peers (p < 0.01) (Lautamo, 2009). The PAGS shows increasing scores with typically developing older children. For interrater reliability all raters fitted the Rasch model expectations, and there was no need to calibrate raters (Lautamo, 2009).
	Availability	https://www.amazon.com.au/RALLA-Skills-Interaction-Observation-Assessment-ebook/dp/B07VVRM7JD
	Comment	The PAGS provides an easy-to-use assessment of a child's social play for professionals who work with occupational therapists such as teachers, nurses, and early childhood workers.
Pretend Play Enjoyment Developmental Checklist Stagnitti (2017)	Purpose	Provide information on the developmental pretend play age of a child, a child's enjoyment of play, and a description of a child's emerging sense of self through play.
	Theoretical orientation	Influenced by the cognitive developmental theories of play, particularly Vygotsky (1966/2016), with pretend play being the mature play of childhood, client-centered approach (Axline, 1947/1974), development of self (Harter, 2012), and play as a meaningful and primary occupation of childhood.
	Age range	12 months to 5 years.
	Area/s assessed	Six areas of pretend play conceptualized as a continuum: play scripts, sequences of play actions, object substitution, doll/teddy play, role play, and social pretend play. Enjoyment of Play Scale provides a scale from 0–6 on a child's enjoyment of play. A description is given of a child's emerging sense of self. A Professional Scoring Booklet and Parent/Carer Scoring Booklet are provided with brief descriptions of play, enjoyment level, and example behaviors reflecting emerging sense of self.
	Time to assess	Depending on the child's age and play ability, 10 minutes to 30 minutes.
	Setting	Observation of a child's play indoors in the home, clinic, hospital, early childhood setting, or preschool. In a one-on-one setting, the parent/carer booklet provides information on social pretend play.

Assessment and Author	Description	
	Play materials	Recommendations in the manual and supplied by the therapist in consultation with parent/carer so play materials are culturally appropriate.
	Reliability and validity	Reliability to be established through research. Parent/carer scoring booklet report used in research (Dadson, Brown, & Stagnitti, 2020) to show manipulation of play objects reduces impact of screen on a child's fine-motor ability. This assessment is a refinement of the Symbolic and Imaginative Play Developmental Checklist (Stagnitti, 1998), which showed validity of object substitution and sequences of play action with Bayley Scales of Infant Development (Mental Scale) developmental age ($r = 0.75$; $p < 0.01$ and $r = 0.69$; $p < 0.01$, respectively) (Coombs, 2002). The Parent/Carer Scoring Booklet used in television series Old People's Home for 4 Year Olds (]https://iview.abc.net.au/show/old-people-s-home-for-4-year-olds by Dr Evan Kidd, who found the parent scores changed positively over the time of the series (personal communication, August 2019), with the series highlighting parents' perception of changes in their child. Used as a pre- and postmeasure for a child who had experienced a motor vehicle accident (Parson, Stagnitti, Dooley, & Renshaw, 2020).
	Availability	https://www.learntoplayevents.com/shop/ Training is available through workshops (see link above).
	Comment	This assessment informs a therapist where to begin intervention. This assessment provides information on the baseline play ability and enjoyment of the child in play before beginning Learn to Play Therapy (Stagnitti, 2021).

Table 3.2 Standardized Play Assessments with No Commercially Available Manual, with Standardized Procedures Published in a Book or Journal

Assessment and Author	Description	
Affect in Play Scale (APS) Russ (2004) Brief Rating Version Cordiano, Russ, and Short (2008) Preschool Version Fehr and Russ (2014) Kaugars and Russ (2009).	Purpose	Assess a child's affective expression and cognition in play.
	Theoretical orientation	Cognitive and affective processes are developed in pretend play. Symbolism and fantasy are core to pretend play. Influenced by Singer's work.

(continues)

Table 3.2 Standardized Play Assessments with No Commercially Available Manual, with Standardized Procedures Published in a Book or Journal _(continued)_

Assessment and Author	Description	
	Age range	5–10 years.
	Area/s assessed	Cognitive dimension scores: organization of play, quality and complexity of play, imagination, comfort, enjoyment. Affective process scores: frequency of affect expression, variety of 11 affective categories, intensity of affect expression.
	Time to assess	5 minutes.
	Setting Play materials	Clinical or school setting. 2 puppets (male and female) and blocks.
	Reliability and validity	Several publications on validity, for example significant correlations for girls' understanding of emotions and APS (r = 0.36 and 0.33; p < .05) (Seja & Russ, 1999). APS scores significantly related to flexible thinking and creativity with APS scores predictive of coping over time (Russ, Robins & Christiano, 1999). Interrater reliability found to be good to excellent (r = 0.67–0.9) (Russ et al., 1999).
	Availability	Information on standardized procedures and scoring for Affect in Play Scale found in Russ, S. W. (2004). Play in child development and psychotherapy: Toward empirically supported practice. Mahwah, NJ: Erlbaum.
	Comment	Russ states that training is needed to score. The APS provides a lot of information on a child's cognition and emotion in play in 5 minutes. Full assessment is videotaped, but brief version is not videotaped.
Assessment of Ludic Behaviors Ferland (1997, 2005)	Purpose	Direct observation of the child's free play behaviors. Designed particularly for children with disabilities, such as children with cerebral palsy.
	Theoretical orientation	Ferland developed the Ludic Model (Ferland, 1997) that defines play as a result of interaction between: action, interest, and attitude (Messier, Ferland, & Majnemer, 2008). This is a model of playfulness as a subjective ludic attitude and includes curiosity, attention and exploration (Ray-Kaeser, Chatelain, Kindler, & Schneider, 2018).
	Age range	0- to 6-year-old children with physical disabilities.

Assessment and Author	Description	
	Area/s assessed	Scores are given for (1) general level of interest and motivation in the environment, (2) ludic (playful) interests in actions and the use of objects and space, (3) ludic abilities with regard to actions, objects, and space, (4) ludic attitude, and (5) communication of needs and feelings. The "Initial Interview with Parents on the Ludic Behavior of Their Child" (Ferland, 2005) is a parent interview to be used with the Assessment of Ludic Behaviors, which gives information on a child's usual play materials, play preferences, play interests, favorite playmates, positions for play, and frequency of play in the home environment (Ray-Kaeser et al., 2018).
	Time to assess	A 1-hour observation of a child's free play.
	Setting	The therapist sets up a playful environment.
	Play materials	Play materials from sensorimotor to pretend play materials are provided by the therapist. Toys are not standard.
	Reliability and validity	Construct validity verified by three groups of experts who used the assessment clinically and in relation to the Pediatric Evaluation of Disability Inventory (Messier et al., 2008). The Assessment of Ludic Behaviors (ALB) and Preschool Play Scale identified different aspects of a child's play (Messier et al., 2008).
	Availability	Ferland, F. (2005). The Ludic Model. Play, children with physical disabilities and occupational therapy. Ottawa: Canadian Association of Occupational Therapists.
	Comment	Specializes in assessment of play for children with physical disabilities. No additional training required.
Children's Developmental Play Instrument (CDPI) Chazan (2009) Chazan and Kuchirko (2017, 2019)	**Purpose**	Use for play observation of typically developing children. It is an adaptation of The Children's Play Therapy Instrument (CPTI, Kernberg, Chazan, & Normandin, 1998) designed to understand the connection between normality and pathology and hence the contribution to psychoanalysis.
	Theoretical orientation	Influenced by psychoanalysis approaches, particularly Anna Freud.
	Age range	Studies report age range from 1 year to 8.5 years (Chazan & Kuchirko, 2017).

(continues)

Table 3.2 Standardized Play Assessments with No Commercially Available Manual, with Standardized Procedures Published in a Book or Journal *(continued)*

Assessment and Author		Description
	Area/s assessed	Measures multiple variables of play activity, which are organized into three steps of analysis. Step 1: segmentation of child's activity (preplay, play activity, nonplay, and interruption). Only data from play activity are analyzed in steps 2 and 3. Step 2: Descriptive analysis and structural components of the play activity (classification, script description, sphere, and affective, cognitive, narrative, and developmental components). Step 3: Functional analysis of play activity (level of play, engagement, symbolic play, play style) (Chazan & Kuchirko, 2019).
	Time to assess	10 minutes of video.
	Setting	Various settings such as: school, day camp, preschool. Child is observed playing during playtime within their natural environment indoors and/or outdoors.
	Play materials	Within the child's environment.
	Reliability and validity	Excellent reliability with Kappa = 0.8 (0.54–0.92, 95% confidence interval) (Chazan & Kuchirko, 2017). Construct validity studies have examined engagement, symbolic functioning. and play styles both empirically (for example, Chazan & Kuchirko, 2017) and qualitatively (Chazan & Kuchirko, 2019). The results support the underlying constructs of the CPDI.
	Availability	Journal articles and books (e.g., Chazan 2002, 2009). Unpublished manual (Chazan, 2005; revised 2010).
	Comment	The CPDI provides multifactorial analysis on children's play for children who are typically developing. This in turn provides information on the continuum of children's play development. It was not developed for children with a clinical diagnosis. However, it provides in-depth analysis through Step 3 on how children are coping.
Play in Early Childhood Evaluation System (PIECES) Kelly-Vance and Ryalls (2005, 2020)	Purpose	Play observation for typically developing children and children with disability. The focus is primarily on cognitive development, with social skills and social communication (Kelly-Vance & Ryalls, 2020). Cognitive development is assessed through observation of a child's exploration of toys and pretend play (Kelly-Vance & Ryalls, 2020).
	Theoretical orientation	Cognitive developmental theorists of play (particularly Piaget) with emphasis on links between play, language, and cognition (Conner, Kelly-Vance, Ryalls, & Friehe, 2014).

Assessment and Author	Description	
	Age range	1 month to 5 years (older children with developmental delays can also be assessed).
	Area/s assessed	Observer records every play behavior, called "play acts," as well as toys used, others involved in the play, and any interfering behaviors (Kelly-Vance & Ryalls, 2020). Observed play behaviors are compared to a developmental guideline called the Play Description and Codes (Kelly-Vance & Ryalls, 2020). This guideline categorizes play as: exploratory, simple pretend play, complex pretend play, nonplay behaviors, and social skills.
	Time to assess	30-minute observation.
	Setting	Free play environment with peers or alone. Environments can be home, childcare, preschool, clinic.
	Play materials	The observer ensures a variety of toys that would elicit exploratory or pretend play, for example, kitchen set, tools, animals, dolls, stacking toys (Kelly-Vance & Ryalls, 2020).
	Reliability and validity	Interrater reliability was reported to be 90% for typically developing children and 100% for children with developmental delays. Test-retest reliability was reported to be r = 0.48 for typically developing children and r = 0.58 for children with developmental delays (Kelly-Vance & Ryalls, 2020). The developmental categories of play have been validated (Kelly-Vance & Ryalls, 2020)
	Availability	www.plaisuno.com
	Comment	The PIECES can be used as a classroom screening tool and can be modified for children with cerebral palsy (Ryalls et al., 2016). Results are used to plan intervention for play skills. The PIECES play assessment is part of a linked assessment and intervention system (PLAIS). The intervention is CLIPS (Children Learning in Play System).
Revised Knox Preschool Play Scale Knox (2008)	Purpose	Developed for research so that a developmental description of play was gained.
	Theoretical orientation	Based on Developmental theory (Schaefer et al., 1991). Knox was influenced by Reilly and the arousal modulation theories.
	Age range	0 to 6 years.

(continues)

Table 3.2 Standardized Play Assessments with No Commercially Available Manual, with Standardized Procedures Published in a Book or Journal   *(continued)*

Assessment and Author	Description	
	Area/s assessed	Play is described in 6-month increments for children up to 3 years and yearly increments for children ages 3 to 6 years. The 12 categories of play are divided among 4 dimensions: space management (gross motor skills, interests); material management (manipulation, construction, purpose, attention); pretense/symbolism (imitation, dramatization); participation (type, cooperation, humor, language).
	Time to assess	2 x 30-minute observations (Pacciulio et al., 2010).
	Setting	Observations of free play in indoor and outdoor familiar environments.
	Play materials	Materials and toys are found within the child's own environment.
	Reliability and validity	Interrater reliability: range from 0.000 to 0.984 for play categories and 0.000 to 0.986 for dimensions of play. Test-retest reliability: 0.000 to 0.918 for play categories, and 0.861 to 0.961 for dimensions of play. Correlations between PPS and Parten's Social Play Hierarchy and Lunzer's Scale of Organisation of Play Behaviour ranged from 0.495 to 0.713. (Bledsoe & Shepherd, 1982; Harrison & Kielhofner, 1986; Shepherd et al., 1994).
	Availability	Chapter by Knox (2008).
	Comment	Produces qualitative play information and a developmental age. Skills assessed are a broad range of skills involved in manipulation of objects and play. Scoring has been unclear and consequently refined by Pacciulio et al. (2010) and Jankovich et al. (2008).
Test of Playfulness (ToP) Bundy (1997, 2005)	Purpose	To assess characteristics of playfulness in the context of children's play.
	Theoretical orientation	Based on the definition of playfulness by Lieberman (1977) and Metacommunicative Theory (Bateson, 1955).
	Age range	6 months to 18 years.
	Area/s assessed	Version 4 consists of 26 items scored on a 4-point scale (Bundy, unpublished manual; Skard & Bundy, 2008). In the context of play, the ToP operationalizes intrinsic motivation, internal locus of control, suspension of reality, and framing (i.e., how the child maintains the play scenario and understands social cues within the play context). These attributes are scored under the headings of extent, intensity, and skillfulness.

Assessment and Author		Description
	Time to assess	15-minute observation; can be videotaped.
	Setting	Observation of free play.
	Play materials	No standardized play materials required.
	Reliability and validity	Rasch person reliability index = 0.91; ToP can reliably discriminate 4, and nearly 5, levels of playfulness (strata = 4.57) (Bundy, unpublished manual). The ToP dataset has been subjected to iterative Rasch analyses over the years. Currently, 24/26 items (92%) show adequate fit to the Rasch model, and 2,831/3,151 children (89.8%) showed adequate fit to the model (Bundy, unpublished manual). Similarities found between typical children and children with physical disabilities (Harkness & Bundy, 2001), differences found between typical children and children with attention-deficit hyperactivity disorder (Cordier, Bundy, Hocking, & Einfeld, 2010) and children with autism spectrum disorder (Kent, Cordier, Joosten, Wilkes-Gillan, & Bundy, 2020), and differences in environment (Rigby & Gaik, 2007). Numerous intervention studies suggest that the ToP is sensitive to change (e.g., Kent et al., 2020, Wilkes-Gillan, Bundy, Cordier, Lincoln, & Chen, 2016).
	Availability	Skard and Bundy, 2008; However, several items have been removed since the publication of this chapter. The website http://www.testofplayfulness.com contains a scoring program useful for generating interval-level measures from ToP data. Training is available for research teams upon request.
	Comments	There are no normative values available for practice (Bundy, 2005). The ToP has subjected to iterative Rasch analyses, spanning more than 3,000 children, both typically developing and with a variety of clinical diagnoses. The instrument demonstrates consistently strong measurement properties.
Westby Symbolic Play Scale Westby (1991)	Purpose	Understand the play development of a child in relation to a child's language development. Original purpose was to determine whether a child should be given priority for language remediation (Westby, 1980). The revision of the assessment aimed to relate children's pretend play ability to performance on standardized cognitive tests (Westby, 1991).

(continues)

Table 3.2 Standardized Play Assessments with No Commercially Available Manual, with Standardized Procedures Published in a Book or Journal *(continued)*

Assessment and Author		Description
	Theoretical orientation	Cognitive developmental theorists of play, particularly Piaget's work, and development of language. The assessment evolved from play observations during a Piagetian-based language program for children with severe intellectual disability (Westby, 1980).
	Age range	8 months to 5 years.
	Area/s assessed	Phase I pre-symbolic—the developmental assessment of symbolic play from 8–17 months. Presymbolic observations occur under the categories of object permanence, means-ends/problem solving, object use, and communication. Symbolic observations occur from 18 months to 5 years under the categories of decontextualization, thematic content, organization, and self-other relations. Language is categorized under function, and form and content. Developmental levels of play scored as: spontaneous, joins with examiner, or imitates examiner.
	Time to assess	Not given; however, allow at least 20 minutes.
	Setting	Ideally in a playroom specifically set up for the assessment.
	Play materials	Westby (1991) recommends a wide variety of toys (high realism) and objects (low realism) grouped by developmental level such as: presymbolic, familiar high-realism toys, small representational toys and objects, gross motor area, and specific thematic play (for example, restaurant, service station).
	Reliability and validity	The play and language dimensions and original age levels were based on 80% of middle-class preschoolers performing the play language behaviors at each level (Westby, 1980).
	Availability	Detailed information given in Westby, C. (1991). A scale for assessing children's pretend play. In C. Schaefer, K. Gitlin, & A. Sandgrund (Eds.), Play diagnosis and assessment (pp. 131–161). New York: John Wiley & Sons Inc. A Revised Concise Symbolic Play Scale (Westby, 2000) can be downloaded from https://www.smartspeechtherapy.com/wp-content/uploads/2017/07/Revised-Concise-Symbolic-Play-Scale.pdf
	Comment	The WSPS has been widely used in speech pathology.

Practical Considerations

This section describes practical considerations when preparing to carry out a formal play assessment. Occupational therapists must consider where and when to complete the assessment. They also need to pay specific attention to setting up the assessment environment.

When and Where to Complete the Assessment

For young children, the morning is a preferable time for a play assessment. Young children often get tired by the afternoon. An assessment of play in the morning provides the optimum time of day to assess a child before they become tired. A child also needs to be feeling well. A child who is sick or coming down with a cold or fever does not feel like playing. If this is the case, the play assessment should be rescheduled, otherwise a "false negative" may be the result. That is, a child may score as having large deficits in play, when in reality, they were not feeling well.

The setting, the "where," for a formal play assessment is also a consideration. For a formal play assessment, the setting is usually indoors in a quiet room. The room should be well lit with toys available based on the assessment's requirements. Children who struggle with the ability to spontaneously play can become overwhelmed with too many toys, so a recommendation is to place out fewer toys initially with further toys close at hand but out of sight of the child. The therapist should also consider other distractions that may be in the room. Sometimes these distractions cannot be taken away (such as a two-way mirror, light switches), and other times they can be taken out of the room or placed under a covering (such as computers, other toys).

For a play assessment, space is required. If the play assessment is being carried out in a school or at a child's home, the space available may not be in control of the occupational therapist. At a school, the allowed space for the play assessment may require the therapist to move desks or chairs aside to allow for a space on the floor for the child to engage with and move the toys. In the home, an open space may also be difficult to organize, so the therapist may need to physically shape a play space (for example, create a "cubby house" such as in the ChIPPA2, or use cushions or cloth). In a home environment, the child can also run to get their own toys, and this allows observations of how the child plays with familiar toys and what the child

has available at home. For children with motor impairments, special equipment may be required to maximize the child's ability to engage in play, such as adapted seating, adapted play materials, or a communication aid (Ray-Kaeser et al., 2018).

Setting Up the Assessment Environment

The majority of formal play assessments require the therapist to set up the environment for the assessment. This takes preparation and consideration of the play materials and how the play materials are set out. A norm-referenced assessment, such as the ChIPPA 2 or Symbolic Play Test, supplies the play materials needed. Other formal play assessments provide lists or suggestions for the types of play materials that will allow observations of the child's play ability (e.g., Assessment of Ludic Behaviors, Westby Symbolic Play Scale, Animated Movie Test). The play materials chosen for the play assessment should not have sharp edges or be too small (the latter being a criticism by Whittaker [1980] of the Symbolic Play Test). Extra consideration is made for children with allergies (for example, many play doughs have gluten to which some children may be allergic), and particular colors, toys, or objects may be thoughtfully chosen so as to be culturally responsive to a child (Drewes, 2009).

How the play materials are set out are also detailed in formal assessments; for example, the ChIPPA 2 requires the therapist to set up a play space and explains how to present the play materials in the manual. The Westby Symbolic Play Scale and Assessment of Ludic Behaviors have play materials grouped according to developmental levels of play or types of play.

Some formal play assessments require minimal environmental setup because they emphasize the natural environment. For example, the Play Assessment for Group Settings (Lautamo & Laaksonen, 2019) and the Test of Playfulness (Bundy, 1997, 2005; Pearton et al., 2014) allow observations of the child in a familiar setting. For these assessments there is minimal setting up of the environment as the environment is a familiar setting to the child, and the child may not be aware that they are being observed. In cases where they are aware, it has been reported that the children, after a short while, "scarcely seemed to notice that they were being filmed" or observed (Pearton et al., 2014, p. 262).

When a child is observed in a familiar setting, the occupational therapist is passively observing and not interacting with the child. The considerations of the therapist in these situations are that the child is comfortable in the familiar environment, the therapist is unobtrusive, and the adults where the child is being observed have arranged a chosen time for the assessment that will allow play behaviors to be observed. If a therapist is approached by a child when observations are being conducted in the child's familiar setting, the therapist responds to the child; however, the therapist does not instruct the child on what or how to play. If the child approaches to enquire why the therapist is there, the therapist provides a generic answer such as "I'm learning how children play."

When Formal Assessment of Play Is and Is Not Appropriate

A formal play assessment is appropriate when knowledge of the play ability of a child is needed to gain insight into a child's functioning within their environment and the occupational therapist has read the manual, been trained in the assessment (if needed and available), and practiced how to administer and score the play assessment before they assess a child. A formal play assessment can reduce the potential for personal biases of the therapist and reduce missed observations that are crucial to understanding a child's play ability (Unsworth, 2000). Standardized play assessments provide a standardized approach from child to child (Unsworth, 2000). Using standardized play assessments over time, sharpens a therapist's observations

to recognize patterns among children in their play ability and also when and where to look for further information to support their growing knowledge of how the child plays. A formal play assessment used by therapists provides common language and understanding of play between therapists. One of the great advantages of using a formal play assessment is that changes in a child's play ability can be measured over time (AOTA, 2020; Unsworth, 2000). Please see **Practice Example 3.3** for an example of the appropriate use of a play assessment.

A formal play assessment is not appropriate when the therapist is ill prepared; the choice of play assessment is inappropriate for the child's age, disability, or culture; or the reason for referral does not relate to the child's play ability. There are a variety of limitations of standardized assessments (Kelly-Vance & Ryalls, 2020; Wallen & Doyle, 1996). For example, cultural relevancy may be an issue as an assessment developed in the United States of America may have play materials, administration, and scoring that is culturally irrelevant for children in the Amazon. Some tools have been poorly constructed and lack reliability and validity studies that limit their usefulness. A formal play assessment is not appropriate if there is poor preparation by the therapist or overinterpretation of results because the therapist misunderstands the scoring system. The choice of the formal play assessment may be inappropriate if it does not include the age range of the child. For example, it is inappropriate to

---

PRACTICE EXAMPLE 3.3 **Joel and an Appropriate Use of a Formal Play Assessment**

Joel is a 6-year-old child with hemiplegia. The referral indicated that Joel sought out social interaction with other children; however, he tended to destroy other children's play scenes. Joel also had a language delay and was struggling in school with literacy.

A play assessment was indicated because of Joel's difficulties with social interaction during play. Play assessments suitable for his age and disability are the Assessment of Ludic Behaviors (Ferland, 1997, 2005), the ChIPPA 2 (Pfeifer, Pacciulio, et al., 2011), and the PIECES version for children with physical disability (Ryalls et al., 2016). The occupational therapist selected the Assessment of Ludic Behaviors and prepared well by reading the relevant literature and practicing the administration and scoring of the assessment. The therapist has practiced the assessment with 10 children prior to the assessment and has attended training. In the practice sessions, the therapist videoed five of the assessments and asked a colleague (also trained in the assessment) to score the assessments from the videos. This allows for consistent scoring of the assessment. As the 6-year-old child's play assessment is the 11th assessment the therapist has carried out, the therapist is beginning to sharpen observations of what to look for and noticing similarities and differences between this child's play ability compared to the other children.

The results of the assessment show that Joel had difficulty self-initiating play, lacked playfulness and enjoyment when playing, had understanding of the functional use of toys (e.g., a truck is to be pushed), and did not engage in pretense. He had learned how to use toys from observing other children (such as push a truck, put a block on another block, or put people in a train and push the train); but he could not extend his play or join in playing with peers because he did not understand what they were playing. The play assessment contributed an understanding of the child's social and language difficulties and behavior within play.

PRACTICE EXAMPLE 3.4 Juan and a Situation Where Formal Play Assessment Was Not Appropriate

Juan is a 7-year-old child with cerebral palsy, referred for an occupational therapy evaluation for swallowing, toileting, and parent education for positioning. A play assessment would not be appropriate, as the immediate needs for this child and the family are based on practical management for daily living. Furthermore, a play assessment would be inappropriate if the therapist:

- Chose a play assessment that was not suited to the child's cultural background.
- Used a play assessment that did not cover the child's age range. (For example, in this case, the Pretend Play Enjoyment Developmental Checklist, the Revised Knox Preschool Play Scale, and PIECES are all for children younger than Juan.)
- Had not prepared how to administer or score the assessment.
- Had not carried out any previous play assessments.
- Had received no training.

This therapist would most likely enter the play assessment with personal biases in their belief about play; have a limited understanding of play; not be in a position to observe Juan and record objective information about his play; and not be able to analyze what is appropriate play ability for Juan's gender, age, and culture.

use the ChIPPA 2 with children under 3 years because it is not suitable for this group of children. However, the Pretend Play Enjoyment Developmental Checklist or the Assessment of Ludic Behaviors would be appropriate for a child under 3 years. The selection of a play assessment tool must also relate to the reason for referral. For example, occupational therapy for a child referred for toileting or burns would not likely prioritize a play assessment at initial consultation. Please see **Practice Example 3.4** for an example of when a play assessment would be inappropriate.

Conclusion

Formally assessing play allows occupational therapists to identify client needs in both a meaningful and objective manner. Performing this important role requires art, skill, professional reasoning, and knowledge. The therapist new to this area of practice may hesitate at the oxymoron of formally assessing the ability to spontaneously initiate play and engage in the enjoyment and fun of play. However, formal assessment of play is possible within occupational therapy practice when the therapist understands the art of how to administer a play assessment. A formal play assessment is a child-initiated or child-directed assessment that fits with client-centered practice in occupational therapy. As such, the therapist's interactions with a child are to create a safe environment and a feeling of safety so that the child feels free to engage with the play materials in any way they are able. Therapists should be aware of the options for formal play assessment described in this chapter and thoughtfully consider their choice of assessment for their work setting and clientele in relation to which aspect of play is a concern. By measuring play, occupational therapists can determine and justify where play intervention is needed as well as document the outcome of services addressing these needs.

References

Allison, K. L., & Rossouw, P. J. (2013). The therapeutic alliance: exploring the concept of "safety" from a neuropsychotherapeutic perspective. *International Journal of Neuropsychotherapy, 1*, 21–29. https://doi.org/10.12744/ijnpt.2013.0021-0029

American Occupational Therapy Association (AOTA). (2020). Occupational therapy practice framework: Domain and process—Fourth Edition (4th ed.). *American Journal of Occupational Therapy, 74*(Supplement 2), 7412410010. https://doi.org/10.5014/ajot.2020.74S2001

Axline, V. (1947/1974). *Play therapy.* New York: Ballantine Books, Random House.

Ayres, A. J. (1975). *Sensory integration and learning disorders.* Los Angeles: Western Psychological Services.

Bateson, G. (1955). A theory of play and fantasy. *Psychiatric Research Reports, 2*, 39–51.

Bergen, D. (2002). The role of pretend play in children's cognitive development. *Early Childhood Research & Practice, 4*, 1–13. http://ecrp.uiuc.edu/v4n1/index.html

Bledsoe, N., & Shepherd, J. T. (1982). A study of reliability and validity of a preschool play scale. *American Journal of Occupational Therapy, 36*, 783–787.

Brown, S., & Vaughan, C. (2009). *Play. How it shapes the brain, opens the imagination, and invigorates the soul.* New York: Penguin Books.

Brown, T., & McDonald, R. (2009). Play assessment. A psychometric overview. In K. Stagnitti & R. Cooper (Eds.), *Play as therapy. Assessment and therapeutic interventions* (pp. 72–86). London: Jessica Kingsley Publishers.

Bulgarelli, D., Bianquin, N., Caprino, F., Molina, P., & Ray-Kaeser, S. (2018). Review of tools for play and play-based assessment. In S. Besio, D. Bulgarelli, & V. Stancheva-Popkostasdinova (Eds.), *Evaluation of children's play* (pp. 57–113). Berlin: De Gruyter Sciendo. https://doi.org/10.1515/9783110610604-005

Bundy, A. (1997). Play and playfulness: What to look for. In L. D. Parham & L. S. Fazio (Eds.), *Play in occupational therapy for children* (pp. 52–66). St. Louis, MO: Mosby.

Bundy, A. (2005). Measuring play performance. In M. Law, C. Baum, & W. Dunn (Eds.), *Measuring occupational performance* (pp. 129–149). Thorofare NJ: SLACK Incorporated.

Bundy, A. C. (1993). Assessment of play and leisure: Delineation of the problem. *American Journal of Occupational Therapy, 47,* 217–222.

Canadian Association of Occupational Therapists (CAOT). (1996). Practice paper: Occupational therapy and children's play. *Canadian Journal of Occupational Therapy, 63,* 1–9.

Chazan, S. E. (2002). *Profiles of play.* London: Jessica Kingsley Press.

Chazan, S. E. (2005; revised 2010). *The Children's Developmental Play Instrument (CDPI). Combined manual and rating sheets.* (Unpublished).

Chazan, S. E. (2009). Observing play activity. The Children's Developmental Play Instrument (CDPI) with reliability studies. *Child Indicators Research, 2,* 417–436. https://doi.org/10.1007/s12187-009-9043-9

Chazan, S. E., & Kuchirko, Y. O. (2017). The children's developmental play instrument (CDPI). An extended validity study. *Journal of Infant, Child, and Adolescent Psychotherapy, 16,* 234–244. https://doi.org/10.1080/15289168.2017.1312880

Chazan, S. E., & Kuchirko, Y. O. (2019). Observing children's play activity using the Children's Developmental Play Instrument (CPDI): A qualitative study. *Journal of Infant, Child, and Adolescent Psychotherapy, 18,* 71–92. https://doi.org/10.1080/15289168.2019.1567447

Chiu, H.-M., Chen, K.-L., Lee, Y.-C., Chen, C.-T., Lin, C.-H., & Lin, Y.-C. (2017). The relationship between pretend play and playfulness in children with autism spectrum disorder. *American Journal of Occupational Therapy, 71*(Supplement), 266–266. https://doi.org/10.5014/ajot.2017.71S1-PO2051

Conner, J., Kelly-Vance, L., Ryalls, B., & Friehe, M. (2014). A play and language intervention for two-year-old children: Implications for improving play skills and language. *Journal of Research in Childhood Education, 28,* 221–237. https://doi.org/10.1080/02568543.2014.883452

Coombs, G. (2002). *Validation of the Symbolic and Imaginative Play Developmental Checklist. (Unpublished master's thesis).* Master of Psychology, Monash University: Melbourne.

Cooper, R. (2009). Play as a transaction: The impact of child maltreatment. In K. Stagnitti & R. Cooper (Eds.), *Play as therapy: Assessment and intervention* (pp. 31–44). London: Jessica Kingsley Publishers.

Cordiano, T. J. S., Russ, S. W., & Short, E. J. (2008). Development and validation of the Affect in Play Scale—Brief Rating Version (APS-BR). *Journal of Personality Assessment, 90,* 52–60. https://doi.org/10.1080/00223890701693744

Cordier, R., Bundy, A., Hocking, C., & Einfeld, S. (2010). Empathy in the play of children with attention deficit hyperactivity disorder. *OTJR: Occupation, Participation and Health, 30*(3), 122–132.

Couch, K. J., Deitz, J. C., & Kanny, E. M. (1998). The role of play in pediatric occupational therapy. *American Journal of Occupational Therapy, 52,* 111–117.

Dabiri Golchin, M., Mirzakhani, N, Stagnitti, K., Dabiri Golchin, M., & Rezaei, M. (2017). Psychometric properties of Persian Version of "Child-Initiated Pretend Play Assessment" for Iranian children. *Iran Journal of Pediatrics, 27*(1), e7053. https://doi.org/10.5812/ijp.7053

Dadson, P., Brown, T., & Stagnitti, K. (2020, January, early view). Relationship between screen-time and hand function, play and sensory processing in children without disabilities aged 4–7 years: An exploratory study. *Australian Occupational Therapy Journal.* https://org/10.1111/1440-1630.12650

Dender, A., & Stagnitti, K. (2011). The development of the Indigenous Child Initiated Pretend Play Assessment: Selection of play materials and administration. *Australian Occupational Therapy Journal, 58,* 34–42. https://doi.org/10.1111/j.1440-1630.2010.00905.x doi.org/10.1300/J006v14n02_01

Dooley, B., Stagnitti, K., & Galvin, J. (2019). An investigation of the pretend play abilities of children with an acquired brain injury. *British Journal of Occupational Therapy, 0,* 1–9. https://doi.org/10.1177/0308022619836941

Drewes, A. (2009). Cultural considerations. In K. Stagnitti & R. Cooper (Eds.), *Play as therapy; assessment and therapeutic interventions* (pp. 159–173). London: Jessica Kingsley Publishers.

Eberle, S. G. (2014). The elements of play. Toward a philosophy and definition of play. *American Journal of Play, 6,* 214–233. https://www.journalofplay.org/sites/www.journalofplay.org/files/pdf-articles/6-2-article-elements-of-play.pdf

Farmer-Dougan, V., & Kaszuba, T. (1999). Reliability and validity of play-based observations: relationship between the PLAY behaviour observation system and standardised measures of cognitive and social skills. *Educational Psychology, 19,* 429–440. https://doi.org/10.1080/0144341990190404

Fehr, K. K., & Russ, S. W. (2014). Assessment of pretend play in preschool aged children: Validation and factor analysis of the Affect in Play Scale—Preschool Version. *Journal of Personality Assessment, 96,* 350–357. https://doi.org/10.1080/10409280802545388

Fein, G. (1981). Pretend play in childhood. *An integrative review. Child Development, 52,* 1095–1118.

Ferland, F. (1997). *Play, children with physical disabilities and occupational therapy: The Ludic Model.* Ottawa: University of Ottawa Press.

Ferland, F. (2005). *The Ludic Model. Play, children with physical disabilities and occupational therapy.* Ottawa: Canadian Association of Occupational Therapists.

Fewell, R. R., & Glick, M. P. (1993). Observing play: An appropriate process for learning and assessment. *Infants and Young Children, 5,* 35–43.

Fiorelli, J. A., & Russ, S. W. (2012). Pretend play, coping, and subjective well-being in children. A follow up study. *American Journal of Play, 5,* 81–103. https://files.eric.ed.gov/fulltext/EJ985605.pdf

Geller, S. M., & Greenberg, L. S. (2002). Therapeutic presence: Therapists' experience of presence in the psychotherapy encounter. *Person-Centered & Experiential Psychotherapies, 1,* 71–86. https://doi.org/10.1080/14779757.2002.9688279

Geller, S. M., & Porges, S. W. (2014). Therapeutic presence: Neurophysiological mechanisms mediating feeling safe in therapeutic relationships. *Journal of Psychotherapy Integration, 24,* 178–192. https://doi.org/10.1037/a0037511

Gitlin-Weiner, K., Sandgrund, A., & Schaefer, C. (2000). *Play diagnosis and assessment* (2nd ed.). New York: John Wiley & Sons.

Goldingay, S., Stagnitti, K., Dean, B., Robertson, N., Davidson, D., & Francis, E. (2020). Storying beyond social difficulties with neuro-diverse adolescents. *The Imagine, Create, Belong social development program.* London: Routledge.

Göncü, A., & Perone, A. (2005). Pretend play as a life-span activity. *Topoi, 24,* 137–147. https://doi.org/10.1007/s11245-005-5051-7

Harkness, L., & Bundy, A. C. (2001). The Test of Playfulness and children with physical disabilities. *Occupational Therapy Journal of Research, 21,* 73–89. https://doi.org/10.1177/153944920102100203

Harrison, H., & Kielhofner, G. (1986). Examining the reliability and validity of the Preschool Play Scale with handicapped children. *American Journal of Occupational Therapy, 40,* 167–173.

Harter, S. (2012). *The construction of the self.* New York: Guilford Press.

Jankovich, M., Mullen, J., Rinear, E., Tanta, K., & Deitz, J. (2008). Revised Knox Preschool Play Scale: Interrater agreement and construct validity. *American Journal of Occupational Therapy, 62*(2), 221–227. https://doi.org/10.5014/ajot.62.2.221

Kaugars, A. S., & Russ, S. W. (2009). Assessing preschool children's pretend play: Preliminary validation of the Affect in Play Scale—Preschool Version. *Early Education and Development, 20,* 733–755. https://doi.org/10.1080/10409280802545388

Kelly-Vance, L., & Ryalls, B. O. (2005). A systematic, reliable approach to play assessment in preschoolers. *School Psychology International, 26,* 398–412. /doi.org/10.1177/0143034305059017

Kelly-Vance, L., & Ryalls, B. O. (2020). Play-based approaches to preschool assessment. In V. C. Alfonso, B. A. Bracken, & R. J. Nagle (Eds.), *Psychoeducational assessment of preschool children* (pp. 160–177). New York: Taylor & Francis.

Kent, C., Cordier, R., Joosten, A., Wilkes-Gillan, S., & Bundy, A. (2020). Can we play together? A closer look at the peers of a peer-mediated intervention to improve play in children with autism spectrum disorder. *Journal of Autism and Developmental Disorders,* 1–14.

Kernberg, P. R., Chazan, S. E., & Normandin, L. (1998). The children's play therapy instrument (CPTI): Description, development and reliability studies. *Journal of Psychotherapy Practice and Research, 7,* 196–207.

Kielhofner, G., & Barris, R. (1984). Collecting data on play: A critique of available methods. *Occupational Therapy Journal of Research, 4,* 151–180.

Knox, S. (2008). Development and current use of the Knox Preschool Play Scale. In L. D. Parham & L.S. Fazio (Eds.), *Play in occupational therapy for children* (2nd ed., pp. 55–70). St. Louis, MO: Mosby.

Lautamo, T. (2009). Assessing play in a social setting. In K. Stagnitti & R. Cooper (Eds.), *Play as therapy: Assessment and therapeutic interventions* (pp. 115–129). London: Jessica Kingsley Publishers.

Lautamo, T., & Laaksonen, V. (2019). *RALLA play skills and peer interaction skills. The observation based assessment tools.* Finland: Ralla Oy.

Lewis, V., & Boucher, J. (1997). *The Test of Pretend Play. Manual.* London: Psychological Services.

Lewis, V., Boucher, J., & Astell, A. (1992). The assessment of symbolic play in young children: A prototype test. *European Journal of Disorders of Communications, 27,* 231–245.

Lexico. (2020). *Definition of oxymoron.* Oxford. https://www.lexico.com/en/definition/oxymoron

Lieberman, J. N. (1977). *Playfulness.* New York: Academic Press.

Lin, S.-K., Tsai, C.-H., Li, H.-J., Huang, C.-Y., & Chen, K.-L. (2017). Theory of mind predominantly associated with the quality, not quantity, of pretend play in children with autism spectrum disorder. *European Child & Adolescent Psychiatry, 26*(10), 1187–1196. https://doi.org/10.1007/s00787-017-0973-3

Lowe, M., & Costello, A. (1988). *The Symbolic Play Test* (2nd ed.). Windsor: NFER-Nelson.

Lucisano, R. V., Pfeifer, L. I., Santos, J. L. F., & Stagnitti, K. (2020). Construct validity of the Child-Initiated Pretend Play Assessment—for 3 year old Brazilian children. *Australian Occupational Therapy Journal.* https://doi.org/10.1111/1440-1630.12697

Lynch, H., Prellwitz, M., Schulze, C., & Moore, A. H. (2018). The state of play in children's occupational therapy: A comparison between Ireland, Sweden and Switzerland. *British Journal of Occupational Therapy, 81*(1), 42–50. https://doi.org/10.1177/0308022617733256

Messier, J., Ferland, F., & Majnemer, A. (2008). Play behaviour of school age children with intellectual disability: Their capacities, interests and attitude. *Journal of Developmental Physical Disabilities, 20,* 193–207. https://doi.org/10.1007/s10882-007-9089-x

Miller Kuhaneck, H., Tanta, K. J., Coombs, A. K., & Pannone, H. (2013). A survey of pediatric occupational therapists' use of play. *Journal of Occupational Therapy, School, & Early Intervention, 6,* 213–227. https://doi.org/10.1080/19411243.2013.850940

Moore, A., & Lynch, H. (2018). Play and play occupation: A survey of paediatric occupational therapy in Ireland. *Irish Journal of Occupational Therapy, 46,* 59–72. https://www.emerald.com/insight/content/doi/10.1108/IJOT-08-2017-0022/full/html

Nicolopoulou, A., & Ilgaz, H. (2013). What do we know about pretend play and narrative development? A response to Lillard, Lerner, Hopkins, Dore, Smith and Palmquist on "The impact of pretend play on children's development: a review of the evidence." *American Journal of Play, 6,* 55–81. https://www.journalofplay.org/sites/www.journalofplay.org/files/pdf-articles/6-1-article-what-do-we-know-about-pretend-play.pdf

O'Connor, C., & Stagnitti, K. (2011). Play, behaviour, language and social skills: The comparison of a play and a non-play intervention within a specialist school setting. *Research in Developmental Disabilities, 32*, 1205–1211. https://doi.org/10.1016/j.ridd.2010.12.037

Pacciulio, A. M., Pfeifer, L. I., & Santos, J. L. F. (2010). Preliminary reliability and repeatability of the Brazilian Version of the Revised Knox Preschool Play Scale. *Occupational Therapy International, 17*, 74–80. https://doi.org/10.1002/oti.289

Parham, L. D., & Fazio, L. S. (2008). *Play in occupational therapy for children* (2nd ed.). St Louis, MO: Mosby

Parham, L. D., & Primeau, L. A. (1997). Play and occupational therapy. In L. D. Parham & L. S. Fazio (Eds.), *Play in occupational therapy for children* (pp. 2–21). St. Louis, MO: Mosby.

Parson, J., Stagnitti, K., Dooley, B., & Renshaw, K. (2020). Play ability: Observing, engaging and sequencing play skills for very young children. In J. Courtney (Ed.), *Infant play therapy: Foundations, models, programs, and practice* (pp. 53–66). London: Routledge.

Patriquin, M. A., Hartwig, E. M., Friedman, B. H., Porges, S. W., & Scarpa, A. (2019). Autonomic response in autism spectrum disorder: Relationship to social and cognitive functioning. *Biological Psychology, 145*, 185–197. https://doi.org/10.1016/j.biopsycho.2019.05.004

Pearton, J. L., Ramugondo, E., Cloete, L., & Cordier, R. (2014). Playfulness and prenatal alcohol exposure: A comparative study. *Australian Occupational Therapy Journal, 61*, 259–267. https://doi.org/10.1111/1440-1630.12118

Pellegrini, A. D., & Perlmutter, J. C. (1987). A re-examination of the Smilansky–Parten Matrix of Play Behavior. *Journal of Research in Childhood Education, 2*(2), 89–96

Perone, A., & Göncü, A. (2014). Life-span pretend play in two communities, *Mind, Culture, and Activity, 21*(3), 200–220. https://doi.org/10.1080/10749039.2014.922584

Pfeifer, L., Pacciulio, A. M., Abrão dos Santos, C., Licio dos Santos, J., & Stagnitti, K. (2011a). Pretend play of children with cerebral palsy. *Physical and Occupational Therapy in Pediatrics, 31*(4), 390–402. https://doi.org/10.3109/01942638.2011.572149

Pfeifer, L., Queiroz Jair, M. A., dos Santos, L., & Stagnitti, K. (2011b). Cross-cultural adaptation and reliability of Child-Initiated Pretend Play Assessment (ChIPPA). *Canadian Journal of Occupational Therapy, 78*(3), 187–195. https://doi.org/10.2182/cjot.2011.78.

Power, T., & Radcliffe, J. (1991). Cognitive assessment of preschool play using the Symbolic Play Test. In C. Schaefer, K. Gitlin, & A. Sandgrund (Eds.), *Play diagnosis and assessment* (pp. 87–111). New York: John Wiley.

Quinn, S., Donnelly, S., & Kidd, E. (2018). The relationship between symbolic play and language acquisition: A meta-analytic review. *Developmental Review, 49*, 121–135. https://doi.org/10.1016/j.dr.2018.05.005

Rakoczy, H. (2008). Pretence as individual and collective intentionality. *Mind & Language, 23*, 499–517. https://doi.org/10.1111/j.1468-0017.2008.00357.x

Ray-Kaeser, S., Chatelain, S., Kindler, V., & Schneider, E. (2018). The evaluation of play from occupational therapy and psychology perspectives. In S. Besio, D. Bulgarelli, & V. Stancheva-Popkostadinova (Eds.), *Evaluation of children's play. Tools and methods* (pp. 19–57). Berlin: De Gruyter;

European Cooperation in Science and Technology. https://doi.org/10.1515/9783110610604-005

Renshaw, K., & Parson, J. (2020). Infant filial therapy—from conception to early years. In J. Courtney (Ed.), *Infant play therapy: Foundations, models, programs and practice*. London: Routledge.

Richardson, P. K. (2001). Use of standardized tests in pediatric practice. In J. Case-Smith (Ed.), *Occupational therapy for children* (pp. 217–245). St. Louis, MO: Mosby.

Rigby, P., & Gaik, S. (2007). Stability of playfulness across environmental settings: A pilot study. *Physical & Occupational Therapy in Pediatrics, 27*(1), 27–43.

Rodger, S. (1994). A survey of assessments used by paediatric occupational therapists. *Australian Occupational Therapy Journal, 41*, 137–142.

Rodger, S., Brown, G. T., & Brown, A. (2005). Profile of paediatric occupational therapy practice in Australia. *Australian Occupational Therapy Journal, 52*, 311–325. https://doi.org/10.1111/j.1440-1630.2005.00487.x

Rodger, S., Brown, G. T., Brown, A., & Roever, C. (2006). A comparison of pediatrics occupational therapy university program curricula in New Zealand, Australia, and Canada. *Physical and Occupational Therapy in Pediatrics, 26*(1/2), 153–180. https://pubmed.ncbi.nlm.nih.gov/16938830/

Rodger, S., & Ziviani, J. (1999).Play-based occupational therapy. *International Journal of Disability, Development and Education, 46*, 337–365.

Rodger, S., & Ziviani, J. (Eds.). (2006). *Occupational therapy with children. Understanding children's occupations and enabling participation*. Melbourne: Blackwell Publishing.

Russ, S. (2014). Pretend play and creativity. An overview. In S. Russ, *Pretend play in childhood: Foundation of adult creativity* (pp. 7–28). Washington, DC: American Psychological Association. https://doi.org/10.1037/14282-000

Russ, S. W., Robins, A. L., & Christiano, B. A. (1999). Pretend play: Longitudinal prediction of creativity and affect in fantasy in children. *Creativity Research Journal, 12*, 129–139.

Russ, S. W. (2004). *Play in child development and psychotherapy: Toward empirically supported practice*. Mahwah, NJ: Erlbaum.

Ryalls, B. O., Harbourne, R., Kelly-Vance, L., Wickstrom, J., Stergiou, N., & Kyvelidou, A. (2016). A perceptual motor intervention improves play behaviour in children with moderate to severe cerebral palsy. *Frontiers in Psychology*. https://doi.org/10.3389/fpsyg.2016.00643

Schaefer, C., Gitlin, K., & Sandgrund, A. (Eds.). (1991). *Play diagnosis and assessment*. New York: John Wiley & Sons.

Seja, A., & Russ, S. W. (1999). Children's fantasy play and emotional understanding. *Journal of Clinical Child Psychology, 28*, 269–277.

Shepherd, J. T., Brollier, C. B., & Dandrow, R. L. (1994). Play skills of preschool children with speech and language delays. *Physical & Occupational Therapy in Pediatrics, 14*, 1–20.

Short-DeGraff, M., & Fisher, A. G. (1993). A proposal for diverse research methods and a common research language. *American Journal of Occupational Therapy, 47*, 295–297.

Skard, G., & Bundy, A. C. (2008). Test of playfulness. In *Play in occupational therapy for children* (pp. 71–93). St. Louis, MO: Mosby.

Smith, P., & Vollstedt, R. (1985). On defining play: An empirical study of the relationship between play and various play criteria. *Child Development, 56*(4), 1042–1050.

Spitzer, S. (2003). Using participant observation to study the meaning of occupations of young children with autism and other developmental disabilities. *American Journal of Occupational Therapy, 57,* 66–76. https://doi.org/10.5014/ajot.57.1.66

Springfield, E., Rodger, S., & Maas, F. (1993). Paediatric occupational therapy services in Queensland. Part 2: methods and patterns. *Australian Occupational Therapy Journal, 40,* 123–136.

Stagnitti, K. (1998). *Learn to play. A program to develop the imaginative play skills of children.* Melbourne: Coordinates Publishing.

Stagnitti, K. (2004). Understanding play: The implications for play assessment. *Australian Occupational Therapy Journal, 51,* 3–12. https://doi.org/10.1046/j.1440-1630.2003.00387.x

Stagnitti, K. (2017). *Pretend Play Enjoyment Developmental Checklist.* Melbourne: Learn to Play.

Stagnitti, K. (2018). *The Animated Movie Test.* Melbourne: Learn to Play.

Stagnitti, K. (2019). *Child-Initiated Pretend Play Assessment 2.* Melbourne: Learn to Play.

Stagnitti, K. (2021). *Learn to Play Therapy. Process, principles and practical activities* (2nd ed.). Melbourne: Learn to Play.

Stagnitti, K., Goldingay, S., & Pepin, G. (2017). A new assessment for adolescents with social difficulties, the Animated Movie Test. *Australian Occupational Therapy Journal, 64* (Supplement 2), 134.

Stagnitti, K., & Lewis, F. M. (2015). The importance of the quality of preschool children's pretend play ability and subsequent development of semantic organisation and narrative re-telling skills in early primary school. *International Journal of Speech-Language Pathology, 17*(2), 148–158. https://doi.org/10.3109/17549507.2014.941934

Stagnitti, K., Rodger, S., & Clarke, J. (1997). Determining gender-neutral toys for play assessment with preschool children. *Australian Occupational Therapy Journal, 44,* 119–131.

Stagnitti, K., & Unsworth, C. (2004). The test-retest reliability of the Child-Initiated Pretend Play Assessment. *American Journal of Occupational Therapy, 58,* 93–99. https://doi.org/10.5014/ajot.58.1.93

Stagnitti, K., Unsworth, C. A., & Rodger, S. (2000). Development of an assessment to identify play behaviours that discriminate between the play of typical preschoolers and preschoolers with pre-academic problems. *Canadian Journal of Occupational Therapy, 67,* 291–303. https://doi.org/10.1177/000841740006700507

Sunderland, M. (2007). *What every parent needs to know.* London: DK Books.

Swindells, D., & Stagnitti, K. (2006). Pretend play and parents' view of social competence: The construct validity of the Child-Initiated Pretend Play Assessment. *Australian Occupational Therapy Journal, 53*(4), 314–324.

Tessier, V. P., Normandin, L., Ensink, K., & Fonagy, P. (2016). Fact or fiction? A longitudinal study of play and the development of reflective functioning. *Bulletin of the Menninger Clinic, 80,* 60–79. https://doi.org/10.1521/bumc.2016.80.1.60

Udwin, O., & Yule, W. (1982). Validational data on Lowe and Costello's Symbolic Play Test. *Child Care Health and Development, 8,* 361–366.

Unsworth, C. (2000). Measuring the outcome of occupational therapy: tools and resources. *Australian Occupational Therapy Journal, 47,* 147–158. https://doi.org/10.1046/j.1440-1630.2000.00239.x

Uren, N., & Stagnitti, K. (2009). Pretend play, social competence and learning in preschool children. *Australian Occupational Therapy Journal, 56,* 33–40. https://doi.org/10.1111/j.1440-1630.2008.0761.x

Vygotsky, L. S. (1966/2016). Play and its role in the mental development of the child. International Research in Early Childhood Education, 7(2), 3–25.

Wallen, M., & Doyle, S. (1996). Performance indicators in paediatrics: The role of standardized assessments and goal setting. *Australian Journal of Occupational Therapy 43,* 172–177.

Westby, C. (1980). Assessment of cognitive and language abilities through play. *Language, Speech and Hearing Services in Schools, 11,* 154–168. https://doi.org/10.1044/0161-1461.1103.154

Westby, C. (1991). A scale for assessing children's pretend play. In C. Schaefer, K. Gitlin, & A. Sandgrund (Eds.), *Play diagnosis and assessment* (pp. 131–161). New York: Wiley.

Westby, C. (2000). A scale for assessing children's play. In K. Gitlin-Weiner, A. Sandgrund, & C. Schaefer (Eds.), *Play diagnosis and assessment* (pp. 15–57). New York: Wiley.

Whitebread, D., & O'Sullivan, L. (2012). Preschool children's social pretend play: Supporting the development of metacommunication, metacognition and self-regulation. *International Journal of Play, 1,* 197–213. https://doi.org/10.1080/21594937.2012.693384

Whittaker, C. A. (1980). A note on developmental trends in the symbolic play of hospitalized profoundly retarded children. *Journal of Child Psychological Psychiatry, 21,* 253–261.

Wilcock, A. (1998). *An occupational perspective of health.* Thorofare, NJ: SLACK Incorporated.

Wilke, R. (1992). *Gender differences in the toy choices of toddlers: validation of the Symbolic Play Test.* (Unpublished honours thesis), University of Queensland, Brisbane, Australia.

Wilkes-Gillan, S., Bundy, A., Cordier, R., Lincoln, M., & Chen, Y. W. (2016). A randomised controlled trial of a play-based intervention to improve the social play skills of children with attention deficit hyperactivity disorder (ADHD). *PLoS One, 11*(8), e0160558.

Wyver, S. R., & Spence, S. H. (1999). Play and divergent problem solving: Evidence supporting a reciprocal relationship. *Early Education and Development, 10,* 419–444. https://doi.org/10.1207/s15566935eed1004_1

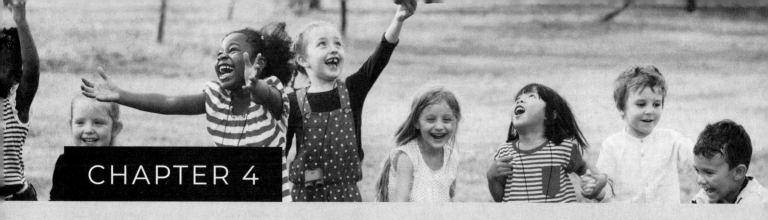

CHAPTER 4

Informal Play Assessment and Activity Analysis

Heather M. Kuhaneck, PhD, OTR/L, FAOTA
Alexia E. Metz, PhD, OTR/L

After reading this chapter, the reader will:

- List possible methods of informal play assessment.
- Describe the benefits of informal play assessment.
- Assess play environments.
- Articulate the importance of activity analysis as a form of ongoing play assessment.
- Complete activity analysis for play activities using the form provided.
- Explain the process for completing an occupational analysis for a child's play.

You see a child play, and it is so close to seeing an artist paint, for in play a child says things without uttering a word. You can see how he solves his problems. You can also see what's wrong.

—Erik Erikson

As a core tenet of this text, examination of the occupation of play should be a critical piece of pediatric occupational therapy evaluation. Occupational therapists routinely complete evaluations as one of the first steps of client-centered practice (American Occupational Therapy Association [AOTA], 2020). The evaluation provides the therapist with information about the client's needs and primary concerns regarding performance in specific occupations in order to determine the various supports and barriers affecting performance. If occupational therapy is recommended, then the therapist must collaborate with the client to determine appropriate goals and outcomes. Often, important goals and outcomes for families and children include having friends,

being able to play and have fun, and enjoying the quality of life and well-being that play provides. Therefore, as a part of the comprehensive pediatric evaluation, the occupational therapist specifically considers play.

Play Assessment

As described in Chapter 3, when the specific assessment of play is included, there are multiple aspects to be attended to. Therapists must consider who the child plays with, what the child would prefer to play, what the child actually plays, what the child plays with, where the child plays, and when the child plays. In addition, because we are working with a child who does not yet have complete autonomy, we absolutely must consider the influence of the child's social context on the answers of each of those questions. Parents, siblings, and teachers have an incredibly important role in shaping the play of children.

As described in earlier chapters, an important feature of play assessment in occupational therapy is the further elaboration of "why." We care about the meaning of play for children and the way in which play impacts their quality of life and well-being. One outcome of a thorough evaluation that includes play will be the generation of plans for children in need of occupational therapy services that target outcomes of importance to children and their families and will not merely list motor skills to learn.

The differing features of play that must be included in our evaluation suggest the use of multiple methods of assessment. Just as we often use multiple tools and methods to evaluate activities of daily living, we may need many tools and methods to examine play. To answer the different "w" questions about play, we must use a variety of methods. There are many from which to choose. There are a variety of formal and structured play assessments, standardized observational assessments with specific procedures and a manual, that were described in the prior chapter. However, there are many informal methods as well. Two cases, of Callie and Gaby, will illustrate the important points of this chapter as we progress and will highlight the differences that may occur between children with difficulties such as cerebral palsy and autism spectrum disorder.

Informal Methods of Play Assessment

Informal assessments, for the purpose of this chapter, include interviews, checklists, parent questionnaires, and naturalistic observation. Many of the available questionnaires will have a manual, and those likely have basic procedures for administration. However, as they are administered verbally or in writing in a question-and-answer format, there is not generally the need for the types of specific and formal procedures for administration that occur with standardized assessments, as outlined in the previous chapter. Additionally, informal observation using occupational analysis is considered here as an important method of occupational therapy assessment both initially and in an ongoing fashion throughout intervention. Occupational analysis during naturalistic observations may be one of our most relevant informal methods of assessing play.

Although formal play assessments are incredibly beneficial and provide a wealth of important information, informal play assessment also has its place in a thorough evaluation. There are times when it may be quite difficult to follow the formal procedures required of the standardized assessments. The child being evaluated may not be able to physically complete what is required for the standardized assessments that the therapist has available. Therapists may be practicing where they do not have access to those tools or the materials needed to complete them. Therapists may be practicing with children who do not fit within the norm group used in the standardization process, thereby hindering reliability and validity. In any of these situations, informal play assessments may provide crucial information. In addition, even when a formal play assessment has been completed with a child, the additional information gathered through informal assessment supports the combined usefulness of both methods.

Purposes and Benefits of Informal Play Assessment

Like all assessment tools, informal play assessments are meant to allow therapists to gather information. However, because of the ways in which the information is gathered, they are not typically used to diagnose and are much more likely to be used for goal setting, treatment planning, and documentation of outcome achievement. Informal play assessments may be more specifically tailored to an individual client, context, or situation. They also may provide access to information not obtained through the formal assessment of play, depending on the tool chosen. They may specifically provide information related to possible intervention methods, as the therapist learns from observation or interview with those who know the child best, what is already working for this child. Informal play assessment can occur almost anywhere, with the typical or usual materials available, requires no formal practice for administration or scoring, and therefore it may require less preparation than more formal play assessments.

Informal Play Assessment to Answer the "Wh" Questions

In any evaluation process, the therapist must make decisions about what information the therapist needs to gather through observation, which must come from the interview, which could come from record review, and so on. Some information does not require complicated methods of discovery, and a simple question posed to the right person will do. There are many answers to the "wh" questions of play that can be gathered quickly and easily by merely asking a caregiver and/or teacher through an informal interview process. Examples of these types of questions are provided in **Table 4.1**.

Table 4.1 Interview Questions to Answer Our "Wh" Questions about a Child's Play

Type of Question	Questions for a Caregiver (and for the child if the child is able to answer)	Questions for a Teacher	Considerations	Possible Targeted Goal Area	Possible Targeted Approach
Who	Who does your child play with in your family? (including extended family) In the neighborhood? In the community? At school? Who would your child prefer to play with? Who gets to decide what your child is playing? Who provides the toys and activities for your child?	Who does the child play with in the classroom? Who generally wants to play with this child? Who, if anyone, teases or bullies this child? Who, if anyone, avoids this child? Who follows this child's suggestions?	Why do we think this child chooses who he chooses to play? What are the characteristics of the preferred playmates? How might we use that knowledge in our therapy?	Increase the number or variety of playmates. Increase acceptance by peers. Improve parent–child play or parent playfulness. Improve autonomy in play.	Establish/ restore—teach new skills needed to improve social connectedness. Modify activities or environments or tasks to promote shared activities. Educate—provide options to generate peer interest.
What	What does your child play when given free choice? What does your child prefer or request to play? What does your child do over and over? What makes this child laugh during play? What is available to play with? What types of toys do you have at home for your child? How much variety is there? How do you feel about the quantity of toys in your home? What toys do you feel are important for children? Are there any toys you do not want the child to play with? Why?	What does this child choose to play with in the classroom? At recess? What does this child do repeatedly if allowed? What does this child try to play that is against school rules? What makes this child laugh during play? What is available to play with? What types of toys and materials are available for play in the child's classroom, recess area, or daycare facility? What quantity of toys are available? Are there enough materials for all the children who attend?	What about these activities are pleasurable for this child? Are these choices developmentally and age appropriate? What sensory inputs do they provide? Are they a "just right challenge for the child"? If they are gendered play, what are the important considerations for the family/social context?	Increase the variety in play forms selected. Increase access to preferred play forms.	Establish/ restore. Modify.

(continues)

(continued)

Table 4.1 Interview Questions to Answer Our "Wh" Questions about a Child's Play

Type of Question	Questions for a Caregiver (and for the child if the child is able to answer)	Questions for a Teacher	Considerations	Possible Targeted Goal Area	Possible Targeted Approach
Where	Where does your child typically play when indoors? When outdoors? Which specific spaces in the home are play spaces? Where does your child play when the weather is good? Bad? Where is your child's favorite place to play in the community? How much access does your child have to commercial play spaces such as at the mall, or restaurants? Where can your child play with peers and where alone? Where does your child have access to play on a regular basis? Where does your child get to play for some special occasions?	Where in the classroom does the child choose to play? Where at the school are children allowed to play (playground with equipment, blacktop, field, etc.)?	How accessible are the play spaces and what variety of activities are available in those spaces? What about the child's preferred spaces might make them preferred?	Improve accessibility and opportunity. Improve variety.	Modify. Educate. Advocate.
When	When does your child get to play, and how often? When does your child have access to the play spaces you indicated are favorites? When is play free vs. structured play? When does your child get to play with the preferred people you indicated?	When do the students get to play during the school day? How often and for how long?	How might the timing of play activity influence the child's behavior, performance, mood, etc.	Alter the child's schedule to allow more time and/or different times for play.	Modify. Educate. Advocate.
Why (meaning)	Does the child indicate feeling powerful or in control? Does this child indicate feelings of success or mastery when playing? Does the child appear to act out emotional issues through play? Does the child seem content when playing? Does this child appear to enjoy the physical or social experience of the play? How engaged in play is this child? How attentive and engrossed is the child?	Does the child appear to engage in certain play activities in order to fit in or belong? Does the child appear to enjoy play with peers? Does the child seem to fit in with peers during play? Does the child seem to use play to manage emotions?	Why might children be playing in the way they are? What might the activity mean for the child? Why might it be preferred? What might the internal experience of the play be for the child?	Improve feelings of mastery Experience joy and contentment. Improve feelings of autonomy, and provide independent choice making. Improve feelings of belonging to the peer culture. Improve persistence in play.	Establish . Restore. Modify. Educate. Advocate.

Adapting those same questions to ask them of a child that is old enough and able to answer for themselves can be a worthwhile use of evaluation time. The child may tell you very different things than the parent or teacher. Follow-up discussions with the family may clarify those differences in perceptions and enlighten both parties about the perspectives of the other.

In the case of young children or children with limited communication, however, alternative approaches must be used. Family and caregiver questionnaires potentially can help in identifying the child's interests; however, caregiver report alone may not accurately indicate a child's preference (Bryze, 2008; Burke, Schaaf, & Hall, 2008; Reid, DiCarlo, Schepis, Hawkins, & Stricklin, 2003; Russo, Tincani, & Axelrod, 2014; Schneider & Rosenblum, 2014; Takata, 1974). Observations and reading of the child's cues can provide indicators of the child's interests and desires (Holloway, 2008; Knox, 2008; Spitzer, 2003a, 2003b), as can alternative assessment methods such as drawing if the child is able (Wiseman, Rossmann, Lee, & Harris, 2019). For those with limited motor control, assistive technology devices and computer-aided assessment tools can be used to examine or help a child express his or her preferences (Besio & Amelina, 2017; Fearnbach et al., 2020; Lane & Mistrett, 2008).

In addition to informal interviews, specific tools that ask about preferences, the "what," and perhaps the "why" of play allow the therapist to determine the child's preferences for play and the meaningfulness of the activities for the child. Several tools assist in this process. One of the newer tools is the My Child's Play (MCP) Questionnaire (Schneider & Rosenblum, 2014). Others include the Children's Assessment of Participation and Enjoyment (King et al., 2004), Preferences for Activities of Children (King et al., 2004), Perceived Efficacy and Goal Setting System (Missiuna, Pollock, & Law, 2004), Kid Play Profile (Henry, 2000, 2008), and Preteen Play Profile (Henry, 2008). The Play Activity Questionnaire (Finegan, Niccols, Zacher, & Hood, 1991) examines play preferences as well and has been used in some studies of gendered play. See **Table 4.2** for more information about these tools.

Informal assessment also can provide information about friendships and the child's peer culture. Research suggests the importance of shared play among children in creating friendships and belonging

Table 4.2 Informal Assessments of Play

Assessment and Author	Type	Description
Adolescent Leisure Interest Profile Henry (1998, 2008)	Self-report questionnaire	A measure of leisure activity, interests, participation, and feelings about leisure.
Child Behaviors Inventory of Playfulness Rogers et al. (1998)	Parent/teacher questionnaire	Two subscales of playfulness and externality (seeking approval, looking to others); 30 items.
Children's Playfulness Scale Barnett (1990) Trevlas, Grammatikopoulos, Tsigilis, and Zachopoulou (2003)	Teacher questionnaire	A measure of spontaneity, joy, and sense of humor; 23 items.
iCan-Play Hui and Dimitropoulou (2020)	Self-report questionnaire using AT	A measure of self-perception of play frequency, desired play activities, and play contexts, for children with severe multiple disabilities.
The Children's Leisure Assessment Scale Rosenblum et al. (2010) Schreuer, Sachs, and Rosenblum (2014)	Self-report questionnaire	Considers variety, frequency, preferences, and desires. Originally created for Israeli children but has been translated to English. Includes 40 leisure activities.
The Experience of Leisure Scale Meakins, Bundy, and Gliner (2005)	Self-report questionnaire	An adult leisure scale (age 19+) rated on 4-point scale for time, ease, and degree of intensity; 23 items.

(continues)

Table 4.2 Informal Assessments of Play *(continued)*

Assessment and Author	Type	Description
MacDonald Play Inventory McDonald and Vigen (2012)	Self-report questionnaire	A measure of the frequency of engagement in play in four categories, play behaviors, and play style. For ages 7–11.
My Child's Play Questionnaire Schneider and Rosenblum (2014)	Parent questionnaire	Considers a variety of aspects of play (persistence, motor control, sharing, preferences, enjoyment); 50 items, for children ages 3–9.
Play History Takata (1974) Taylor, Menarchek-Fetkovich, and Day (2000) Bryze (2008)	Semistructured interview format with play observation	Examines a child's history of play, skills used during play, and choices made for play.

within the peer culture of a classroom (Coelho, Torres, Fernandes, & Santos, 2017; Elgas, Klein, Kantor, & Fernie, 1988; Goldman & Buysse, 2007; Whaley & Rubenstein, 1994; Wohlwend, 2017). The importance of friendships for a child's well-being cannot be over-stated (Caine, 2014; Cuadros & Berger, 2016; Miething et al., 2016) and an important outcome for occupational therapy may be assisting a child in being able to play with peers in order to form friendships. Therefore, we must determine if the child being assessed has friends, is able to play with friends, and is able to show friendship cues through a variety of means. This type of assessment is often informal as well, for example through classroom observation or completion of a parent questionnaire such as the Friendships and Social Skills Test (Whiteside, et al., 2016).

Occupational therapists should be attuned to the child's ability to specifically imitate others in play as more than merely a "play stage" (parallel play, associative play) to go through. The ability of young children to engage with peers through play and imitate their peers' actions in play may be one important indicator of their early development of friendships (Bertran, 2015; Engdahl, 2012; Olsson, Sand, & Stenberg, 2020; Whaley & Rubenstein, 1994). In many children with disabilities, however, physical limitations can inhibit the ability to carefully imitate favored peers. In children with sensory integration dysfunction, deficits in motor planning may limit that ability as well. Although in children, imitation is frequently seen with many other individuals, in toddlers, "friend" imitation is often exact and leads to synchrony between friends (Whaley & Rubenstein, 1994).

Occupational therapists should be aware of and assess the features of friendship that occur through play. In addition to imitation, other important features of early friendships include sharing, helping, separating from others in the friendship pair, and loyalty. Therapists can readily observe these characteristics of young friendships through play in natural settings. We must evaluate our clients' ability to engage in peer play that fosters the growth of friendships and allows them access into their peer culture.

An important aspect of a thorough evaluation of play is to examine the relationships between the who, what, where, when, and why of play. For example, we must consider how the way a child plays (the what) may affect whom the child plays with (who). A second example is considering the person-–environment fit. Many features of the child's play context need to be evaluated in relation to the way in which they impact the child's play options, access, and abilities. These types of questions are often best answered through informal means.

See **Practice Examples 4.1** and **4.2** for the types of important information that can be gained through informal means such as interviews. This information will be explored later in the text as these cases are revisited for intervention planning.

Assessing Environmental Factors and Person Environment Fit

Occupational therapists have an important role in evaluating the environmental factors that influence play performance of the children that we work with (AOTA, 2020). In relation to play and play spaces, the Person Environment Occupation (PEO) approach to occupational therapy (**Figure 4.1**) can be applied (Law, Cooper, Steward, Rigby, & Letts, 1996), examining the player (the person), play spaces, playthings, playmates (the environment),

PRACTICE EXAMPLE 4.1 Callie's Initial Play Assessment and Findings

Callie is a 5-year-old girl with a strong character and personality, who is quite adamant about what she wants to play and how she wants to play it. Her father states he finds it difficult to engage her in play, and he is concerned about how she will do with peers when she begins school in the fall. They have come to the outpatient clinic for an occupational therapy evaluation for both play and self-care concerns. Callie has recently been diagnosed with autism spectrum disorder, yet she is quite verbal and wants to engage socially with others. Her thorough occupational therapy evaluation included the Pediatric Evaluation of Disability Inventory, the Vineland, the Sensory Processing Measure–Home Form, a draw-a-person assessment, and informal play observation. A parent and child interview was also part of the evaluation process. The questions for the interview included a variety of topics related to self-care and play. The play questions were drawn from those listed in Table 4.1. Because of Callie's diagnosis and the reason for her evaluation, questions centered a bit more on the "what" and "who" than on the "where" or "when."

Callie was specifically asked about who she preferred to play with, what she liked to play, and also about the things she did not prefer. She was asked about what she wished she could play or play better. She was also asked about who she played with, who she would like to play with and who she didn't like to play with. She indicated her preferences to be coloring, playing with Legos, and doing puzzles. She played primarily with her younger brother and indicated that she did not have many friends or peers to play with. She said she sometimes liked to play with mommy and daddy. She wanted to be able to play basketball in the neighbor's driveway but she stated that she wasn't able to make any baskets and that the children who lived next door didn't often let her play with them.

Callie's father was asked about the types of games and activities he tried to play with his daughter and then was asked to elaborate about the sequences that occurred when he attempted these activities. He indicated that he frequently tried to build with Legos with her; but that she would identify an object to build, such as a house or a specific type of store, and then she would try to build it with the idea that he would help as well. Inevitably, she would have difficulty making her idea come out the way she envisioned in her mind. He would try to help, she would become upset, and she would yell at him to stop because he wasn't doing it right. She would also yell at the Lego pieces for not coming together the way she wanted. These episodes ended with frustration on both sides. Callie's father indicated that when Callie played with her brother, she similarly bossed him around. Sibling play times often ended in fighting and separation by the parents to their individual rooms. When Callie and her father tried to color together, he reported that she would be very prescriptive. She told him which picture to color, what colors to use, and how to color each picture. She was so worried about how he colored that she would barely color her own. However, she frequently broke the crayons as she colored, and then would become extremely upset and often would either throw the crayon or occasionally crumple or rip up her coloring page and stomp off.

PRACTICE EXAMPLE 4.2 Gaby's Initial Play Assessment and Findings

Gaby is a 9-year-old girl with severe cerebral palsy, no verbal language, and minimal sign language who is being evaluated in the home at the request of the parents. Her evaluation was primarily for home modifications for independence with self-care; however, the parents were also hoping to engage her in greater levels of activity and play/leisure. Her evaluation was completed through observation and a home assessment, along with a parent interview. Gaby has minimal functional active range of motion and limited independent mobility. However, she has a passion for music and singing and a wonderfully happy demeanor. Gaby is able to sign yes with a modified sign the family created with her. Gaby is able to grossly grasp soft toy objects and is able to wave or shake objects with some active movement at the shoulder with one arm. She has very limited fine motor control but could grossly extend her fingers to release objects she had grasped. Gaby is able to roll when placed on the floor, but could not sit independently. She has a wheelchair that was motorized but also had low vision so she was not independent with mobility. She has an AAC device that she was just learning to use, and she was not consistent nor independent with it yet. The family lives in a private home, very intentionally a one-level ranch at the end of a dead-end road with a cul-de-sac. They had felt this would allow Gaby some level of ability to play outside in the driveway with her sister and friends. Because of Gaby's diagnosis and evident motor control issues, the parent interview focused quite a bit on the "what" of Gaby's play but also the interaction of the "what" with the "who, where, and when."

Gaby's mother was the primary informant, although Gaby's 8-year-old sister, Megan, was present and joined in as well. Gaby's mother and sister Megan were asked about what made Gaby laugh and smile, how they thought Gaby preferred to spend her time, and if there were any games or activities they were certain Gaby enjoyed. They agreed that listening to music was Gaby's number one activity. Gaby also enjoyed plush toys and toys that vibrated

(continues)

PRACTICE EXAMPLE 4.2 Gaby's Initial Play Assessment and Findings *(continued)*

or made noise when she touched them. They were asked about Gaby's access to the community and any local playgrounds that were accessible. Both Gaby's mother and Megan commented with apparent dismay that there were not accessible playgrounds nearby, and that limited their ability to access that form of play. Gaby was noted to enjoy the swings when she was able to access them. They did report that there was an accessible community pool and that was a favorite playspace for the entire family during the summer months. In investigating the relationships between what, where, and when Gaby played and who Gaby played with, it became clear that Megan was Gaby's primary playmate and that at times, that limited Megan's play with peers in the neighborhood as she sought to stay with Gaby and try to include her as much as possible. When Megan wasn't available, Gaby played alone, listening to music while lying on the floor and snuggling with her plush toys. Gaby was reported to prefer to get out of her wheelchair when she arrived home, after having been in it all day at school.

Her sister, Megan, reported that her neighborhood friends thought Gaby was too old to play with stuffed toys, and that they sometimes made fun of her and wouldn't let Gaby and Megan play with them in the neighborhood, even when they were playing in areas that were accessible to the wheelchair. Megan clearly felt torn at times between wanting to play with peers and her fierce loyalty to her sister. She tried to get the neighborhood children to play games that Gaby might be able to play too, such as balloon volleyball, or popping large bubbles that they all could make, but with varying success.

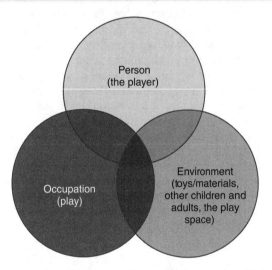

Figure 4.1 The Person Environment Occupation Model applied to play

Data from Law, M., Cooper, B., Strong, S., Stewart, D., Rigby, P., & Letts, L. (1996). The person-environment-occupation model: A transactive approach to occupational performance. *Canadian Journal of Occupational Therapy*, 63(1), 9–23; and Metz, A. E. (2020). Applying a task-person-environment approach to designing play studies. *Play for All Conference Presentation*. Online April 26, 2020. https://usplaycoalition.org/playconference2020

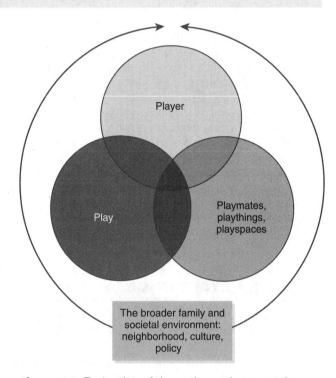

Figure 4.2 Evaluation of the entire environmental context for play allows for broader consideration of potential interventions

and play (the occupation). Occupational therapy practitioners can specifically evaluate the elements of the environment and adjust them to maximize the person–environment fit to promote play (**Figure 4.2**; Metz, 2020). In this model, multiple areas need to be assessed, including characteristics of the child and characteristics of the desired play. For the purposes of this section, we will focus on how to assess the play spaces, playmates, and playthings. It is important to consider and also assess the broader context for play, as issues outside the immediate home or school environment may also provide potential avenues for interventions to promote play. The assessments

in **Table 4.3** can be used as measures of various elements of the play environment.

Other aspects of the environment may need to be assessed through observation or parent interview. Assessment of the home environment might look for features such as spaces that allow movement and exploration, limited noise and confusion, the ratio of space to people, and the presence or absence of toys. Occupational therapists analyze environmental supports and barriers to determine how to intervene with

Table 4.3 Assessments for Play Environments

Tool	Purpose and Type	Availability
Craig Hospital Inventory of Environmental Factors (CHIEF) Whiteneck et al. (2004)	A measure of the things that keep a person from doing what he or she wants to do. This tool examines frequency and severity of these barriers.	https://craighospital.org/uploads /CraigHospital.ChiefManual.pdf
The Child and Adolescent Scale of Environment (CASE) Bedell (2011)	An adaptation of the CHIEF, the CASE is an 18-item parent report measure of the perceived impact of environmental features of the home, school, or community related to needs for services. Designed originally for those with brain injuries, it has been used with individuals with other diagnoses.	https://www.canchild.ca/en /resources/226-the-child-and -adolescent-scale-of-environment -case
European Child Environment Questionnaire (ECEQ) Dickinson et al. (2011)	A parent-report questionnaire with three domains (physical environment, social support, and attitude) developed initially for children with cerebral palsy in Europe. It has now been translated into other languages for use in other countries.	https://research.ncl.ac.uk/sparcle /Publications_files/Published%20 article%20ECEQ%20development.pdf
The HOME Inventory Caldwell and Bradley (2016)	Measures the quality and quantity of stimulation and support available for a child in the home. There are versions from infancy to late adolescence.	https://thesanfordschool.asu.edu /home-inventory
The Affordances in the Home Environment for Motor Development (AHEMD) Cacola et al. (2011)	A parent questionnaire assessing the quantity and quality of affordances in the home of infants ages 3–18 months. This tool has now been translated into multiple languages and has been used in multiple countries.	http://www.ese.ipvc.pt/dmh/AHEMD /ahemd_5.htmx
Test of Environmental Supportiveness Skard and Bundy (2008)	A 17-item observation tool that rates elements of the environment that help or hinder playfulness. Used with children 15 months to 12 years.	Contact authors
Parent/Caregiver's Support of Young Children's Playfulness Scale Waldman-Levy and Bundy (2016)	A 24-item observation tool for children 6 months to 6 years that rates the quality and frequency of parental supportive behavior.	Contact authors

each individual. Environmental supports and barriers may be assessed through activity analysis during the evaluation of the child. The therapist will specifically want to observe or ask about each of the types of environmental factors that could influence the child's play (AOTA, 2020). This could include specific interview questions for parents such as those provided in Table 4.1. The occupational therapist may also wish to use a tool such as the Environmental Restriction Questionnaire (ERQ), which measures parental perceptions regarding environmental features that restrict their child's participation (Rosenberg et al., 2010, 2012).

If at all possible, the therapist should also interview the child. The child may be able to provide important information about preferences, reasons for the preferences, and insights into desires for play, important to client-centered practice. Methods for eliciting information from children may include verbal questioning alone, questioning with photos or pictures, allowing the child to take pictures of preferred spaces, asking them what they want for their birthday, or some other holiday that may include gift giving for children, or using toy catalogs to have the child point to preferred items and explain why.

Observation of Play Spaces. Occupational therapists frequently use observation as part of an evaluation (AOTA, 2020). Although observations may lack the reliability and validity of standardized assessment, there are ways to quantify some of the observations. For example, one scheme for considering the complexity of classroom materials was developed by Getz and Berndt (1982). They examined preschool classrooms, described specific classroom areas, and then labeled "play units" (toys that belong together) as either simple, complex, or super based on the affordances of the materials in that area. **See Box 4.1.** This type of method could be expanded upon for occupational therapy observations and perhaps used as a way to quantify room changes following occupational therapy consultation.

Occupational therapists may also be able to observe and assess playgrounds using methods described by Woolley and Lowe (2013). These authors rated playgrounds for their play value, providing scores based on:

- Range and number of fixed play equipment
- Number of pieces of moveable equipment
- Open space allowing for movement/activities
- Different sizes and types of spaces
- Vegetation/trees
- Landform changes
- Access to loose materials
- Access to natural materials
- Water and sand access
- Obvious physical boundaries such as fencing
- Seating opportunities
- Range of surfacing materials

Box 4.1 Examining the Complexity of Classroom Materials

Compute a room score by totaling the play units in a room and dividing by the number of children in attendance (Getz & Berndt, 1982)

- 1 point for Simple Units—materials allow just one type of activity such as rocking on a rocking horse.
- 4 points for Complex Units—one resource that allows multiple uses or things to occur such as paint, or blocks
- 8 points for Super Units—materials that provide three or more elements together that can be combined to create multiple activities, such as a sand table with items within it like shovels, animals, etc.

The spaces are also scored based on the level of challenge and learning opportunities the space could provide for a variety of age groups and how enticing and stimulating the area is (Woolley & Lowe, 2013).

Other ways to assess playground spaces through observation would include examining the inclusiveness of the space (Playworld Systems, 2013). For example, the therapist might consider if the playground allows for various motor activities for multiple age levels and levels of competence, or if it provides ways for children of all abilities to maneuver through it. The therapist could consider the surfacing and whether children with mobility devices will have any difficulty. The therapist might also want to examine if all children are visible by an adult from any spot on the playground. There should be comfortable spots for the adults as well, with shade and benches. Children should be able to find places to retreat when they become overwhelmed. There must be enough variety of height and challenge for children, and for children who cannot climb or slide, there must be other things to do. Those things to do should be things that all children will want to do, so that they can all play together.

A variety of playground safety checklists exist such as the one from the National Program for Playground Safety (NPPS, 2020). Please see **Appendix 4.1** for one example adapted from Chandonnet, Elam, and Lucas (2013). There is also the Environmental Assessment of Public Recreation Spaces (Saelens, Frank, Auffrey, Whitaker, Burdette, & Colabianchi, 2006) and the Playable Space Quality Assessment Tool (PlayEngland, 2009). The Americans with Disabilities Act (ADA) National Network provides a checklist for assessing accessibility as well (ADA, 2016).

Although the occupational therapist may provide services in one specific setting, it may also be important to assess the child's other environments and the child's performance in relation to those other environments. Children have been shown to exhibit different levels of play performance and playfulness in their different environments (Rigby & Gaik, 2007). Occupational therapists may also become involved in assessing outside community environments and contribute to assessment of play spaces, advocating for inclusivity on behalf of a population or a community.

See **Practice Examples 4.3** and **4.4** for assessment of Callie's and Gaby's play environments.

Assessment of Risk and Tolerance for Risk. Distinct from danger, play spaces may promote thrill, joy, and a sense of accomplishment if they

PRACTICE EXAMPLE 4.3 Assessing Callie's Play Environment

In the outpatient setting for Callie's evaluation, a home evaluation was not possible. Therefore, Callie's father was asked about the home in relation to the spaces available to play, the objects and toys available, and other aspects of "where and when" Callie was able to play in addition to "with what." The information gathered was meant to assist the therapist with intervention planning. It can be very helpful to know what is available, what has been tried and worked, and what has been tried but has not worked. It is also important to determine how play is valued in the home and what amount of space and materials are devoted to it.

Callie lived in a condo with three bedrooms, so she had her own room, separate from her brother. There was not a dedicated playroom, but she was able to play in her room or in the family room with her brother. There was also a playground for the condo complex that had what he called "the basics." There were things to climb on, a slide, a sandbox area, but no swings.

Callie's father reported that he felt there were "plenty" of toys available for his children to play with. The interview with Callie's father also uncovered that Callie's mother primarily purchased the toys for the home and did so based on her online discoveries. She frequently chose the toys recommended highly by other parents, or those listed as helping learning or development. Callie rarely had the opportunity to go to the store to pick out toys because her behavior when they had last attempted this had been quite difficult, and they had to remove Callie from the store screaming. Neither parent wished to repeat that scene. Additional toys came from Callie's grandparents as gifts. Callie's father reported that these gifts to Callie often were dolls and that she had a room full of dolls she never played with.

PRACTICE EXAMPLE 4.4 Assessing Gaby's Play Environment

In Gaby's case, the therapist was able to view the home and assess the play spaces. Gaby had her own room. Gaby's bed was elevated to make transfers easier from the wheelchair. In the bed were many plush toys. On a table in the room was a radio, as well as wireless speakers that played music from Gaby's mother's phone. On a shelf were some bubbles, a few switch-activated toys and one "Big Red" switch. There was a Tickle Me Elmo in the closet as well.

Her sister, Megan, had a closet full of board games and craft activities and also preferred to play games on her iPad and to use YouTube as well. She preferred to make things, though, and was becoming engaged more and more with an after-school program with a maker-space.

Gaby often spent after-school time on her favorite blanket on the floor in the family room, where she could see and hear her mother and sister as they prepared dinner and did Megan's homework. She had access there to playing music and often had one or two toys lying nearby.

offer opportunity to take risk. Mastery of risk leads to self-efficacy. Therapists might follow the guidelines of Brussoni (2015), Kleppe (2018), and Sandseter (2009) to assess the extent to which play spaces support risky play (**Table 4. 4**).

One aspect that influences the range of play opportunities available for children is the parent's or teacher's toleration of risk. The Tolerance of Risk in Play Scale (Hill & Bundy, 2014) assesses an adult's tolerance of risky child play. Another tool, the Risk Engagement and Protection Survey (Olsen, Ishikawa, Mâsse, Chan, & Brussoni, 2018), was initially developed with fathers and has been examined with mothers as well (Olsen, Lin, Ishikawa, Mâsse, & Brussoni, 2019). This tool measures parental views on risk taking and safety for their children and is meant to inform parenting programs and allow for evaluation.

See **Practice Examples 4.5** and **4.6** for consideration of how Callie's and Gaby's parental toleration of risk impacted their ability to access and engage in play.

Assessment of Toys and Objects. Toys in the play environment should be assessed for their safety as well as their play potential, variety, and usability.

Safety Some physical characteristics of toys can cause injury, and the occupational therapist must examine and assess safety risks. See **Box 4.2** for a list of possible risks associated with toys. The largest burden for maintaining toy safety remains on the side of the consumer, including occupational therapy practitioners. Therapists should therefore evaluate all play objects through a lens of safety. Therapists must stay informed of product recalls as well. When the Consumer Product Safety Commission (CPSC)

Table 4.4 Opportunities and Affordances for Risky Play

Affordance/Feature of Object, Item, or Piece of Equipment	Allows	Risk
Climbable and jump-down-off-able	Getting to great heights, jumping down from heights,	Possibility of injury with landing or possibility of falling, crashing
Balance-on-able	Balancing	Possibility of falling
Stand or walk-on-able (flat, smooth, grassy surfaces)	Cycling, running, skating, skiing, chasing, and play fighting/high-speed and rough-and-tumble play	Possibility of falls, collisions
Slide-downable	Sliding, rolling, sledding, running, cycling, skiing/ high-speed	Possibility of collisions, abrasions
Swing-on-able	Moving through space with ability to gain high-speed and great heights	Possibility of falls or collisions
Graspable (including sticks, soft hammers, plastic shovels, can include other dangerous tools)	Throwing or striking, whittling, sawing, axing	Possibility of injuries from collision with objects, being poked or cut, bruised
Wrappable or tie-able	Tying up others,	Possibility of injury through rope burns, dragging, strangulation, impingement
Bounce-able (mattresses, sofas, trampolines)	Jumping	Possibility of injury via impact or falls
Land-able (mattresses, sofas, pillows, soft grounds, and soft walls)	Falling, crashing	Possibility of injury via impact or falls
Move-able, lift-able	Carrying, pushing, sliding	Possibility of bruising or impingement

---

PRACTICE EXAMPLE 4.5 Assessment of Risk in Callie's Play

Callie's father was asked generally about his feelings related to the types of play he would and would not allow Callie to engage in, in relation to how dangerous he felt they were. At Callie's age, her diagnosis, and because of where they lived, he reported she was always supervised in her play outdoors, but that he would sit on the bench and watch from a distance as opposed to being "right on top of her all the time." He also mentioned the need to be able to watch both Callie and her brother at the playground and stated he trusted Callie not to hurt herself with carelessness more than he trusted her younger brother. There were no activities on the nearby playground that he would not let her attempt. He stated he thought the playground was "pretty tame." He did specify that the family had rules about sticks and rocks, that were meant to stop Callie's brother, who seemed to always want to pick up and use rocks and sticks as weapons in his play. The one area of more risky play that was currently an area of difficulty was bike riding in the neighborhood. Callie was just learning to ride with training wheels and he did not feel she was at all safe unless he were there right next to her. He said she was still watching her feet and the ground and not yet looking where she was going, so he wouldn't let her ride without him beside her, even in the back parking lot of the complex that was hardly used.

PRACTICE EXAMPLE 4.6 Assessment of Risk in Gaby's Play

Gaby's mother reported herself to be a "fairly laid back mom." She described how much freedom she had as a child and how it makes her sad that the children now don't have that opportunity to learn to manage for themselves a bit. She also noted that she trusted Megan immensely. She said Megan was her "old soul" and stated she felt ok about letting Gaby and Megan play in the back or front of the house without her, as long as they didn't leave the cul-de-sac area. Her main concern for Gaby was for her safety with cars, as she wasn't able to maneuver out of the way quickly in her motorized wheelchair. She was also slightly concerned about the wheelchair getting stuck or tipping over after perhaps striking the curb the wrong way. She felt that Megan was able to watch Gaby enough to give Gaby and Megan both some measure of freedom that she was allowed at that age.

Box 4.2 Risk Possibilities to Assess or Consider with Specific Toys and Playthings

- Sharp areas that could puncture or cut
- Areas that heat up and could burn
- Electrical features that could shock or electrocute
- Any lengthy cords that could strangle
- Any plastic coverings that could suffocate
- Extremely loud decibel level that could damage hearing
- Toys that propel objects with force and can damage an eye or cut or puncture
- Areas that move or bend and could pinch skin or crush digits
- Toys that move or have height where a fall could occur
- Toys with small pieces that could pose a choking hazard

Box 4.3 Assessment of the Dimensions of Play Provided by a Specific Toy

- Does the toy lead to a child demonstrating thinking and learning behaviors (exploration, facial expressions of concentration, commenting on discoveries)?
- Does the toy lead to child problem solving?
- Does the toy lead the child to show curiosity by asking questions about it or showing facial expressions of puzzlement?
- Does the toy sustain a child's interest?
- Does a toy lead the child to creativity, by using the toy in a novel way or conveying a new or unique idea?
- Does the toy lead a child to use symbolism, such as using it for pretend?
- Does the toy lead a child to interact, collaborate, and/or communicate with peers?
- Is the toy something the child can use independently without frustration or assistance?
- Does the toy impact the child's mood, create enjoyment?

---

recommends or mandates a product recall, the information is posted to a searchable list online: https://www.cpsc.gov/Recalls. Occupational therapy practitioners working with children should review the list regularly. Toys on the list should be removed from clinical practice settings. If a therapist is aware that a family has a listed toy in a client's home, particularly if it was a therapist-recommended purchase, the therapist should alert them to the recall.

Play Potential and Variety Occupational therapists can work with parents or teachers to develop a toy inventory in homes or classrooms. Therapists can provide a list of categories of toys (see Chapter 1) and example toys for each category and ask the parents/teachers to report on the variety of toys available. Individual toys can be rated using methods developed for research purposes (Trawick-Smith et al., 2014). A toy score is compiled by rating dimensions of play as listed in **Box 4.3**. AOTA (2011) created a checklist to assess the characteristics of toys for their suitability for play, comprising yes/no questions addressing toy safety, appeal, affordances, uses, appeal, and worth. Together, these assessments of toys can provide a basis for parent or teacher education, leading to improved play spaces for individuals or groups of children.

Based on an evaluation of what the child can do and what the child needs or wants to do with objects, the occupational therapist determines which and how many objects in the environment support play for that child (see **Practice Examples 4.7** and **4.8** Callie and Gaby). The occupational therapist may help select toys to create a home play environment (AOTA, 2011; Morozini, 2015).

Usability According to the International Organization for Standardization (ISO), the term *usability* means that a product can be used by a user to achieve specific goals both efficiently and effectively and that the user will be satisfied with the product within a specific context of use (Ekin, Çağiltay, & Karasu, 2018; ISO 9241-11, 1998). Most studies of usability have focused on technology and web applications more so than toys (Sherwin & Nielsen, 2019). However, usability is now a feature being considered in toy design (Ekin et al., 2018). Specifically, usability for a toy often means a few specific things (Crafts, 2013.). First, that the toy can be accessed and played with, without any instruction. Think of a ball, for example. For most children, there would not need to be instructions for how to approach and begin to play with a ball. Usable toys also provide some form of intrinsic "reinforcement" for their use. This may be as simple as the texture of a plush toy that feels good to the touch, or an electronic doll that smiles when it is picked up. Highly usable toys enable play across many ages and abilities. Think of a toy like playdough or Legos that can be used many different ways by different children. These toys are highly usable. Lastly, for children, the toys should be unbreakable. Some had added the additional consideration of child self-efficacy to toy usability (Martin, 2007).

PRACTICE EXAMPLE 4.7 Assessment of Callie's Toys

Callie's father's answers about Callie's toys were illuminating. Callie had many toy objects that she never used; and the objects that she played with the most, the Legos, were difficult enough for her to manipulate that they led to frustration rather than feelings of success and enjoyment. Her crayons, a favorite play object, were hard for her to keep in "good working order" as she broke them often. She disliked using the broken pieces so they had to keep replacing her crayons.

The occupational therapist noted that although Callie reported that she wished to play basketball, she did not have a basketball or hoop, or a nerf basketball or hoop to practice with. Callie's play objects were not items that she could use without frustration and they didn't necessarily promote her problem-solving ability.

PRACTICE EXAMPLE 4.8 Assessment of Gaby's Play Objects

Gaby had many play objects available to her that she reportedly preferred, as well as many items tucked away in a closet that she was no longer using. The therapist noted the earlier attempts at using technology to help Gaby play, but also noted that there were no new technology-related play items and no computer with appropriate books or games for Gaby.

The occupational therapist noted that many of Gaby's preferred items were those that would more typically be chosen and used by a child much younger than Gaby. The toy objects available to her, although preferred, did not lend themselves to sustained interest, nor were they age appropriate to potentially support communication with peers or neighborhood children.

In occupational therapy, examining usability for a specific child is based on an occupational analysis, but we may also consider an instrument such as the *Toys and Games Usability Evaluation Tool* (TUET; Costa, Périno, & Ray-Kaeser, 2018). The purpose of the tool, according to the site where it is freely available, is to help "toy companies, education and rehabilitation professionals, toy librarians, teachers and parents . . . design, select and adapt toys and games to the needs of all children, including those with hearing, visual, or motor impairments" (TUET, 2018) In terms of motor impairment, the tool specifically targets upper limb impairments.

Activity Analysis and Occupational Analysis as Informal Methods of Play Assessment

Occupational therapists use both activity analysis and occupational analysis as tools for assessment (AOTA, 2020). In activity analysis, the therapist seeks to understand the basic components of activities that can be used in therapeutic ways or that can be readily altered to provide greater therapeutic benefit. In occupational analysis the therapist is examining "the specific situation of the client and therefore . . . the specific occupations the client wants or needs to do in the actual context in which these occupations are performed" (Schell et al., 2019, p. 322). Activity analysis is one of the earliest tools of the profession, and both are fundamental skills occupational therapists possess. Although some elements of activity analysis are used by a few other professionals, both activity analysis and occupational analysis are used in a unique way by occupational therapists to look holistically at their complexity and individuality (Spitzer, 2020). Over the years, many therapists have written about the process, and as stated by Buckley and Poole (2004), it is often difficult to determine where specific ideas originated. However, for those interested, **Appendix 4.2** provides information about the lengthy history of activity analysis within occupational therapy and how these changes were expressed through the curriculum to train occupational therapists of the time **(Appendix 4.3)**.

Activity Analysis. There have been multiple definitions of activity analysis throughout the years, but a common element within the definitions is the careful observation of an activity to identify the features of the activity that may be adapted and/or used therapeutically. Fidler and Velde (1999, p. 48) described activity analysis as follows:

> [A] process that assesses the elements or characteristics of an activity for the purpose of identifying and defining the dimensions of its performance requirements and its social and cultural significance and meanings. It is a process of looking at parts as these relate to the whole.

Mosey (1981, 1986) described activity analysis as the process of distinguishing the parts of an activity via careful observation to then select the most appropriate activities for use in intervention. Llorens (1993) added the dimension of client desires and motivations in her description of activity analysis. Over time, the term *occupational analysis* came to be used to mean the process of focusing on the specific consideration of the client in a particular context, and the meaning of the occupation for that client.

Activity analysis is the process through which occupational therapists learn to analyze specific activities in great detail. This type of activity analysis is often done by novice occupational therapists or more experienced therapists encountering a novel activity. Typically, a student will engage in an activity and then complete a full analysis for the express purpose of learning the process of activity analysis, whereas a therapist more skilled in the process will complete an activity analysis to learn the essential features of a novel activity. Activity analysis allows us to determine the demands of an activity.

Activity analysis is used to "arrive at an understanding of the activity's inherent qualities and characteristics, its meaning in and of itself, irrespective of a performer" (Fidler & Velde, 1999, p. 47). This knowledge then is used in the clinical reasoning process of the therapist to select appropriate activities as possibilities for intervention (see Chapter 7). Part of this process is the ability to compare activity A with activity B to consider the features of each and determine which is best for a client to meet a particular goal. The knowledge gained through completing activity analysis with multiple activities and the ability to do so quickly and thoroughly in one's head, allows us to later select appropriate and meaningful therapeutic activities for a client to achieve specific aims. In relation to play, this is used most frequently when we are using play as a tool.

We want to stress here that although experienced practicing therapists typically do not complete formal activity analyses and do not typically fill out lengthy paper forms, activity analysis remains a crucial process for occupational therapists. We constantly are reevaluating and completing informal activity analyses in our heads. We consider this process to be essential to pediatric occupational therapy.

Occupational Analysis. Occupational analysis is a fundamental component of occupational therapy evaluation and intervention. During an evaluation, it allows a therapist to observe a client during the completion of a task and create hypotheses regarding the causes for a client's difficulties in performance, as well as hypotheses regarding how to alter or modify activities to increase client success and personal meaning. During occupational analysis, the therapist must consider the activity in the context in which it is typically performed.

Occupational analysis allows us to modify the activity or engage the client in the appropriate activity with the just-right challenge that provides therapeutic value and a match to the client's current capabilities (see Chapter 8). The outcome of occupational analysis specifically is the therapist's ability to adapt, alter, or modify an activity to allow a client to participate and to rapidly grade components of activities to increase or decrease their difficulty for a client. In relation to play, this skill allows us to create the just right challenge, make work into play, and maintain a playful collaborative atmosphere with pediatric clients. In working with clients, occupational analysis becomes second nature to the seasoned occupational therapist. However, it is a skill that must be learned, and it takes practice to become adept. So, let us now turn to how to do activity analysis.

The Process of Activity Analysis. Although a multitude of variables need to be considered during an activity analysis, the steps to completing one are relatively simple. The process for an activity analysis is to observe or engage in an activity until one has a good understanding of what the activity entails. Next, one considers all aspects of the activity and the context within which the activity typically occurs. For those who require a written format such clinicians analyzing an unfamiliar activity and students, the activity is then described on paper or by digital means. See **Figure 4.3** for an activity analysis form you can use to guide your thinking as you begin to develop this skill. This downloadable form is provided in the Navigate 2 digital offering that comes with purchase of this text.

There are specific considerations and questions to ask of yourself about the activity to complete the form. First, you enter the name of the activity and provide a general description of what the activity consists of. For some activities you may be able to pull a definition right from a dictionary. For example, for the activity of playing soccer, a quick Internet search suggests that a description of soccer is "a game played by two teams of eleven players with a round ball that may not be touched with the hands or arms during play except by the goalkeepers. The object of the game is to score goals by kicking or heading the ball into the opponents' goal" (Lexico, 2020). However, for many activities you will write your own brief description.

Next you will consider the global demands of the activity. Each activity has certain demands or requirements that stand out. For example, playing with

Name

Description

Global Demands

Materials and Supplies Needed

Safety Concerns

Space Needed

Time Needed

Figure 4.3 Activity analysis form

Steps or Processes to Complete the Activity

Movements Needed for Each Step

Coordination and Balance Needed

Sensory Input Provided or Experienced

Thinking Skills Needed

Social Interaction Required

Possible Emotional Responses or Associations

Figure 4.3 (Continued)

puzzles has primarily visual-perceptual-motor and fine-motor demands but little requirements in terms of strength and balance if completed while sitting or lying prone. Alternatively, riding a bike has intense visual-motor-coordination and balance demands and very little in the way of fine-motor skill requirements. For the global demands section of the form, think about the primary areas of skill that the activity requires, and focus on those. Those primary demands would be the reason you might select an activity to encourage development of specific skills (using play as a tool), so those are the most important to consider. If you wanted to work on eye–hand coordination in play, you would select something like catching or throwing a ball as opposed to something like winding up a windup toy. However, if you wanted to work on pinch and bilateral hand use, you might select the windup toy. You would not likely select balloon volleyball to work on hand strength, but you might select it to work on endurance or active range of motion at the shoulder and elbow.

For the box on the form labeled materials and supplies needed, you should list everything required to complete the activity from start to finish. Then you must consider the cost and ease of access to those materials and supplies. Does it require special paint that you have to order in advance? Does it use only simple household materials that are readily available? Does it require special equipment such as helmets or padding? Does it require payment to attend or participate?

As you consider the materials and supplies, at the same time consider their safety. Is there a potential for physical harm, allergic reaction, dust, fumes, skin irritations, poisons, or injury with tools? As you continue to consider safety, think about the potential for falling, being hit with something, or psychological distress from the process. Some activities such as bungee jumping are more inherently dangerous than others, such as making pom-poms with yarn.

As you consider the space requirements for the activity, think about whether the activity needs a large or small space, a quiet or noisy space, an open uncluttered space, a well-lit space, or a darkened space. Consider who else might be in the space where this activity occurs.

In relation to the time the activity takes, consider the entire time from beginning to completion, but also consider whether or not the activity can be started and stopped. If someone is unable to finish, can the product to that point be saved? Do any of the steps require a specific period of time?

Next consider all of the steps to complete the activity. Some activities have very few steps, while others have many. See **Table 4.5** for a comparison of the number and complexity of steps for four different play activities. It is important to list each step individually and consider each step individually, as each step may require very different motor skills, cognitive skills, perceptual skills, and so on.

The movement portion of the activity analysis is specifically important when using one of the frames of reference related to sensory-motor skill. You can identify exactly which motions are required, which joints are used for each, which specific muscles must contract to perform that motion, and with how much strength required to complete the motion for each step. What position must the activity be completed in? Is the motion against gravity or gravity assisted? Is the motion against resistance? Is the motion weighted, for example, by needing to hold onto a heavy object? Is the full range of motion required? You also consider the number of times that the motion must be repeated and how much endurance is therefore required. Consider how much smoothness and accuracy is required for the motion. Is it important to have good timing to complete this activity? Is the activity unilateral or bilateral? If bilateral, is it symmetrical or asymmetrical? If asymmetrical, is it reciprocal? Is crossing midline required? What type of eye–hand or eye–foot coordination is required? What posture and balance is required? Does the activity require movement through space, and if so, how? How novel is the motion for the step? Will completing the novel motion require significant praxis for most people?

Next consider the specific sensory experiences provided by and required for the activity. Does the activity have a smell, does it make noise, does it require touching varied objects or textures, does it require experiencing hot or cold temperatures? Does it provide opportunities to experience joint and muscle input through pulling, pushing, carrying, hanging, kicking, jumping. Does it provide opportunities to experience the joy or fear of motion through space? Is it required that the participant taste something for this activity? What colors, patterns, or other visual experiences are provided? In terms of sensory perception, does this activity require one to be able to identify or match by color, size, shape/form? Must one know right from left, up from down? Is figure-ground perception required? Is depth perception required? Does the activity require stereognosis? Is it

Table 4.5 Comparison of Number and Complexity of Steps for Four Selected Play Activities

Step	Playing Peek-a-Boo	Blowing Bubbles	Playing Puzzles	Bike Riding
1	Face someone	Get container of bubbles	Collect desired puzzle	Pick up bike by grasping handlebars
2	Place hands over face, covering eyes	Open the bubbles	Open puzzle box	Put one leg over bike, straddle seat
3	Slowly remove hands while saying peek-a-boo	Remove the bubble wand	Remove puzzle pieces from box	Sit on bike seat
4	Repeat as desired	Blow into the end of the wand with the open area for the "bubble juice" to create bubbles	Separate puzzle pieces from each other	Lift leg to put one foot on one pedal
5		Put wand back into jar and repeat until finished playing	Spread out puzzle pieces on the table or floor	Lift other leg and begin to push pedal with the first foot
6		Place cap back on container	Look for matching pieces and place them one at a time. Repeat until all pieces are in or attached, or you are finished playing	Alternate feet, pushing one pedal first, then the next
7		Put the bubbles away	Place puzzle pieces back in the box	Maintain handlebars in appropriate position to direct the bike to where you want to go, avoiding obstacles
8			Put puzzle away	Apply brakes to stop the bike when ready
9				Put one or both feet down on the ground
10				While still holding onto the handlebars, lift one leg/foot over the bike to rest on the ground next to the other
11				Place bike down on the ground or put kickstand down and rest bike on kickstand

important to have a good body scheme to be able to complete this activity?

In terms of the thinking skills required, consider all the cognitive requirements of the activity (Chapparo, 2010). How much does one need a good attention span and strong concentration? What are the memory requirements of this activity? How much monitoring is required while completing the activity? How much planning is required? What is the nature of problem solving required to this activity? Is logic required? Must one be fully oriented to person, place, and time? What level of arousal is required? How much independent choice making is required? Does one need good judgment for this activity? Is safety awareness an issue? Does the activity require symbolic or abstract thinking? Does the activity require categorization? What technical knowledge is required? How much new learning is required? How much sequencing is required? Are there few or multiple steps?

Next, consider the social interaction required. Some activities can be done alone. Others require interaction in order to complete them. Think about how much interaction is needed for the activity and the nature of the interaction. Is cooperation required? Sharing? Turn taking? Is conversation required? Is there an aspect of competition? How much dependence on others is required?

Finally, consider the emotional aspect of the activity. What motivating factors are there in this activity? How much does this activity provide a sense of control, a sense of productivity, a sense of competence, and a sense of achievement? How challenging is the activity, and how much opportunity is there for success? Is this activity structured or unstructured? Does it have a predictable or unpredictable outcome? How much creativity and expression is allowed? How much choice is allowed? How much delay of gratification is needed? How much does this activity allow individuality? Are the motions aggressive (hammering, banging), or destructive? Are there other outlets in this activity for aggression? What could the materials symbolize or represent for an individual? What is the potential for positive or negative associations with the activity? For example, is the activity typically considered gendered? Or associated with a certain age group? Are there cultural associations?

As you will note, our format does not specifically follow the occupational therapy practice framework (OTPF) (AOTA, 2020). Although prior activity analysis literature has incorporated first the Uniform Terminology (Cottrell, 1996) and, then the OTPF in writings about activity analysis (Crepeau, 2003; Hersch, Lamport, & Coffey, 2005), Fidler and Velde (1999) warned about the use of such documents to guide activity analysis. They stated that it was difficult to translate certain portions of the Uniform Terminology into the analysis of an activity. The same could be said of the OTPF. There are areas of the OTPF, for example, that focus on the client rather than the activity. Using such documents could lead therapists to miss some essential aspect of the activity's character. Additionally, while the OTPF is an important document for our profession, some of the terminology may be hard to understand for our pediatric clients, their parents,

or the teachers we work with. For our purposes, we suggest you consider the OTPF where it is applicable, but our process and format for the activity analysis does not strictly follow its terminology, and we have chosen to use regular everyday language. In chapters that follow, we will describe how it can be helpful to teach parents how to do aspects of activity analysis, to help them problem solve at home with their children when the therapist is not available. To do so, we need to use terminology they will understand.

The Process of Occupational Analysis.

Once an occupational therapist has mastered the art of completing activity analyses, the next task is to integrate that skill into practice with clients. Skill with occupational analysis is useful for practitioners in their initial evaluations of client performance and throughout client intervention. The difference between the activity analysis and occupational analysis is that when completing occupational analysis, the therapist must consider information not only about the activity and the specific context but also about the client. Often, this information is gathered during the initial evaluation as the therapist creates the occupational profile (AOTA, 2020). This information can also be gathered by using occupational analysis while observing an individual client completing a specific activity in an evaluation or treatment, which allows the occupational therapist to determine what aspects of the activity are difficult for the client and to generate hypotheses regarding why. Typically, experienced occupational therapists perform this analysis in their head. **Box 4.4** briefly lists the steps therapists perform to complete occupational analyses, and **Box 4.5** lists some of the aspects of the occupation and the client that therapists must consider. Generally, this process is guided by a particular frame of reference or multiple frames of reference. Often, this process occurs quickly during a session with a client and allows the therapist to make immediate adjustments or to rapidly select alternatives to allow the client success.

Assessing Play through Observation with Activity and Occupational Analysis

One important method of informal play assessment is completed through the process of observing play in natural situations. The therapist uses the knowledge gained through activity analysis to understand

> **Box 4.4** Steps to Completing Occupational Analyses
>
> - The therapist observes a client completing an occupation by watching the performance of each individual step.
> - The therapist considers which frame of reference is appropriate to use based on what is known about the client through evaluation.
> - The therapist observes specific features of performance based upon the frame(s) of reference chosen.
> - The therapist notes the client's difficulty and hypothesizes the possible cause(s).
> - The therapist compares what is required (what is known about the activity from activity analysis) with the client's skills, abilities, likes, and dislikes gathered from the evaluation process to note discrepancies that could be removed or diminished through careful grading or modification.
> - The therapist assesses and considers ways to improve the meaningfulness of the occupation for the child. (See Box 4.5.)

> **Box 4.5** Therapist Considerations about Occupational Analysis
>
> - What does this child like, enjoy, prefer?
> - What motivates this child to perform (intrinsic or extrinsic motivations; praise, high-fives, treats, choice of preferred activity, own personal challenge, competition with others, adult reactions)?
> - What memories might this child have in regard to this activity?
> - Has the child had past success or failure with this activity or a similar activity?
> - How does the child's family feel about this activity?
> - Do the child's friends or siblings participate in this activity?
> - How is the child's frustration tolerance? Does the child exhibit self-efficacy in relation to play activities such as this one?
> - Is the child afraid of this activity or similar activities?
> - What about this context supports or hinders the child's performance?
> - Might the child be more willing to participate in an altered context (for example, more or less observation by peers, more or less competition with others, parent watching or not, different size room, room with different sensory features—quieter/louder, dimmer/brighter)?

the properties and characteristics of a broad variety of play activities. The play activity analysis informs the process of occupational analysis while observing a child playing in a typical context for that child to understand play as an occupation. This process may occur in a classroom, at a home, at a playground, or elsewhere in the community. It may occur during solo play or during play with peers or adults. The therapist follows the process described earlier to consider specific activity characteristics and demands, determine the specific aspects of play the child may be struggling with, and identify the individual meaning of play for a particular client as seen in Callie and Gaby.

Conclusion

Within a comprehensive occupational therapy evaluation, specific assessment of play may be accomplished through a variety of informal means. Interviews of caregivers, teachers, and children provide fruitful information while available questionnaires elaborate on specific aspects of children's preferences and perceptions of performance ability. Using activity analysis with play activities should play a crucial role in understanding the play activity characteristics of preferred activities as well as generating the proper activity–child match. Skill with both activity analysis and occupational analysis are needed in order for the therapist to create the just right challenge for a child in play. All of these methods of informal play assessment allow the occupational therapy to gather the information needed to collaborate with families and children to generate important goals about play. We invite the student, novice therapist, and experienced therapist alike to practice the skill of activity analysis and apply occupational analysis creatively to their intervention planning and implementation with pediatric clients as described in the chapters that follow.

References

Accreditation Council for Occupational Therapy Education (ACOTE). (2008). *Standards and interpretive guidelines*. Retrieved from http://www.aota.org/Educate/Accredit/StandardsReview /guide/42369.aspx

Accreditation Council for Occupational Therapy Education (ACOTE®). (2018). Standards and interpretive guide. *American Journal of Occupational Therapy*. https://doi.org/10.5014 /ajot.2018.72S217

American Medical Association. (1943). Essentials of an acceptable school of occupational therapy. *Journal of the American Medical Association, 122*, 541–542.

American Occupational Therapy Association (AOTA). (1975). Essentials of an accredited educational program for the occupational therapist. *American Journal of Occupational Therapy, 29*, 485–496.

American Occupational Therapy Association (AOTA). (2008). Occupational therapy practice framework: Domain & process. *American Journal of Occupational Therapy, 62*, 625–683.

American Occupational Therapy Association (AOTA). (2011). *How to pick a toy: Checklist for Toy Shopping*. Retrieved from https://www.aota.org/About-Occupational-Therapy/Patients -Clients/ChildrenAndYouth/Toy-Shopping.aspx

American Occupational Therapy Association (AOTA). (2020). Occupational therapy practice framework: Domain and process. *American Journal of Occupational Therapy, 74*(Suppl. 2), 7412410010. https://doi.org/10.5014/ajot.2020.74S2001

Americans with Disabilities Act (ADA). (2016). *Research of the National Network*. ADA National Network. https://adata.org /research.

Barnes, R. M. (1949). *Motion and time study* (3rd ed.). New York: John Wiley & Sons.

Barnett, L. A. (1990). Playfulness: Definition, design, and measurement. *Play & Culture, 3*, 319–336

Bedell, G. (2011). *The Child and Adolescent Scale of Environment (CASE): Administration and scoring guidelines*. Medford, MA: Author.

Bertran, M. (2015). Factors that influence friendship choices in children under 3 in two schools: An approach towards child culture in formal settings in Barcelona. *Childhood, 22*(2), 187–200.

Besio, S., & Amelina, N. (2017). Play in children with physical impairment. In S. Besio, D. Bulgarelli, & V. Stancheva-Popkostadinova (Eds.), *Play development in children with disabilities*. Warsaw, Poland: De Gruyter.

Brussoni, M., Gibbons, R., Gray, C., Ishikawa, T., Sandseter, E. B., Bienenstock, A., Chabot, G., Fuselli, P., Herrington, S., Janssen, I., Pickett, W., Power, M., Stanger, N., Sampson, M., & Tremblay, M. S. (2015). What is the relationship between risky outdoor play and health in children? A systematic review. *International Journal of Environmental Research and Public Health, 12*(6), 6423–6454. https://doi.org/10.3390/ijerph120606423

Bryze, K. C. (2008). Narrative contributions to the play history. In L. D. Parham & L. S. Fazio (Eds.), *Play in occupational therapy for children* (2nd ed., pp. 43–54). St. Louis, MO: Mosby Elsevier.

Buckley, K., & Poole, S. (2004). Activity analysis. In J. Hinohosa & M. Blount (Eds.), *Texture of life* (pp. 69–114). Bethesda, MD: AOTA Press.

Burke, J. P., Schaaf, R. C., & Hall, T. B. L. (2008). Family narratives and play assessment. In L. D. Parham & L. S. Fazio (Eds.), *Play in occupational therapy for children* (2nd ed., pp. 195–215). St. Louis, MO: Mosby Elsevier.

Cacola, P., et al. (2011). *AHEMD Project Affordances in the home environment for motor development*. http://www.ese.ipvc.pt /dmh/AHEMD/ahemd_5.htm

Caine, B. (2014). *Friendship: A history*. London: Routledge.

Caldwell, B. M., & Bradley, R. H. (2016). *Home Observation for Measurement of the Environment: Administration manual*. Tempe, AZ: Family & Human Dynamics Research Institute, Arizona State University.

Chandonnet, K., Elam, E., & Lucas, L. (2013). Analysis of playground equipment at Muskegon Public Schools: A needs assessment. *Grand Valley State University ScholarWorks@GVSU*.

Chapparo, C. (2010). Perceive, recall, plan and perform: Occupational centred task-analysis and intervention system. In S. Rodger (Eds.), *Occupation centred practice with children: A practical guide for occupational therapist* (pp. 183–202). Hoboken, NJ: Wiley-Blackwell.

Coelho, L., Torres, N., Fernandes, C., & Santos, A. J. (2017). Quality of play, social acceptance and reciprocal friendship in preschool children. *European Early Childhood Education Research Journal, 25*(6), 812–823.

Collins English Dictionary. (2020). *Collins English Dictionary | Definitions, translations, example sentences and pronunciations*. https://www.collinsdictionary.com/us/dictionary/english

Colman, W. (1990). Evolving educational practices in occupational therapy: The war emergency courses, 1936–54. *American Journal of Occupational Therapy, 44*, 1028–1036.

Colman, W. (1992). Structuring education: Development of the first educational standards in occupational therapy, 1917–1930. *American Journal of Occupational Therapy, 46*, 653–660.

Costa, M., Périno, O., & Ray-Kaeser, S. (2018). *TUET toys & [and] games usability evaluation tool (No. BOOK)*. Alicante, Spain: AIJU.

Cottrell, R. (1996). *Perspectives on purposeful activity: Foundation and future of occupational therapy*. Bethesda MD: AOTA Press.

Crafts, T. (2013). *What a child's toy can teach us about usability and design principles*. Ayantek. https://www.ayantek.com/what-childs -toy-can-teach-us-about-usability-and-design-principles/

Creighton, C. (1992). The origin and evolution of activity analysis. *American Journal of Occupational Therapy, 46*, 45–48.

Crepeau, E. B. (2003). Analyzing occupation and activity: A way of thinking about occupational performance. In E. B. Crepeau, E. S. Cohn, & B. B. Schell (Eds.), *Willard & Spackman's occupational therapy* (10th ed., pp. 189–202). Philadelphia: Lippincott, Williams & Wilkins.

Cuadros, O., & Berger, C. (2016). The protective role of friendship quality on the wellbeing of adolescents victimized by peers. *Journal of Youth and Adolescence, 45*(9), 1877–1888.

Dickinson, H. O., Colver, A., & Sparcle Group. (2011). Quantifying the physical, social and attitudinal environment of children with cerebral palsy. *Disability and Rehabilitation, 33*(1), 36–50.

Ekin, C. Ç., Çağiltay, K., & Karasu, N. (2018). Usability study of a smart toy on students with intellectual disabilities. *Journal of Systems Architecture, 89*, 95–102.

Elgas, P. M., Klein, E., Kantor, R., & Fernie, D. E. (1988). Play and the peer culture: Play styles and object use. *Journal of Research in Childhood Education, 3*, 142–153.

Engdahl, I. (2012). Doing friendship during the second year of life in a Swedish preschool. *European Early Childhood Education Research Journal*, 20(1), 83–98.

Fearnbach, S. N., Martin, C. K., Heymsfield, S. B., Staiano, A. E., Newton, R. L., Garn, A. C.,... Finlayson, G. (2020). Validation of the Activity Preference Assessment: A tool for quantifying children's implicit preferences for sedentary and physical activities. *International Journal of Behavioral Nutrition and Physical Activity*, 17(1), 1–13.

Fidler, G. S., & Fidler, J. W. (1963). *Occupational therapy: A communication process in psychiatry*. New York: Macmillan.

Fidler, G. S., & Velde, B. P. (1999). *Activities: Reality and symbol*. Thorofare, NJ: Slack.

Finegan, J. K., Niccols, G. A., Zacher, J. E., & Hood, J. E. (1991). The play activity questionnaire: A parent report measure of children's play preferences. *Archives of Sexual Behavior*, 20, 393–408.

Getz, S., & Berndt, E. G. (1982). A test of a method for quantifying amount, complexity, and arrangement of play resources in the preschool classroom. *Journal of Applied Developmental Psychology*, 3(4), 295–305.

Gilbreth, F. B. (1904). Science in management for the one best way to do work. In H. F. Merrill (Ed.), *Classics in management* (pp. 245–294. New York: American Management Association.

Goldman, B. D., & Buysse, V. (2007). Friendships in very young children. In O. N. Saracho & B. Spodek (Eds.), *Contemporary perspectives on socialization and social development in early childhood education* (pp. 165–192). Charlotte, NC: Information Age.

Haas, L. J. (1925). *Occupational therapy for the mentally and nervously ill*. Milwaukee, WI: Bruce.

Heaton, L. D. (Ed.). (1968). *Army medical specialist corps*. Washington, DC: Office of the Surgeon General, Department of the Army.

Henry, A. (2008). Assessment of play and leisure in children and adolescents. In L. D. Parham & L. S. Fazio (Eds.), *Play in occupational therapy for children* (2nd ed., pp. 95–193). St. Louis, MO: Mosby Elsevier.

Henry, A. D. (2000). *Kid play profile*. San Antonio, TX: Therapy Skill Builders.

Hersch, G. I., Lamport, N. K., & Coffey, M. S. (2005). *Activity analysis: Application to occupation*. Thorofare, NJ: Slack.

Hill, A., & Bundy, A. C. (2014). Reliability and validity of a new instrument to measure tolerance of everyday risk for children. *Child: Care, Health and Development*, 40(1), 68–76.

Holloway, E. (2008). Fostering early parent–infant playfulness in the neonatal intensive care unit. In L. D. Parham & L. S. Fazio (Eds.), *Play in occupational therapy for children* (2nd ed., pp. 335–350). St. Louis, MO: Mosby Elsevier.

Hui, S., & Dimitropoulou, K. (2020). iCan-Play: A practice guideline for assessment and intervention of play for children with severe multiple disabilities. *The Open Journal of Occupational Therapy*, 8(3), 1–14. https://doi.org/10.15453/2168-6408.1696

International Standardization for Organization (ISO) 9241-11. (1998). Ergonomic requirements for office work with visual display terminals—part 11: Guidance on usability. *International Organization for Standardization*.

Kearney, P. (2004). *The influence of competing paradigms on occupational therapy education: A brief history*. Retrieved June 27, 2007, from http://www.newfoundations.com/History/OccTher.html

King, G., Law, M., King, S., Hurley, P., Hanna, S., Kertoy, M., et al. (2004). *Children's Assessment of Participation and Enjoyment (CAPE) and Preferences for Activities of Children (PAC)*. San Antonio, TX: Harcourt Assessment.

Kleppe, R. (2018). *One-to-three-year-olds' risky play in early childhood education and care*. Oslo: Oslo Metropolitan University.

Knox, S. (2008). Development and current use of the revised Knox Preschool Play Scale. In L. D. Parham & L. S. Fazio (Eds.), *Play in occupational therapy for children* (2nd ed., pp. 55–70). St. Louis, MO: Mosby Elsevier.

Lane, S. J., & Mistrett, S. (2008). Facilitating play in early intervention. In L. D. Parham & L. S. Fazio (Eds.), *Play in occupational therapy for children* (2nd ed., pp. 413–425). St. Louis, MO: Mosby Elsevier.

Law, M., Cooper, B., Strong, S., Stewart, D., Rigby, P., & Letts, L. (1996). The person-environment-occupation model: A transactive approach to occupational performance. *Canadian Journal of Occupational Therapy*, 63(1), 9–23.

Lexico Dictionaries. (2020). Soccer: Definition of soccer by Oxford Dictionary on Lexico.com also meaning of soccer. *Lexico Dictionaries | English*. https://www.lexico.com/definition/soccer

Licht, S. (1967). The founding and the founders of the American Occupational Therapy Association. *American Journal of Occupational Therapy*, 21, 269–278.

Llorens, L. A. (1973). Activity analysis for cognitive-perceptual-motor dysfunction. *American Journal of Occupational Therapy*, 27, 453–456.

Llorens, L. A. (1986). Activity analysis: Agreement among factors in a sensory processing model. *American Journal of Occupational Therapy*, 40, 103–110.

Llorens, L. A. (1993). Activity analysis: Agreement between participants and observers on perceived factors in occupation components. *Occupational Therapy Journal of Research*, 13, 198–211.

Martin, C. V. (2007). The importance of self-efficacy to usability: Grounded theory analysis of a child's toy assembly task. In *Proceedings of the Human Factors and Ergonomics Society Annual Meeting* (Vol. 51, No. 14, pp. 865–868). Los Angeles, CA: SAGE Publications.

McDaniel, M. L. (n.d.). *Occupational therapists before World War II (1917–40)*. Retrieved July 18, 2007, from http://history.amedd.army.mil/booksdocs/histories/ArmyMedicalSpecialistCorps/chapter4.htm#f

McDonald, A. E., & Vigen, C. (2012). Reliability and validity of the McDonald Play Inventory. *American Journal of Occupational Therapy*, 66(4), e52–e60.

Meakins, C. R., Bundy, A. C., & Gliner, J. (2005). Validity and reliability of the experience of leisure scale (TELS). F. F. McMahon, D. E. Lytle, & B. Sutton-Smith (Eds.), *Play. An interdisciplinary synthesis (Play and Culture Studies*, 6, pp. 255–267). Lanham, MD: University Press of America.

Metz, A. E. (2020). Applying a task-person-environment approach to designing play studies. Play for All Conference Presentation. Online April 26, 2020. https://usplaycoalition.org/playconference2020

Miething, A., Almquist, Y. B., Östberg, V., Rostila, M., Edling, C., & Rydgren, J. (2016). Friendship networks and psychological well-being from late adolescence to young adulthood: A gender-specific structural equation modeling approach. *BMC Psychology*, 4(1), 34.

Missiuna, C., Pollock, N., & Law, M. (2004). *The perceived efficacy and goal setting system*. San Antonio, TX: PsychCorp.

Morozini, M. (2015). Exploring the engagement of parents in the co-occupation of parent-child play: An occupational science's perspective. *International Journal of Prevention and Treatment*, 4(2A), 11–28. https://doi.org/10.5923/s.ijpt.201501.02

Mosey, A. C. (1981). *Occupational therapy: Configuration of a profession*. New York: Raven Press.

Mosey, A. C. (1986). *Psychosocial components of occupational therapy*. New York: Raven Press.

Nadworny, M. J. (1957). Frederick Taylor and Frank Gilbreth: Competition in scientific management. *Business History Review*, 31, 23–34.

National Program for Playground Safety (NPPS). (2020). *Playground safety checklist*.

Olsen, L., Ishikawa, T., Mâsse, L., Chan, G., & Brussoni, M. (2018). Risk Engagement and Protection Survey (REPS): Developing and validating a survey tool on fathers' attitudes towards child injury protection and risk engagement. *Injury Prevention*. https://doi.org/http://dx.doi.org/10.1136/injuryprev-2017-042413

Olsen, L. L., Lin, Y., Ishikawa, T., Mâsse, L. C., & Brussoni, M. (2019). Comparison of risk engagement and protection survey (REPS) among mothers and fathers of children aged 6–12 years. *Injury Prevention*, 25(5), 438–443.

Olsson, I., Sand, M. L., & Stenberg, G. (2020). Teachers' perception of inclusion in elementary school: The importance of imitation. *European Journal of Special Needs Education*, 35(4), 567–575.

PlayEngland. (2009). *Playable Space Quality Assessment Tool*.

Reid, D. H., DiCarlo, C. F., Schepis, M. M., Hawkins, J., & Stricklin, S. B., (2003). Observational assessment of toy preferences among young children with disabilities in inclusive settings: Efficiency analysis and comparison with staff opinion. *Behavior Modification*, 27, 233–250.

Rigby, P., & Gaik, S. (2007). Stability of playfulness across environmental settings: A pilot study. *Physical & Occupational Therapy in Pediatrics*, 27(1), 27–43.

Rogers, C. S., Impara, J. C., Frary, R. B., Harris, T., Meeks, A., Semanic-Lauth, S., & Reynolds, M. (1998). Measuring playfulness: Development of the Child Behavior Inventory of Playfulness. In M. Duncan, G. Chick, & A. Aycock (Eds.), *Play and cultural studies* (Vol. 4, pp. 121–136). Greenwich, CT: Ablex Publishing Corp.

Rosenberg, L., Ratzon, N. Z., Jarus, T., & Bart, O. (2010). Development and initial validation of the Environmental Restriction Questionnaire (ERQ). *Research in Developmental Disabilities*, 31, 1323–1331. https://doi.org/10.1016/j.ridd.2010.07.009

Rosenberg, L., Ratzon, N. Z., Jarus, T., & Bart, O. (2012). Perceived environmental restrictions for the participation of children with mild developmental disabilities. *Child: Care, Health and Development*, 38, 836–843. https://doi.org/10.1111/j.1365-2214.2011.01303.x

Rosenblum, S., Sachs, D., & Schreuer, N. (2010). Reliability and validity of the Children's Leisure Assessment Scale. *American Journal of Occupational Therapy*, 64(4), 633–641

Russo, S. R., Tincani, M., & Axelrod, S. (2014). Evaluating open-ended parent reports and direct preference assessments to identify reinforcers for young children with autism. *Child & Family Behavior Therapy*, 36(2), 107–120.

Saelens, B. E., Frank, L. D., Auffrey, C., Whitaker, R. C., Burdette, H. L., & Colabianchi, N. (2006). Measuring physical environments of parks and playgrounds: EAPRS instrument development and inter-rater reliability. *Journal of Physical Activity and Health*, 3(s1), S190–S207.

Sandseter, E. B. H. (2009). Affordances for risky play in preschool: The importance of features in the play environment. *Early Childhood Education Journal*, 36(5), 439–446.

Schell, B. A. B., Gillen, G., Crepeau, E., & Scaffa, M. (2019). Analyzing occupations and activity. In B. A. B. Schell & G. Gillen (Eds.), *Willard and Spackman's occupational therapy* (13th ed., pp. 320–333). Philadelphia, PA: Wolters Kluwer.

Schneider, E., & Rosenblum, S. (2014). Development, reliability, and validity of the My Child's Play (MCP) questionnaire. *American Journal of Occupational Therapy*, 68(3), 277–285.

Schreuer, N., Sachs, D., & Rosenblum, S. (2014). Participation in leisure activities: Differences between children with and without physical disabilities. *Research in Developmental Disabilities*, 35(1), 223–233.

Sherwin, K., & Nielsen, J. (2019). *Children's UX: Usability issues in designing for young people*. Nielsen Norman Group. https://www.ngroup.com/articles/childrens-websites-usability-issues/

Skard, G., & Bundy, A. C. (2008). Test of playfulness. In L. D. Parham & L. S. Fazio (Eds.), *Play in occupational therapy for children* (2nd ed., pp. 71–93). St. Louis, MO: Mosby Elsevier.

Spitzer, S. L. (2003a). Using participant observation to study the meaning of occupations of young children with autism and other developmental disabilities. *American Journal of Occupational Therapy*, 57(1), 66–76.

Spitzer, S. L. (2003b). With and without words: Exploring occupation in relation to young children with autism. *Journal of Occupational Science*, 10(2), 67–79.

Spitzer, S. (2020). Observational assessment and activity analysis. In J. O'Brien & H. Kuhaneck (Eds). *Case-Smith's Occupational Therapy for Children* (8th ed.). Elsevier. 136-157.

Spriegel, W. R., & Myers, C. E. (1953). *The writings of the Gilbreths*. Homewood, IL: Richard D. Irwin.

Takata, N. (1974). Play as a prescription. In. M. Reilly (Ed.), *Play as exploratory learning* (pp. 209–246). Los Angeles: Sage.

Taylor, F. W. (1904). Principles of scientific management. In H. F. Merrill (Ed.), *Classics in management* (pp. 82–116). New York: American Management Association.

Taylor, K., Menarchek-Fetkovich, M., & Day, C. (2000). The play history interview. In K. Gitlin-Weiner, A. Sandgrund, & C. Schafer (Eds.), *Play diagnosis and assessment* (2nd ed., pp 114–139). New York: John Wiley & Sons.

Trawick-Smith, J., Wolff, J., Koschel, M., & Vallarelli, J. (2014). Which toys promote high-quality play? Reflections on the five-year anniversary of the TIMPANI study. *YC Young Children*, 69(2), 40.

Trevlas, E., Grammatikopoulos, V., Tsigilis, N., & Zachopoulou, E. (2003). Evaluating playfulness: Construct validity of the children's playfulness scale. *Early Childhood Education Journal*, 31, 33–39.

TUET. (2018). *What is TUET and why has it been created?* TUET Web. https://www.tuet.eu/

Waldman-Levi, A., & Bundy, A. (2016). A glimpse into co-occupations: Parent/caregiver's support of young children's playfulness scale. *Occupational Therapy in Mental Health*, 32(3), 217–227. https://doi.org/10.1080/0164212X.2015.1116420

Whaley, K. L., & Rubenstein, T. S. (1994). How toddlers "do" friendship: A descriptive analysis of naturally occurring friendships in a group child care setting. *Journal of Social and Personal Relationships, 11,* 383–400.

Whiteneck, G., Meade, M. A., Dijkers, M., Tate, D. G., Bushnik, T., & Forchheimer, M. B. (2004). Environmental factors and their role in participation and life satisfaction after spinal cord injury. *Archives of Physical Medicine and Rehabilitation, 85*(11), 1793–1803.

Whiteside, S. P. H., McCarthy, D. M., Sim, L. A., Biggs, B. K., Petrikin, J. E., & Mellon, M. W. "Development of the Friendships and Social Skills Test (FASST): A parent report measure," *Journal of Child and Family Studies,* 25 (6), 2016, pp. 1777–1788.

Wiseman, N., Rossmann, C., Lee, J., & Harris, N. (2019)."It's like you are in the jungle": Using the draw-and-tell method to explore preschool children's play preferences and factors that shape their active play. *Health Promotion Journal of Australia, 30,* 85–94.

Wohlwend, K. E. (2017). Who gets to play? Access, popular media and participatory literacies. *Early Years, 37*(1), 62–76.

Woolley, H., & Lowe, A. (2013). Exploring the relationship between design approach and play value of outdoor play spaces. *Landscape Research, 38*(1), 53–74. https://doi.org/10.1080/01426397.2011.640432

APPENDIX 4.1 Safety and Accessibility Checklist

Playground Location: _____

Assessment Completed by: _____ Date: _____

Playground Safety
Surfacing
☐ Yes ☐ No ☐ N/A Is surfacing material safe? (i.e., woodchips, bark, mulch, engineered wood fiber, sand gravel, shredded rubber, or other synthetic product)

☐ Yes ☐ No ☐ N/A Does surfacing extend a minimum of 6 feet past all equipment that comprises the use zone?

☐ Yes ☐ No ☐ N/A Does surfacing for slides extend a minimum of the slide's height + 4 feet.?

☐ Yes ☐ No ☐ N/A Does the surfacing for swings extend a minimum distance of twice the height of the pivot point?

Maintenance
☐ Yes ☐ No ☐ N/A Is all of the equipment securely anchored into the ground?

☐ Yes ☐ No ☐ N/A Is all of the equipment free of chipping paint?

☐ Yes ☐ No ☐ N/A Is all of the hardware free of corrosion?

☐ Yes ☐ No ☐ N/A Is all of the hardware secured?

☐ Yes ☐ No ☐ N/A Are the hooks closed with a gap no greater than 0.4 inches?

General Hazards

☐ Yes ☐ No ☐ N/A   If equipment is wood, is it smooth and free from splinters?

☐ Yes ☐ No ☐ N/A   Is all equipment free of sharp points, corners, and edges?

☐ Yes ☐ No ☐ N/A   Is all equipment free of protrusions and projections?

☐ Yes ☐ No ☐ N/A   Is all equipment free of pinch, crush, and shearing points?

☐ Yes ☐ No ☐ N/A   Are all openings between 3.5 inches and 9 inches to prevent head entrapment?

☐ Yes ☐ No ☐ N/A   Is the playground free of tripping hazards?

☐ Yes ☐ No ☐ N/A   Are suspended cables, ropes, and wires away from high traffic areas?

Stairways

☐ Yes ☐ No ☐ N/A   Is step width at least 16 inches?

☐ Yes ☐ No ☐ N/A   Is tread depth on an open or closed step at least 8 inches?

☐ Yes ☐ No ☐ N/A   If steps are closed, do they prevent accumulation of sand, water, or other materials between steps?

Handrails

☐ Yes ☐ No ☐ N/A   Do handrails extend the full length on both sides of stepladders and stairways?

☐ Yes ☐ No ☐ N/A   Is the vertical distance from the top edge of steps to the top of handrails between 22 inches and 38 inches?

☐ Yes ☐ No ☐ N/A   Is the diameter of the handrail between 0.95 inches and 1.55 inches?

Platforms, Guardrails, and Protective Barriers

☐ Yes ☐ No ☐ N/A   Does the platform have openings to allow for drainage?

☐ Yes ☐ No ☐ N/A   Are guardrails or protective barriers present on elevated surfaces ≥ 30 inches?

☐ Yes ☐ No ☐ N/A   Are protective barriers present on elevated surfaces ≥ 48 inches?

Guardrails

☐ Yes ☐ No ☐ N/A   Is the top guardrail surface at least 38 inches high and the lower edge no more than 28 inches above the platform?

Protective Barriers

☐ Yes ☐ No ☐ N/A   Is the top surface of the protective barrier at least 38 inches high?

Stepped Platforms

☐ Yes ☐ No ☐ N/A   Is the maximum difference in height between stepped platforms no more than 18 inches?

Ladders and Rings
Rung Ladders

☐ Yes ☐ No ☐ N/A   Are the rungs on the ladder evenly spaced?

☐ Yes ☐ No ☐ N/A   Are spaces between rungs between 3.5 inches and 9 inches?

☐ Yes ☐ No ☐ N/A   Are width of rungs at least 16 inches?

☐ Yes ☐ No ☐ N/A   Is rung diameter between .95 inches and 1.55 inches?

Stepladders

☐ Yes ☐ No ☐ N/A   Is tread width at least 16 inches?

☐ Yes ☐ No ☐ N/A   Is tread depth on an open step at least 3 inches?

☐ Yes ☐ No ☐ N/A   Is tread depth on a closed step at least 6 inches?

☐ Yes ☐ No ☐ N/A   If steps are closed, do they prevent accumulation of sand, water, or other materials between steps?

Horizontal Ladders and Overhead Rings

☐ Yes ☐ No ☐ N/A   Is the space between adjacent rungs of overhead ladders greater than 9 inches?

☐ Yes ☐ No ☐ N/A   Is the center-to-center spacing of horizontal ladder rungs no more than 15 inches?

Sliding Poles

☐ Yes ☐ No ☐ N/A   Is the sliding pole continuous with no protruding welds or seams?

☐ Yes ☐ No ☐ N/A   Is the horizontal distance between the pole and platform used for access at least 18 inches?

☐ Yes ☐ No ☐ N/A   There is no point on the sliding pole that is more than 20 inches away from the edge of the access structure?

☐ Yes ☐ No ☐ N/A   Is the pole at least 60 inches above the level of the access platform?

☐ Yes ☐ No ☐ N/A   Is the diameter of the sliding pole no greater than 1.9 inches?

Climbing Ropes

☐ Yes ☐ No ☐ N/A   Is the climbing rope secured at both ends and not able to loop back on itself creating a loop with a perimeter greater than 5 inches?

Balance Beams

☐ Yes ☐ No ☐ N/A   Does the height of the balance beam not exceed 16 inches?

Merry-Go-Round

☐ Yes ☐ No ☐ N/A   Is the rotating platform continuous and circular?

☐ Yes ☐ No ☐ N/A   Are their adequate hand grips available that meet handrail guidelines?

☐ Yes ☐ No ☐ N/A   Does the surfacing for swings extend a minimum distance of twice the height of the pivot point?

Seesaws and Rockers
Seesaws

☐ Yes ☐ No ☐ N/A   Is there shock-absorbing material embedded in the ground underneath the seesaw seats (e.g., partial car tires)?

☐ Yes ☐ No ☐ N/A   Are there handholds are provided at each seating position?

☐ Yes ☐ No ☐ N/A   Is the maximum attainable angle between a line connecting the seats and the horizontal 25 degrees?

Spring Rocker

☐ Yes ☐ No ☐ N/A Is the spring rocker equipped with handgrips and footrests?

Slides
Slide Platform (for all slides)

☐ Yes ☐ No ☐ N/A Is the length of the platform on the freestanding slide a minimum of 22 inches?

☐ Yes ☐ No ☐ N/A Is the slide surrounded by protective barriers and guardrails?

☐ Yes ☐ No ☐ N/A Are no spaces present between the platform and start of the slide chute?

☐ Yes ☐ No ☐ N/A Are there handhelds available?

☐ Yes ☐ No ☐ N/A Is there an aid to facilitate the user to a sitting position at the beginning of the slide (for example, handholds)?

Sliding Section of Straight Slide

☐ Yes ☐ No ☐ N/A Is the average incline no more than 30 degrees?

☐ Yes ☐ No ☐ N/A Does the flat open chute have sides with a 4-inch minimum extending up on both sides the entire length of the slide?

Exit Region of Slides

☐ Yes ☐ No ☐ N/A Is the exit region horizontal and parallel to the ground and have a minimum length of 11 inches?

☐ Yes ☐ No ☐ N/A Does a slide over 4 feet in height have an exit region between 7 and 15 inches above the protective surfacing?

☐ Yes ☐ No ☐ N/A Are the slide edges rounded or curved?

Embankment Slide

☐ Yes ☐ No ☐ N/A Does the chute have a maximum height of 12 inches above the ground surface?

Tube Slide

☐ Yes ☐ No ☐ N/A Is the internal diameter of the tube no less than 23 inches?

Roller Slide

☐ Yes ☐ No ☐ N/A Is the space between adjacent rollers and between the end of rollers less than 3/16 of an inch?

Swings
General Swings

☐ Yes ☐ No ☐ N/A Can all structures only be removed with the use of tools?

☐ Yes ☐ No ☐ N/A Are all hooks pinched closed?

Single-Axis Swings

☐ Yes ☐ No ☐ N/A Are each of the use zones free from other equipment's use zones?

☐ Yes ☐ No ☐ N/A Is there no more than two single axis swings hung in each bay of the supporting structure?

☐ Yes ☐ No ☐ N/A Is the vertical distance from the underside of an occupied swing seat no less than 16 inches from the protective surface?

☐ Yes ☐ No ☐ N/A Are the swing hangers spaced no less than 20 inches apart?

Tot Swing

☐ Yes ☐ No ☐ N/A Are all the criteria for single-axis swings followed?

☐ Yes ☐ No ☐ N/A Is the vertical distance from the underside of an occupied tot swing no less than 24 inches from the protective surfacing?

☐ Yes ☐ No ☐ N/A Is the maximum attainable angle between a line connecting the seats and the horizontal 25 degrees?

Multi-Axis Tire Swings

☐ Yes ☐ No ☐ N/A Is the tire swing suspended using three suspension chains connected to a single swivel mechanism?

☐ Yes ☐ No ☐ N/A Is the tire swing in a bay without any other swings?

☐ Yes ☐ No ☐ N/A When pushed to its highest point is the tire swing a minimum of 30 inches from the side supports?

Playground Accessibility Checklist

Playground Component Information

Indicate the number of components for each category.

Ground Level Play Components:____

Ground Level Component on Accessible Route: ____

Different Types of Ground-Level Play Components: ____

Elevated Play Components: ____

Elevated Components on Accessible Route: ____

Ground-Level Accessible Routes

☐ Yes ☐ No ☐ N/A Are routes at least 60 inches wide?
☐ Yes ☐ No ☐ N/A Are any slopes 1:16 or less?
☐ Yes ☐ No ☐ N/A Are slopes at boundary transition 1:12 or less?

Ramps and Landings

Ramps

☐ Yes ☐ No ☐ N/A Are ramps at least 60 inches wide?
☐ Yes ☐ No ☐ N/A Is the slope 1:12 or less?
☐ Yes ☐ No ☐ N/A Do the ramps rise less than 12 inches?

Landings

☐ Yes ☐ No ☐ N/A Are landings at least 60 inches long?
☐ Yes ☐ No ☐ N/A Are landings as wide as the ramp they are connected to?

Maneuvering Space Where Ramps Are Provided

☐ Yes ☐ No ☐ N/A Is there one maneuvering space on the same level of the play component?
☐ Yes ☐ No ☐ N/A Is the slope less than 1:48 in all directions?

Handrails

☐ Yes ☐ No ☐ N/A Are there handrails located on *both* sides of the ramp connecting the play component?
☐ Yes ☐ No ☐ N/A Are the handrails 20 to 28 inches above the ramp surface?

Transfer-Related Items
Transfer Systems

☐ Yes ☐ No ☐ N/A Are transfer systems at least 24 inches wide?

Transfer Platforms

☐ Yes ☐ No ☐ N/A Are transfer platforms 11 to 18 inches high?
☐ Yes ☐ No ☐ N/A Are transfer platforms at least 24 inches wide?
☐ Yes ☐ No ☐ N/A Are the sides of the transfer platforms free of obstructions?

Transfer Steps

☐ Yes ☐ No ☐ N/A Are transfer steps at least 24 inches wide?
☐ Yes ☐ No ☐ N/A Are transfer steps at least 14 inches deep?
☐ Yes ☐ No ☐ N/A Are transfer steps less than 8 inches high?

Transfer Supports

☐ Yes ☐ No ☐ N/A Are transfer supports present at transfer platforms and transfer steps?

Space-Related Items
Clear Floor or Ground Space

☐ Yes ☐ No ☐ N/A Are clear floor spaces at least 30 inches by 48 inches?
☐ Yes ☐ No ☐ N/A Is the slope less than 1:48 in all directions?

Maneuvering Space

☐ Yes ☐ No ☐ N/A Is at least one maneuvering space present at the same level as an elevated playground component?
☐ Yes ☐ No ☐ N/A Is the turning circle at least 60 inches in diameter?
☐ Yes ☐ No ☐ N/A Is the slope less than 1:48 in all directions?

Entry Points

☐ Yes ☐ No ☐ N/A Are entry points at least 11 inches high?
☐ Yes ☐ No ☐ N/A Are entry points no higher than 24 inches?

Play Tables

☐ Yes ☐ No ☐ N/A Are play tables at least 24 inches high?
☐ Yes ☐ No ☐ N/A Are play tables at least 30 inches wide?
☐ Yes ☐ No ☐ N/A Are play tables at least 17 inches deep?

Reach Range

☐ Yes ☐ No ☐ N/A Are items to be reached for in the range 18 to 40 inches from the ground?

Modified from Chandonnet, K., Elam, E., & Lucas, L. (2013). *Analysis of playground equipment at Muskegon Public Schools: A needs assessment.* Grand Valley State University ScholarWorks@GVSU.

APPENDIX 4.2 History of Activity Analysis

Two men associated with the concepts that led to the eventual emergence of activity analysis in occupational therapy are Frederick Taylor and Frank Gilbreth (Gilbreth 1904; Nadworny, 1957; Taylor, 1904). Both men were involved in the field of management, and both were ultimately interested in improving the efficiency of workers and the productivity of human labor (Nadworny, 1957). Taylor, the "Father of Scientific Management," is best known for the use of time study, recording the time needed to complete tasks with a stopwatch, with the ultimate goal of "increasing output per unit of human effort" (Taylor, 1904, p. 86). Gilbreth, a contemporary of Taylor's, was also interested in increasing worker productivity but believed that the way to achieve this end was to analyze work methods and motions to achieve economy of effort. He therefore focused on fatigue study and motion study using photographic film analysis to carefully observe the methods and motions workers used while performing their tasks (Barnes, 1949; Gilbreth, 1904; Nadworny, 1957). Gilbreth advocated surveying multiple people performing the same task to systematically examine differences and determine the one best way (i.e., most efficient way) of completing the activity. As early as 1904, Gilbreth was labeling this type of analysis a science, calling motion study "the science of determining and perpetuating the scheme of perfection; the performing of the one best way to do work" (pp. 273–274).

Gilbreth and his wife were the first authors to publish information linking motion study specifically to work with the handicapped. In their papers, "The Re-Education of the Crippled Soldier" and "Motion Study for Crippled Soldiers," presented at conferences in 1915, 1916, and 1917 (Spriegel & Myers, 1953), the Gilbreths discussed how their studies of efficient methods could and should be transferred to the education of the wounded soldiers returning from war. These writings did not mention occupational therapy specifically, but their statements sounded quite similar to the philosophy of occupational therapy that was developing during the same time period. For example, the Gilbreths stated the importance of "arousing interest in the discovery, invention, or adaptation of devices that will make it possible for the [individual with a disability] not only to have a productive and paying occupation but also to 'fit back' into all of the ordinary activities of daily life" (Spriegel & Myers, 1953, p. 280). They also spoke about the way in which motion study created

solutions and inventions necessary to allow soldiers to relearn and complete desired tasks. They discussed all aspects of activity analysis as occupational therapists currently use it: adapting methods to the soldier, choosing appropriate activities for the soldier based on what he could do, and modifying or adapting activities for the individual soldier. In these early writings, one can see the beginnings of activity analysis as occupational therapists still use it today.

The Gilbreths were quite influential in early occupational therapy. Mr. Gilbreth influenced the work of both Barton and Dunton, the first two presidents of the National Society for the Promotion of Occupational Therapy, and he presented his work at the new society's first annual meeting, where the influential founders of the profession were present (Creighton, 1992; Licht, 1967). A paper by Mrs. Gilbreth was presented in absentia at the initial meeting of the Society in 1917 at Consolation House (Licht, 1967). The ideas of the Gilbreths thus spread throughout our early occupational therapy leaders.

Not surprisingly, because activity analysis emerged from motion analysis in management, early discussions of this process in occupational therapy focused heavily on the analysis of *motions* for rehabilitation of clients. The first publication that discussed activity analysis with consideration of physical and social-emotional aspects of performance was disseminated in 1925 by Haas. Haas focused on therapists' careful consideration of which activity to choose for a patient because just "being busy is not necessarily therapeutic" (Haas, 1925, p. 25). In Haas's book, written for therapists working in the field of mental health, the term *activity analysis* is not used specifically, but the author described the therapeutic application of crafts and processes similar to our current conception of activity adaptation and grading specifically for clients whose difficulties were mental more than physical.

Although motion analysis continued to be important, the cognitive, sensory–perceptual, and psychological facets of activity became more routinely included in activity analysis as a variety of frames of reference were delineated in occupational therapy (Creighton, 1992; Fidler & Fidler, 1963; Llorens, 1973). Fidler, a strong advocate and passionate occupational therapist who often wrote about mental health issues, proposed an outline for activity analysis that carefully examined the psychodynamic aspects of the activity for the client (Fidler & Fidler, 1963).

As occupational therapy's knowledge base grew and our own theoretical orientations developed, activity analysis began to be linked with specific frames of reference. Llorens (1973, 1986) described different forms of activity analysis, highlighting the aspects of the activity that needed to be considered in relation to the particular frame of reference chosen. Recent history has adapted the formats and processes of activity analysis to new occupational therapy terminology and concepts. For example, Hersch et al. (2005) and Buckley and Poole (2004) promoted a process for activity analysis that has integrated the OTPF (AOTA, 2008). With the increased emphasis on consideration of context throughout occupational therapy, both works consider contextual features of activities as well.

APPENDIX 4.3 Training of Students in Activity Analysis

Early records of occupational therapy from the military suggest that activity analysis was first used and taught to reconstruction aides during World War I. The early military training for these occupational therapy aides focused on a variety of specific crafts and motion analysis of each. The social-emotional or psychological impact of activities did not yet appear to be a strong consideration in training and intervention (Heaton, 1968). However, a large variety of crafts were taught, suggesting that military educational practice considered it important to have a variety of activities available to allow for individual preferences and needs. An examination of the curriculum changes between the 6-month occupational therapy course at Walter Reed in 1924–1925 to the 9-month course taught in 1932–1933 shows the increased emphasis on the use of activities in treatment and the increased focus on activity analysis as well (McDaniel, n.d.).

Early curricula in occupational therapy outside of the military were highly varied, and no standards of education existed until 1924 (Colman, 1992). Even then, the standards adopted were minimum standards, which were very flexible and had little real enforcement. Much debate occurred in our early years regarding the content and the focus of occupational therapy education (Colman, 1990, 1992). The term *activity analysis* does not appear to be specifically mentioned in curriculum in our early years. The American Medical Association, in their "Essentials of an Acceptable School of Occupational Therapy" (1943), recommended first 25, and then 30, semester hours of instruction in a variety of therapeutic activities, but there was no specification of courses in activity analysis per se. In the 1950s, the military training of occupational therapists included in their discussions and demonstrations "the adaptations of activities for patient treatment and the analysis of activities for interest, exercise, and motion potential (fig. 137)" (Heaton, 1968).

An increased emphasis on the medical model, with a concurrent decrease in emphasis on specific activities in training for occupational therapy, was evident in the 1965 essentials and the curriculum study completed in the early 1960s that recommended de-emphasizing traditional arts and crafts (Kearney, 2004). In the 1970s, the first indication of the importance of training students to use activity analysis as a tool surfaced in the Essentials (AOTA, 1975; Kearney, 2004). According to the essentials developed in the 1970s, upon completion of an accredited occupational therapy program, a student should be able to complete activity analysis and relate the specific components of tasks to the needs of a client (AOTA, 1975; Kearney, 2004). In 2008, the standard in occupational therapy (B.2.7) stated that students must "Exhibit the ability to analyze tasks relative to areas of occupation, performance skills, performance patterns, activity demands, context(s), and client factors to formulate an intervention plan" (Accreditation Council for Occupational Therapy Education, 2008). The current standard B.3.6 states that students must "demonstrate activity analysis in areas of occupation, performance skills, performance patterns, context(s) and environments, and client factors to formulate the intervention plan" (Accreditation Council for Occupational Therapy Education, 2018).

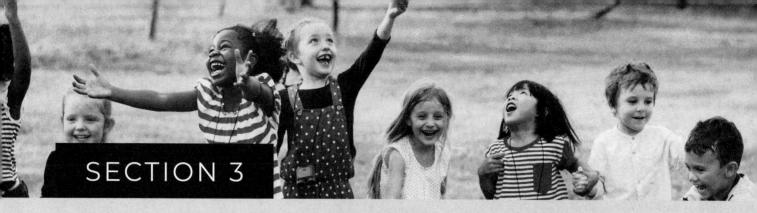

SECTION 3

And How To Apply Them

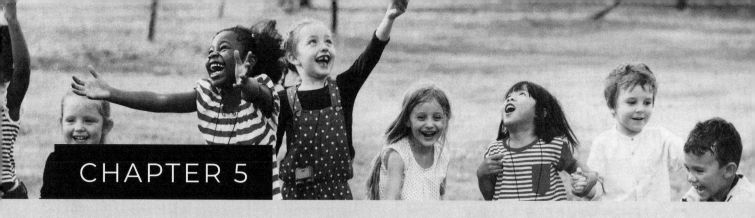

CHAPTER 5

The Occupational Therapist as a Tour Guide to the Land of "PLAY"

Heather M. Kuhaneck, PhD, OTR/L, FAOTA
Elissa Cunningham, OTD, OTR/L

After reading this chapter, the reader will:

- Consider the metaphor of a tour guide to enhance one's ability to promote play in children.
- Create goals for and about play.
- Describe the varied intervention approaches used in occupational therapy to promote play.

Play, while it cannot change the external realities of children's lives, can be a vehicle for children to explore and enjoy their differences and similarities and to create, even for a brief time, a more just world where everyone is an equal and valued participant.

—Patricia G. Ramsey

In this chapter we ask you to consider PLAY as an important destination, one that most children discover on their own, but one that many of the children receiving therapy have difficulty finding and enjoying as fully as other children who are typically developing. Imagine the occupational therapy practitioner as a tour guide for a child to visit PLAY. A good tour guide as well as a good therapist must have knowledge of the "area," passion and enthusiasm, skill for storytelling and good communication, as well as a variety of personal characteristics such as flexibility and adaptability, dependability, and a willingness to learn about others. A good tour guide and therapist will focus on the experience of the client rather than their own. That does not mean

that the tour guide or therapist does not also enjoy the experience. PLAY is a great place, and the tour guide might love this trip as well. But the guide must remain clear that although a constant part of the tour and a collaborator in the eventual adventure, the therapist guide and the client have different roles.

The guide or therapist is the one responsible for the client and all aspects of this adventure. Good tours are well planned, and although the route may be alterable, they generally arrive at the intended destination. Tour guides and therapists make that happen, while managing a variety of anticipated and unanticipated external forces occasionally beyond their immediate control. Each of these specific actions occurs at different times, some prior to the tour, some during the tour, and some afterwards. Some actions must occur throughout all of those phases.

The client taking the tour, of course, wants to have a positive experience, wants to have fun and try new things, but likely does not want to be too scared or forced to try undesirable things. The person taking the tour perhaps wants to enjoy the company of the guide.

The person taking the tour probably wants to feel important to the guide, or at least feel that the guide (therapist) cares about the client's well-being. The person taking the tour likely wants to have some level of autonomy and choice about how the tour unfolds. The same can be said for occupational therapy with children to promote play.

Getting to the Land of PLAY

A tour guide must plan, select the methods of travel for the tour, determine the destination, and map the route. There must be sufficient supplies. Logistics must be considered. And, at times, things may need to be altered or adapted.

Planning the Journey

Any good tour guide has likely created some sort of itinerary, has procured maps, and has a solid idea of the overall plan in order to reach the desired destination(s). In occupational therapy, we use intervention plans to guide therapy to desired outcomes. Thorough intervention plans for children may be quite global in nature, including many different areas of occupation. It is up to each therapist and team to orchestrate the order and timing of intervention for specific occupations, and the use of specific intervention approaches and activities across the child's entire program to tailor the intervention specifically for each individual. Certain intervention methods used by occupational therapy practitioners are not unique to our profession, but our combined theory base, philosophy, and focus on occupation is distinct. This unique philosophy and domain of practice is outlined in the American Occupational Therapy Association's Occupational Therapy Practice Framework (OTPF; AOTA, 2020). Although this document provides a description of the occupational therapy process, it is not meant to be a specific blueprint for creating an intervention plan for a child. This chapter will provide an overview of the specific strategies and methods of intervention that occupational therapists might use to travel toward the land of PLAY. These methods are then explored in greater depth in the chapters that follow. First, let us review the methods of occupational therapy intervention, and then we will apply the idea of the tour guide to what we do in occupational therapy to get to "PLAY." Let us consider what specifically can occur with a child to promote play using the metaphor of a tour guide whose success is based on efforts prior to, during, and after each trip. Much of the work of good intervention occurs outside the actual session with the child. The therapist, like the tour guide, must extensively plan for success.

Selecting the Methods for the Journey

Tours have methods of moving from location to location, and these are selected to be the most efficient or effective or the most desirable based upon personal preferences. Occupational therapy intervention includes selecting goals, approaches, and service delivery methods. The approaches to intervention identified in the OTPF (AOTA, 2020) include (1) create or promote, (2) establish or restore, (3) maintain, (4) modify, and (5) prevent. Occupational therapists provide therapeutic use of occupations and activities; provision of interventions to support occupation, education, training, advocacy, and self-advocacy; and group or virtual interventions. Intervention may also include providing recommendations or referral to others.

Occupation is both a means and an end (AOTA, 2020). This means that occupation may be used as an intervention method, and it is also the important outcome of occupational therapy intervention. In terms of play, it may be both the desired outcome of occupational therapy and also a method used in occupational therapy sessions. For example, in occupational therapy, play is often used as a tool to help a child improve in fine-motor or gross-motor skills (Tanta & Kuhaneck, 2020). Play also may be used as a reward for doing other "work" of the session, such as handwriting. Usually when used in this way, play is meant to help a child manage behavior and attention to complete difficult tasks, knowing there is a favored activity to follow. When play is the end goal, occupational therapy may focus on learning social skills needed for playing with peers or may be provided directly within the context of playing board games with siblings during a home session. See **Figure 5.1** for a visual depiction of these approaches.

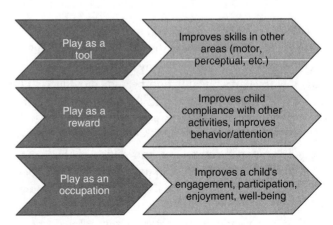

Figure 5.1 Approaches to using play in occupational therapy and their possible outcomes

Data from Tanta, K. J., & Kuhaneck, H. (2020). Assessment and treatment of play. In J. C. O'Brien & H. Kuhaneck (Eds.), *Case-Smith's occupational therapy for children and adolescents* (8th ed., pp. 239–266). Elsevier.

The OTPF divides the primary occupation of play into components of play exploration and play participation. Therefore, therapeutic activities with clients can be focused on their exposure to different forms of play or geared toward increasing their access and ability to engage with play activities. Incorporating playful activities can occur within all five approaches, (AOTA, 2020), as seen in **Table 5.1**

with examples for Callie and Gaby, children first introduced in Chapter 4."

Mapping the Destination

The first important consideration is whether or not to BE a tour guide to PLAY. Therapists have many things they may address. The OTPF provides us with pages

Table 5.1 Incorporating Play within Each of the Occupational Therapy Practice Framework Intervention Approaches

OTPF Intervention Approach (AOTA, 2020)	General Pediatric Play Activity Examples	Example for Callie and Gaby[1]
Create/Promote—an approach that provides enrichment through environment and activities that enhance performance in those with and without disability.	Play groups, parent/caregiver child classes, toy libraries, parent/caregiver resources for play and development.	A therapist might work with Callie and her family to find a play group of children who enjoy coloring, basketball, or construction play like she does for Callie to expand her play network and be able to practice socializing with others through play. Gaby and her family might be encouraged to visit a toy lending library to try new electronic toys within Gaby's physical abilities to allow her more independent play as well as play with her sibling or peers.
Establish/Restore—an approach aimed at remediating or restoring skills and abilities that have not been developed yet or have been lost through impairment or disability.	Playful activities and toys and games that promote movement, strength, and endurance. Games and activities that challenge motor planning and provide sensory experiences. Visual schedules and games and play activities that promote problem solving and strategy use.	Callie might work with the therapist on improving her ability to throw accurately, during play, so that she could play basketball with the neighbors. Gaby might be enticed to play games that improve her grasp, release, and fine-motor skill so that she could better access other toys and computer activities more independently. Gaby might work in therapy to begin to do simple pretend play. Callie might work in therapy to establish her ability to join her peers in games she has not yet tried.
Maintain—an approach meant to keep skills that have been learned or regained through provision of supports.	Provide toy and home program recommendations to families to maintain skills gained in therapy sessions.	Callie can be encouraged to play basketball at home to practice the skills she is learning in therapy. Gaby can play activities with her sister on the computer to maintain her ability to access computer play applications. Gaby's family can be coached to allow Gaby to make her own choices of play activities as much as possible to maintain her independent choice and autonomy.

(continues)

[1] The cases of Callie and Gabby were introduced in Chapter 4.

Table 5.1 Incorporating Play within Each of the Occupational Therapy Practice Framework Intervention Approaches
(continued)

OTPF Intervention Approach (AOTA, 2020)	General Pediatric Play Activity Examples	Example for Callie and Gaby[1]
Modify/Compensate/Adapt—an approach focused on modifying activity demands and/or context to support occupational performance.	Modify toys and games to support play and participation. Provide modified tools and utensils to support play participation. Provide sensory environments and sensory rich activities to maintain regulation for playing.	Callie can be provided with different building toys other than the Legos that seem too difficult for her. The new building toys (such as magnetic building tiles) should require less refined fine-motor skill and judgment of force, so that she can be more successful in building her imagined creations.
	Build or identify external supports to promote participation in play. Modify the environment or advocate for environmental modifications that provide accessible play spaces. Educate others in the context to support the child's play.	Callie can be presented with a modified game of basketball such as the use of a large trash can for a basket so that she can participate successfully immediately. Gaby may need to be provided with alternative computer access methods such as switches, joysticks, etc. so that she can participate in computer games with her sister and neighborhood peers. Megan and the neighborhood peers can be taught how to select and modify specific computer applications and games to allow Gaby to participate with them.
Prevent—an approach to providing supports and intervention directed toward at-risk clients to prevent further disability.	Provide technology or other equipment to prevent progression of disability.	Callie is at risk of social isolation due to her behavior with peers. The therapist might reduce this risk through social skill interventions during adult-led play groups. Gaby is at risk of learned helplessness, social isolation, and frequent participation in activities that are not of her choosing. The therapist may seek to prevent these outcomes through fostering Gaby's active choices and provision of access to a variety of play opportunities to try and explore.

and pages of ways we can engage with clients and perform our duties as occupational therapists. Making a decision to be a tour guide to PLAY requires a deep conviction that PLAY is an important place to visit for all children. For many children with disabilities, PLAY is not considered a top priority and is used merely to measure other areas, reinforce other skills, or as therapy to promote development of other areas (Claughton, 2015). Choosing to be a tour guide to PLAY also means that we are open to detouring to specific destinations in PLAY that the child chooses, even if they may be unexpected. Last, choosing to be a tour guide to PLAY means we actively seek to get there at least some of the time in our therapy sessions.

If we would like the destination to be "PLAY," we need a road map or travel plan to get us to "play." Therapists must carefully plan the intervention for the child both across the span of time the child will be in therapy and within each specific therapy session. As client-centered and evidence-based practice is essential (AOTA, 2020), this professional reasoning is based on information from the occupational profile, the analysis of occupational performance, and the evidence, as well as a clear understanding of the realities of the context.

Fill in this chart by listing information in bullet form to help you plan your tour.

Client Factors to Consider (Gathered from Assessment)			Mapping the Plan			Play Destination
Strengths	Difficulties	Preferences and Favorites	Toys and materials therapeutic for this child	Strategies matched to assist or prompt this child	Possible play activities or themes for this child	Child's play goals and skills to target

Therapist "To-Do" List: *(This may include items to procure or purchase, items that need to be adapted prior to intervention, information to provide to educate others, research the therapist needs to do to learn about a new technique or strategy, or characters and play themes the therapist needs to learn such as watching a new animated film the child prefers.)*

Figure 5.2 Format for planning a tour to PLAY

We must also know specifically what we want to see and do when we arrive at "PLAY." This requires knowledge about the child's desires, preferences, and favorites. It also requires goals that focus on the aspects of play to be addressed. Goals pinpoint our specific PLAY destination. See **Figure 5.2** for a form to use with specific clients to map out your plan to get to PLAY.

If we as occupational therapists value play as an occupation, play should be an explicit goal of occupational therapy (Bundy, 1993). Therapists may not be accustomed to writing play goals and objectives. Some may feel better equipped to be tour guides to handwriting than to PLAY. Others may feel they are unable to write goals for play for a variety of reasons. Although there are many "how-to" guides for writing measurable goals and objectives, there is limited information available to help pediatric therapists write goals and objectives for play. Research suggests that some therapists feel play is not their role, that it will not be covered by insurance, for example (Miller Kuhaneck, Tanta, Coombs, & Pannone, 2013). We urge you to question that assumption and stretch yourself to make changes to your evaluation processes and goal writing. It may be helpful to start with small changes over time to slowly build your repertoire of appropriate play-related goals that may be included where you practice. **Table 5.2** provides examples that may help you to begin to write goals and objectives in this area. If payment and funding is a primary concern, **Table 5.3** explores potential CPT® codes that therapists can use for multitasking play with other areas. The case of Callie (see **Practice Example 5.1**) illustrates how play goals can foster better engagement in play as an important outcome.

Logistics and Supplies

No matter the setting the therapist is working in, one important role is to provide what is needed to get to "PLAY." This may mean ordering or purchasing appropriate play materials for a clinic or outpatient space. It may mean at times providing therapy outside during recess or during after school activities for school-based practitioners (Bazyk & Bazyk, 2009; Grady, Seidle, & Bundy, 2020; Jarus, Anaby, Bart, Engel-Yeger, & Law, 2010). It may mean providing specific objects that are props for favorite specific pretend play themes (Howe, Abuhatoum, & Chang-Kredl, 2014; Lewis & Boucher, 1995). It may mean modeling how to make play happen with typical household items, if working in a home with limited appropriate toy availability. It may mean creating wish lists and advocating for budget increases for therapy materials. Or, it may mean collecting used items that can be carefully sanitized, or "junk objects" for loose parts play outdoors (Gibson, Cornell, & Gill 2017; Maxwell, Mitchell, & Evans, 2008).

Once the materials are available, it is also up to the therapist to decide which materials are appropriate for each session. The therapist decides which should be visible and which should be hidden away. The therapist determines which should be within reach and accessible to the child independently and which should be out of reach and require adult assistance. The therapist decides how many choices are available to a child at any one time

Table 5.2 Example of Possible Play Goals

Targeted Area	Possible Verb Words	Sample Goals*
Play participation: Increase engagement with specific forms of play or use toys/objects in a specific way (functional play, symbolic play).	Play Participate Demonstrate Engage in Attempt Interact Use Pretend Try Act like Make believe Verbally indicate imagined Role play Decide	_____ will attempt to play ball games with siblings. _____ will interact in play with peers daily at the afterschool program. _____ will engage in parallel play while seated next to a peer with similar materials. _____ will use toy figures to engage in three novel actions. _____ will pretend to be at least one character from a favorite book.
Play variety: Play with a variety of objects, toys, partners, themes; increase the variety of play themes or type.	Play Select Choose Decide Initiate Vary Change Alter Modify Transform Create	_____ will play with at least three new peers during recess. _____ will select at least three different play activities during each recess period.
Play complexity: Increase the number of steps, the length of the sequence, or the difficulty level.	Play Select Choose Complete Alter Vary Sequence Suggest Direct	_____ will choose play activities with at least three steps. _____ will independently alter a play activity to make it more difficult. _____ will direct the creation of a three-step game.
Play creativity: Increase the ability to come up with new ideas and combine old ideas in new ways, use a toy in a novel way.	Originate Invent Combine Create Describe Associate Merge Incorporate Direct	_____ will independently create one new character to act out during pretend play in the "pirate ship" at the playground. _____ will describe how to merge two games together into a new game.
Playfulness: Increase the ability to engage playfully with persons or objects (any of the specific characteristics of playfulness could become areas for goals).	Demonstrate Engage in Participate Indicate Joke	_____ will joke with peers while playing. _____ will indicate to others that play is occurring through _____ play cue.
Play activity level: Increase willingness to engage in active or physically challenging play.	Engage in Participate Allow Choose Select Tolerate Accept	_____ will engage in play on the climbing wall. _____ will accept a peer's offer to play catch.

Targeted Area	Possible Verb Words	Sample Goals*
Play persistence: Increase the length of time the child plays or the child's persistence.	Engage in Participate Continue Play Persist Sustain	_____will sustain engagement in puzzle play until free play time is complete. _____will play family games for at least 5 minutes without giving up.
Play success: Increase a child's feelings of competence / self-efficacy.	Express State Identify Indicate Say Specify	_____ will independently identify improvements in play performance. _____ will verbally indicate pleasure at his performance during constructional play.
Play transitions: Increase ability to shift engagement and focus from one activity to another.	Conclude Stop Shift Transition Convert Change Alter Tolerate	_____ will conclude playing video games when the allotted time is up. ____ will willingly shift from one game to another when requested by a peer.
Play manners: Share, take turns in play, or wait for playmate's response/turn.	Wait Take turns Delay Postpone Pause Share Exchange Split Divide Give Negotiate	_____will take turns with a peer for at least three turns. ____ will independently give a peer a portion of the play materials available when requested.
Play initiation and choice: Increase ability for a child to initiate play activity of own choice, and express choices to others.	Initiate Start Begin Commence Instigate Ask Request Inquire Invite	_____ will independently begin playing with his chosen toys. _____ will ask a peer to play a specific game of his choice.
Play acceptance: Increase a child's ability to be accepted by peers, enter into an activity with playmates without disrupting the play process.	Join Enter Request Engage with Allow Accept Admit Negotiate	_____will successfully join peers in an ongoing neighborhood game. _____ will be admitted by peers to a play activity at least once per recess.

Based on ideas from Baranek, Reinhartsen, & Wannamaker (2001), Florey & Greene (2008), Miller & Kuhaneck (2008), and Miller-Kuhaneck (2008).

* As settings vary extensively in the specifics of how they write measurable short-term goals/objectives, these are just meant to provide ideas for you to modify to meet your setting's specific needs.

Table 5.3 Functional Goals Related to CPT® Codes That Can Promote Play

Sample Possible Goals	Possible CPT® code (AMA, 2021)	CPT® Code Explanation (AMA, 2021)	Rationale
_____ will independently make a choice between two opportunities available in the home/school environment in 75% of trials. _____ will independently choose an achievable activity from a variety of at least three activity options, in 75% of opportunities. When encountering a problem, _____ will independently identify two options to solve the problem in 75% of opportunities. _____will sustain attention to an enjoyable task for at least XYZ # of minutes in 75% of opportunities. _____ will independently initiate engagement in a chosen activity at least once per week in 2 out of 4 weeks per month. _____will independently alter engagement in an activity by changing it or by allowing a peer to change it without protest, in 75% of opportunities observed at recess. _____ will independently use strategies to regulate behavior when frustrated in 75% of opportunities during enjoyable activities. _____ will engage in a chosen activity with a peer for at least 5 minutes at a time, in 75% of opportunities. _____ will share materials with a peer when asked in 75% of opportunities. _____ will take turns with a peer for at least three turns without adult prompting in 75% of opportunities. _____ will independently indicate preferences (verbally/with body language/using a device) in 75% of opportunities. _____ will participate in one novel activity chosen by a peer for at least 5 minutes, in 75% of opportunities. _____ will indicate feelings of success (verbally/with body language) during self-selected challenging activities in 50% of opportunities.	97129 97130	Therapeutic interventions that focus on cognitive function (e.g., attention, memory, reasoning, executive function, problem solving, and/or pragmatic functioning) and compensatory strategies to manage the performance of an activity (e.g., managing time or schedules, initiating, organizing, and sequencing tasks).	All of these are important functional outcomes that can be achieved through sessions that focus on play. Play naturally includes making choices related to play preferences, materials, and settings. Play also typically includes opportunities to solve problems, manage frustration, sustain attention, and initiate, alter, and terminate activities.
_____ will use XYZ AT device with minimal assistance to engage with peers for at least 3 minutes in 75% of opportunities. _____ will independently don XYZ clothing in 75% of opportunities.	97535	Self-care/home management training (e.g., activities of daily living (ADLs) and compensatory training, meal preparation, safety procedures, and instructions in use of assistive technology devices/adaptive equipment).	For children who need to use AT devices, there are a variety of play activities that can support their engagement, participation, and interaction with peers.

Sample Possible Goals	Possible CPT® code (AMA, 2021)	CPT® Code Explanation (AMA, 2021)	Rationale
			For children who enjoy dress-up and make-believe, and choose to engage in that form of play, play sessions may provide naturally occurring opportunities for children to begin to participate in ADL skills without the therapist focusing specifically on "learning to button."
_____ will independently and safely maneuver his/her/their wheelchair while outdoors at recess (at the park) in 75% of opportunities.	97542	Wheelchair management (e.g., assessment, fitting, training).	For children who use wheelchairs, any play session that includes play away from a table will naturally provide opportunities for wheelchair training.

PRACTICE EXAMPLE 5.1 Callie's Goals and Treatment Plan

Callie was an imaginative, creative, and intelligent 5-year-old with ASD. However, she was struggling with dyspraxia, tactile defensiveness, and issues with self-esteem. She was a very "bossy" play partner with her family and her peers, insisting on having everything her way. When things did not go as planned, which, because of her dyspraxia, was often, or when peers wanted to play something differently than she did, she would become extremely upset. This often resulted in removing herself from the situation, sometimes in extreme ways such as hiding under the bed for an hour. These types of situations meant that play was frequently not enjoyable for anyone. Her parents were often on edge, trying to coax success, but constantly fearful of the next outburst. Peers were beginning to refuse to play with her, and Callie's self-esteem, already a problem, was getting worse. Because of this, although Callie also had a variety of motor concerns and difficulties with academic and self-care performance, Callie's parents agreed that it was important to help Callie play better. While they also wanted her motor skills to improve, they knew that merely improving motor skills would not necessarily equate to these important peer and social skills improving on their own. (See Chapter 4 for Callie's evaluation results.)

One of Callie's goals, therefore, became to participate fully and to completion in activities chosen by peers. This goal allowed the therapist to work toward improvement in a wide range of play activities and focused a portion of the intervention plan on this specific aspect of peer play that Callie was struggling with. It also meant that during therapy, peers needed to be available for at least portions of the sessions in order to practice needed skills during play. This was not an impossibility, but it required a therapist tour guide, who planned ahead or who was ready to take advantage of peer opportunities when they presented themselves. Although a therapist can be an important play partner, if peer play is a goal, then peers need to be included as well.

A second goal, more focused on the enjoyment portion of play, was for Callie to be better able to identify activities that were "just right" for herself and to identify new activities she would like to try to play. She tended to have wonderful play ideas that were too challenging, ending in extreme frustration. The therapist planned to work with Callie toward better understanding about each person's range of abilities, as well as the specific range of activities within her own ability level AND ways to modify her activities and her approach to them so that over time, she would enjoy her play more and end up in frustration less. For example, the therapist made up a variety of "Goldilocks" games. Each game had three tries, and the games were set up so that one trial would be too hard, one would be too easy, and one would be just right. Callie knew the story of the three bears, and this theme made it ok that sometimes she would not be successful in the activity they were doing because one out of three was expected to be too difficult. The therapist occasionally played too, setting up the game so that one trial would be too hard for her as well. After each game, the therapist and Callie playfully talked about what made it easier or harder for each of them. They talked about the

(continues)

differences and similarities in their performance and about the differences that age, strength, height, weight, limb length, vision, and dexterity could mean to performance in certain games. (Who do you think this game would be harder for, someone who wears glasses or someone who was very small? Why?) Games or activities that worked well for the "Goldilocks" approach were ones that were able to be graded up and down easily such as ball games, building games, and craft activities. The therapist also instructed Callie in the basics of activity analysis at a level she could understand (Does this game need you

to have good vision? Does this game need you to have good balance? Does this game need you to be able to throw really far?). They then began to consider a variety of new games and talk about which might be good for Callie, noting what she WAS good at. ("You are really creative. Which of these needs someone to be really creative?"). Then they started to talk about why certain things might be harder for her and using the prior Goldilocks game as the basis for changing the difficulty level of activities. Eventually Callie was asked to try to make things easier and harder for herself.

(Metz, Imwalle, Dauch, & Wheeler, 2017). These are all important "tour guide" duties, and many of these decisions should be made before the session begins. However, setup is one area that with practice, therapists are able to manage in the moment, adding more materials to the mix during sessions when needed and quickly removing objects that seem to be problematic.

So how does the therapist make these decisions? Safety always comes first! Beyond safety, then the therapist considers the child's preferences and goals. There should be materials and toys available that the child enjoys and seeks out. Then the therapist may think about whether a focus of the session should be on autonomy and choice making in play, cooperation and collaboration in play, sharing, taking turns, initiating, sustaining play, or any of a number of specific elements of play. Please also see Chapter 9 for more information on setting up play spaces.

Adapt for Access

Prior to a session, the therapist determines if specific materials need to be adapted in order for them to be successful. For example, the therapist might know that in order for an independent dress-up activity to occur, the costume needs to have the buttons removed and Velcro sewn on. Or, perhaps a board game needs to have different pieces created that are easier to grasp, or easier to see on the game board. Or, perhaps a tricycle needs to have a different braking mechanism in order for a child with physical disabilities to ride safely with peers. All of these would require the thoughtful planning of the tour guide prior to any therapy session that would use these materials. These types of modifications cannot typically be completed during therapy. Please also

see Chapter 8 for more information on adaptations including modifications.

"On Tour": During a Session

Once the therapist and child have entered into the therapy session, there will be a variety of additional items for the therapist to attend to, in order to ensure that the tour arrives at "PLAY." One important thing to remember is that just because the tour has been well planned, there may still be detours, barriers, or fortuitous events that must be dealt with, with flexibility and an eye for the opportune.

Consider One's Role and Modify Interaction Style

There is nothing to be done about the fact that the therapist is an adult. As a result, there will always be that power dynamic and the possibility that the therapist can slip into an authoritative and supervisory role rather than the playmate role. The more the therapist does this, the less likely the child will be able to see the therapist as a playmate when it is time to focus on play. However, there are many ways the therapist can alter engagement to become a playmate. Tone of voice matters, physical location in relation to the child matters, humor and silliness matters. Allowing choice matters. The skills required for therapeutic use of self during play are described thoroughly in Chapter 6. What is important is that the therapist actively considers the power dynamic and strives to be a playmate when trying to arrive at "PLAY." It is a conscious choice of the therapist. The focus shifts away from "I decide how we spend our therapy time and I will tell you what to do, how to do it, and make you do it" to "Let's play (together)." Also see **Practice**

Opportunity 5.1 for an example of how one adult's creativity and playfulness as a "tour guide to play" promoted inclusive play in a camp.

Select Activities

Within each session at PLAY, there may be an almost infinite list of possible activities that could occur; therefore, an important role of the therapist tour guide is to select proper activities to present as options. This selection and presentation process is different from the more traditional therapeutic experience of "here is what we are going to do today." If you watch children playing together, they do often take turns making suggestions for what to play. So being a playmate does not mean you cannot offer ideas, it just means you are exploring possibilities with your client and will not impose your ideas. The experienced tour guide to PLAY knows the lay of the land and the many different ways through difficult terrain and scenic landscapes and thus is able to rapidly think through a variety of available play options that are both therapeutic and fun so that a fluid and engaging session occurs that meets the child's play goals. The excellent tour guide also is willing to deviate from plans when amazing opportunities present themselves. See Chapter 7 for more detail about how therapists select appropriate play activities using theory and professional reasoning and a case example about how to consider one's response to those unexpected opportunities.

Practice Opportunity 5.1 Children as the Experts on Inclusivity

Ariana Brazier, PhD, and Julia Brazier
ATL Parent Like A Boss, Inc.

While working with the multigrade combo group in the summer camp, I noticed that most of the group enjoyed volleyball and kickball inside the gym.[2] The multigrade combo consisted of a small group of students with behavioral challenges from across the third- to fifth-grade range. The group frequently had one student with a physical disability that necessitated elbow or forearm crutches whenever walking; so, while he often participated, he often sat out also.

One day, he and I were sitting on the cheerleading mats in the gymnasium when we started silently smacking a foam ball back and forth from opposite ends of the mat. While we tried to keep the ball from touching the floor, it was not an imperative; no one was removed from the game for any reason. Quickly, this informal game became a modified seated/crawling form of volleyball without the net, scorekeeping, or referees—no rules. We were having so much fun that the other kids joined.

About 2 weeks later, the group instructor informed me that the students had begun playing the floor game every day (even in my absence) and named the game after my fellow student initiator. This was exciting news, as the game was likely a self-esteem boost as he had created a game that everyone liked and was able to play. Thereby, this created new opportunities not only for his equitable inclusion, but also for his leadership and expertise.

As this group demonstrated, child-directed play can facilitate the development of their own brand of inclusivity and learn the value of accessibility. No prompting or coaching was necessary for them to be inclusive. In addition to the immense value of learning in mixed-age groups, the children of various ages were learning how to accommodate differences—significantly, in this specific instance, the other children were appreciative of his differences as they were the reason for the new game.

Each time the group engaged in his game, they were able to view him through an asset- or strengths-based lens. As an adult in their company, we should develop a habit of revisiting these teachable moments via informal dialogue. Revisiting the game through dialogue allows us the opportunity to challenge children to recreate this kind of cooperative play and learning with available resources. In turn, we can highlight and remind each of them of their existing creative, community-building skills.

Moreover, instead of leaning into our inclination toward ableism that would have us challenge or expect this child to perform according to someone else's capacities or participate in a game structured according to an arbitrary conceptualization of able-bodiedness, we avoid subjecting our students to play deprivation. This form of deprivation might ordinarily occur because of our personal ignorance, biases, negligence, or insecurity with regard to ability, race, class, gender, and so forth. Intentional or not, this student was receiving individualized attention. Following his lead, I was able to facilitate this play experience instead of hindering it, and I could effectively encourage him to perform at his capacity. This success cofacilitation ultimately necessitated that the I, the adult in the group, *be within* the group, *not above or outside* the group.

---

[2] Ariana Brazier was conducting ethnographic research on the ways Black children in this school/summer camp cluster play. Her point of view is the "I" in the narrative, while the latter "we" refers to all adults.

Grade Activities

No matter how adept a therapist is at collaborating with a child to create a play activity, occasionally things will go wrong. The activity might be too easy and boring, or too hard and frustrating. When this happens, the therapist must be ready to jump in, take responsibility, and fix it by grading the activity. Like all good tour guides, the therapist is responsible for ensuring everything is as ideal as it can be and for fixing problems when they occur. The therapist may tell the child outright that the problem is the therapist's fault, such as with a comment like "Wow, I put that WAY too far away from you." Then the therapist would grade the activity by moving the item slightly closer, just close enough to make the challenge the right level of difficulty (Ayres, 1972).

The types of fixes we call grading may include changing the weight, size, or color contrast of objects; changing the distance of targets; changing the location of the game or activity, such as by varying its height or angle; changing the speed or direction or type of motion of the child or the objects; or changing the strength, endurance, or coordination required to complete the play activity. See Chapter 8 for more in-depth guidance on grading during play.

Modify or Alter Materials

Therapists may need to quickly change materials during sessions. Sometimes the therapist will need to add materials based on the way a specific play theme is emerging. For example, during a game a child might say, "Oh no, the alligator is coming." The therapist may quickly look for something available nearby, appropriate to "be" an alligator. The child may only want to play with a specific color item, requiring the therapist grab the blue ball instead of the red one. The child might be particular about characters, or refuse a race car but prefer a truck, or insist that there MUST be a rubber duck if they are going to pretend bath time.

Other times, the therapist may need to remove something. A child may not like the texture of something, or may refuse to play with items that remind them of something they dislike. The therapist can be playful about this. For example, the child may become upset with a specific object they are struggling with, and the therapist can take it away and put it in "Oscar the Grouch's trash can."

Sometimes the therapist must simultaneously do both removing and providing materials. The child may not want to use tools given to play the game, and the therapist may need to provide different tools, for example, removing tongs while handing the child tweezers instead, or suggesting beanbags instead of Nerf® balls, while swapping them.

The well-stocked and organized play space will allow for these rapid alterations without disrupting the play. We cannot stress enough how important it is to have a variety of play materials readily available. The well-stocked play space allows play to grow, shift, and morph into whatever it is going to be that day. The excellent tour guide has lots of possible options in each location to manage any possible dilemma.

Assist

At times, all that might be required to help a child play is a slight bit of assistance. Assistance can occur in many forms such as providing something needed, holding something still, moving something out of the way, moving something closer, opening something to allow access, or providing support for a body part or limb. Assistance could take the form of pushing children to go faster or higher than they could on their own. Assistance could also mean reading instructions out loud for a child who cannot yet read. Specific examples in a therapeutic context could be providing a hand to hold briefly as the child traverses an obstacle such as a log in an outdoor play space, quietly and unobtrusively holding something still for a child who is struggling to balance on it, or holding the pillowcase open wide as the child tries to throw objects into it. The aim of this type of assistance is to allow for successful performance and fluid continuation of the play experience.

Demonstrate, Prompt, and Teach

All good tour guides also inform their clients about the places they are visiting. Children who are having difficulty getting to "PLAY" may need to be encouraged to play, but they may also need to be taught why to go there at all. The therapist may need to demonstrate that play is fun and enjoyable. The therapist may need to encourage the child to try new games or experiences. See **Box 5.1** for specific strategies.

Box 5.1 Strategies to Encourage Play

- Use one's own childhood as an example (i.e., "When I was a child, I loved to play _____ because_____. Would you like to play this with me?")
- Sit down and start playing something with gusto and enjoyment, allowing the child to watch and eventually join in.
- Model silly behaviors, and express your joy over the fun they provide.
- Describe why certain things are fun for you and ask the child, "You try, is this fun for you too?"
- Suggest to a child, "I know you like the TV show X, I wonder if we could use this to act like the character Y."
- Ask, "Show me how _(favorite character)___ would do this?"
- Prompt pretend play with the use of enticing props for preferred themes such as costumes, hats, crowns, clown or genie shoes, or Star Trek™ communicators.
- Purposely omit necessary objects for a play theme, and provide some possible objects for substitutions. For example, while pretending "rock band" make sure there is no toy drum or drumstick and instead provide a Tupperware or upside-down bowl for the drum, or an unsharpened pencil for the drumstick (Lee, Qu, Hu, Jin, & Huang, 2020).
- Imitate what the child is doing. This can be one method to enter into their play activity and social space, and it can be a successful method of engaging them and improving play skills (Ingersoll, 2012; Kuhaneck, Spitzer, & Bodison, 2020).

Sometimes on tour to new places, one gets an opportunity to learn a new skill. Teaching specific play skills, such as how to use specific toys, or how to use props for pretending, may occur through a variety of cognitive problem-solving strategies, specific use of verbal, visual, or manual cues, demonstration or modeling, or physical guidance. The literature on specific forms of prompting suggest different prompting strategies are best for different children (Seok & DaCosta, 2021). Physical prompting such as hand over hand or "doing for" should be used sparingly and only when it is critical to allow the child success and safety. Hand over hand approaches can be quite intrusive. However, therapists can encourage greater skill during play activities in a variety of other ways. The therapist may encourage children to talk aloud to themselves to guide their own play as they engage in it (Winsler, Abar, Feder, Schunn, & Rubio, 2007). Therapists may cue specific required movements by touching a body part while verbalizing "place this up here" and then tapping the desired location. The therapist may question the child to point their focus in the correct area ("Which foot do you think should move up first?"). The therapist may merely talk to the child about what the child is doing, providing commentary and noting specific methods and approaches the child takes that are successful. "When you do that with your arm outstretched, it works much better." Therapists may teach using other children as guides, for example commenting to a child, "My friend Johnny plays this game too, and he always does X."

A variety of specific interventions could be included in occupational therapy sessions to help assist children to achieve specific play skills such as video modeling (Kent et al., 2020; Kossyvaki & Papoudi, 2016; Park, Bouck, & Duenas, 2019; Sancho, Sidener, Reeve, & Sidener, 2010), peer-supported or peer-mediated play (Kent, Cordier, Joosten, Wilkes-Gillan, & Bundy, 2018; Wolfberg & Schuler, 1993), social stories (Barry & Burlew, 2004; Quirmbach, Lincoln, Feinberg-Gizzo, Ingersoll, & Andrews, 2009), Lego therapy (Lindsay, Hounsell, & Cassiani, 2017), Reciprocal Imitation Training (Ingersoll & Schreibman, 2006), and perhaps even the use of robots (Wainer, Robins, Amirabdollahian, & Dautenhahn, 2014).

Be Flexible and Follow the Desires of the Client When Possible

Any good tour guide knows that sometimes things will go wrong, and they will need to be flexible and agile in coming up with workable alternatives. A bridge may be out requiring a different route, or a planned excursion may need to be cancelled because of bad weather. In terms of therapy, you may find yourself doing intervention in a space you had not planned on, or find that something you always do with child X is now broken. Sometimes a client may refuse to do the suggested activity. You will need to drop your plans and do something else. Other times, a client will express an interest to do something that was not preplanned. To enhance the client's experience, show that you accept their choices, and acknowledge their expression of internal motivation. It can be very important to determine some method of using their idea in a creative way that also is therapeutic. This may also change your plans. The ability to be flexible in the moment of the session is a critical skill. This topic will be elaborated upon in Chapter 8.

Posttour

After a travel adventure, the tour company typically gathers feedback from its clients regarding their enjoyment of the tour and the ways in which the tour could be improved. Therapists rarely ask children about what might make the session more fun next time, but it can be a useful exercise for learning about what is most important to the child. For children who are nonverbal, careful observation will be required to glean these insights (Spitzer, 2003). Therapists should also regularly check in with parents, other caregivers, and teachers about the way in which the child is playing outside of the therapy sessions, to determine if there is carryover from therapy to outside life. This ongoing assessment provides the necessary information for a tour guide to PLAY to increase effectiveness and enhance the voyage and for the therapist to improve the therapy.

Educate

Outside of the therapy sessions, therapists must educate others in the child's life if there is to be any carryover or follow-through. Even with the best levels of service delivery possible in our current system of health care and education, children are with their therapists just a fraction of each week. Whatever is working during therapy needs to be taught to others to use outside of therapy. Therapists may want to specifically target their teaching to a child's parents, caregivers, siblings, or grandparents, or to important peers. Teachers can be important allies in promoting play as well. Please also see Chapters 10 and 11 for more information about play with families and at school.

What Happens When You Can't Reach the Destination of PLAY?

Some of you may have read this and thought to yourself that in your setting or situation you would not be able to guide a tour to PLAY for various reasons. If you believe PLAY is an important destination, then any small steps

toward it that are achievable are worthwhile. You may be able to add in a variety of more playful approaches, use play more frequently as a tool or a reward, or promote and advocate for play outside of your therapy sessions. Going back to the travel metaphor, the journey along the way is also important, and not only the final destination may be enjoyable. And just like most adults cannot be on perpetual vacation traveling on tours, children will not ONLY tour to PLAY. As occupational therapists, we often have to guide children to other destinations as well. But perhaps as we travel with children to destinations like "handwriting" or "feeding," we can also take more small detours that get us closer to PLAY or allow us to go through PLAY for a time on our way to other areas. We have found that the more we know about, value, and prioritize play, the more we find ways of including play during all aspects of therapy with children.

Conclusion

The Land of PLAY is an important destination in childhood and one that some children may need assistance to reach. While PLAY is not always the chosen terminus of pediatric occupational therapy practitioners, if therapists believe it is an important place to visit, they must be intentional about guiding their clients to and through that experience. Getting to PLAY is unlikely to occur without the specific desire or the decision of the therapist, client, family, and perhaps other team members that getting to PLAY is an important outcome of therapy. Functioning as a tour guide, the occupational therapist can be systematic but flexible in reaching that "location." Getting to PLAY will require appropriate planning, the inclusion of very specific strategies and methods, as well as specific ways of being therapeutic with the child. If the therapist has done a good job as tour guide to "PLAY," the child should experience therapy as enjoyable and should want to be with the therapist and engage in more play and therapy. This chapter was meant as an overview of the more in-depth chapters to follow. Each will explore aspects of the occupational therapy process, methods, or contexts, and their importance in reaching PLAY.

References

American Medical Association (AMA). (2021). *Current Procedural Terminology (CPT®)*. Chicago, IL: American Medical Association.

American Occupational Therapy Association (AOTA). (2020). Occupational therapy practice framework: Domain and process (4th ed.). *American Journal of Occupational Therapy*, 74(Suppl. 2), 7412410010. https://doi.org/10.5014/ajot.2020.74S2001

Ayres, A. J. (1972). *Sensory integration and learning disorders*. Los Angeles, CA: Western Psychological Services.

Baranek, G. T., Reinhartsen, D., & Wannamaker, S. (2001). Play: Engaging children with autism. *Sensorimotor Interventions in Autism*, 311–351.

Barry, L. M., & Burlew, S. B. (2004). Using social stories to teach choice and play skills to children with autism. *Focus on Autism and Other Developmental Disabilities*, 19(1), 45–51.

Bazyk, S., & Bazyk, J. (2009). Meaning of occupation-based groups for low-income urban youths attending after-school care. *American Journal of Occupational Therapy*, 63(1), 69–80.

Bundy, A. C. (1993). Assessment of play and leisure: Delineation of the problem. *American Journal of Occupational Therapy*, 47, 217–222.

Claughton, A. (2015). Choosing time: Supporting the play of students with a dis/ability. In T. Corcoran, J. White, & B. Whitburn (Eds.), *Disability studies: Innovations and Controversies* (pp. 89–102). Rotterdam: Brill Sense.

Florey, L. L., & Greene, S. (2008). Play in middle childhood. In L. D. Parham & L. S. Fazio (Eds.), *Play in occupational therapy for children* (2nd ed., pp. 279–299). St. Louis, MO: Mosby Elsevier.

Gibson, J. L., Cornell, M., & Gill, T. (2017). A systematic review of research into the impact of loose parts play on children's cognitive, social and emotional development. *School Mental Health*, 9(4), 295–309.

Grady, P., Seidle, J. S., & Bundy, A. (2020). Wrapped in cotton wool: Using implementation science to examine unexpected results in a recess-based intervention study for children with autism spectrum disorder (ASD). *American Journal of Occupational Therapy*, 74(4_Supplement_1), 7411520482p1–7411520482p1.

Howe, N., Abuhatoum, S., & Chang-Kredl, S. (2014). "Everything's upside down. We'll call it Upside Down Valley!": Siblings' creative play themes, object use, and language during pretend play. *Early Education and Development*, 25(3), 381–398.

Ingersoll, B. (2012). Brief report: Effect of a focused imitation intervention on social functioning in children with autism. *Journal of Autism and Developmental Disorders*, 42(8), 1768–1773.

Ingersoll, B., & Schreibman, L. (2006). Teaching reciprocal imitation skills to young children with autism using a naturalistic behavioral approach: Effects on language, pretend play, and joint attention. *Journal of Autism and Developmental Disorders*, 36(4), 487.

Jarus, T., Anaby, D., Bart, O., Engel-Yeger, B., & Law, M. (2010). Childhood participation in after-school activities: What is to be expected? *British Journal of Occupational Therapy*, 73(8), 344–350.

Kent, C., Cordier, R., Joosten, A., Wilkes-Gillan, S., & Bundy, A. (2018). Peer-mediated intervention to improve play skills in children with autism spectrum disorder: A feasibility study. *Australian Occupational Therapy Journal*, 65(3), 176–186.

Kent, C., Cordier, R., Joosten, A., Wilkes-Gillan, S., Bundy, A., & Speyer, R. (2020). A systematic review and meta-analysis of interventions to improve play skills in children with autism spectrum disorder. *Review Journal of Autism and Developmental Disorders*, 7(1), 91–118.

Kossyvaki, L., & Papoudi, D. (2016). A review of play interventions for children with autism at school. *International Journal of Disability, Development and Education*, 63(1), 45–63.

Kuhaneck, H., Spitzer, S. L., & Bodison, S. C. (2020). A systematic review of interventions to improve the occupation of play in children with autism. *OTJR: Occupation, Participation and Health*, 40(2), 83–98.

Lee, G. T., Qu, K., Hu, X., Jin, N., & Huang, J. (2020). Arranging play activities with missing items to increase object-substitution symbolic play in children with autism spectrum disorder. *Disability and Rehabilitation*, 1–13.

Lewis, V., & Boucher, J. (1995). Generativity in the play of young people with autism. *Journal of Autism and Developmental Disorders*, 25(2), 105–121.

Lindsay, S., Hounsell, K. G., & Cassiani, C. (2017). A scoping review of the role of Lego® therapy for improving inclusion and social skills among children and youth with autism. *Disability and Health Journal*, 10(2), 173–182.

Maxwell, L. E., Mitchell, M. R., & Evans, G. W. (2008). Effects of play equipment and loose parts on preschool children's outdoor play behavior: An observational study and design intervention. *Children Youth and Environments*, 18(2), 36–63.

Metz, A., Imwalle, M., Dauch, C., & Wheeler, B. (2017). The influence of the number of toys in the environment on play in toddlers. *American Journal of Occupational Therapy*, 71(4_Supplement_1), 7111505079p1–7111505079p1.

Miller, E., & Kuhaneck, H. (2008). Children's perceptions of play experiences and play preferences: A qualitative study. *American Journal of Occupational Therapy*, 62, 407–415.

Miller, E., & Miller-Kuhaneck, H. (2008). Application of the dynamic model for play choice. Paper presented at the annual conference of the American Occupational Therapy Association, Long Beach, CA.

Miller Kuhaneck, H., Tanta, K. J., Coombs, A. K., & Pannone, H. (2013). A survey of pediatric occupational therapists' use of play. *Journal of Occupational Therapy, Schools, & Early Intervention*, 6(3), 213–227.

Park, J., Bouck, E., & Duenas, A. (2019). The effect of video modeling and video prompting interventions on individuals with intellectual disability: A systematic literature review. *Journal of Special Education Technology*, 34(1), 3–16.

Quirmbach, L. M., Lincoln, A. J., Feinberg-Gizzo, M. J., Ingersoll, B. R., & Andrews, S. M. (2009). Social stories: Mechanisms of effectiveness in increasing game play skills in children diagnosed with autism spectrum disorder using a pretest posttest repeated measures randomized control group design. *Journal of Autism and Developmental Disorders*, 39(2), 299–321.

Sancho, K., Sidener, T. M., Reeve, S. A., & Sidener, D. W. (2010). Two variations of video modeling interventions for teaching play skills to children with autism. *Education and Treatment of Children*, 33(3), 421–442.

Seok, S., & DaCosta, B. (2021). A systematic review of the use of prompting for preschoolers with developmental delay. In A. Singh, J. Yeh, S. Blanchard, & L. Anunciação (Eds.), *Handbook of research on critical issues in special education for school rehabilitation practices* (pp. 47–65). Hershey, PA: IGI Global.

Spitzer, S. L. (2003). Using participant observation to study the meaning of occupations of young children with autism and other developmental disabilities. *American Journal of Occupational Therapy*, 57(1), 66–76.

Tanta, K. J., & Kuhaneck, H. (2020). Assessment and treatment of play. In J. C. O'Brien & H. Kuhaneck (Eds.), *Case-Smith's occupational therapy for children and adolescents* (8th ed. pp. 239–266). St. Louis, MO: Elsevier.

Wainer, J., Robins, B., Amirabdollahian, F., & Dautenhahn, K. (2014). Using the humanoid robot Kaspar to autonomously play triadic games and facilitate collaborative play among children with autism. *IEEE Transactions on Autonomous Mental Development*, 6(3), 183–199.

Winsler, A., Abar, B., Feder, M. A., Schunn, C. D., & Rubio, D. A. (2007). Private speech and executive functioning among high-functioning children with autistic spectrum disorders. *Journal of Autism and Developmental Disorders*, 37(9), 1617–1635.

Wolfberg, P. J., & Schuler, A. L. (1993). Integrated play groups: A model for promoting the social and cognitive dimensions of play in children with autism. *Journal of Autism and Developmental Disorders*, 23(3), 467–489.

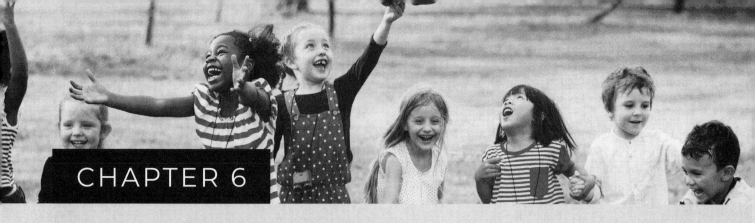

Being Playful: Therapeutic Use of Self in Pediatric Occupational Therapy

Susan L. Spitzer, PhD, OTR/L

After reading this chapter, the reader will:

- Define therapeutic use of self and explain its core concepts.
- Communicate the value of a playful therapeutic use of self.
- Recognize challenges to implementing therapeutic use of self in play.
- Describe and apply strategies to interact playfully with a pediatric client.
- Match strategies for therapeutic use of self to a child's characteristics.
- Manage practitioner's own needs, attitudes, and roles in pediatric occupational therapy.
- Relate therapeutic use of self to diverse caregiver relationships to support play.
- Discuss the research supporting playful therapeutic use of self.

Whoever wants to understand much must play much.
—Gottfried Benn

Occupational therapy practitioners implement therapeutic use of self in a playful manner to harness the power of play. Playful occupational therapy sessions encourage clients to be active participants in the valued occupation of play. Playful sessions start with the personal dynamics of the child and the occupational therapy practitioner. If children have a strong sense of playfulness and a predisposition to play, then therapists need make few adaptations in their demeanor for that client. If, however, as is more likely the case, a child's playfulness is restricted in some way, the therapist must take professional responsibility for creating a playful environment. The child's own playfulness may be limited. Or, the therapeutic activities that address our clients' needs may be, by their nature, more effortful than playful (Hellendoorn, 1994). Playful sessions do not always occur spontaneously. When adults get involved in play activities without understanding and valuing play, they tend to focus on managing and monitoring children rather than supporting their play and development (McInnes et al., 2011). Yet therapy and play need not be at odds with each other. To reconcile the two, occupational therapy practitioners use their knowledge of play and skill in activity analysis to shape play activities as well as therapeutic use of self to promote the child's experience of the activities as play so that individual playfulness and play can emerge.

The occupational therapy practitioner embodies and models playfulness for the client. The therapist draws on therapeutic use of self to communicate to children that therapy can be fun and to therapeutically engage children, their families, and others. The therapist constantly attends to and adjusts his or her style and responses to each child's developmental level and unique characteristics. This chapter illustrates the process of playful therapeutic use of self along with its core components, its importance to rewarding and effective pediatric occupational therapy, and strategies for managing implementation challenges. Multiple clinical examples of various styles of playful therapeutic interaction are provided to help you envision and develop yourself as a therapeutic tool with pediatric clients.

Therapeutic Use of Self: An Artful Tool of Practice

The therapist is crucial to intervention (King, 2017). When an occupational therapy practitioner interacts with a client in a planned and thoughtful manner designed to maximize the client's therapeutic outcome, this is known as therapeutic use of self. As occupational therapists engage in therapeutic use of self, they become a *tool* of practice (Mosey, 1986). This tool is relevant in all practice areas including pediatrics (American Occupational Therapy Association [AOTA], 2016; King, 2017). In pediatrics, therapeutic use of self enables greater attunement to the individual developmental level of each client (Fusco, 2012). Skills that must be adapted to manage pediatric practice demands include therapeutic communication, which provides a base for relating with pediatric clients, and the use of empathy and rapport to cement therapeutic relationships. The practitioner creatively applies these skills for individual clients within their particular occupational circumstances.

Required Skills for Therapeutic Use of Self

Every response and interaction is potentially therapeutic if the occupational therapy practitioner makes a conscious effort to act in a way that best meets the client's needs and facilitates the therapeutic process. As such, therapeutic use of self is highly valued by practitioners (Taylor, Lee, Kielhofner, & Ketkar, 2009). The occupational therapist must be very sensitive to the client's feelings and needs with a view toward future therapeutic goals (O'Brien & Taylor, 2020; Taylor, 2008). Practitioners exercise a high degree of self-control to manage their feelings, needs, and values to refrain from responding spontaneously. Clinicians cannot allow themselves to be distracted by workload pressures or personal stressors (Sharma & Clark, 2018). This conscious work is enacted in a relaxed, informal manner for the client (Mosey, 1986; Palmadottir, 2006) so that it is perceived as playful. Therapeutic use of self requires analytical forethought and careful professional reasoning to determine a skilled response that matches the client's therapeutic needs and provides opportunities for therapeutic gain (O'Brien & Taylor, 2020; Taylor, 2008).

Creating individualized responses moment by moment is an artful aspect of practice (Price, 2009; Williams & Paterson, 2009). Dramatic variations in therapeutic use of self are required for different clients and at different points in time with the same client (Peloquin, 1990; Price, 2009; Taylor, 2008). The occupational therapist cannot rely exclusively on routine or standardized protocols and instead must attend to the individual client's needs and interactions (Hinojosa, 2007; King, Chiarello, Phoenix, D'Arrigo, & Pinto, 2021).

Creative, individualized responses to clients consist of specific interpersonal skills that are intentionally applied to promote engagement in occupations (Taylor, 2008). Taylor identified the following nine categories of interpersonal skills that are involved in therapeutic use of self: therapeutic communication; establishing relationships; interviewing and questioning; understanding families, social systems, and group dynamics; working effectively with supervisors, employers, and other professionals; understanding and managing difficult interpersonal behavior; resolving empathic breaks and conflicts; professional behavior, values, and ethics; and therapist self-care and professional development. Each skill is described in great detail in Taylor's original source, which is highly recommended to those readers not yet familiar with this pivotal work on therapeutic use of self. Here, the focus is on the detailed application of therapeutic communication and relationships for unleashing the power of play in pediatric occupational therapy and on the importance of creativity in using these skills with children.

Creativity

Creativity is an intrinsic part of the philosophy of occupational therapy (Schmid, 2004) and is especially linked to play and spirituality in occupational therapy (Toomey, 2003). At its essence, creativity identifies novel approaches that are useful (Mayer, 2010). Creativity is how we meet the diverse challenges of practice. Whatever you may believe about your intrinsic creative ability, everyone has the potential to be creative (Mayer, 2010).

Creativity is an intentional choice a person makes, a potential fulfilled by choosing to exercise it in everyday activities through mindful and creative actions rather than assumptions and routine actions (Mullaney, 2018; Runco, 2007; Schmid, 2004). Creativity in occupational therapy practitioners is a developmental process, which facilitates our skills while reinvigorating and refining our practice (Blanche, 1992; Fletcher, 2010; Mullaney, 2018). The use of problem solving, the ability to generate and integrate new ideas, and the disciplined work to apply knowledge, all of which are critical to creativity, must be learned and cultivated (Feldhusen & Goh, 1995; Sapp, 1995). Research indicates that clients are the impetus for creativity in occupational therapy (Oven & Lobe, 2019). When we consciously approach each clinical challenge as an opportunity for new ideas and new ways of applying knowledge, we promote our own creativity. Detailed suggestions for enhancing creativity in occupational therapy are provided in **Box 6.1**.

Box 6.1 Methods for Enhancing Creativity in Occupational Therapy

- Change physical location to give new perspective.
- Redefine the problem (for example, reconsider a problem of a child not wanting to play as a problem of not knowing how to play, not feeling successful in play, or being overwhelmed by the sensory features of play).
- Simplify a complex situation into a core problem or issue.
- Consider the broader, bigger problem.
- Consider slight alternatives and variations to a problem.
- Find or apply an analogy of how this situation is similar to something else you know about.
- Consider similarities/analogies in nature.
- Borrow or adapt other similar approaches from others (e.g., from this book, from other occupational therapy practitioners).
- Experiment with different ideas such as using familiar items in new ways.
- Question assumptions.
- Consider an approach that is contrary to conventionally accepted ideas.
- Find ways to change restrictive rules or the environment to allow other options.
- Keep an open mind.
- Entertain multiple possibilities rather than searching for one right answer.
- Be persistent because effort is required for creativity to emerge.
- Believe in your creative potential.

Data from Blanche, E. (1992). Creativity in sensory integrative treatment. *Sensory Integration Special Interest Section Newsletter, 15*(1), 3–4; Runco, M. A. (2007). *Creativity theories and themes: Research, development, and practice.* San Diego, CA: Elsevier Academic Press.

Communication to Frame Play

Communication, both verbal and nonverbal, is an important part of therapeutic use of self (Burke, 2010; O'Brien & Taylor, 2020; Taylor, 2008) and is essential to establishing a playful environment. For treatment activities to be experienced as play, they must be marked by the therapist and child as play and as distinctly different from work or other activities (Goodhall & Atkinson, 2017; Howard & McInnes, 2013; Skard & Bundy, 2008). This is quite similar to the typical process described in Chapter 1, where both animals and children send play signals to potential playmates. When communicating in play, infant and adult brains synchronize together, creating a connection between them (Piazza et al., 2020). Adults can be a very powerful support if they can be interactive play partners (Brodin, 2018; Zappaterra, 2018). If they are going to play with children, adults must understand children's signals about what they want to play, send clear signals that they want to play, and adapt to potential negative responses and miscommunication.

Understanding the Communication Signals of a Pediatric Client

The different communication patterns and perspectives between adult and child can make it difficult for the adult therapist to understand the pediatric client. Some children share their ideas and solicit the engagement of the clinician (Holland & Thompson, 2018; Lawlor, 2012). Some children can be interviewed effectively by asking about what they like to do, what they do well, and what they want to do (Curtin, 2017). Nonetheless, in many cases, pediatric clients do not articulate enough detail and insight about their play and other occupations. This is especially true in the case of younger children and those who do not have access to an effective language-based communication system. Children do not possess the same language and communication skills as adults, and children with disabilities may have additional limitations in their communication abilities (Curtin, 2001; Doussard-Roosevelt et al., 2003; Festante, Antonelli, Chorna, Corsi, & Guzzetta, 2019; Warren & Brady, 2007). Some children with disabilities may provide limited or unclear feedback for our actions (Doussard-Roosevelt et al., 2003; Warren & Brady, 2007). Their bodies may limit their abilities to react, or they may process information in a slow or altered way, which reduces the amount and clarity of communication signals. For example, young children with significant cognitive and motor delays rarely initiate social interaction (Van keer et al., 2019), and children with autism spectrum disorder (ASD) are less likely to respond to adult invitations (Williams, Costall, & Reddy, 2018). They may use a communication style and social interaction pattern that differs from practitioners who do not share their diagnosis as in the case of individuals with ASD (Crompton, Sharp, Axbey, Fletcher-Watson, Flynn, & Ropar, 2020; Chen, Senande, Thorsen, & Patten, 2021). Further complicating the therapist's attempts to understand the pediatric client is that children, in general, experience the world differently from adults because of differences in development and social position (Corsaro & Eder, 1990; Fine & Sandstrom, 1988; Kaplan, 1997). Children with disabilities may have sensory perceptual and motor differences that change their experiences of the world (i.e., Durig, 1996; Frank, 2000; Grandin, 1995; Delafield-Butt, 2021). A child's play interests often differ from an adult's and may differ from many other children (Lynch & Stanley, 2018; Spitzer, 2003a, 2003b). Because of these substantial differences between occupational therapists and their pediatric clients, understanding the child as an occupational being can be very challenging (Spitzer, 2003a, 2003b).

In order to understand occupational meaning, the occupational therapist must observe, listen, and interpret a child's cues to determine the child's interests and motivation (Curtin, 2017; Holloway, 2008; Knox, 2008; Lynch & Stanley, 2018 Spitzer, 2003a). For children who do not explicitly communicate their desires, occupational therapists rely on their observation skills as well as their in-depth knowledge of body movement and activity analysis to interpret nonverbal cues. Possible nonverbal indicators of engagement and interest in an activity include self-initiated interaction, enthusiasm, greater frequency and/or duration of eye contact, positive affect, focused attention, full participation, behavior modulation, and vocalizations and/or communication (Brown et al., 2008; D'Arrigo, Copley, Poulsen, & Ziviani, 2020). Even children with significant speech and motor impairments can communicate subtle preference for a toy, material, or sensation through orienting (noticing and looking or listening), affective responses (smiling, swinging arms, or verbalizations), and leaning toward a preferred object (D'Arrigo et al., 2020; Van Tubbergen, Warschausky, Birnholz, & Baker, 2008). Specific strategies for understanding the pediatric client's perspective are listed in **Box 6.2**.

Box 6.2 Strategies to Enhance Understanding of Nonverbal Pediatric Clients

- Suspend your adult assumptions to identify the child's perspective (Curtin, 2001; Fine & Sandstrom, 1988; Tortora, 2006).
- Avoid being an authority figure—minimize stopping and directing of the client (Curtin, 2001, 2017; Fine & Sandstrom, 1988).
- Look for the effect/impact of your presence (Fine & Sandstrom, 1988).
- Assume all actions are potentially communicative (Curtin, 2017; Durig, 1996; Tortora, 2006).
- Attend to communication through occupational engagement, especially shared occupations (Grandin & Scariano, 1986; Morozini, 2015; Spitzer, 2003a; Williams, 1992).
- Look for individualized communication strategies around shared routines, physical environment, likes and dislikes, and bodily expressions (Goode, 1980, 1994; Spitzer, 2003a).
- Develop a shared history with the client—understand their favorite objects and preferences, and participate in activities with them (Goode, 1980, 1994; Spitzer, 2003a; Tortora, 2006).
- Interview other people knowledgeable about the client's interests, preferences, and dislikes, and how the child indicates these (Curtin, 2017).
- Follow the client's directions—"passive obedience" (Goode, 1980).
- Imitate, physically simulate, or imagine the individual's sensory experience of the occupation to "feel" what the child's experience might be when moving, touching, listening, and looking in that specific manner (Goode, 1980; Spitzer, 2003a; Tortora, 2006).
- Sharpen conscious awareness of various auditory, visual, tactile, and kinesthetic sensations to which the child may be responding in the moment (Spitzer, 2003a).

Data from Curtin, C. (2001). Eliciting children's voices in qualitative research. American Journal of Occupational Therapy, 55, 295–302. https://doi.org/10.5014/ajot.55.3.295; Fine, G. A., & Sandstrom, K. L. (1988). Knowing children: Participant observation with minors. Newbury Park, CA: Sage; Tortora, S. (2006). The dancing dialogue: Using the communicative power of movement with young children. Baltimore, MD: Paul H. Brookes Publishing Co.; Curtin, C. (2017). Strategies for collaborating with children: Creating partnerships in occupational therapy and research. Thorofare, NJ: Slack Incorporated; Durig, A. (1996). Autism and the crisis of meaning. Albany: State University of New York Press; Grandin, T., & Scariano, M. M. (1986). Emergence: Labeled autistic. Novato, CA: Arean Press; Morozini, M. (2015). Exploring the engagement of parents in the co-occupation of parent–child play: An occupational science's perspective. International Journal of Prevention and Treatment, 4, 11–28. https://doi.org/10.5923/s.ijpt.201501.02; Spitzer, S. L. (2003a). Using participant observation to study the meaning of occupations of young children with autism and other developmental disabilities. American Journal of Occupational Therapy, 57(1), 66–76. https://doi.org/10.5014/ajot.57.1.66; Williams, D. (1992). Nobody nowhere: The extraordinary autobiography of an autistic. New York: Times Books; Goode, D. A. (1980). The world of the congenitally deaf-blind. In J. Jacobs (Ed.), Mental retardation: A phenomenological approach (pp. 187–207). Springfield, IL: Charles C. Thomas; Goode, D. (1994). A world without words: The social construction of children born deaf and blind. Philadelphia, PA: Temple University Press.

When attempting to understand the child's perspective, the occupational therapist must operate "as if" the child provided intentional communication, assuming the child meant something by his or her actions. The occupational therapist must interpret and act as if the child's actions have meaning regardless of the child's ability and intentionality to conceptualize and communicate that point. This positive responsiveness is not based on an "objective" assessment of the child's skill level but a focus on the child's *potential* and attempts to become skilled. For example, the child might make a vocalization that sounds almost like a word. The adult then acts as if the child "talked" (Brazelton, Koslowski, & Main, 1974; Trevarthen, 1980). The adult takes the next step of relating a child's sounds to the most likely word or phrase and then reacts as if this was the word the child intended despite not knowing definitively (see **Practice Example 6.1**). Many children do not develop in a step-by-step linear fashion. If the therapist incorporates what he or she thought the child "said," the therapist must still allow the child the opportunity to accept or reject this interpretation. In another case, the child might look at or reach in the direction of a toy, and the occupational therapist can offer to include the toy. Again, the occupational therapy practitioner must also be open to the child's reactions as to whether the child truly was interested in the toy. In this way, the occupational therapist is actively part of both understanding and demonstrating this understanding of the child. It is a reciprocal, shared process of relating to each other, the foundation for a therapeutic relationship.

When the occupational therapy practitioner uses information about interests and preferences to develop individually tailored activities and approaches, it allows the pediatric client to feel understood (D'Arrigo et al., 2020; Mattingly & Fleming, 1994; Price & Miner, 2007). This engages a child in therapy (King et al., 2021). A clinician can use these specific details to transform the same physical materials with similar motor actions into dramatically different play activities for different individual children (see **Figure 6.1**). For example, one child interested in construction might be offered fuzzy balls to pick up with tongs like a crane, whereas another child might be offered the same materials as special eating tools in an outer-space diner (see Chapter 8 for details on how to create individualized therapeutic play activities). These personalized games demonstrate the occupational therapists' knowledge of and valuing of the client. This communication is the beginning of developing empathy and rapport in the therapeutic relationship.

"This Is Fun!": Sending Play Messages Through Nonverbal and Verbal Communication

Playfulness is communicated with both verbal and nonverbal strategies. Whether occupational therapists are responding to a child or initiating interaction, they can mark therapy as fun and frame therapy as play (Curtin, 2017; Parham, 1992). Creating play starts in the first session with a warm greeting directly to the child and caregivers, followed by actions that

---

PRACTICE EXAMPLE 6.1 Phoebe and As If to Say

Phoebe was a 2-year-old with cerebral palsy and severe speech apraxia. To indicate she was done or did not like an activity, Phoebe cried, turned her head away, or moved into full trunk flexion. Her other communication was inconsistent. About 30% of the time, a vocalization, look at, touch of, or reach toward an object indicated an interest or need, in that she would engage with the item. The remaining 70% of the time when offered an object that appeared to be of possible interest, Phoebe would cry, turn her head away, or move into full trunk flexion to indicate that she was not interested in the object at that time. One of Phoebe's favorite play activities that she always enjoyed and never protested was getting tickles on her upper body, which her foster parents did while playfully and repeatedly saying "I got you."

During home visit, Phoebe suddenly vocalized different sounds, which sounded like "ga-ooo." Surprised, the occupational therapy practitioner mentally noted that this was a longer and more complicated utterance and considered its meaning. Then, quickly the practitioner recognized its similarity to the "got you" sounds involved in Phoebe's favorite play activity. Given that requesting a "got you" game was well beyond previously observed skills and abilities, the provider knew that the sounds could just as likely be a random vocalization. Nonetheless, the practitioner creatively questioned this assumption as a real possibility and acted as if this was intentional functional communication to initiate play. The practitioner responded playfully by wiggling his fingers in the air and saying "got you?! You want to play *got you*?" and then coached the foster parents to play their tickling "got you" game. The practitioner explained to the foster parents, "I don't know for sure that is what Phoebe meant but it really sounded like 'got you' so we want to respect any possible attempts made." These sounds were not heard again for several weeks but gradually became more common, allowing Phoebe to initiate her favorite play.

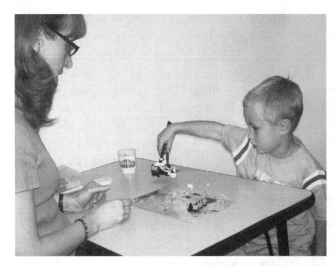
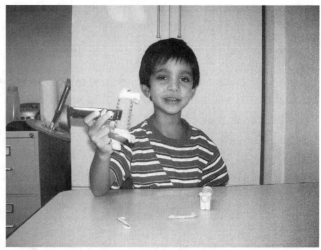
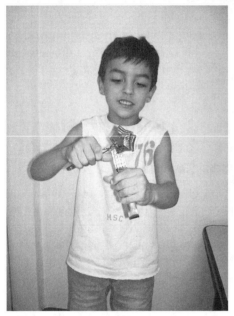
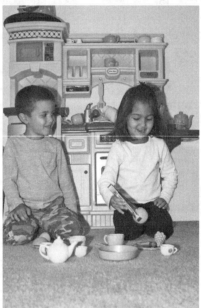
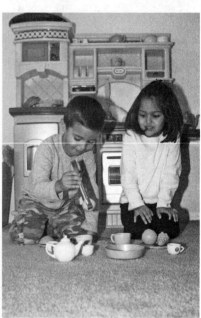

Figure 6.1 The occupational therapy practitioner creates personalized games and activities by using the same materials in different ways based on the child's individual interests and goals. For example, tongs can be used as a "crane" to pick up vehicles, as a way to transport animals to food, as a "weapon," or as a utensil for "eating."

Top left: Courtesy of Cameron Flanagan. Top right and bottom left: Courtesy of Susan L. Spitzer. Bottom middle and bottom right: Courtesy of David A. Morales.

communicate you are a nice, friendly person and want to partner with the child in fun activities (Curtin, 2017; O'Connor, Butler, & Lynch, 2020). This is a graded process individualized to the child's own cognitive, social, and self-regulatory abilities. When matched to the child, this message of play helps the child *anticipate* and expect that the activity will be fun. This playful approach helps transform the activity into play. With repeated fun experiences, the child begins to associate occupational therapy with play.

This is not an automatic process because the mere presence of adults can predispose children to view activities as more work than play (Howard, Jenvey, & Hill, 2006; McInnes, 2019) until a clear and consistent play setting has been created (Goodhall & Atkinson, 2017; McInnes et al., 2011). Additionally, adults often have difficulty framing play for

children with disabilities when activities are difficult and require more effort (Román-Oyola et al., 2018). Children with anxiety and oppositionality may resist and distrust messages of play because of concerns and even fears about being manipulated into activities that are not truly play. Applying these strategies in pediatrics requires special consideration of how adults send playful communication signals that can be understood by clients of differing developmental abilities.

Research on parent–child play communication, when integrated with occupational therapy literature, together provide rich information regarding specific strategies that occupational therapy practitioners can use with their pediatric clients to communicate that occupational therapy is play (see **Table 6.1** for a summary and **Appendix 6.1** for a worksheet to use for

Table 6.1 Strategies to Communicate Playfulness

Practitioner Sources of Communication	Specific Strategies/Techniques
Eyes	■ Look at the child. ■ Look between the child and a potential toy/play object.
Face	■ Smile. ■ Exaggerate and hold positive emotional expressions. ■ Imitate the child's expression.
Body	■ Turn, lean, and move toward the child. ■ Imitate the child's actions. ■ Exaggerate and slow body movements such as head nodding, head wagging, or head cocking. ■ Hold out, manipulate, hide, or point to toys/objects.
Touch	■ Touch the child with an object to show it to them. ■ Use touch to get attention (as appropriate for the context).
Voice (vocalizations)	■ Use a playful tone. ■ Vary pitch, loudness, rhythm. ■ Repeat sounds. ■ Imitate sounds and ways that sounds are used by child.
Language	■ Match language to child's development. ■ Use the words *play* and *choice*. ■ Minimize the word *work* and directing/correcting language ("let's play __" instead of "do __" and "let's try __" instead of "that's too __"). ■ Use language in song, melody, rhythm, or different voices (e.g., accent). ■ Imitate child's words. ■ Use "kid play" words, phrases, and sounds. ■ Use humor, jokes, and mischievous tone. ■ Talk as if toys or body parts were alive and thinking.

implementation). Developmentally, nonverbal strategies tend to dominate initially in parent-infant play. The adult gives visual, auditory, and physical stimuli to the infant. As the child develops, the play is more cooperative and collaborative, with the child taking an increasingly more active role, reflected in a greater use of language for communication. Similar developmental considerations are reflected in practice. In general, occupational therapists rely heavily on their nonverbal communication and voice characteristics (Langthaler, 1990, as cited by Mattingly & Fleming, 1994).

It is important to note that the amount of adult communication must be graded carefully for the child's timing and arousal. Many children with disabilities such as ASD, learning disabilities, and cognitive impairment require more time to process and respond, so adults often need to slow down and wait in order to provide adequate opportunity for communication. Providing the opportunity to communicate without demanding communication can help create a playful environment for a child who struggles to communicate (Curtin, 2017). A balanced level of communication maintains an arousal state that enables continued engagement in

play (Curtin, 2017; Greenspan & Weider, 1997; Parham, 1992; Power, 2000). Although a certain level of excitement and enthusiasm often accompanies play, too much stimulation, even of a positive sort, can overload a child into a state of disorganization. This is usually a bigger concern in typically developing children during infancy (Feldman, 2009), but self-regulation difficulties may continue throughout childhood in children with disabilities. Adults must be sensitive to a child's need to withdraw, partially or completely, at times after a period of engagement (Lillas, TenPas, Crowley, & Spitzer, 2018; see **Figure 6.2**).

These moments of allowing a child time to regulate and communicate require the practitioner to attend very closely to the child to determine the child's participation. These moments can feel uncomfortable to a new therapist because therapists are used to motor action. The lack of action can feel awkward. At this point, the practitioner's action is mental effort along with inhibition of physical action. In the presence of a parent, caregiver, or other observer, the therapist can feel self-conscious that unobservable action may be misinterpreted as inaction, as "doing nothing." In the face of these emotions,

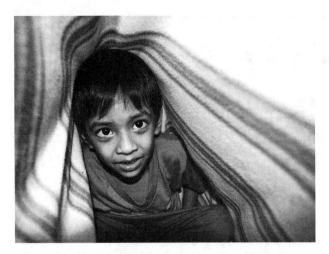

Figure 6.2 Sometimes children need practitioners to allow them time to take a break from play in order to regulate and be ready to re-engage
© Waty Shariff/EyeEm/Getty Images.

it takes intense conscious effort to maintain confidence and heightened attentiveness to the child to offer opportunities for participation and to determine the best way to educate others about these moments.

Communicating Play Nonverbally

Adult nonverbal communication that initiates and sustains play in children with and without disabilities includes eye gaze, facial expressions, and body language/movements, which are common for occupational therapists (Power, 2000; Taylor, 2008; Van keer et al., 2019). The use of nonverbal communication by adults is associated with increases in interaction for children with significant cognitive and motor delays (Van keer et al., 2019). Occupational therapists carefully control their own actions to convey an effective message to their clients (Mattingly & Fleming, 1994). Such nonverbal communication usually occurs in close but comfortable proximity (Hall, 1966/1982). Proximity of the adult to the play activity has been found to cue children that the activity is play (Howard, 2002; Wing, 1995). If the adult is too far away, the child is less likely to notice these subtle actions in the distance and less likely to view the activity as play.

Gaze. In newborns and young children with disabilities, the adult looks at the child extensively and usually initiates the gaze (Messer & Vietze, 1984; Van keer et al., 2019). The child is more likely to look at the adult if the adult is looking at the child, and playful interactions are more likely to occur when the adult is looking at the child (Messer & Vietze, 1984; Stern, 1974; Van keer et al., 2019). Mutual gaze is best when the adult moves to the child's eye level such as through kneeling or sitting down (Curtin, 2017). This adult–child gaze

is almost continuous, in violation of adult Western cultural standards for a more intermittent pattern (Stern, 1974). As the child develops, the adult may also look back and forth between the child and a potential play object/toy to communicate shared interest in that toy (Deák, Krasno, Jasso, & Triesch, 2018).

Similarly, the occupational therapist's eye gaze can communicate that the therapist is ready and open to play. Eye contact has been associated with joking and fun for children in occupational therapy using a sensory integration approach (Holland et al., 2018). Eye gaze is included within joint attention interventions, which have strong research support for improving communication and interactive engagement in children with ASD (Kasari, Gulsrud, Wong, Kwon, & Locke, 2010; Wong, 2013). However, the occupational therapy practitioner must also be cautious because some individual children can tolerate only limited amounts of stimulation from eye gaze and may not look much at the therapist directly (Miller, 1996; Sivberg, Jakobsson, & Lundqvist, 2019). Furthermore, it may be a less effective strategy if the play activity requires greater postural or motor effort to attain mutual gaze (Franchak, Kretch, & Adolph, 2018).

Facial Expressions. Adult facial expressions that initiate or sustain play include mock surprise, smiling, and concern/sympathy (Power, 2000; Stern, 1974). Mostly, the adult's facial expressions are positive. Smiling helps the child perceive the adult as friendly (Curtin, 2017; see **Figure 6.3**). As the child

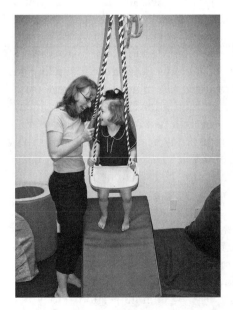

Figure 6.3 The occupational therapy practitioner communicates an openness and willingness to play by looking at, turning toward, getting close to, and smiling at the child
Courtesy of Emilie Baribault and Ellie Baribault.

begins to demonstrate clear facial expressions, the adult may also imitate the child's expressions to continue play (Murray, De Pascalis, Bozicevic, Hawkins, Sclafani, & Ferrari, 2016). Facial expressions with children tend to be significantly more exaggerated and maintained for a longer time period than facial expressions used in adult communication. Exaggerated expressions communicate that the activity is fun in such a clear way that the child is more likely to register the message and respond in play. For the occupational therapist, holding positive exaggerated facial expressions can promote a playful environment (Holland et al., 2018; Parham, 1992).

Body Language. The adult's body movements that encourage play in children include imitating the child's hand and body movements; moving the head, such as nodding up and down, wagging side to side, and head cocking; facing and leaning toward the child; and holding out, manipulating, hiding, or pointing to toys/objects (Pawlby, 1977; Stern, 1974). The strongest research support is for imitating the child's actions for children with ASD (Field et al., 2014; Kuhaneck, Spitzer, & Bodison, 2019) and object manipulation for infants (Deák et al., 2018). As with facial expressions, these actions tend to be exaggerated and slowed down in comparison with adult communication. Similar body language can be used by the occupational therapist to show that he or she is involved with the child's interests (Curtin, 2017).

Touch. Pediatric occupational therapists rate therapeutic touch as important to their practice (Cole & McLean, 2003). Positive social touch has been found to communicate positive emotions and promote positive relationships (Cascio, Moore, & McGlone, 2019; Hertenstein, Veerkamp, Kerestes, & Holmes, 2006). Touch is used heavily in playful interactions with infants and with young children with disabilities (Moszkowski & Stack, 2007; Van keer et al., 2019)—tickling, crawling fingers up and down arms and legs, starting and stopping a light tap, and physically assisted games. Tickling games often involve joyous laughter in humans and appear to have a biological basis that may be shared with other species (Panksepp & Burgdorf, 2003). Many play themes such as play fighting or peek-a-boo may include touch. Even a tap to show an object or direct attention may be very effective to cue a child indirectly about what to do or how to do something without explicitly directing him or her or breaking up the flow of play. As children get older, similar types of touch remain but may decrease in frequency.

Sometimes practitioners are uncomfortable with using touch to communicate because, among adults, touch tends to have connotations of affection, intimacy, and even sexuality (Aldis, 1975; Taylor, 2008). In some settings, touch is not allowed or is devalued. When done in a conscious way, however, positive social touch can be an effective therapeutic strategy. Pediatric occupational therapy practitioners must use touch in a way that is both careful and respectful but also caring. Patting, stroking, tickling, and physically guiding the child are examples of touch that promote children's psychological development (Cascio et al., 2019; Hertenstein et al., 2006). It is safest to touch on the hand and arm and within the client's visual range, asking permission or giving notification when possible (Taylor, 2008). Nonetheless, the therapist must be alert for possible negative perceptions of touch especially due to trauma, tactile hyperresponsiveness, or cultural norms. In some cases, pediatric occupational therapists may need to advocate institutional changes so that caring touch can be used with their clients.

Communicating Play Verbally and with Vocalizations

Occupational therapists can use sounds and words in a playful way while still addressing therapeutic outcomes (Parham, 1992). Vocalizations and language are matched to the child's developmental level to communicate playfulness.

Sounds. As children develop, adult and child communication in play tends to become increasingly verbal (Power, 2000). Initially, with infants, voice is used without much language. The adult uses vocal sounds to communicate playfulness. These communicative sounds are marked by sudden changes in pitch, rhythm, and stress and by elongated vowel sounds (Aldis, 1975; Stern, 1974). The ranges of pitch and loudness are broader than the ranges typically used in adult conversation (Power, 2000). Sounds and nonsense words may be repeated frequently (Aldis, 1975). At times, the adult's vocalizations may sound similar to features the child uses (Pawlby, 1977). The occupational therapist determines if and what sounds may be appropriate for a client's developmental level and to communicate playfulness.

Words. As the child develops and interacts more with the adult, the adult tends to use more language. The adult commonly asks questions, praises the child, imitates the child's "words," and gives words to the child's utterances and actions (Delafield-Butt, Zeedyk,

Harder, Væver, & Caldwell, 2020; Halliday & Leslie, 1986; Shine & Acosta, 1999). Language becomes increasingly more complex and collaborative as the adult initiates, prompts, structures, and provides ideas to expand play, especially pretend play (Damast, Tamis-LeMonda, & Bornstein, 1996; Dunn, Wooding, & Hermann, 1977). Typically, the adult's language is at a developmental level equal to or slightly higher than the child's development (Damast et al., 1996).

Matching language to a pediatric client's development requires ongoing adjustment (for resources on typical communication development, see https://identifythesigns.org/communicating-with-baby-toolkit/; https://www.cdc.gov/ncbddd/actearly/milestones/index.html; and https://pathways.org/topics-of-development/communication/). Many children with disabilities have difficulties with auditory or language processing. Disabilities may obscure children's ability to demonstrate what they understand. Uneven development in different aspects of cognitive, regulation, behavior, and communicative abilities can blur the picture further. Similarly, the occupational therapy practitioner must modify the selection and use of language. It is important to use words selectively and monitor to ensure that the child understood what was said. Words that are used by the child and family may be better understood because they are more familiar as well as personally or culturally meaningful such as "flopsy" instead of "rabbit" for a favorite toy. Simple words and shorter sentences are often helpful (Curtin, 2017). Pairing words with clear and consistent intonation and body language provides a message that the child is more likely to understand. Additionally, at times, the occupational therapist will need to limit talking to avoid disrupting the child's focused engagement in the flow of play (Parham, 1992). Selecting affirming words judiciously, playing with alternative words and sounds, and using a light tone can shift the session to being more fun and less serious.

Affirming Words Choosing words that affirm a playful therapeutic use of self requires thoughtful attention and creativity to minimize directive and negative language. Adults often use language to exert control and direct children how to behave, which research indicates is a threat to play (Holland & Thompson, 2018; Shine & Acosta, 1999). If the session is going to be playful, the occupational therapy practitioner generally must avoid using language to "direct" or "teach." Research suggests that if we use the words *play* and *choice* more frequently and avoid the word *work*, we can support play more effectively (McInnes et al., 2011).

Obviously, this is difficult because we often need to direct or guide our clients to promote therapeutic outcomes. At these times, we must be especially thoughtful about whether and how we should give them feedback about their performance, encourage them to try or persist in a challenging task, or change how they are doing the activity and eliminate the need for performance feedback. Sometimes we elect to hold commentary when a child experiences an error as frustrating or degrading to allow the child to "save face" and sustain engagement (Curtin, 2017). For example, an embarrassed child might blame the therapist for setting up the toys in the wrong way. In this case, the therapist considers the child's goals to determine if it is best to confront this incorrect perception or allow the child a way out such as acknowledging "maybe you are right." At other times, the therapist might focus on a positive admonition that focuses on what the child can be or wants to be such as "I like the way you ____" rather than "don't forget to ____" or reminding a client to use "grown-up hands" or "kind hands" instead of criticizing "too rough" or directing "hands down." We strive to use words that promote therapeutic relationships and focus on the possibilities of play, even in the midst of negative behaviors and occupational challenges.

Same Words, Different Way A directive can sound more playful when said in an unconventional way, such as singing directions, repeating key words in a melodic rhythm, or using a voice different from one's normal speech pattern. In this way, the practitioner's use of speech is more like the way children themselves play with the sounds of language (Nilsen & Nilsen, 1978). Consider an occupational therapist who wants a child to work on fastening buttons and zippers. The occupational therapist can announce, "Come sit down and do your buttons," "It is time for buttons and zippers," or "Let's do buttons and zippers." Despite differing levels of directedness, all these announcements send a similar message about an effortful activity on which the child needs to "work." But it can be transformed when the therapist sings these same words to a common children's song like "The Farmer in the Dell," where the statement is punctuated with "Hi-ho the-dairy-oh." Emphasizing particularly fun sounds and repeating the sounds in a rhythm can also change the way the child views this direction. For example, the occupational therapist can alter speed between slow and fast in saying, "It's time for button-zzzzz and zzz-ipper-zzzzz, and zzz-ipper-zzzzz and button-zzzzz. Button-zzzzz and zzz-ipper-zzzzz, and zzz-ipper-zzzzz and button-zzzzz." The activity can also become more playful by announcing in a slow robotic accent: "It is time for bu-ttons and zi-pper-s." The direction becomes so fun that children often like to repeat these phrases themselves in similar and modified ways, and sometimes even as they do the transformed work, as a self-talk strategy. For some children, the sounds themselves become reinforcing, and getting to hear the sound becomes a motivating reason to do an activity, as elements of work and play blend together.

Kid Play Words and Sound Effects Utilizing words and sounds commonly used by children provides feedback that facilitates a playful process in therapy, where the focus is on participation. This differs from serious, realistic, grown-up words that remind the child that he or she is working on something for which the quality of the performance is important. When mistakes happen, words and sound effects like "bonk," "oops," "oops-a-daisy," "ut-oh," or "ut-oh spaghetti-o-s" sound fun, helping to incorporate errors into play rather than stopping play to focus on the error. When the child misbehaves, words like "Hey silly goose, let's __!" keep the session playful, rather than stopping to chastise the child or insisting on compliance (e.g., "no, come here.")

Positive feedback can also be incorporated into play. Standard adult comments of "good job" or "good work" may suggest that the adult is there to monitor and judge the quality of the child's performance. Words like "yeah," "wow," "yahoo," "zoom," "incredible," and "amazing" provide positive feedback in a way that maintains the flow of the play experience. Such an approach is especially helpful for clients with perfectionistic and anxious tendencies to minimize performance concerns.

Children are often most interested in words that adults have been socialized not to use, such as "poop." Such "potty talk" or bathroom humor, while common in younger children, is nonetheless strongly reacted to by many adults who object to such inappropriate language (American Academy of Pediatrics, 2003). Children find the words' novelty and adult reactions to be funny. If an occupational therapist wants to be playful, he or she may decide to go against adult social taboos and use these words in therapeutic ways (see **Practice Example 6.2**).

Kidding Around Adding humor, jokes, and mischievousness can help build therapeutic relationships and lighten up otherwise serious work (Crepeau & Garren, 2011; Curtin, 2017; Leber & Vanoli, 2001). Humor can be an especially important type of play for children with significant physical disabilities (Graham et al., 2019) and has been associated with increased tool learning in young children (Esseily, Rat-Fischer,

---

> **PRACTICE EXAMPLE 6.2**
> **Jacob and Word Play**
>
> **Heather M. Kuhaneck, PhD, OTR/L**
>
> Jacob was a 7-year-old diagnosed with oppositional defiant disorder who was fascinated with the word *poop*. He would frequently say "poop" and loved to watch adults get upset when he said it. He used this as a strategy to avoid and escape adult demands because it distracted adults from the activity at hand. His occupational therapist creatively redefined the problem of poop after being sure to explain her reasoning to Jacob's mother and getting her agreement. The occupational therapist began to incorporate the word and the concept of "poop" into activities such as drawing pictures of poop, tracing, coloring, cutting, writing the word *poop*, and playing obstacle course games with brown bean-bag poop, and movements such as pretending to jump into the poop. Jacob quickly realized that saying "poop" was not upsetting to his therapist, and it therefore lost its power. He quickly tired of the word and soon wanted to play new games.

Somogyi, O'Reagan, & Fagard, 2016; Fagard, Rat-Fischer, Esseily, Somogyi, & O'Regan, 2016). Even work elements can be overly exaggerated to be playful elements. For example, the occupational therapy practitioner may present a challenge with mock concern or mischievousness, such as, "This is pretty tricky. Hmmm, do you think you can do this? Oh, no, this is too hard. What if you fall? I don't know if you can do it." A therapist might "conspire" with a child to scare or surprise mommy. Even when a child tries to avoid a challenge, the atmosphere can be kept playful by a mock chastisement of something like "Hey, no cheating-g-g-g." Children with ADHD may be very engaged to attend to what a therapist says to catch the therapist trying to "trick" them with incorrect statements. The laughter that follows can build attachment bonds among client, therapist, and others involved (Nelson, 2008). When the therapist laughs at him- or herself or allows him- or herself to look silly, the therapist communicates a commitment to playfulness and an acceptance of his or her own shortcomings.

Because humor involves a more complicated understanding of reality and pretense, the occupational therapist must exercise caution in making sure that the level of humor is appropriate for the child's development. If not, children may misunderstand and believe they are being made fun of (laughed at) or teased, an obviously unintended outcome. Clear, simple forms of joking actions accompanied by laughter can be understood at 19 months of age

developmentally and require less cognitive understanding than pretend play (Hoicka & Gattis, 2008). A child can find something humorous if he or she recognizes both that something is being said or done that is "wrong" and that it is *intentionally* done incorrectly. For example, putting a spoon on one's head when the person knows that a spoon is for eating is humorous if knowingly and intentionally done but is a mistake if done during meal time when trying to eat. The impossibility of the idea "Why don't you jump *under* the ball?" can be very funny for a 6-year-old who understands such language. Sometimes mistakes can have unintended funny consequences, such as tossing an eraser to a child and it lands in a nearby cup of water. A young teenager may even enjoy "opposite day," where both client and therapist must say the opposite of what they mean (e.g., "do" for "don't"); the opposites can be funny in themselves, and it can be amusing when one person forgets and the other does the opposite of what was expected. When the adolescent asks, "Why do I have to do this?" the occupational therapist may be able to say jokingly, "Because I am so mean." Certainly, this level of humor requires a client's cognitive understanding and emotional tolerance to see something as funny and not real. Clear, simple jokes of doing or saying what the child clearly knows "should not be" as well as smiling, laughing, or marking the humor as "I'm just joking or being silly" are usually good ways to introduce humor in order to prevent misunderstandings when there are concerns about cognitive understanding.

With maturity, children understand more subtle and ambiguous forms of humor. At this level, children's joke books and websites can be good sources of additional ideas. A sense of humor may be less present in the play of children with intellectual disabilities (Messier, Ferland, & Majnemer, 2008) or may take a different form. Because cognitive development can be difficult to assess in some children with disabilities, it is usually best to follow the child's lead in using humor. When the child laughs, this provides a good example of the type of humor the occupational therapy practitioner may use.

Personification Extending communication to inanimate objects can change the communication dynamics. Children commonly employ this approach when they use words to respond to and address inanimate objects, acting as if they are alive. They talk to a toy like it is a person who might do what they say or answer them (e.g., "good night toys" as the toys are put away, or "dollie wants to play "). This can have an element of pretend play; or, it can be a particular type of humor if the child sees it as funny or comical.

An occupational therapy practitioner can use language in this alternate way to create a playful mode, especially for otherwise serious challenges. For example, Baron (1991) described using a client's favorite toy, a Pee Wee Herman figure, in occupational therapy to help with power struggles in a child with oppositional defiant disorder. Limit-setting and feedback were given to the child by Pee Wee Herman via the therapist's voice. The child accepted this input because he could pretend it "came from" his favorite toy instead of the adult authority figure.

Such a strategy can also be used to make mistakes more playful and lighthearted. For example, if the child misses an attempt to throw a ball or put an object into a container, the occupational therapist can begin a pseudo-conversation with the ball: "Ball, you need to behave. He was putting you inside. You need to listen and go inside. Be a good ball and do what you are told. We'll give you another chance." Such humorous behavior on the part of the occupational therapist marks this activity as playful. This strategy also works well without toys. For example, the occupational therapist who is working on in-hand manipulation skills with a child often faces the challenge of the child compensating in various less-than-therapeutic ways. The child may try to use the other hand to help or may push one hand against his or her body or the table to aid with the tasks, thereby defeating the activity's therapeutic purpose. If the occupational therapist directs the child not to do that or to do it a different way, the activity's hard work is highlighted for the child. Instead, the occupational therapist can use a similar directive oriented toward the child's hand: "It's not your turn, hand. Let that other hand have his turn," or "Hey, hand, get to work. No cheating. You know the rules." Suddenly even chastisement can become play in this mock serious tone. The child is no longer being corrected directly but can join the adult therapist in "chastising" his hand. Furthermore, it frees the pediatric client to switch temporarily from the worker role into an empowered director of "others" with agency to impact the environment, consistent with the research that playfulness can be a predictor of self-efficacy in children with developmental challenges (Román-Oyola et al., 2017).

Handling Negative Responses and Miscommunication

Whenever people communicate, there is always potential for negative reactions and miscommunication. You can be assured that miscommunication occurs in therapy as well (Holland & Thompson, 2018; Taylor, 2008). It is important to be watchful and recognize when it does occur. By monitoring the child's perspective and reactions, you can quickly repair any unintended problems and tension in a therapeutic way (Horvath et al., 2011; King et al., 2021; Taylor, 2008) and resend the message so that it is more likely to be registered correctly. It is the therapist who must take responsibility for miscommunication, including explicit and sincere apologies, and find ways to move forward.

To determine if the child received the intended message about play, the occupational therapy practitioner must read the child's cues and reactions. When a practitioner is playful, the child usually is agreeable to the therapeutic activity at hand (Terr et al., 2007). Some children provide clear feedback that they understand the message of play. They may begin to be more playful through laughing, smiling, pretending, or extending the therapist's play ideas. Or, the child may disengage or react negatively through affect, statements, agitation, resistance, or destructive actions, suggesting that the practitioner's attempts to communicate playfulness have not been accepted. Common ways that children use to show that they find something unpleasant (not playful) include actively withdrawing, pushing away, ignoring, distractibility, looking away, turning away, slumping, decreasing responses, avoiding participation, and fussing/crying as was seen in the case of Phoebe (see Practice Example 6.1; Brazelton et al., 1974; D'Arrigo et al., 2020). If a child has misunderstood the communication, then the strategies need to be modified until they match the individual child's needs.

Persisting with communication efforts in the face of a child's negative reactions taxes therapeutic use of self. Aggressive, destructive, or defiant behavior can easily trigger adult emotions such as frustration, pain, or judgment about the "bad" behavior that we just want to stop. Sometimes it is hard to understand or face these emotions and behaviors, especially when they can seem like personal attacks. A tantrum or "meltdown" can be exhausting. This is precisely when the clinician relies on therapeutic use of self to consciously set aside those emotions and instead focus on what the child is communicating with the so-called bad behavior because this is a stressful experience for clients (Curtin, 2017; Delahooke, 2020). Horvath et al. (2010) have noted that "responding nondefensively to a client's hostility or negativity is critical to establishing and maintaining a strong alliance." Given the high prevalence of psychosocial trauma, maintaining control of our own emotions and attending to the child's therapeutic needs enables us to carry out our ethical commitment to not traumatize or retraumatize a client experiencing stress (Champagne, 2011). The more practitioners

value therapeutic use of self, the more likely they are to report feelings of positive regard for clients (Taylor et al., 2009). Consider how this applies in a session when a child suddenly drops to the ground crying as another child picks up a ball to carry out to the playground. To avoid chastising this emotionally distressed child, the occupational therapist uses this opportunity for the child to build emotional awareness (for example, "It looks like you are sad because you did not get to carry the ball") and skills (for example, "Do you want to ask for a turn or see if you can carry it next time?"). Offering choices is essential to maintain play (Graham et al., 2019; King & Howard, 2014b). Negotiating through play can also be a successful strategy (Olli, Salanterä, Karlsson, & Vehkakoski, 2021). When a therapist focuses on the central concern of what does the upset child not like and why, it is easier to be empathetic and respond therapeutically without becoming distracted by personal feelings of discomfort, disappointment, and judgment. The therapeutic outcome builds client skill development while avoiding power struggles (Curtin, 2017).

Empathy and Rapport for a Playful Therapeutic Relationship

Empathy and rapport allow the occupational therapy practitioner to engage in playful alliance with the child. Empathy is a deep understanding and caring about the child as an occupational being. With empathy, the occupational therapist can demonstrate genuine respect for the child so that therapeutic rapport can emerge (Peloquin, 1995; Price, 2009; Schwartzberg, 1993). The therapist's empathy and rapport facilitate personal agency, enabling the child and family to play (Ferland, 2005; Lindström & Isaksson, 2017).

Empathy in Occupational Therapy

Empathy in occupational therapy is an informed caring, where thinking and feeling occur simultaneously (Peloquin, 1995). It is informed by knowing the child as a person, beyond a disability or diagnosis. The therapist identifies and feels the specific fears, doubts, hopes, and desires of the child and family (Price, 2009; Taylor, 2008). Understanding is based on accepting the client as an equal person (Crepeau, 1991). By understanding the child and family, the occupational therapist is able to share their perspective and have a sense of what their world feels like (Abreu, 2011). This understanding informs caring about the child (Peloquin, 1995). Specifically, occupational therapists care about a client's growth, development, function, and adaptation (Gilfoyle, 1980; Mosey, 1981, 1986). Caring is part of the therapeutic process (Peloquin, 1990, 1993) and is especially important to clients (McCorquodale & Kinsella, 2015). Caring humanizes the science of therapy (Gilfoyle, 1980). Without caring, clients are depersonalized (Peloquin, 1990, 1993). This is not providing care *to* or taking care *of* but caring *for* clients (Gilfoyle, 1980). Mayeroff (1971, p. 1) defined caring as helping another person "grow and actualize" the self. Rather than simply saying we care, occupational therapists demonstrate we care by doing things for and with clients (Gahnstrom-Strandqvist, Tham, Josephsson, & Borell, 2000; Mattingly & Fleming, 1994). Occupational therapists help patients to care about themselves, what they can do, and what they might be able to do (Devereaux, 1984; Gilfoyle, 1980). Research has found that clients experience a positive relationship if the occupational therapist demonstrates a caring attitude by paying attention to their feelings and showing interest in them (Palmadottir, 2006). The therapist's demonstration of empathy correlates with client motivation and participation (Fan & Taylor, 2018).

Sometimes a therapist naturally wants to care for a client on a personal basis, whereas at other times, a therapist does not have an immediate connection with emotional caring. In these latter situations, Sharma and Clark (2018) suggested using imagination to visualize how clients participate in occupations and what this means to them. Activity analyses can be a rich source of understanding elements of meaning and challenge. Wright-St. Clair (2001) recommended that therapists focus on the general professional ideal and moral obligation to care for clients' well-being. This general focus on a philosophy of caring allows us to "ethically care" for individual clients for whom we might not otherwise innately care (Wright-St. Clair, 2001).

Rapport in a Therapeutic Occupational Therapy Relationship

The therapeutic relationship is essential to client-centered occupational therapy (D'Arrigo et al., 2020; Hinojosa, 2007; McCorquodale & Kinsella, 2015; Tickle-Degnen, 2002) and is highly valued by occupational therapists (Taylor et al., 2009). Based on a survey of 129 practicing occupational therapists, Cole and McLean (2003) defined a therapeutic relationship as "a trusting connection and rapport established between therapist and client through collaboration, communication, therapist empathy and mutual understanding and respect" (pp. 33–34).

The therapeutic relationship is developed in stages (Lloyd & Maas, 1991; Price, 2009). Moments of rapport along with demonstrations of empathy build an increasingly stronger therapeutic relationship. Rapport is a working alliance or bond between the occupational therapist and client (Tickle-Degnen, 2002), where therapists value a client's perspective as much as their own (Crepeau & Garren, 2011). In occupational therapy, rapport can be central to the client's experience of meaning whether this be cocreation of meaning, shared social meaning, or social validation of meaning (Aiken et al., 2011; Arntzen, 2018; Peloquin, 1995; Tasker & Higgs, 2017). The therapeutic relationship is an emotional bond (Horvath et al., 2011; Shirk, Karver, & Brown, 2011) and the outcome of working relationally (Fusco, 2012; Morrison & Smith, 2013). Trust is also critical to the therapeutic relationship. Clients trust that their occupational therapist is competent and will help them achieve meaningful outcomes (Gahnstrom-Strandqvist et al., 2000; Guidetti & Tham, 2002; Price, 2009). In Palmadottir's (2003) study, clients described occupational therapy as a having a strong positive impact when the therapist–client relationship was characterized by trust and respect. When the child and family feel confident and trust the occupational therapist, they can take on greater challenges and greater risks, and even confront the potential for failure (Price, 2009).

Occupational therapists are responsible for creating an environment that promotes a therapeutic relationship (Crepeau & Garren, 2011; Morrison, 2013). Practitioners use a variety of specific strategies to build rapport in a therapeutic relationship (**Box 6.3**). Strategies may vary by setting and client (King et al., 2021). For example, occupational therapists rated rapport and counseling skills significantly higher in developing a therapeutic relationship in adult practice areas than in pediatric settings (Cole & McLean, 2003). In contrast, pediatric and geriatric occupational therapists rated therapeutic touch significantly higher for developing a therapeutic relationship. In pediatrics, building rapport can be more effective when embedded in play than when focused on in isolation (Leach, 2005). Strategies must be personalized for each child to create a positive relationship and therapeutic engagement (King et al., 2021).

Demonstrating Empathy and Rapport Through Play

With a foundational understanding of the child, the occupational therapist is able to demonstrate empathy and rapport therapeutically by playing *with* the child (Blanche, 2008; Price & Miner, 2007; Spitzer, 2008). A practitioner's presence and engagement with the client

Box 6.3 Strategies Used by Occupational Therapy Practitioners to Build Rapport

- Provide clients with choices.
- Include client in joint problem solving.
- Individualize activities and approaches to client's needs.
- Convey belief in client's potential.
- Emphasize children's strengths by discussing them.
- Structure opportunities for success.
- Joke/use humor.
- Share personal stories judiciously (without shifting focus from the client's concerns).
- Touch therapeutically.
- Engage in casual everyday conversational topics.
- Provide ongoing attention to feelings, needs, and desires.

Data from Cole, M. B., & McLean, V. (2003). Therapeutic relationships re-defined. *Occupational Therapy in Mental Health*, 19(2), 33–56. https://doi.org/10.1300/J004v19n02_03; Crepeau, E. B., & Garren, K. R. (2011). I looked to her as a guide: The therapeutic relationship in hand therapy. *Disability and Rehabilitation*, 33(10), 872–881. https://doi.org/10.3109/09638288.2010.511419; Curtin, C. (2017). *Strategies for collaborating with children: Creating partnerships in occupational therapy and research*. Thorofare, NJ: Slack Incorporated; Morrison, T. (2013). Individual and environmental implications of working alliances in occupational therapy. *British Journal of Occupational Therapy*, 76(11), 507–514. https://doi.org/10.4276/030802213X13833255804676; D'Arrigo, R. G., Copley, J. A., Poulsen, A. A., & Ziviani, J. (2020). The engaged child in occupational therapy. *Canadian Journal of Occupational Therapy*, 87(2), 127–136. https://doi.org/10.1177/0008417420905708; Gahnstrom-Strandqvist, K., Tham, K., Josephsson, S., & Borell, L. (2000). Actions of competence in occupational therapy practice. *Scandinavian Journal of Occupational Therapy*, 7, 15–25. https://doi.org/10.1080/110381200443580; Guidetti, S., & Tham, K. (2002). Therapeutic strategies used by occupational therapists in self-care training: A qualitative study. *Occupational Therapy International*, 9, 257–276. https://doi.org/10.1002/oti.168; and Taylor, R. R. (2008). *The intentional relationship: Occupational therapy and use of self*. Philadelphia, PA: F. A. Davis.

in therapy are important factors by which clients experience a therapeutic relationship (McCorquodale & Kinsella, 2015). Often pediatric clients cannot conceptually understand an acknowledgment of empathy, and thus, empathy must be demonstrated. Through the therapist's actions, the child can experience empathy and develop feelings of rapport. Playfulness and the social aspect of play promote a relationship between adult and child and therapist and pediatric client because they are engaged together in play (Karver et al., 2018; Román-Oyola, Fiueroa-Feliciano, et al., 2017; Román-Oyola, Reynolds, et al., 2019; Schaefer & Drewes, 2011). Engaging in play with the child demonstrates the therapist's understanding of the joyful experience of play (Bracegirdle, 1992). As an adult, the occupational therapist may demonstrate playfulness by being gregarious, uninhibited, comedic, dynamic, creative, and spontaneous (Barnett, 2007; Guitard, Ferland, & Dutil, 2005). The occupational therapy practitioner can share in play by taking a full role as a player—taking turns; being a character; and being a play partner who assists, supports, encourages the child, and expresses/mirrors the child's reactions in ways that promote play (see

Figure 6.4). The occupational therapist can enlist family members and peers to participate with playful activities. By playing, the occupational therapist creates a playful environment where pediatric clients can play as well (Ferland, 2005). To create a playful therapeutic relationship with a pediatric client, the occupational therapist shares in the control, spontaneity, challenge, and possibility of play.

Sharing Control

In assuming a play partner role, the occupational therapy practitioner builds rapport and creates play by sharing control with the pediatric client and family. The occupational therapist minimizes directedness to the extent possible for each individual child because research indicates that exerting control is incompatible with adult–child play (Holland & Thompson, 2018; Howard, 2002; Olli, et al., 2021; Shine & Acosta, 1999; Wing, 1995). Many adults are reluctant to share their control with children and give them choices (McInnes et al., 2011). Choice is important for the child to experience play, and yet children tend to perceive less choice when adults are present (King & Howard, 2010, 2014a, 2014b). Therefore, the therapist must actively work to counter this tendency. An occupational therapist can share control through flexibly offering choices (what, when, how) and encouraging and accepting the child's reactions to and feelings expressed about the activities (D'Arrigo et al., 2020; Fleming, 1994; Karver et al., 2018; Mattingly & Fleming, 1994; Parham, 1992; Price & Miner, 2007). For example, a child who is feeling fatigued or taxed during a session may lie down and pretend to be "asleep." Sometimes giving

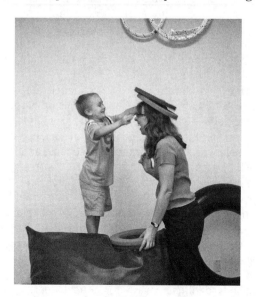

Figure 6.4 When playing with the child, the occupational therapist is a full partner in the activity
Courtesy of Cameron Flanagan.

those children the break they need by allowing them to "sleep" or by "sleeping" next to them for a few seconds until the "alarm" goes off is just what they need. In this way, the occupational therapist shares a playful rest moment rather than allowing avoidance or directing the child back to work. The practitioner can also share control with family members or other caregivers who may contribute some wonderful ideas for play with this child. When the occupational therapist shares control with clients, clients also can have some sense of internal control and experience the freedom to participate in the spontaneous process of play (Henricks, 1999).

Spontaneity and Flexibility

Although the occupational therapy practitioner has an intervention plan and enters each treatment session with plans guided by goals, he or she must remain very flexible in how these plans may be adjusted in the moment of therapy. The occupational therapist must be willing to adjust an intervention plan in the moment to allow spontaneous play opportunities to emerge (Blanche, 2008). Because play is a spontaneous process, and in therapy, a social process as well, the practitioner must be open to adapting to the child's response and to seizing upon playful opportunities. The occupational therapist must have a "playful eye" to recognize playful possibilities, as seen in **Practice Example 6.3** with Michael.

Managing Challenge

The playful occupational therapy practitioner demonstrates empathy for the challenges as well as the joys of play. The occupational therapist can model playful acceptance of mistakes, errors, trips, falls, and so on. In these circumstances, an adult tends to simply clean up, pick up, fix the mistake, or try again in a quick manner and continue on with the activity at hand. This often happens so swiftly that the child fails to notice it. By slowing down and explicating the process, the occupational therapist can use this as an opportunity to model a sharing of frustration: "Oops, I dropped it" and an "Oh well, that's okay, let's keep playing" attitude. The occupational therapist deliberately reacts in words and actions to demonstrate empathy with the child. The degree of these actions must be graded and matched with the child's developmental level so as not to be interpreted as belittling. The objective is to persist with the playful process rather than become overly preoccupied with the observable product or performance, an extrinsic standard that tends to be inconsistent with play.

Focusing on Future Possibilities

The playful occupational therapy practitioner also builds rapport with a child by focusing on the transformative possibility of play. The therapist acts "as if" the pediatric client is not disabled, especially not

---

PRACTICE EXAMPLE 6.3 Michael and Playful Therapeutic Opportunities

Michael was a 4-year-old diagnosed with autism spectrum disorder. One of his goals for occupational therapy was to write horizontal, vertical, and circular lines. When he was given a writing utensil, he often threw it; at most, he would scribble briefly. Michael threw tantrums when adults would direct control of the writing utensil. He preferred to use nontoy objects and resisted the therapist's suggestions. He seemed most interested in seeing things fall apart or making another big impact—such as throwing, kicking, stepping on, or dumping toys from bins and boxes. His occupational therapist was having difficulty finding a way to work on his prewriting goal because all efforts so far had been unsuccessful.

Unexpectedly one session, Michael picked up a spray bottle of water and began spraying it repetitively on the table. At first, his occupational therapist thought she should stop this action because it seemed to be perseverative and to serve no therapeutic purpose. But she carefully ran through his goals in her head for possible ways of intersecting therapeutic goals and this sudden interest. She quickly and creatively realized that spraying water on the table was similar to cleaning the table and that they could use a pencil on the laminated table and then clean it with the water. She dried the table off with a quick sweep and managed to get Michael to wait momentarily while she quickly drew a line on the table. "Zip!" she said. Then she pointed to the table and said, "Spray it." He did, and she wiped off the water with a towel. "It's gone! Magic," she said. "Yeah!" he said. Then she offered him a pencil, demonstrating and encouraging him to make different lines, which he did, "erasing" them with water between trials with great exclamations of enjoyment. He kept indicating a desire to continue practicing in this manner.

Michael's occupational therapist found herself surprised by the spontaneous direction the session had gone because she had never anticipated such a therapeutic treatment activity. She also felt a great sense of satisfaction and confidence in her abilities. It was moments like these that affirmed her skill in and belief in the profession. Her flexibility identified a way for Michael to learn a skill that he needed in a creative way that affirmed his interests. This was the first time he drew lines; later, he began practicing on fogged-up windows of the car and other surfaces, and eventually paper.

in the social sense in which disability is understood. The playful occupational therapist is not limited by the realities of current time and space, but feels free to act as if things were different. Thus, the occupational therapist maintains a future orientation (Price & Miner, 2007; Schafer, 1994). This happens most frequently when a child with a significant disability is enabled to take on an extraordinary role. For example, a child with spastic cerebral palsy who is usually the receiver of help for most activities helps the therapist with creative ideas for decorating a new tray table. A child with autism who rarely initiates ideas or social interaction or engages in pretend play suddenly repetitively says "Power Rangers," her brothers' favorite television show, and the occupational therapist then acts as if the child is a Power Ranger. A child with ADHD who frequently hurts other children and breaks toys because of her poor body awareness and difficulty grading force becomes a superhero who saves people from the "bad guys." When the occupational therapy practitioner uses a playful approach, pediatric clients can imagine and explore a different occupational identity of "What if I were _____, what if I could do _____," which are typical play experiences.

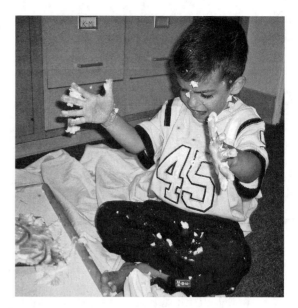

Figure 6.5 With messy play, occupational therapy practitioners must be prepared and must be able to suspend rules about neatness and any negative attitudes about messiness and its inconvenience
Courtesy of Susan L. Spitzer.

Managing Therapist and Player Roles

Implementing a playful therapeutic use of self involves a level of work for the occupational therapy practitioner, more so when first learning its practice. Reconciling role conflict in that of adult therapist with that of a child's play partner is not easy (see **Figure 6.5**). A strong knowledge about play provides a foundation for grounding these roles. Specifically, clinicians must be aware of and manage their internal attitudes and beliefs about play, handle external constraints, learn to have fun and play, and engage in ongoing reflective analysis. The more knowledge we have about play, the easier it is to separate our attitudes and beliefs from the evidence.

Managing Therapist Attitudes and Beliefs About Play

For the play that occurs in a session to be therapeutic, occupational therapists must also know themselves and control their own responses within the session (Schwartzberg, 1993). Responses based on the therapists' own needs and interests may not be therapeutic for the child. The therapist must stay focused on the child, determine what response is therapeutic for the child in that moment, and respond accordingly. By being aware of who he or she is, the occupational therapy practitioner can control his or her impulses and attune behaviors to approach clients in a consciously therapeutic manner that builds a therapeutic relationship.

Self-awareness should include reflection on one's attitudes, abilities, limitations, and needs. An occupational therapist must be aware of his or her own attitudes and biases to keep them in check when working with clients (Lloyd & Maas, 1991; Punwar, 2000; Taylor, 2008). Occupational therapists must know what their abilities are in order to have confidence in their abilities and demonstrate competence (Frank, 1958; Lloyd & Maas, 1991; Schultz-Krohn, 2019). Likewise, occupational therapists must be aware of their limitations to experience and demonstrate humility about their limitations and their relative role in the therapeutic process (Frank, 1958; Mosey, 1986). They must have knowledge of their own needs to address and meet these needs outside of therapy sessions so they do not interfere with focusing on the client's needs within therapy (Lloyd & Maas, 1991; Mosey, 1986; Taylor, 2008). Reflective discussion and observation with experienced and skilled occupational therapists can also yield insight in developing your own therapeutic use of self. The reader is referred to Taylor (2008) and Gorenberg (2013) for detailed guidance on developing self-awareness for promoting therapeutic use of self.

Shaped by personal experiences and values, occupational therapy practitioners have their own attitudes about different types of play—about what is and what is not appropriate and about what children should and should not do. Research indicates that many adults are not comfortable with play, child-led activities, and allowing children choice (McInnes et al., 2011). Attitudes about power and willingness to share power with clients must be examined to develop a genuine partnership with clients (Palmadottir, 2006), including the child, parents, teachers, and other caregivers. Adults may have a range of beliefs about what their role should be. Biases about the child's behavior, parenting approaches, culture, and teaching style must be critically examined and controlled so that clients can be approached in a nonjudgmental manner (McCorquodale & Kinsella, 2015; Punwar, 2000).

Recognizing these attitudes and beliefs as stemming from one's internal sense of self rather than the research evidence can give therapeutic focus when various types of play emerge in therapy sessions. For example, Jacob's occupational therapist did not believe that it was generally appropriate for children to play with "poop," and Michael's occupational therapist did not believe it was generally appropriate for children to write on tables (see earlier), but both were willing to accept these unconventional actions for their individual therapeutic value in the context of play. Other play areas that commonly challenge us to analyze our attitudes and beliefs include humor, gender, and aggression.

Attitudes About Humor in Play

Because humor is relative, many people have different attitudes about what constitutes humor. For example, using a made-up robotic "accent" may be funny, but using an accent typical for a particular social class, geographical region, or ethnic group may be seen as objectionable. A child may focus purely on the difference in sound and be unaware of social attitudes or political backgrounds. Or, the child may be attempting to make sense of social differences. Occupational therapy practitioners must be able to set aside their own attitudes to judge objectively the child's intent and others' reception of potentially humorous actions.

Attitudes About Gender and Play

Various attitudes abound about gender and play. As described in Chapter 1, research indicates that boys and girls tend to play different activities and with different toys; however, this is not absolute and may vary to greater and lesser degrees in local

sociocultural contexts (Davis & Hines, 2020; Pawlowski et al., 2015; Tietz & Shine, 2001; Todd, Fischer, Di Costa, Roestorf, Harbour, Hardiman, & Barry, 2018; Van Rheenen, 2001). The context is important because adults influence play through their own gender perceptions (Chapman, 2016; Josephidou, 2019). Furthermore, gender boundaries are often negotiated in play (Thorne, 1993; Van Rheenen, 2001). Some people feel most comfortable when children play in traditional gender-based activities, but some find it objectionable. Some people feel comfortable with and even prefer to see girls playing with stereotypically masculine toys, games, and physical activities, but some people object to girls doing some or all aspects of "boy play." Some people enjoy seeing boys play with stereotypically feminine toys, games, and activities (such as dolls, dance, and jump rope), and some are troubled by this. Some people's attitudes vary based on the particular activity or the child's disability. Some worry about a child being limited or stigmatized by engaging in gendered or cross-gendered play and prefer gender-neutral play. People may have such attitudes based on their experiences, values, or concerns about society's reactions. Notably, the child may prefer a type of play based on the understanding of its social typology or may not even be aware of such constructs (Pawlowski et al., 2015).

Occupational therapy practitioners need to recognize that gendered play does exist but is also negotiated in the local social context of the family and on the playground. We have a responsibility to analyze our own attitudes and recognize how they may differ from the available knowledge base (see Chapter 1; **Figure 6.6**). This enables us to focus on the child, the family, and the social context in an informed manner when analyzing the therapeutic benefits and challenges of gendered, cross-gendered, or gender-neutral play for an individual client.

Attitudes About Aggressive-Themed Play

Aggressive-themed play is another type of play that can evoke strong attitudes. Although many adults are quick to condemn aggression in any form, it is important to note that aggressive behavior and themes are common in typically developing children's play. As described in Chapter 1, there are patterns of aggressive-themed play. Researchers have suggested a variety of potential beneficial functions of aggressive play, but there is no agreement about whether aggressive play should be allowed or discouraged. Adults tend to have negative attitudes about aggressive play and at best

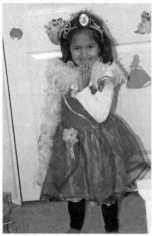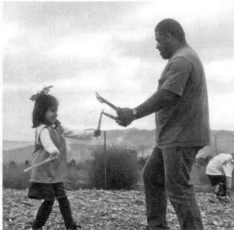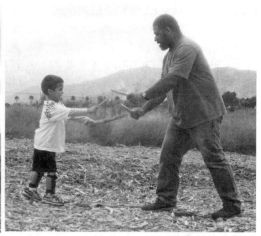

Figure 6.6 Occupational therapy practitioners must examine their own attitudes regarding gendered, cross-gendered, and aggressive-themed play, which commonly occur in children

Left: Courtesy of David A. Morales. Middle and Right: Courtesy of Susan L. Spitzer.

tolerate it but rarely encourage it (Goldstein, 1995; Johnson, Welteroth, & Corl, 2001). Adult attitudes tend to be related to their educational status, their play memories, presence of siblings, and the child's gender (Goldstein, 1995; Johnson et al., 2001). Recognizing the difference between our attitudes and the knowledge base allows us to focus on individual cases of aggressive play and whether to allow, encourage, discourage, or shape its form.

Managing Physical and Social Constraints

When acting as a child's play partner in an occupational therapy session, the therapist must be aware of and adjust to physical and social constraints. A therapeutic alliance involves an interaction of therapist, client, and the environmental context (Morrison, 2013). For example, a child may want to engage in physical play with the therapist, but the therapist must be mindful of his or her own body mechanics to ensure personal safety. Some children want to take risks without recognizing the almost certain danger involved. Another child may find it a game to make large chalk drawings all over the sidewalk, but the school administration may only have designated a particular area for this purpose. The child may find it fun to smear paint all over her body, getting it on her clothes and surrounding furniture, but a parent, other caregiver, or program administrator may not be amused given the temporary, if not permanent, damage to physical property. The child may be drawn to loud noises and a loud, excited voice from the therapist, but this may be disruptive to others. Weather and light may limit safety and accessibility of play. In these and similar

cases, the occupational therapy practitioner might have to leave the play partner role to redirect and set limits for the child to protect self, client, property, or professional relationships in order to safeguard the future of therapy sessions. Morozini (2015) identified the following adult options for these situations:

- Distract the child's attention to another play activity or toy.
- Draw the child's attention to the inappropriate behavior.
- Give firm directions of what to do.
- Move a toy away from the child.
- End a play activity.

However, she also noted that adults then must make concerted efforts to repair the impact of controlling behaviors and recreate play. For repeated challenges that disrupt play, some children may need the therapist to set respectful limits that reduce the occurrence of these challenges (Curtin, 2017).

Learning to Play and Have Fun in Your Work

It is difficult for the child to have fun if the occupational therapist is not having fun. Play is about having fun, a pleasurable emotional state (Eberle, 2014; Guitard et al., 2005; Schaefer & Drewes, 2011; Skard & Bundy, 2008; see also Chapter 1). Adults experience playfulness as "the predisposition to frame (or reframe) a situation in such a way as to provide oneself (and possibly others) with amusement, humor, and/or entertainment" (Barnett, 2007, p. 955). Research indicates that adults who are more playful may have stronger self-efficacy (Román-Oyola et al., 2017). The effort of therapy feels less like work for both parties when embedded in a therapeutic relationship. The occupational therapist can have fun within the therapy session by adopting key features of playfulness: intrinsic motivation, internal control, and freedom to suspend reality (Skard & Bundy, 2008).

Practitioner Intrinsic Motivation

At times, it can be difficult to hold onto one's intrinsic motivation in the face of the external work aspects of being a therapist. To tap into their own intrinsic motivation, occupational therapy practitioners must identify what they themselves enjoy about being a practitioner and what they like about their individual clients. Practitioners must understand play and value a play-based approach in order for it to be intrinsically motivating (McInnes et al. 2011; Schaefer & Greenberg, 1997). To be playful, it is especially important to identify and seek out the fun aspects (Shen et al., 2014). Then, practitioners can keep these ideas foremost in their thinking to promote a playful disposition, a real enjoyment of their chosen profession. Specifically identifying the fun characteristics and reminding oneself of these can help the occupational therapist maintain a genuine playful orientation and a desire to be engaged in the session.

The intrinsic motivation of play is not exclusive in the therapeutic context as it is juggled with the necessity of goal attainment. Certainly, it is the clinician's professional responsibility to promote progress toward the client's goals. The intrinsically motivated therapist is also focused on the process of play involved in furthering those end goals. This is akin to playing sports, where players enjoy the game even when they are not scoring and find the game worth playing even if they do not win (Shen et al., 2014). Similarly, the playful clinician enjoys the child's strengths and foundational gains that support later goal achievement. When we see our clients engaged in play, we see deep concentration, strong motivation, satisfaction, and positive energy that propels the therapeutic process, which is also very meaningful for the therapist (Aiken et al., 2011; Howard & McInnes, 2013). Establishing goals directly addressing play or goals that align with play can better harness the power of intrinsic motivation. Play goals can connect the intrinsic process of playing in therapy with the extrinsic product of participating in play.

Practitioner Internal Control

Internal control is not to be confused with having total control of the session because control must be shared with the client as well. Internal control is having confidence in the therapeutic process and one's self as a therapeutic agent, which allows the occupational therapy practitioner comfort with sharing control with the child. Each therapist must examine his or her abilities and doubts to identify a plan to build a sense of internal control. With a foundation of theory, research, training, and mentoring, you will know what to do, when to do it, and why to do it. The practitioner's role for how, when, and whether they intervene in children's play is critical for having confidence in implementing a play-based approach (Howard & McInnes, 2013; McInnes, 2019). Although the details may be specifically enacted with individual clients, the guiding principles and techniques remain stable. With your growing knowledge of play, you will have the ability to make well-reasoned clinical decisions and determine when modifications to a standard practice are needed. With skill in activity analysis, the cornerstone of therapy, you will have the internal control you need in order to be spontaneous and playful as you share control with your pediatric clients.

Practitioner Suspension of Reality

Occupational therapy practitioners who adopt a playful style temporarily suspend their own reality. Play creates a protective frame (Apter, 1991). The players act "as if" free from their own worries, from social conventions, from the apparent limits of clinical "disability," and from planned activities (Spitzer, 2008). The focus is on the child's capacity to do despite disability (Hasselkus & Dickie, 1994). Play is a transformative process where players transform themselves and their environments, either physically or symbolically, creating meaning for their lives (Henricks, 1999). When implemented, the players are free to be spontaneous and creative (Guitard et al., 2005); however, suspending reality has been identified as a more difficult factor for adults to implement with children with disabilities (Román-Oyola et al., 2018).

As seen in the example of Michael and writing on the table, the playful occupational therapist acts as if free from social conventions—conventional ideas about both play for the child and appropriate adult–therapist behavior. Michael's occupational therapist was able to suspend social rules about "not writing on the table," enabling him to develop the skills to write, and she opted to work on conventional rules later. Conventional ideas often involve demonstrating good disciplined behavior, which is polite and respectful to adults. But if the occupational therapy practitioner is going to play with the child, then some of these social rules may have to be held in abeyance. Crawling around on the floor, making exaggerated facial expressions, talking in a singsong fashion, taking turns in a game, getting dressed up, and many other strategies are not generally accepted as mature professional behavior, and the occupational therapist cannot be overly preoccupied with these social normative ideas during sessions. The playful practitioner is free to be silly and laugh without worrying about looking silly, even in front of parents, other caregivers, student interns, or other professionals. Instead, the playful occupational therapist recognizes that using these strategies in the context of a playful session is masterful.

The occupational therapy practitioner must also distance oneself from the realities of life outside the session. The therapist cannot allow him- or herself to be preoccupied with personal finances, an upcoming vacation, family relationships, health, chores, work relationships, productivity demands, and so forth. All these distractions need to stay outside the session because they take away from the here-and-now quality of the play process.

When occupational therapists play on the boundary of reality and possibility, they take calculated risks. This is part of the creative process (Schmid, 2004). Schafer (1994) argued that this can be very therapeutic because of the potential for reality to be transformed by possibility. However, there is a risk that the potential for growth and development will not materialize. Furthermore, there is always a risk that things might even go "wrong." What might happen if the child gets too disappointed, too frustrated, too disorganized, too angry, or too active? In consideration, the occupational therapist grades and modifies the activity to better ensure success as described in Chapter 8. This is a balancing act because activities that are too predictable or too safe are unlikely to be very playful or therapeutic (Burke, 1977).

The occupational therapist must calculate the risk that both therapist and client can manage. The practitioner is able to abandon neither the reality of the child's life nor the reality of professional responsibility. In other words, the occupational therapist must also remain a therapist and balance therapist and play partner roles (see **Practice Example 6.4**).

PRACTICE EXAMPLE 6.4 Sarah and a Calculated Risk

Sarah was a 5-year-old client with a seizure disorder and developmental delays who resisted wet, sticky textures in food and in art and learning projects. The occupational therapist suggested she and Sarah play with toy animals, which Sarah liked, in the "mud" (a bowl of chocolate pudding). Sarah appeared excited, repeating the phrase "play with the animals in the mud" until she saw the pudding. She pulled away and directed the therapist, "You do it." The occupational therapist carefully dipped the just-washed animals in the pudding, modeling positive emotions and statements. Soon Sarah came closer and gradually began playing too. At first, she was very careful not to actually touch the pudding, but then it kept happening accidentally. She asked to wipe it off, and the therapist helped her so that she would continue playing. After a few times of wiping the pudding off, the occupational therapist suggested, "You can lick it," and pretended to lick her fingers. Sarah laughed and tried licking the pudding off an animal, deliberately dunking and licking each animal like a spoon. They both laughed. When the occupational therapist described the session to Sarah's mom, Sarah's mom responded, "Yuck!" (pause) "Cool!" This was the first time Sarah had eaten pudding. From then on, Sarah willingly ate pudding with a spoon.

Sarah's occupational therapist planned for this session by washing the animals and wearing gloves, anticipating that maybe Sarah might be coaxed into sticking her finger in the pudding and then licking her fingers. However, it was in the therapeutic moment that the occupational therapist envisioned a slight modification and allowed Sarah's own creative and unconventional activity modification of using a familiar item in a new way. The occupational therapist took a calculated risk. She knew the toys were clean and thus safe. She knew this was of great interest to Sarah. She knew this could help promote Sarah's tolerance of tactile sensation. She also knew that many people would frown on a child Sarah's age licking toys that are not meant for licking, especially when she was too old to be mouthing toys (her mother's initial "yuck" response). Her colleagues might even believe it inappropriate, but Sarah's mom was pretty open-minded, frequently commenting that she was willing to try anything that might help Sarah.

Sarah's occupational therapist had a playful eye to see this as a therapeutic opportunity. She acted as if free from social rules that might have stopped this activity and its positive therapeutic outcome. This activity also worked because Sarah's occupational therapist considered the fit within Sarah's family context. The therapist was able to recognize the difference between her general social attitudes and the family's and consciously act in a way that was therapeutic. The outcome would not have been so therapeutic if Sarah's family had strict rules about not putting toys in one's mouth, especially if Sarah wanted to play it again.

Continuing Development of Your Playful Therapeutic Use of Self

Although the development of therapeutic use of self begins with the formal educational training of occupational therapy practitioners, it is a lifelong, reflective, demanding, and yet satisfying process. Research indicates that improved therapeutic use of self is developed over time through mentoring and reflective practice (Bonsaksen, 2013; Carstensen & Bonsaksen, 2017; Hussain, Carstensen, Yazdani, Ellingham, & Bonsaksen, 2018; Maloney & Griffith, 2013; Price, 2009; Taylor, 2008). For example, initially occupational therapy students tend to rely more heavily on a problem-solving mode, and with time and experience, occupational therapists use more collaborating, empathizing, and advocating modes (Bonsaksen, 2013; Carstensen & Bonsaksen, 2017). Each therapist must find and hone his or her own therapeutic style. You will need to integrate the tools in this book with your personal abilities. Even with decades of experience, we constantly reflect on practice and find ways to improve each session. Although this process is work, play helps sustain our efforts, and the benefits of a satisfying career are well worth the effort. This is the way occupational therapists elevate practice to an art (Hinojosa, 2007; Mosey, 1981). "Without art, the occupational therapy process is only the application of scientific knowledge in a sterile vacuum" (Mosey, 1981, p. 25).

Although some of us may have personal traits that are naturally more or less helpful in healing, our therapeutic use of self is a conscious role that we create and enact (Taylor, 2008). This therapeutic role can be influenced by, but is not dependent on, who we are (D'Arrigo et al., 2020; Frank, 1958). Each therapist may have a preferred style that is consistent with their personality; however, it is important that we become comfortable and able to adjust therapeutic modes for different clients and different situations (Mosey, 1986; Taylor, 2008). For some of us, these play strategies feel very comfortable and natural with children. For others, with a different predisposition, such strategies may be more challenging to assume. Even caring is a skill to be developed (Gilfoyle, 1980). You may need to learn or relearn to play as an adult. You must learn to play with a range of children. Bracegirdle (1992) suggested interacting with playful children, who will teach you to play if you are open to their directions and enticements, and watching playful parents play with their young children, especially babies. By paying conscious attention to developing your skills,

trying them, and reflecting on their outcome, you will develop an understanding of the nuances of matching strategies to clients and will hone your skills. With ongoing practice and analytical reflection, occupational therapists can develop these skills regardless of their individual comfort level and innate disposition.

Therapeutic use of self is quite demanding. Most of the work is internal and thus is not visible to others until the therapist acts. Therapists employ a high degree of unfaltering attention to observe the details of each child and the environment to analyze these in relation to the current activity and overall goals before individually adjusting their responses to the child. Occupational therapists may not always get clear positive feedback for these actions because children with disabilities cannot always provide this (Adamson et al., 2012; Doussard-Roosevelt et al., 2003; Warren & Brady, 2007). Without this external reinforcing validation, our efforts can feel more like work and cause us to doubt our efficacy or to become discouraged with our attempts.

Therapeutic use of self also involves emotional work (Andonian, 2017; McKenna & Mellson, 2013). Occupational therapists work with people who may be experiencing very difficult emotions such as anxiety, anger, and depression or who may have other challenging interpersonal characteristics (Taylor, 2008; Taylor et al., 2009). Confronted with repeated exposure to the challenges of life, illness, disability, trauma, and sometimes death, occupational therapists often struggle alongside clients and families to make sense of negative events, pain, and suffering (McColl, 2003). Amidst these strong emotions, it takes great effort to manage our own feelings, responses, and behaviors to focus on the client's therapeutic needs and goals. Sustaining a playful style despite these challenges definitely involves a strong therapeutic use of self for the pediatric occupational therapy practitioner.

The intense work of therapeutic use of self is clearly very important and necessary for effective therapy, but it can also cause exhaustion and burnout if occupational therapists do not find ways to care for themselves outside of work (Schlenz, Guthrie, & Dudgeon, 1995; Stoffel, 2013; Taylor & Peloquin, 2008). Emotional exhaustion may compromise professional reasoning (Winters, 2016). Therapist strategies of caring for themselves are very individual but may include exercise, mindfulness, guided imagery, time with a friend or family member, reading fiction, cooking a favorite meal, and humor (Gupta et al., 2012; Luken & Sammons, 2016; Taylor, 2008; Winters, 2016). For some practitioners, counseling or psychotherapy may be helpful to manage feelings ignited in the course of being a therapist. Caring for ourselves helps provide occupational therapists with the energy and positive self-concept to care for our clients (Devereax, 1984).

The benefits of the work of therapeutic use of self are tremendous in terms of satisfying practice. Occupational therapists report deep satisfaction with establishment of therapeutic relationships (Williams & Patterson, 2009). Occupational therapists feel competent when working together with clients as partners focused on personally meaningful goals (Gahnstrom-Strandqvist et al., 2000). Occupational therapists believe that the therapeutic relationship, empathy, and rapport help bring about functional outcomes across practice settings (Cole & McLean, 2003; Taylor et al., 2009). Once an occupational therapist is able to behave playfully and creatively, he or she is more likely also to experience play while working as a therapist (Ferland, 2005) and increased job enjoyment (Vergeer & MacRae, 1993). Occupational therapists also feel successful when they "find the key" to helping a child (Case-Smith, 1997, p. 140), which is often a playful relationship.

It can be helpful to remind ourselves that by embracing the complexities of therapeutic use of self, we realize that the challenges fend off boredom and offer opportunity for a dynamic and rewarding practice. In play we focus on the joy of our jobs, which can support our professional resilience and well-being (Hildenbrand, 2019; Perlo et al., 2017). Then, we can enjoy the pleasure of the activity as well (Greenspan & Wieder, 1997).

Therapeutic Use of Self and Caregiver Relationships

Although this book is committed to the use of play with pediatric clients, pediatric practice is incomplete without also applying therapeutic use of self with the child's family and other adult caregivers in diverse family forms (Karver et al., 2018; Shirk et al., 2011)[1]. Known as family-centered practice, supporting and including families in treatment planning and intervention are best practices in pediatric occupational therapy and overall health care (Dunn, 2000; Kuo et al., 2012) and essential for building resilience in children (Masten & Barnes, 2018). Families want to feel that professionals support them, listen, and understand their needs as a family and without judging them (Kruijsen-Terpstra et al., 2014). A good parent–practitioner relationship

and clinician responsiveness to parent needs and emotions has been found to influence parent engagement in therapy (D'Arrigo et al., 2019). Establishing a good therapeutic relationship with the child's family, teachers, and other caregivers ensures that they too will feel comfortable, trust the therapist, work openly and honestly with the therapist, and be willing to try different activities with their children (O'Brien & Taylor, 2020). Furthermore, by focusing on play and playfulness, the occupational therapy practitioner helps build relationships that reinforce and empower the family (Kruijsen-Terpstra et al., 2016; Román-Oyola et al., 2018; Waldman-Levi & Weintraub, 2015; see Chapter 11 for more details on promoting family play).

In practice, the inclusion of families varies, especially across practice settings (Fingerhut et al., 2013; King, Williams, & Hahn Goldberg, 2017). Brown, Humphry, and Taylor (1997) found that occupational therapists use a hierarchical continuum of the following levels of family-therapy involvement, with each level requiring more knowledge and skill: no family involvement, family as informant, family as therapist's assistant, family as coclient, family as consultant, family as team collaborator, and family as director of service. Occupational therapy practitioners have an obligation to commit to supporting and including families at the latter, higher levels. This is not an expectation that families must be involved, but rather that families are welcomed and supported to be as involved as they desire and are able. Family-centered care emphasizes the role of parents as partners and ultimate decision makers for their children (Kuo, 2012; U.S. Department of Health and Human Services, 2014). To include parents and other caregivers, therapists must actively focus on interactions with parents and caregivers as well as their children (An, Palisano, Yi, Chiarello, Dunst, & Gracely, 2019a, 2019b).

Families have individual experiences, routines, strengths, needs, and hopes for the future that shape the environment for our clients and therapy (Masten & Barnes, 2018; U.S. Department of Health and Human Services, 2014). Occupational development in children has been linked to the opportunities and resources in the environment and parental views and values in addition to personal motivation (Wiseman et al., 2005). The family's context may or may not support play and treatment outcomes. Such diverse factors make therapist–caregiver relationships quite complex (Tasker & Higgs, 2017). When addressing play, therapeutic interactions often intersect with caregivers' emotional responses and their cultural and societal context. Sensitivity to a family's

---

[1] Because families come in diverse forms, the use of the word *parent* throughout this book is intended to encompass all people in parental roles, including guardians, caregivers, and so on.

values and customs is essential to family-centered care (Kuo et al., 2012; U.S. Department of Health and Human Services, 2014).

Family Emotional Responses

Sometimes a family's emotions and behaviors can present obstacles to play and therapy. As parents and other caregivers adjust to the child's disability, they may experience doubts and guilt about their parenting abilities, stress and anxiety about their child's future, and other negative and complex emotions that change with each stage of the child's development (Anderson & Hinojosa, 1984). Whenever the occupational therapist presents evaluation results or mentions the child's needs, the parent or other caregiver may experience a resurgence in distress or mourning over the child's deficits. Parents may have negative attitudes about play or struggle with their own difficulties playing with their children (Graham et al., 2015; Morozini, 2015; Waldman-Levi, Bundy, & Katz, 2015). As a result of their feelings, parents and other caregivers may be overprotective or highly directive with their children which can disrupt play. Parents often need to express these feelings. If they trust the occupational therapy practitioner, parents may be comfortable sharing these feelings with the practitioner. Some parents may need additional support and can be referred to counseling or parent support groups (King et al., 2017). Sometimes a parent's emotions and behaviors trigger attitudes in the practitioner, who may overly identify with the child or the caregiver. This is another aspect of pediatric practice that necessitates that the therapist reflect on and consciously check his or her own emotions in order to remain therapeutic. Specifically, playful and positive interactions have been found to be most effective in creating a therapeutic relationship with caregivers that promotes the child's participation in play (see **Box 6.4**).

Family Cultural and Societal Context

A family's or other caregiver's values and behaviors regarding play and occupational therapy can also be influenced by their cultural and socioeconomic background (Morozini, 2015), which may be both similar to and different from the therapist's personal and professional values. Unchecked, a lack of familiarity, a lack of understanding, or conflict with a family's background can result in negative assumptions, devaluation, and bias (AOTA, 2020). We must be open to recognize unique family strengths and values as well as power dynamics, which influence a family's ability to support their child. This process also requires constant humility

---

Box 6.4 Strategies for Therapeutic Use of Self with Families and Other Caregivers of Pediatric Clients

- Allow parents and caregivers to express feelings without judgment—listening without ignoring or interrupting.
- Reflect on and consciously check own reactions to caregiver emotions and behaviors.
- Provide nurturing and support regarding the challenges they are facing.
- Encourage optimism by sharing positive, productive thoughts focused on the child's potential.
- Give positive feedback about what they are doing well to reinforce their competence.
- Engage in joint problem solving to promote their own experience of mastery.
- Present information as suggestions to be evaluated collaboratively (avoid giving advice).
- Incorporate a playful approach to emphasize the pleasure of sharing play.
- Involve in play activities to build parental/caregiver playfulness and enhance the parent/caregiver–child relationship.
- Use verbal and nonverbal communication to cue the adult how to be involved in play.
- Refer to counseling or support groups when caregiver needs go beyond the practitioner's abilities to address.

Data from Anderson, J., & Hinojosa, J. (1984). Parents and therapists in a professional partnership. *American Journal of Occupational Therapy*, 38, 452–461. https://doi.org/10.5014/ajot.38.7.452; Burke, J. P. (2010). What's going on here? Deconstructing the interactive encounter (Eleanor Clarke Slagle Lecture). *American Journal of Occupational Therapy*, 64, 855–868. https://doi.org/10.5014/ajot.2010.64604; Downs, M. L. (2008). Leisure routines: Parents and children with disability sharing occupation. *Journal of Occupational Science*, 15, 105–110. https://doi.org/10.1080/14427591.2008.9686616; Durand, V. M., Hieneman, M., Clarke, S., & Zona, M. (2009). Optimistic parenting: Hope and help for parents with challenging children. In W. Sailor, G. Dunlap, G. Sugai, & R. Horner (Eds.), *Handbook of positive behavior support: Issues in clinical child psychology* (pp. 233–256). Boston, MA: Springer. https://doi.org/10.1007/978-0-387-09632-2_10; Ferland, F. (2005). *The Ludic model: Play, children with physical disabilities and occupational therapy* (2nd ed.). Ottawa, Ontario: Canadian Association of Occupational Therapists. https://search.proquest.com/docview/213007487?accountid=143111; Morozini, M. (2015). Exploring the engagement of parents in the co-occupation of parent–child play: An occupational science's perspective. *International Journal of Prevention and Treatment*, 4, 11–28. https://doi.org/10.5923/s.ijpt.201501.02; Román-Oyola, R., Reynolds, S., Soto-Feliciano, I., Cabrera-Mercader, L., & Vega-Santana, J. (2017). Child's sensory profile and adult playfulness as predictors of parental self-efficacy. *American Journal of Occupational Therapy*, 71, 7102220010. https://doi.org/10.5014/ajot.2017.021097; and Steiner, A. M. (2011). A strength-based approach to parent education for children with autism. *Journal of Positive Behavior Interventions*, 13, 178–190. http://dx.doi.org/10.1177/1098300710384134.

---

and reflection to avoid assumptions as well as flexibility to be responsive to family strengths and needs. We can use family-specific knowledge to adapt therapy and our interactions for genuine respect and collaboration.

The expression, form, meaning, and uses of play have a cultural basis (Rentzou et al., 2019). Culture shapes play, and children learn about culture through play (Kinkead-Clark, 2019). Ethnic differences may be expressed in gender expectations, childrearing practices, and views of disability, while socioeconomic status may influence access and expectations for activities and experiences (Jaffe, Cosper, & Fabrizi, 2020). For example, different cultures may value different types of play (e.g., Little, 2010; Suizzo & Bornstein, 2006). Parents who experience intergenerational poverty may not view playing with their children as part of their parenting role and may not seek support because parenting is viewed as a private matter (Smith et al., 2015). Traditional gender role attitudes in parents are negatively related to cross-gender-typed toys (Kollmayer et al., 2018). Higher education and socioeconomic status have been associated with more responsive and less directive parenting, which in turn are associated with increased adult–child play (Morozini, 2015). Cultures may have different strengths demonstrated in play such as Mayan children's observation of ongoing interactions and children's creativity and resourcefulness in Zanzibar (Berinstein & Magalhaes, 2009; Correa-Chávez & Rogoff, 2009). Weather, neighborhood violence, racial profiling, and other safety concerns impact parent attitudes and behaviors about outdoor, physical play, especially in families of color and lower income (Dias & Whitaker, 2013; Holt et al., 2016; Kepper et al., 2019; Pinckney, Outley, Brown, & Theriault, 2018; Tandon et al., 2017). Socioeconomic factors and racism may impact a family's time, space, and materials for play. These factors then interact with specific skills, health, and needs of the child with a disability (Sterman et al., 2016). Notably, the functional impact of cultural difference often is connected with inequities in social power relations, where dominant cultures are supported and marginalized cultures stressed, where some have power and privilege and others face racism, discrimination, and oppression (Agner, 2020; Beagan, 2015; Castro et al., 2014; dos Santos & Spesny, 2016).

Our own cultural assumptions based on our individual variables as well as our profession's may conflict with our clients' (Agner, 2020; Beagan, 2015). Occupational therapy has its own culture with values based in predominantly Western, Anglo-American, middle- and upper-class values such as autonomy, personal achievement, and goal-directed individual independence (Awaad, 2003; Beagan, 2015; Castro et al., 2014; dos Santos & Spesny, 2016). Even the research and conceptual development of therapeutic use of self have been predominately American (Solman & Clouston, 2016), and most research on culture in occupational therapy has been done by English-speaking researchers (Castro et al., 2014). The medical culture, in which occupational therapists practice, values the professional as expert, measurable and clearly defined procedures and outcomes, and fragmented and specialized service—a

culture that tends to conflict with developing family partnerships (Fingerhut et al., 2013; Lawlor & Mattingly, 1998). In contrast, some cultures value religion, family honor, societal welfare, and social occupations (Awaad, 2003; Zango Martín et al., 2015). We must recognize our own values and any position of privilege we may have.

Occupational therapists must build self-awareness of their own personal and professional culture as well as knowledge about others' cultures (Awaad, 2003; Beagan, 2015; Chiang & Carlson, 2003; Munoz, 2007; Wittman & Velde, 2002). However well-intentioned we may be, we must recognize our own unconscious bias. Karver et al.'s (2018) research indicates that therapists should "expect and honor divergent views about treatment goals and how to accomplish them" (p. 351) in order to build a productive therapeutic relationship. To be therapeutic, occupational therapists should strive to attain cultural humility and to provide cultural safety for families and caregivers (Agner, 2020; Beagan, 2015).

As we educate ourselves about other cultures, we must refrain from developing rules or stereotypes about different cultural groups because cultures can change over time, and individuals within the group may have unique experiences and values, which differ from others in a culture (Agner, 2020; Awaad, 2003; Castro et al., 2014; Chiang & Carlson, 2003). Cultural learning is an ongoing process where openness, curiosity, and critical self-reflection are essential (Agner, 2020; Beagan, 2015). The focus must be on determining each person's individual occupational meanings and preferences without any cultural assumptions and making occupational therapy relevant to each family (Beagan, 2015; Lindsay, Tétrault, Desmaris, King, & Piérart, 2014). It is not enough to recognize differences but also to consciously respect these differences (Awaad, 2003; Chiang & Carlson, 2003; Munoz, 2007; Wittman & Velde, 2002). By getting to know the children and caregivers with whom we work, valuing and leveraging their strengths, and recognizing inequities, we can work together as collaborators, not adversaries (Ng et al., 2020).

In order to understand a specific family's culture, the occupational therapist may ask the family about their background and request that they notify the therapist if there is something about therapy and play that does not feel right or fit in with their culture and values (Munoz, 2007). Given that culture cannot be seen or assumed, it is wise to consistently address culture in this direct manner with all families regardless of whether they seem culturally similar or dissimilar. However, the therapist may also need to respectfully ask for clarification when observing unexpected actions or unfamiliar practices. Awaad (2003) notes that if we do a good activity analysis of occupational meaning, cultural meaning will also be identified. We need to understand what is not working for a family and anticipate the barriers a family faces. Points of similarity must also be recognized for effective therapeutic use of self. For example, in her research with African American families who have children with medical illnesses and disabilities, Mattingly (2006) found that themes from children's popular play culture, such as Disney characters, can create a shared point for healthcare providers to interact with children and their families, despite differences in race, culture, and class. Knowledge about cultural differences and similarities is used to adapt various aspects of care from evaluation, goals, intervention, and research (Beagan, 2015; Reid & Chiu, 2011). Cultural elements such as specific materials, language, and customs can be included or adapted as valued aspects of play and therapy.

Family–Child Cultural Conflicts over Play

Culture is complex, often composed of multiple identities, and often marked by diversity within as well as across groups. Therefore, children and parents/caregivers do not always agree on the value of play in general or on specific types of play. Parents and other caregivers may disapprove of, discourage, or disallow their children's play preference. Therapists may also need to help advocate for children by sharing relevant information for parents and caregivers to consider (see **Figure 6.7**). Families may not want their children to play themes related to holidays they do not celebrate even if the child wants to play Halloween characters, Santa Claus, Easter Bunny, or pretend birthday parties; aggressive play themes (guns, war, killing, etc.); dark or dangerous themes (e.g., monsters); television shows or videos (e.g., Disney), or cross-gendered play. Families may disapprove of the child's play interest as inappropriate or as a sign of disability. In fact, some families do not value play for their child or themselves, perhaps because they are so focused on the child's disability and are committed to working hard to minimize the effects of the disability (Knox, 1993), or they simply value hard work (McConkey, 1994). In such cases, occupational therapists may want to discuss why play in general or a specific play theme may be helpful therapeutically for the child and the parent–child relationship (Ferland, 2005). With a strong knowledge about play (see Chapters 1 and 2), the occupational therapist is prepared to engage in such health conversations. The therapist may advocate for the child or help negotiate a compromise. We must simultaneously weigh our ethical responsibilities to the child, respect the family's culture, look for common ground, and focus on our

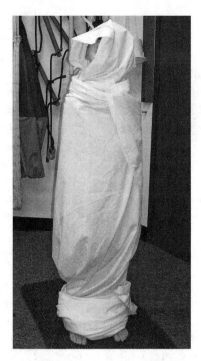

Figure 6.7 Being a mummy can be a new form of pretend play that allows the child to explore danger and fear themes. Although this can be especially culturally and temporally relevant at Halloween in some families, other families may object because of cultural values, religious beliefs, or personal opinions about appropriate play. The occupational therapist may discuss with the family the pros and cons of different forms of play for the child
Courtesy of Susan L. Spitzer.

therapeutic use of self to help the family facilitate the child's occupational performance.

Outcomes Research on Playful Therapeutic Use of Self

The research on therapeutic use of self and adult–child play supports the strategies detailed in this chapter. The bulk of the research on what playful therapeutic use of self is and how to implement it has been embedded throughout this chapter. This section presents additional research on the outcomes of therapeutic use of self and the relationship of adult–child play to children's play participation and development. These bodies of primarily descriptive and correlational research do have limitations with regard to causality. Given the limitations of the research, clinical experience is essential to supplement this research base, and professional reasoning is required to determine which strategies are a good match for individual children. Although future research certainly will clarify this process, current evidence does support the use of playful therapeutic use of self as an effective tool within pediatric occupational therapy.

Therapeutic relationships, the outcome of therapeutic use of self, are consistently associated with positive outcomes in occupational therapy (Taylor & Peloquin, 2008). Therapeutic relationships have been associated with perceptions of quality care, treatment adherence, client satisfaction, and occupational performance (Babatunde et al., 2017; Gunnarsson & Eklund, 2009; Hall et al., 2010; Kayes & McPherson, 2012). Therapeutic relationships have been correlated with client participation (Fan & Taylor, 2018; Pan & Liu, 2016). A meta-analysis found a positive correlation between therapeutic alliance and therapeutic outcomes for children and adolescents in psychotherapy (Karver et al., 2018). Collaboration between therapists and pediatric clients in a sensory integration approach has been associated with child engagement and social reciprocity (Holland et al., 2018). Parents report that therapists' relational skills with their children are more important than technical skills in pediatric rehabilitation because they want their children to feel safe (Crom et al., 2019). While supportive, this body of research is limited primarily in that (1) most of these studies are with adult clients and (2) they are not experimental studies in occupational therapy.

Given limitations of the direct research on therapeutic use of self, it is beneficial to consider the wealth of related research on adult–child interaction, which indicates that adult interaction can influence children's play and development. An adult's developmentally based responsiveness to a child's interest, body language, communication, and activities has been associated with advances in children's play and social skills (Belsky, Goode, & Most, 1980; Bornstein & Tamis-Lemonda, 1997; Landry et al., 2000). Infants, toddlers, and preschoolers play for longer time and in more complex ways when their mothers interact with them (Fiese, 1990; Haight & Miller, 1992; Slade, 1987; Sorce & Emde, 1981). Children 1–5 years of age are more playful when their mothers focus on the process of play such as self-exploration, decision making, and creativity (Waldman-Levi, Grinion, & Olson, 2019). When adults create play activities, children display increased participation and emotional well-being than when engaged in nonplay activities (Howard & McInnes, 2013; Wainwright et al., 2019). Experimental studies have demonstrated that approaching a task as play enhances children's problem solving and performance (McInnes et al., 2009; Thomas et al., 2006). Reciprocity in interpersonal relationships has been found to be important from infancy through adolescence to shape social competence (Feldman, Bamberger, & Kanat-Maymon, 2015). Even within a play-based approach, young children have significantly higher levels of engagement in activities that children select themselves (Wainwright et al., 2019).

Similar increases in play and development for children with disabilities have been associated with general and specific adult interactions. Play has been positively associated with caregiver interaction for young children who were born premature, who were institutionalized, and who have Down syndrome (Daunhauer, Coster, Tickle-Degnen, & Cermak, 2007; de Falco et al., 2010; Lawson, Parrinello, & Ruff, 1992). Playfulness in young children with motor delay has been associated with both the child's developmental abilities and the parents' responsiveness (Chiarello, Huntington, & Bundy, 2006). Evans and Meyer (1999) found that modifying adult interactions to use social and playful communication strategies was effective in decreasing negative behaviors in a 3-year-old with Rett syndrome. Recent research on adult interaction with children with ASD consistently demonstrates that increasing the quality of the adult's developmentally based responsiveness to the child's interest, body language, communication, and activities increases the child's play participation, play diversity, and communication (Flippin & Watson, 2015; Godin et al., 2019; Kasari et al., 2010; Shire, Gulsrud, & Kasari, 2016). Parental responsiveness to the child's interest (rather than redirecting or ignoring the child) has been associated with a higher level of object play and increased time in joint activity engagement for children with ASD (Flippin & Watson, 2011; Patterson et al., 2014; Ruble et al., 2008). Young children with ASD look at, approach, and touch adults more frequently when the adult looks at the child, smiles at the child, moves toward the child, has a relaxed body tone, makes sounds, imitates the child, and is playful (Nadel, Martini, Field, Escalona, & Lundy, 2008).

In sum, research findings to date support the use of therapeutic adult-child play-based interactions to facilitate children's play; however, more experimental research is needed. Researchers are focused on this valuable research in order to demonstrate the value of therapeutic use of self, ascertain how best to do it, and determine how to train clinicians in its use (Solman & Clouston, 2016; Taylor, 2008). The recent development of tools to measure therapist–client interactions (such as Babatunde et al., 2017; Fan & Taylor, 2016; Hall et al., 2010; Vegni, Mauri, D'Apice, & Moja, 2010) is promising for the future of research in this area. Hinojosa (2007) argued that innovation in occupational therapy requires concentrated study of therapeutic use of self and professional relationships. Specifically, we need more studies on therapeutic use of self with children and experimental studies that measure actual practices and dependent outcome variables for play (**Box 6.5**).

Box 6.5 **Research Questions for Future Studies of Playful Therapeutic Use of Self in Pediatric Occupational Therapy**

- Is playful therapeutic use of self an effective intervention tool for therapeutic participation, occupational participation, and play in pediatric occupational therapy?
- Is playful therapeutic use of self more effective than a nonplayful approach?
- Which therapeutic use of self strategies are most effective and for which specific groups of children?
- What factors are related to the development of more playful practitioners?
- How can classroom professors or fieldwork educators best promote playfulness as an outcome in occupational therapy practitioners through their educational activities?

Conclusion

The value of play is actualized through a playful therapeutic use of self. This powerful tool enables the occupational therapy practitioner to artfully adjust skilled interactions to match the individual child's interests, strengths, and challenges. It is a critical skill for all aspects of pediatric practice. Play knowledge informs how we are with clients. This chapter provides you with core knowledge, considerations, and strategies to get you started on developing your own playful therapeutic use of self and to help you reflect on your developing skills. A number of specific strategies are presented for communicating and building a playful therapeutic relationship with a pediatric client and their family. To apply the principles and concepts from this chapter into your practice, you will need to incorporate these strategies in practice and build your skills with thoughtful reflection. We hope that you may revisit this material over time to build and revitalize your playful therapeutic use of self. As you do, you are likely to experience how this playful approach engages the client and therapist despite the often-difficult work of therapy. With a playful therapeutic use of self, both practitioner and child can have fun as they unleash the power of play in occupational therapy.

References

Abreu, B. C. (2011). Accentuate the positive: Reflections on empathic interpersonal interactions (Eleanor Clarke Slagle Lecture). *American Journal of Occupational Therapy*, 65, 623–634. https://doi.org/10.5014/ajot.2011.656002

Adamson, L. B., Bakeman, R., Deckner, D. F., & Nelson, P. B. (2012). Rating parent–child interactions: Joint engagement, communication dynamic, and shared topics in autism, Down syndrome, and typical development. *Journal of Autism and Developmental Disorders*, 42, 2622–2635. https://doi.org/10.1007/s10803-012-1520-1

Aiken, F. E., Fourt, A. M., Cheng, I. K. S., & Polatajko, H. J. (2011). The meaning gap in occupational therapy: Finding meaning in our own occupation. *Canadian Journal of Occupational Therapy*, 78, 294–302. https://doi.org/10.2182/cjot.2011.78.5.4

Agner, J. (2020). The issue is—moving from cultural competence to cultural humility in occupational therapy: A paradigm shift. *American Journal of Occupational Therapy*, 74, 7404347010. https://doi.org/10.5014/ajot.2020.038067

Aldis, O. (1975). *Play fighting*. New York: Academic Press.

American Academy of Pediatrics. (2003). *Guide to toilet training*. https://healthychildren.org/English/ages-stages/toddler/toilet-training/Pages/Potty-Talk.aspx

American Occupational Therapy Association (AOTA). (2016). Occupational therapy services in the promotion of mental health and well-being. *American Journal of Occupational Therapy*, 70, 7012410070. http://dx.doi.org/10.5014/ajot.2016.706S05

American Occupational Therapy Association (AOTA). (2020). *AOTA's guide to acknowledging the impact of discrimination, stigma, and implicit bias on provision of services*. https://www.aota.org/-/media/Corporate/Files/Practice/Guide-Acknowledging-Impact-Discrimination-Stigma-Implicit-Bias.pdf

An, M., Palisano, R. J., Yi, C. H., Chiarello, L. A., Dunst, C. J., & Gracely, E. J. (2019a). Effects of a collaborative intervention process on parent empowerment and child performance: A randomized controlled trial. *Physical & Occupational Therapy in Pediatrics*, 39(1), 1–15. https://doi.org/10.1080/01942638.2017.1365324

An, M., Palisano, R. J., Yi, C. H., Chiarello, L. A., Dunst, C. J., & Gracely, E. J. (2019b). Effects of a collaborative intervention process on parent–therapist interaction: A randomized controlled trial. *Physical & Occupational Therapy in Pediatrics*, 39(3), 259–275. https://doi.org/10.1080/01942638.2018.1496965

Anderson, J., & Hinojosa, J. (1984). Parents and therapists in a professional partnership. *American Journal of Occupational Therapy*, 38, 452–461. https://doi.org/10.5014/ajot.38.7.452

Andonian, L. (2017). Emotional intelligence: An opportunity for occupational therapy. *Occupational Therapy in Mental Health*, 33(4), 299–307. https://doi.org/10.1080/0164212X.2017.1328649

Apter, M. J. (1991). A structural-phenomenology of play. In J. H. Kerr & M. J. Apter (Eds.), *Adult play: A reversal theory approach* (pp. 13–29). Amsterdam: Swets & Zeitlinger.

Arntzen, C. (2018). An embodied and intersubjective practice of occupational therapy. *OTJR: Occupation, participation and health*, *38*(3), 173–180. https://doi.org/10.1177/1539449217727470

Awaad, T. (2003). Culture, cultural competency, and occupational therapy: A review of the literature. *British Journal of Occupational Therapy*, *66*, 356–362. https://doi.org/10.1177/030802260306600804

Babatunde, F., MacDermid, J., & MacIntyre, N. (2017). Characteristics of therapeutic alliance in musculoskeletal physiotherapy and occupational therapy practice: A scoping review of the literature. *BMC Health Services Research*, *17*(1), 375. https://doi.org/10.1186/s12913-017-2311-3

Barnett, L. A. (2007). The nature of playfulness in young adults. *Personality and Individual Differences*, *43*, 949–958. https://doi.org/10.1016/j.paid.2007.02.018

Baron, K. B. (1991). The use of play in child psychiatry: Reframing the therapeutic environment. *Occupational Therapy in Mental Health*, *11*(2/3), 37–56. https://doi.org/10.1300/J004v11n02_04

Beagan, B. L. (2015). Approaches to culture and diversity: A critical synthesis of occupational therapy literature (des approches en matière de culture et de diversité: une synthèse critique de la littérature en ergothérapie). *Canadian Journal of Occupational Therapy*, *82*(5), 272–282. https://doi.org/10.1177/0008417414567530

Belsky, J., Goode, M. K., & Most, R. K. (1980). Maternal stimulation and infant exploratory competence: Cross-sectional, correlational, and experimental analyses. *Child development*, *51*(4), 1168-1178. https://doi.org/10.2307/1129558

Belsky, J., & Most, R. K. (1981). From exploration to play: A cross sectional study of infant-free play behavior. *Developmental Psychology*, *17*, 630–639. https://doi.org/10.1037/0012-1649.17.5.630

Berinstein, S., & Magalhaes, L. (2009). A study of the essence of play experience to children living in Zanzibar, Tanzania. *Occupational Therapy International*, *16*(2), 89–106. https://doi.org/10.1002/oti.270

Blanche, E. (1992). Creativity in sensory integrative treatment. *Sensory Integration Special Interest Section Newsletter*, *15*(1), 3–4.

Blanche, E. I. (2008). Play in children with cerebral palsy: Doing with—not doing to. In L. D. Parham & L. S. Fazio (Eds.), *Play in occupational therapy for children* (2nd ed., pp. 375–393). St. Louis, MO: Mosby Elsevier.

Bonsaksen, T. (2013). Self-reported therapeutic style in occupational therapy students. *British Journal of Occupational Therapy*, *76*(11), 496–502. https://doi.org/10.4276/030802213X13833255804595

Bornstein, M. H., & Tamis-LeMonda, C. A. (1997). Maternal responsiveness and infant mental abilities: Specific predictive relations. *Infant Behavior and Development*, *20*, 283–296. https://doi.org/10.1016/S0163-6383(97)90001-1

Bracegirdle, H. (1992). The use of play in occupational therapy for children: How the therapist can help. *British Journal of Occupational Therapy*, *55*, 201–202. https://doi.org/10.1177/030802269205500512

Brazelton, T. B., Koslowski, B., & Main, M. (1974). The origins of reciprocity: The early mother–infant interaction. In M. Lewis & L. A. Rosenblum (Eds.), *The effect of the infant on its caregiver* (pp. 49–76). New York: John Wiley & Sons.

Brodin, J. (2018). "It takes two to play": Reflections on play in children with multiple disabilities. *Today's Children: Tomorrow's Parents: An Interdisciplinary Journal*, *47–48*, 28–39.

Brown, A. M., Humphry, R., & Taylor, E. (1997). A model of the nature of family–therapist relationships: Implications for education. *American Journal of Occupational Therapy*, *51*, 597–603. https://doi.org/10.5014/ajot.51.7.597

Brown, M., Christensen, K., Schroer, L., Steffan, J., Carlson, A., Giraud, A., et al. (2008, April). *Perceived indicators of engagement in children with autism spectrum disorders participating in sensory-based activities*. Poster presented at the annual conference of the American Occupational Therapy Association, Long Beach, CA.

Burke, J. P. (1977). A clinical perspective on motivation: Pawn versus origin. *American Journal of Occupational Therapy*, *31*(4), 254–258.

Burke, J. P. (2010). What's going on here? Deconstructing the interactive encounter (Eleanor Clarke Slagle Lecture). *American Journal of Occupational Therapy*, *64*, 855–868. https://doi.org/10.5014/ajot.2010.64604

Carstensen, T., & Bonsaksen, T. (2017). Differences and similarities in therapeutic mode use between occupational therapists and occupational therapy students in Norway. *Scandinavian Journal of Occupational Therapy*, *24*(6), 448–454. https://doi.org/10.1080/11038128.2016.1261940

Cascio, C. J., Moore, D., & McGlone, F. (2019). Social touch and human development. *Developmental Cognitive Neuroscience*, *35*, 5–11. https://doi.org/10.1016/j.dcn.2018.04.009

Case-Smith, J. (1997). Variables related to successful school-based practice. *Occupational Therapy Journal of Research*, *17*, 133–153. https://doi.org/10.1177/153944929701700208

Castro, D., Dahlin-Ivanoff, S., & Mårtensson, L. (2014). Occupational therapy and culture: A literature review. *Scandinavian Journal of Occupational Therapy*, *21*(6), 401–414. http://dx.doi.org/10.3109/11038128.2014.898086

Champagne, T. (2011). Attachment, trauma, and occupational therapy practice. *OT Practice*, *16*(5), C1–C8.

Chapman, R. (2016). A case study of gendered play in preschools: How early childhood educators' perceptions of gender influence children's play. *Early Child Development and Care*, *186*(8), 1271–1284, https://doi.org/10.1080/03004430.2015.1089435

Chen, Y. L., Senande, L. L., Thorsen, M., & Patten, K. (2021). Peer preferences and characteristics of same-group and cross-group social interactions among autistic and non-autistic adolescents. *Autism*, *25*(7), 1885-1900. https://doi.org/10.1177/13623613211005918

Chiang, M., & Carlson, G. (2003). Occupational therapy in multicultural contexts: Issues and strategies. *British Journal of Occupational Therapy*, *66*, 559–567. https://doi.org/10.1177/030802260306601204

Chiarello, L. A., Huntington, A., & Bundy, A. (2006). A comparison of motor behaviors, interaction, and playfulness during mother–child and father–child play with children with motor delay: Implications for early intervention practice.

Occupational & Physical Therapy in Pediatrics, *26*(1/2), 129–152. https://doi.org/10.1080/J006v26n01_09

Cole, M. B., & McLean, V. (2003). Therapeutic relationships re-defined. *Occupational Therapy in Mental Health*, *19*(2), 33–56. https://doi.org/10.1300/J004v19n02_03

Correa-Chávez, M., & Rogoff, B. (2009). Children's attention to interactions directed to others: Guatemalan Mayan and European American patterns. *Developmental Psychology*, *45*(3), 630–641. https://doi.org/10.1037/a0014144

Corsaro, W. A., & Eder, D. (1990). Children's peer cultures. *Annual Review of Sociology*, *16*, 197–220.

Crepeau, E. B. (1991). Achieving intersubjective understanding: Examples from an occupational therapy treatment session. *American Journal of Occupational Therapy*, *45*, 1016–1025. https://doi.org/10.5014/ajot.45.11.1016

Crepeau, E. B., & Garren, K. R. (2011). I looked to her as a guide: The therapeutic relationship in hand therapy. *Disability and Rehabilitation*, *33*(10), 872–881, https://doi.org/10.3109/0963 8288.2010.511419

Crom, A., Paap, D., Wijma, A., Dijkstra, P. U., & Pool, G. (2019): Between the lines: A qualitative phenomenological analysis of the therapeutic alliance in pediatric physical therapy. *Physical & Occupational Therapy in Pediatrics*, *40*(1), 1–14. https://doi .org/ 10.1080/01942638.2019.1610138

Crompton, C. J., Sharp, M., Axbey, H., Fletcher-Watson, S., Flynn, E. G., & Ropar, D. (2020). Neurotype-matching, but not being autistic, influences self and observer ratings of interpersonal rapport. *Frontiers in psychology*, *11*, 2961. https://doi.org /10.3389/fpsyg.2020.586171

Curtin, C. (2001). Eliciting children's voices in qualitative research. *American Journal of Occupational Therapy*, *55*, 295–302. https://doi.org/10.5014/ajot.55.3.295

Curtin, C. (2017). *Strategies for collaborating with children: Creating partnerships in occupational therapy and research*. Thorofare, NJ: Slack Incorporated.

Damast, A. M., Tamis-LeMonda, C. S., & Bornstein, M. H. (1996). Mother–child play: Sequential interactions and the relation between maternal beliefs and behaviors. *Child Development*, *67*, 1752–1766. https://doi.org/10.1111/j.1467-8624.1996.tb01825.x

D'Arrigo, R., Copley, J. A., Poulsen, A. A., & Ziviani, J. (2019). Parent engagement and disengagement in paediatric settings: An occupational therapy perspective. *Disability and Rehabilitation*, 1–12. https://doi.org/10.1080/09638288.2019 .1574913

D'Arrigo, R. G., Copley, J. A., Poulsen, A. A., & Ziviani, J. (2020). The engaged child in occupational therapy. *Canadian Journal of Occupational Therapy*, *87*(2), 127–136. https://doi .org/10.1177/0008417420905708

Davis, J. T. M., & Hines, M. (2020). How large are gender differences in toy preferences? A systematic review and meta-analysis of toy preference research. *Archives of Sexual Behavior*, *49*, 373–394. https://doi.org/10.1007/s10508-019-01624-7

Daunhauer, L. A., Coster, W. J., Tickle-Degnen, L., & Cermak, S. A. (2007). Effects of caregiver–child interactions on play occupations among young children institutionalized in Eastern Europe. *American Journal of Occupational Therapy*, *61*, 429–440. https://doi.org/10.5014/ajot.61.4.429

Deák, G. O., Krasno, A. M., Jasso, H., & Triesch, J. (2018). What leads to shared attention? Maternal cues and infant responses during object play. *Infancy*, *23*(1), 4–28. https://doi.org/10.1111 /infa.12204

de Falco, S., Esposito, G., Venuti, P., & Bornstein, M. H. (2010). Mothers and fathers at play with their children with Down syndrome: Influence on child exploratory and symbolic activity. *Journal of Applied Research in Intellectual Disabilities: JARID*, *23*(6), 597–605. https://doi.org/10.1111/j.1468 -3148.2010.00558.x

Delafield-Butt, J. T., Zeedyk, M. S., Harder, S., Væver, M. S., & Caldwell, P. (2020). Making meaning together: Embodied narratives in a case of severe autism. *Psychopathology*, 1–14. https://doi.org/10.1159/000506648

Delafield-Butt, J. (2021). Autism and panpsychism: Putting process in mind. *Journal of Consciousness Studies 28*(9-10), 76-90. https://doi.org/10.53765/20512201.28.9.076

Delahooke, M. (2020). *Beyond behaviours: Using brain science and compassion to understand and solve children's behavioural challenges*. London: Hachette UK.

Devereaux, E. B. (1984). Occupational therapy's challenge: The caring relationship. *American Journal of Occupational Therapy*, *38*, 791–798. https://doi.org/10.5014/ajot.38.12.791

Dias, J. J., & Whitaker, R. C. (2013). Black mothers' perceptions about urban neighborhood safety and outdoor play for their preadolescent daughters. *Journal of Health Care for the Poor and Underserved*, *24*(1), 206–219. 10.1353/hpu.2013.0018

Dos Santos, V., & Spesny, S. L. (2016). Questioning the concept of culture in mainstream occupational therapy (Questionando o conceito de cultura nas linhas de terapia ocupacional dominantes). *Cadernos Brasileiros de Terapia Ocupacional*, *24*(1), 185–190. http://dx.doi.org/10.4322/0104-4931 .ctoRE0675

Doussard-Roosevelt, J. A., Joe, C. M., Bazhenova, O. V., & Porges, S. W. (2003). Mother–child interaction in autistic and nonautistic children: Characteristics of maternal approach behaviors and child social responses. *Development and Psychopathology*, *15*, 277–295. https://doi.org/10.1017 /S0954579403000154

Downs, M. L. (2008). Leisure routines: Parents and children with disability sharing occupation. *Journal of Occupational Science*, *15*, 105–110. https://doi.org/10.1080/14427591.2008.9686 616

Dunn, J., Wooding, C., & Hermann, J. (1977). Mothers' speech to young children: Variation in context. *Developmental Medicine & Child Neurology*, *19*, 629–638. https://doi.org /10.1111/j.1469-8749.1977.tb07996.x

Dunn, W. (2000). *Best practice occupational therapy in community service with children and families*. Thorofare, NJ: Slack.

Durand, V. M., Hieneman, M., Clarke, S., & Zona, M. (2009). Optimistic parenting: Hope and help for parents with challenging children. In W. Sailor, G. Dunlap, G. Sugai, & R. Horner (Eds), *Handbook of Positive Behavior Support: Issues in Clinical Child Psychology* (pp. 233–256). Springer, Boston, MA. https://doi.org/10.1007/978-0-387-09632-2_10

Durig, A. (1996). *Autism and the crisis of meaning*. Albany: State University of New York Press.

Eberle, S. G. (2014). The elements of play: Toward a philosophy and a definition of play. *American Journal of Play*, *6*(2), 214–233.

Esseily, R., Rat-Fischer, L., Somogyi, E., O'Reagan, K. J., & Fagard, J. (2016). Humor production may enhance observational learning of a new tool-use action in 18-month-old infants.

Cognition and Emotion, *30*(4), 817–825. https://doi.org / 10.1080/02699931.2015.1036840

Evans, I. M., & Meyer, L. H. (1999). Modifying adult interactional style as positive behavioural intervention for a child with Rett syndrome. *Journal of Intellectual & Developmental Disability*, *24*, 191–205. https://doi.org/10.1080/13668259900033981

Fagard, J., Rat-Fischer, L., Esseily, R., Somogyi, E., & O'Regan, J. K. (2016). What does it take for an infant to learn how to use a tool by observation? *Frontiers in Psychology*, *7*, 267. http://doi .org/10.3389/fpsyg.2016.00267

Fan, C. W., & Taylor, R. R. (2016). Assessing therapeutic communication during rehabilitation: The Clinical Assessment of Modes. *American Journal of Occupational Therapy*, *70*, 7004280010. http://dx.https://doi.org/org/10.5014/ajot.2016 .018846

Fan, C. W., & Taylor, R. (2018). Correlation between therapeutic use of self and clients' participation in rehabilitation. *The American Journal of Occupational Therapy*, *72*(4), 1. doi: http://dx .doi.org/10.5014/ajot.2018.72S1-PO5001

Feldhusen, J. F., & Goh, B. E. (1995). Assessing and accessing creativity: An integrative review of theory, research and development. *Creativity Research Journal*, *8*, 231–247. https:// doi.org/10.1207/s15326934crj0803_3

Feldman, R. (2009). The development of regulatory functions from birth to 5 years: Insights from premature infants. *Child Development*, *80*, 544–561. https://doi.org/10.1111/j.1467 -8624.2009.01278.x

Feldman, R., Bamberger, E., & Kanat-Maymon, Y. (2015). Parent-specific reciprocity from infancy to adolescence shapes children's social competence and dialogical skills. *Attachment and Human Development*, *15*, 407–423. https://doi.org/10.108 0/14616734.2013.782650

Ferland, F. (2005). *The Ludic model: Play, children with physical disabilities and occupational therapy* (2nd ed.). Ottawa, Ontario: Canadian Association of Occupational Therapists. Retrieved from https:// search.proquest.com/docview/213007487?accountid=143111

Festante, F., Antonelli, C., Chorna, O., Corsi, G., & Guzzetta, A. (2019). Parent–infant interaction during the first year of life in infants at high risk for cerebral palsy: A systematic review of the literature. *Neural Plasticity*, *2019*. https://doi .org/10.1155/2019/5759694

Field, T., Hernandez-Reif, M., Diego, M., Corbin, J., Stutzman, M., Orozco, A., . . . Allender, S. (2014). Imitation can reduce repetitive behaviors and increase play behaviors in children with ASD. *Psychology*, *5*, 1463–1467. https://doi.org/10.4236 /psych.2014.512157

Fiese, B. H. (1990). Playful relationships: A contextual analysis of mother–toddler interaction and symbolic play. *Child Development*, *61*, 1648–1656. https://doi.org /10.1111/j.1467-8624.1990.tb02891.x

Fine, G. A., & Sandstrom, K. L. (1988). *Knowing children: Participant observation with minors*. Newbury Park, CA: Sage.

Fingerhut, P. E., Piro, J., Sutton, A., Campbell, R., Lewis, C., Lawji, D., & Martinez, N. (2013). Family-centered principles implemented in home-based, clinic-based, and school-based pediatric settings. *American Journal of Occupational Therapy*, *67*, 228–235. http://dx.doi.org/10.5014/ajot.2013.006957

Fleming, M. H. (1994). Conditional reasoning: Creating meaningful experiences. In C. Mattingly & M. H. Fleming

(Eds.), *Clinical reasoning: Forms of inquiry in a therapeutic practice* (pp. 197–235). Philadelphia: F. A. Davis.

Fletcher, T. S. (2010). A grounded theory analysis of the relationship between creativity and occupational therapy. (Publication No. 3405818). [Doctoral dissertation, Texas A & M University-Commerce]. *ProQuest Dissertations Publishing*. Retrieved from https:// search.proquest.com/docview/251013499?accountid=143111

Flippin, M., & Watson, L. R. (2011). Relationships between the responsiveness of fathers and mothers and the object play skills of children with autism spectrum disorders. *Journal of Early Intervention*, *33*(3), 220–234. 10.1177/1053815111427445

Flippin, M., & Watson, L. R. (2015). Fathers' and mothers' verbal responsiveness and the language skills of young children with autism spectrum disorder. *American Journal of Speech-Language Pathology*, *24*(3), 400–410. https://doi.org/10.1044/2015 _AJSLP-13-0138

Franchak, J. M., Kretch, K. S., & Adolph, K. E. (2018). See and be seen: Infant–caregiver social looking during locomotor free play. *Developmental Science*, *21*(4), e12626. https://doi .org/10.1111/desc.12626

Frank, G. (2000). *Venus on wheels*. Berkeley: University of California Press.

Frank, J. D. (1958). The therapeutic use of self. *American Journal of Occupational Therapy*, *12*, 215–225.

Fusco, D. (2012). Use of self in the context of youth work. *Child & Youth Services*, *33*(1), 33–45. https://doi.org/10.1080/01459 35X.2012.665323

Gahnstrom-Strandqvist, K., Tham, K., Josephsson, S., & Borell, L. (2000). Actions of competence in occupational therapy practice. *Scandinavian Journal of Occupational Therapy*, *7*, 15–25. https://doi.org/10.1080/110381200443580

Gilfoyle, E. M. (1980). Caring: A philosophy for practice. *American Journal of Occupational Therapy*, *34*, 517–521.

Godin, J., Freeman, A., & Rigby, P. (2019). Interventions to promote the playful engagement in social interaction of preschool-aged children with autism spectrum disorder (ASD): A scoping study. *Early Child Development and Care*, *189*, 10, 1666–1681. https://doi.org/10.1080/03004430.2017.1404999

Goldstein, J. (1995). Aggressive toy play. In A. D. Pellegrini (Ed.), *The future of play theory* (pp. 127–147). Albany: State University of New York Press.

Goode, D. A. (1980). The world of the congenitally deaf-blind. In J. Jacobs (Ed.), *Mental retardation: A phenomenological approach* (pp. 187–207). Springfield, IL: Charles C. Thomas.

Goode, D. (1994). *A world without words: The social construction of children born deaf and blind*. Philadelphia, PA: Temple University Press.

Goodhall, N., & Atkinson, C. (2017). How do children distinguish between "play" and "work"? Conclusions from the literature. *Early Child Development and Care*, *189*(10), 1695–1708. https://doi.org/10.1080/03004430.2017.1406484

Gorenberg, M. (2013). Instructional Insights: Continuing Professional Education to Enhance Therapeutic Relationships in Occupational Therapy. *Occupational Therapy In Health Care*, *27*(4), 393-398. https://doi.org/10.3109/07380577.2013.834404

Graham, N., Mandy, A., Clarke, C., & Morriss-Roberts, C. (2019). Play experiences of children with a high level of physical disability. *American Journal of Occupational Therapy*, *73*, 7306205010. https://doi.org/10.5014/ajot.2019.032516

Graham, N. E., Truman, J., & Holgate, H. (2015). Parents' understanding of play for children with cerebral palsy. *American Journal of Occupational Therapy*, *69*, 6903220050. http://dx.doi.org/10.5014/ajot.2015.015263

Grandin, T. (1995). *Thinking in pictures and other reports from my life with autism*. New York: Doubleday.

Grandin, T., & Scariano, M. M. (1986). *Emergence: Labeled autistic*. Novato, CA: Arean Press.

Greenspan, S. I., & Wieder, S. (1997). An integrated developmental approach to interventions for young children with severe difficulties in relating and communicating. *Zero to Three*, *17*, 5–17.

Greenspan, S. I., Wieder, S., & Simons, R. (1998). *The child with special needs: Encouraging intellectual and emotional growth*. Reading, MA: Addison-Wesley/Addison Wesley Longman.

Guidetti, S., & Tham, K. (2002). Therapeutic strategies used by occupational therapists in self-care training: A qualitative study. *Occupational Therapy International*, *9*, 257–276. https://doi.org/10.1002/oti.168

Guitard, P., Ferland, F., & Dutil, É. (2005). Toward a better understanding of playfulness in adults. *OTJR: Occupation, Participation and Health*, *25*(1), 9–22. https://doi.org/10.1177/153944920502500103

Gunnarsson, A. B., & Eklund, M. (2009). The tree theme method as an intervention in psychosocial occupational therapy: Client acceptability and outcomes. *Australian Occupational Therapy Journal*, *56*, 167–176. http://dx.doi.org/10.1111/j.1440-1630.2008.00738.x

Gupta, S., Paterson, M. L., Lysaght, R. M., & von Zweck, C. M. (2012). Experiences of burnout and coping strategies utilized by occupational therapists. *Canadian Journal of Occupational Therapy*, *79*, 86–95. https://doi.org/10.2182/cjot.2012.79.2.4

Haight, W. L., & Miller, P. J. (1992). The development of everyday pretend play: A longitudinal study of mothers' participation. *Merrill-Palmer Quarterly*, *38*, 331–349. https://www.jstor.org/stable/23087259

Hall, A. M., Ferreira, P. H., Maher, C. G., Latimer, J., & Ferreira, M. L. (2010). The influence of the therapist–patient relationship on treatment outcome in physical rehabilitation: A systematic review. *Physical Therapy*, *90*, 1099–1110. https://doi.org/10.2522/ptj.20090245

Hall, E. T. (1982). *The hidden dimension*. Garden City, NY: Doubleday. (Original work published 1966).

Halliday, S., & Leslie, J. C. (1986). A longitudinal cross-sectional study of the development of mother–child interaction. *British Journal of Developmental Psychology*, *4*, 211–222. https://doi.org/10.1111/j.2044-835X.1986.tb01013.x

Hasselkus, B. R., & Dickie, V. A. (1994). Doing occupational therapy: Dimensions of satisfaction and dissatisfaction. *American Journal of Occupational Therapy*, *48*, 145–154. https://doi.org/10.5014/ajot.48.2.145

Hellendoorn, J. (1994). Imaginative play training for severely retarded children. In J. Hellendoorn, R. van der Kooij, & B. Sutton-Smith (Eds.), *Play and intervention* (pp. 113–122). Albany: State University of New York Press.

Henricks, T. S. (1999). Play as ascending meaning: Implications of a general model of play. In S. Reifel (Ed.), *Play & culture studies: Vol. 2. Play contexts revisited* (pp. 257–277). Westport, CT: Ablex.

Hertenstein, M. J., Veerkamp, J. M., Kerestes, A. M., & Holmes, R. M. (2006). The communicative functions of touch in humans, nonhuman primates, and rats. A review and synthesis of the empirical research. *Genetic, Social, and General Psychology Monographs*, *132*, 5–94. https://doi.org/10.3200/MONO.132.1.5-94

Hildenbrand, W. C. (2019). Inaugural Presidential Address, 2019—Let's start here: Relationships, resilience, relevance. *American Journal of Occupational Therapy*, *73*, 7306130010. https://doi.org/10.5014/ajot.2019.736004

Hinojosa, J. (2007). Becoming Innovators in an era of hyperchange (Eleanor Clarke Slagle Lecture). *American Journal of Occupational Therapy*, *61*, 629–637. https://doi.org/10.5014/ajot.61.6.629

Hoicka, E., & Gattis, M. (2008). Do the wrong thing: How toddlers tell a joke from a mistake. *Cognitive Development*, *23*(1), 180–190. https://doi.org/10.1016/j.cogdev.2007.06.001

Holland, C., & Thompson, B. (2018). Mechanisms of co-constructing play between preschool-age children and novel adults. *American Journal of Occupational Therapy*, *72*(4_Supplement_1), 7211520319p1. https://doi.org/10.5014/ajot.2018.72S1-PO5026

Holland, C., Yay, O., Gallini, G., Blanche, E., & Thompson, B. (2018). Relationships between therapist and client actions during sensory integration therapy for young children with autism. *American Journal of Occupational Therapy*, *72*(4_Supplement_1), 7211515250p1. https://https://doi.org/org/10.5014/ajot.2018.72S1-PO4034

Holloway, E. (2008). Fostering early parent–infant playfulness in the neonatal intensive care unit. In L. D. Parham & L. S. Fazio (Eds.), *Play in occupational therapy for children* (2nd ed., pp. 335–350). St. Louis, MO: Mosby Elsevier.

Holt, N. L., Neely, K. C., Spence, J. C., Carson, V., Pynn, S. R., Boyd, K. A., . . . Robinson, Z. (2016). An intergenerational study of perceptions of changes in active free play among families from rural areas of Western Canada. *BMC Public Health*, *16*(1), 829. https://doi.org/10.1186/s12889-016-3490-2

Horvath, A. O., Del Re, A. C., Flückiger, C., & Symonds, D. (2011). Alliance in individual psychotherapy. *Psychotherapy*, *48*(1), 9. https://doi.org/10.1037/a0022186

Howard, J. (2002). Eliciting young children's perceptions of play, work and learning using the activity apperception story procedure. *Early Child Development and Care*, *172*, 489–502. https://doi.org/10.1080/03004430214548

Howard, J., Jenvey, V., & Hill, C. (2006). Children's categorization of play and learning based on social context. *Early Child Development and Care*, *176*, 379–393. https://doi.org/10.1080/03004430500063804

Howard, J., & McInnes, K. (2013). The impact of children's perception of an activity as play rather than not play on emotional well-being. *Child: Care, Health and Development*, *39*, 737–742. https://doi.org/10.1111/j.1365-2214.2012.01405.x

Hussain, R. A., Carstensen, T., Yazdani, F., Ellingham, B., & Bonsaksen, T. (2018). Short-term changes in occupational therapy students' self-efficacy for therapeutic use of self. *British Journal of Occupational Therapy*, *81*(5), 276–284. https://doi.org/10.1177/0308022617745007

Jaffe, L., Cosper, S., & Fabrizi, S. (2020). Working with families. In J. O'Brien and H. Kuhaneck (Eds.), *Case-Smith's occupational therapy for children* (8th ed., pp. 46–75). St. Louis, MO: Elsevier.

Johnson, J. E., Welteroth, S. J., & Corl, S. M. (2001). Attitudes of parents and teachers about play aggression in young children. In S. Reifel (Ed.), *Play & culture studies: Vol. 3. Theory in context and out* (pp. 335–354). Westport, CT: Ablex.

Josephidou, J. (2019): A gendered contribution to play? Perceptions of Early Childhood Education and Care (ECEC) practitioners in England on how their gender influences their approaches to play. *Early Years*, 1–14. https://doi.org/10.1080/09575146.2019.1655713

Kaplan, E. B. (1997). *Not our kind of girl: Unraveling the myths of Black teenage motherhood*. Los Angeles: University of California.

Karver, M. S., De Nadai, A. S., Monahan, M., & Shirk, S. R. (2018). Meta-analysis of the prospective relation between alliance and outcome in child and adolescent psychotherapy. *Psychotherapy*, 55(4), 341–355. https://doi.org/10.1037/pst0000176

Kasari, C., Gulsrud, A. C., Wong, C. Kwon, S., & Locke, J. (2010). Randomized controlled caregiver mediated joint engagement intervention for toddlers with autism. *Journal of Autism and Developmental Disorders*, 40, 1045–1056. https://doi.org/10.1007/s10803-010-0955-5

Kayes, N. M., & McPherson, K. M. (2012). Human technologies in rehabilitation: 'Who' and 'How' we are with our clients. *Disability and Rehabilitation*, 34(22), 1907–1911. https://doi.org/10.3109/09638288.2012.670044

Kepper, M. M., Staiano, A. E., Katzmarzyk, P. T., Reis, R. S., Eyler, A. A., Griffith, D. M., Michelle, L. Kendall, M. L., ElBanna, B., Denstel, K. D., & Broyles, S. T. (2019). Neighborhood Influences on Women's Parenting Practices for Adolescents' Outdoor Play: A Qualitative Study. *International Journal of Environmental Research and Public Health*, 16(20), 3853. https://doi.org/10.3390/ijerph16203853

King, G. (2017). The role of the therapist in therapeutic change: How knowledge from mental health can inform pediatric rehabilitation. *Physical & Occupational Therapy in Pediatrics*, 37(2), 121–138. https://doi.org/10.1080/01942638.2016.1185508

King, G., Chiarello, L. A., Phoenix, M., D'Arrigo, R., & Pinto, M. (2021). Co-constructing engagement in pediatric rehabilitation: A multiple case study approach. *Disability and Rehabilitation*, 1–12. https://doi.org/10.1080/09638288.2021.1910353

King, G., Williams, L., & Hahn Goldberg, S. (2017). Family-oriented services in pediatric rehabilitation: A scoping review and framework to promote parent and family wellness. *Child: Care, Health and Development*, 43, 334–347. https://doi.org/10.1111/cch.12435.

King, P., & Howard, J. (2010). Understanding children's free play at home, in school and at the after school club: A preliminary investigation into play types, social grouping and perceived control. *The Psychology of Education Review*, 34(1), 32–41.

King, P., & Howard, J. (2014a). Children's perceptions of choice in relation to their play at home, in the school playground and at the out-of-school club. *Children & Society*, 28(2), 116–127. https://doi.org/10.1111/j.1099-0860.2012.00455.x

King, P., & Howard, J. (2014b). Factors influencing children's perceptions of choice within their free play activity: The impact of functional, structural and social affordances. *Journal of Playwork Practice*, 1(2), 173–190. https://doi.org/10.1332/205316214X14114616128010

Kinkead-Clark, Z. (2019). Exploring children's play in early years learning environments; What are the factors that shape children's play in the classroom? *Journal of Early Childhood Research*, 17(3), 177–189. https://doi.org/10.1177/1476718X19849251

Knox, S. (2008). Development and current use of the revised Knox Preschool Play Scale. In L. D. Parham & L. S. Fazio (Eds.), *Play in occupational therapy for children* (2nd ed., pp. 55–70). St. Louis, MO: Mosby Elsevier.

Knox, S. H. (1993). Play and leisure. In H. L. Hopkins & H. D. Smith (Eds.), *Willard and Spackman's occupational therapy* (8th ed., pp. 260–268). Philadelphia: Lippincott.

Kollmayer, M., Schultes, M. T., Schober, B., Hodosi, T., & Spiel, C. (2018). Parents' judgments about the desirability of toys for their children: Associations with gender role attitudes, gender-typing of toys, and demographics. *Sex Roles*, 79(5–6), 329–341. https://doi.org/10.1007/s11199-017-0882-4

Kruijsen-Terpstra, A. J. A., Ketelaar, M., Boeije, H., Jongmans, M. J., Gorter, J. W., Verheijden, J., Lindeman, E., & Verschuren, O. (2014). Parents' experiences with physical and occupational therapy for their young child with cerebral palsy: A mixed studies review. *Child: Care, Health and Development*, 40(6), 787–796. https://doi.org/10.1111/cch.12097

Kruijsen-Terpstra, A., Verschuren, O., Ketelaar, M., Riedijk, L., Gorter, J. W., Jongmans, M. J., . . . LEARN 2 MOVE 2-3,Study Group. (2016). Parents' experiences and needs regarding physical and occupational therapy for their young children with cerebral palsy. *Research in Developmental Disabilities*, 53–54, 314–322. https://doi.org/http://dx.doi.org/10.1016/j.ridd.2016.02.012

Kuhaneck, H., Spitzer, S. L., & Bodison, S. C. (2019). *A systematic review of interventions to improve the occupation of play in children with autism*. OTJR: Occupation, Participation and Health. https://doi.org/10.1177/1539449219880531

Kuo, D. Z., Houtrow, A. J., Arango, P., Kuhlthau, K. A., Simmons, J. M., & Neff, J. M. (2012). Family-centered care: Current applications and future directions in pediatric health care. *Maternal and Child Health Journal*, 16(2), 297–305. DOI 10.1007/s10995-011-0751-7

Landry, S. H., Smith, K. E., Swank, P. R., & Miller-Loncar, C. L. (2000). Early maternal and child influences on children's later independent cognitive and social functioning. *Child Development*, 71, 358–375. https://doi.org/10.1111/1467-8624.00150

Lawlor, M. C. (2012). The particularities of engagement: Intersubjectivity in occupational therapy practice. *OTJR: Occupation, Participation and Health*, 32(4), 151–159. https://doi.org/http://dx.doi.org/10.3928/15394492-20120302-01

Lawlor, M. C., & Mattingly, C. F. (1998). The complexities embedded in family-centered care. *American Journal of Occupational Therapy*, 52, 259–267.

Lawson, K. R., Parrinello, R., & Ruff, H. A. (1992). Maternal behavior and infant attention. *Infant Behavior and Development*, 15, 209–229. https://doi.org/10.1016/0163-6383(92)80024-O

Leach, M. J. (2005). Rapport: A key to treatment success. *Complementary therapies in clinical practice*, 11(4), 262–265. https://doi.org/10.1016/j.ctcp.2005.05.005

Leber, D., & Vanoli, E. (2001). Therapeutic use of humor: Occupational therapy clinicians' perceptions and practices. *American Journal of Occupational Therapy, 55*(2), 221–226.

Lillas, C., TenPas, H., Crowley, C., & Spitzer, S.L. (2018). Improving regulation skills for increased participation for individuals with ASD. In R. Watling and S.L. Spitzer (Eds)., *Autism Across the Lifespan: A Comprehensive Occupational Therapy Approach* (4th Edition, pp. 319-338). Bethesda, MD: AOTA press.

Lindsay, S., Tétrault, S., Desmaris, C., King, G. A., & Piérart, G. (2014). The cultural brokerage work of occupational therapists in providing culturally sensitive care (Le travail de médiation culturelle effectué par des ergothérapeutes offrant des soins adaptés à la culture). *Canadian Journal of Occupational Therapy, 81*(2), 114–123. https://doi.org/10.1177/0008417413520441

Lindström, L., & Isaksson, G. (2017). Personalized occupational transformations: Narratives from two occupational therapists' experiences with complex therapeutic processes. *Occupational Therapy in Mental Health, 33*(1), 15–30. https://doi.org/10.1080/0164212X.2016.1194243

Little, H. (2010). Relationship between parents' beliefs and their responses to children's risk-taking behaviour during outdoor play. *Journal of Early Childhood Research, 8*(3), 315–330. https://doi.org/10.1177/1476718X10368587

Lloyd, C., & Maas, F. (1991). The therapeutic relationship. *British Journal of Occupational Therapy, 54,* 111–113. https://doi.org/10.1177/030802269105400309

Luken, M., & Sammons, A. (2016). Systematic review of mindfulness practice for reducing job burnout. *American Journal of Occupational Therapy, 70,* 7002250020. https://doi.org/10.5014/ajot.2016.016956

Lynch, H., & Stanley, M. (2018). Beyond words: Using qualitative video methods for researching occupation with young children. *OTJR: Occupation, Participation and Health, 38*(1), 56–66. https://doi.org/10.1177/1539449217718504

Maloney, S. M., & Griffith, K. (2013). Occupational therapy students' development of therapeutic communication skills during a service-learning experience. *Occupational Therapy in Mental Health, 29*(1), 10–26. https://doi.org/10.1080/0164212X.2013.760288

Masten, A., & Barnes, A. (2018). Resilience in children: Developmental perspectives. *Children, 5*(7), 98. https://doi.org/10.3390/children5070098

Mattingly, C. (2006). Pocahontas goes to the clinic: Popular culture as Lingua Franca in a cultural borderland. *American Anthropologist, 108,* 494–501. https://doi.org/10.1525/aa.2006.108.3.494

Mattingly, C., & Fleming, M. H. (1994). Interactive reasoning: Collaborating with the person. In C. Mattingly & M. H. Fleming (Eds.), *Clinical reasoning: Forms of inquiry in a therapeutic practice* (pp. 178–196). Philadelphia: F. A. Davis.

Mayer, E. R. (2010). Fifty years of creativity research. In R. J. Sternberg (Ed.), *Handbook of creativity* (pp. 449–461). Cambridge, UK: Cambridge University Press.

Mayeroff, M. (1971). *On caring.* New York: Harper Perennial.

McColl, M. A. (2003). Spirituality and disability. In M. A. McColl (Ed.), *Spirituality and occupational therapy* (pp. 19–30). Ottawa, Ontario, Canada: Canadian Association of Occupational Therapists.

McConkey, R. (1994). Families at play: Interventions for children with developmental handicaps. In J. Hellendoorn, R. van der Kooij, & B. Sutton-Smith (Eds.), *Play and intervention* (pp. 123–132). Albany: State University of New York Press.

McCorquodale, L., & Kinsella, E. A. (2015). Critical reflexivity in client-centred therapeutic relationships. *Scandinavian Journal of Occupational Therapy, 22*(4), 311–317. https://doi.org/10.3109/11038128.2015.1018319

McInnes, K. (2019). Playful learning in the early years—through the eyes of children. *Education 3–13, 47*(7), 796–805. https://doi.org/10.1080/03004279.2019.1622495

McInnes, K., Howard, J., Miles, G. E., & Crowley, K. (2009). Behavioural differences exhibited by children when practising a task under formal and playful conditions. *Educational & Child Psychology, 26,* 31–39.

McInnes, K., Howard, J., Miles, G. E., & Crowley, K. (2011). Differences in practitioners' understanding of play and how this influences pedagogy and children's perceptions of play. *Early Years: An International Journal of Research and Development, 31,* 121–133. https://doi.org/10.1080/09575146.2011.572870

McKenna, J., & Mellson, J. (2013). Emotional intelligence and the occupational therapist. *British Journal of Occupational Therapy, 76*(9), 427–430. https://doi.org/10.4276/030802213X13782044946382

Messer, D. J., & Vietze, P. M. (1984). Timing and transitions in mother–infant gaze. *Infant Behavior and Development, 7,* 167–181. https://doi.org/10.1016/S0163-6383(84)80056-9

Messier, J., Ferland, F., & Majnemer, A. (2008). Play behavior of school age children with intellectual disability: Their capacities, interests and attitude. *Journal of Developmental and Physical Disabilities, 20,* 193–207. https://doi.org/10.1007/s10882-007-9089-x

Miller, H. (1996). Eye contact and gaze aversion: Implications for persons with autism. *Sensory Integration Special Interest Section Newsletter, 19*(2), 1–3.

Morozini, M. (2015). Exploring the engagement of parents in the co-occupation of parent–child play: An occupational science's perspective. *International Journal of Prevention and Treatment, 4,* 11–28. https://doi.org/10.5923/s.ijpt.201501.02

Morrison, T. (2013). Individual and environmental implications of working alliances in occupational therapy. *British Journal of Occupational Therapy, 76*(11), 507–514. https://doi.org/10.4276/030802213X13833255804676

Morrison, T. L., & Smith, J. D. (2013). Working alliance development in occupational therapy: A cross-case analysis. *Australian Occupational Therapy Journal, 60*(5), 326–333. https://doi.org/http://dx.doi.org/10.1111/1440-1630.12053

Mosey, A. C. (1981). *Occupational therapy: Configuration of a profession.* New York: Raven Press.

Mosey, A. C. (1986). *Psychosocial components of occupational therapy.* New York: Raven Press.

Moszkowski, R. J., & Stack, D. M. (2007). Infant touching behaviour during mother–infant face-to-face interactions. *Infant and Child Development, 16,* 307–319. https://doi.org/10.1002/icd.510

Mullaney, R. J. (2018, November). Intentional use of creativity from OT school to OT practice. *OT Practice, 23*(19), 24–25.

Munoz, J. P. (2007). Culturally responsive caring in occupational therapy. *Occupational Therapy International, 14,* 256–280. https://doi.org/10.1002/oti.238

Murray, L., De Pascalis, L., Bozicevic, L., Hawkins, L., Sclafani, V., & Ferrari, P. F. (2016). The functional architecture of mother–infant communication, and the development of infant social expressiveness in the first two months. *Scientific Reports, 6*(1), 39019. https://doi.org/10.1038/srep39019

Nadel, J., Martini, M., Field, T., Escalona, A., & Lundy, B. (2008). Children with autism approach more imitative and playful adults. *Early Child Development and Care, 178*, 461–465. https://doi.org/10.1080/03004430600801699

Nelson, J. K. (2008). Laugh and the world laughs with you: An attachment perspective on the meaning of laughter in psychotherapy. *Clinical Social Work Journal, 36*(1), 41–49. https://doi.org/10.1007/s10615-007-0133-1

Ng, S. L., Mylopoulos, M., Kangasjarvi, E., Boyd, V. A., Teles, S., Orsino, A., Lingard, L., & Phelan, S. (2020). Critically reflective practice and its sources: A qualitative exploration. *Medical Education.* https://doi.org/10.1111/medu.14032

Nilsen, D. L. F., & Nilsen, A. P. (1978). *Language play: An introduction to linguistics.* Rowley, MA: Newbury House.

O'Brien, J., & Taylor, R. (2020). The intentional relationship: Working with children and families. In J. O'Brien and H. Kuhaneck (Eds.), *Case-Smith's occupational therapy for children* (8th ed., pp. 122–134). St. Louis, MO: Elsevier.

O'Connor, D., Butler, A., & Lynch, H. (2020). Partners in play: Exploring "playing with" children living with severe physical and intellectual disabilities. *British Journal of Occupational Therapy, 0308022620967293.* https://doi.org/10.1177/0308022620967293

Olli, J., Salanterä, S., Karlsson, L., & Vehkakoski, T. (2021). Getting into the Same Boat: Enabling the Realization of the Disabled Child's Agency in Adult–Child Play Interaction. *Scandinavian Journal of Disability Research, 23*(1), 272-283. https://doi.org/10.16993/sjdr.790

Oven, A., & Lobe, B. (2019). Occupational therapists' creativity: Tapping into client centeredness using a novel creativity questionnaire. *American Journal of Occupational Therapy, 73*, 7304205110. https://doi.org/10.5014/ajot.2019.032680

Palmadottir, G. (2003). Client perspectives on occupational therapy in rehabilitation services. *Scandinavian Journal of Occupational Therapy, 10*, 157–166. https://doi.org/10.1080/11038120310017318

Palmadottir, G. (2006). Client–therapist relationships: Experiences of occupational therapy clients in rehabilitation. *British Journal of Occupational Therapy, 69*, 394–401. https://doi.org/10.1177/030802260606900902

Pan, A., & Liu, L. (2016). Therapeutic relationship and treatment outcome. *American Journal of Occupational Therapy, 70* (4_Supplement_1), 7011510234p1. https://doi.org/10.5014/ajot.2016.70S1-PO7019

Panksepp, J., & Burgdorf, J. (2003). "Laughing" rats and the evolutionary antecedents of human joy? *Physiology & Behavior, 79*, 533–547. https://doi.org/10.1016/S0031-9384(03)00159-8

Parham, L. D. (1992). Strategies for maintaining a playful atmosphere during therapy. *Sensory Integration Special Interest Section Newsletter, 15*(1), 2–3.

Patterson, S. Y., Elder, L., Gulsrud, A., & Kasari, C. (2014). The association between parental interaction style and children's joint engagement in families with toddlers with autism. *Autism: International Journal of Research and Practice, 18*, 511–518. https://doi.org/10.1177/1362361313483595

Pawlby, S. J. (1977). Imitative interaction. In H. R. Schaffer (Ed.), *Studies in mother–infant interaction* (pp. 203–224). London: Academic Press.

Pawlowski, C. S., Ergler, C., Tjørnhøj-Thomsen, T., Schipperijn, J., & Troelsen, J. (2015). "Like a soccer camp for boys": A qualitative exploration of gendered activity patterns in children's self-organized play during school recess. *European Physical Education Review, 21*(3), 275–291. https://doi.org/10.1177/1356336X14561533

Peloquin, S. M. (1990). The patient–therapist relationship in occupational therapy: Understanding visions and images. *American Journal of Occupational Therapy, 44*, 13–21. https://doi.org/10.5014/ajot.44.1.13

Peloquin, S. M. (1993). The depersonalization of patients: A profile gleaned from narratives. *American Journal of Occupational Therapy, 47*, 830–837. https://doi.org/10.5014/ajot.47.9.830

Peloquin, S. M. (1995). The fullness of empathy: Reflections and illustrations. *American Journal of Occupational Therapy, 49*, 24–31. https://doi.org/10.5014/ajot.49.1.24

Perlo, J., Balik, B., Swensen, S., Kabcenell, A., Landsman, J., & Feeley, D. (2017). *IHI framework for improving joy in work. IHI White Paper.* Cambridge, MA: Institute for Healthcare Improvement. http://www.ihi.org/resources/Pages/IHIWhitePapers/Framework-Improving-Joy-in-Work.aspx

Piazza, E. A., Hasenfratz, L., Hasson, U., & Lew-Williams, C. (2020). Infant and adult brains are coupled to the dynamics of natural communication. *Psychological Science, 31*(1), 6–17. https://doi.org/10.1177/0956797619878698

Pinckney, H. P., Outley, C., Brown, A., & Theriault, D. (2018). Playing while black. *Leisure Sciences, 40*(7), 675–685. https://doi.org/10.1080/01490400.2018.1534627

Power, T. G. (2000). *Play and exploration in children and animals.* Mahwah, NJ: Erlbaum.

Price, P. (2009). The therapeutic relationship. In E. B. Crepeau, E. S. Cohn, & B. A. Boyt Schell (Eds.), *Willard & Spackman's occupational therapy* (11th ed., pp. 328–341). Philadelphia, PA: Lippincott Williams & Wilkins.

Price, P., & Miner, S. (2007). Occupation emerges in the process of therapy. *American Journal of Occupational Therapy, 61*, 441–450. https://doi.org/10.5014/ajot.61.4.441

Punwar, A. J. (2000). The art and science of practice. In A. J. Punwar & S. M. Peloquin (Eds.), *Occupational therapy principles and practice* (3rd ed., pp. 93–108). Philadelphia, PA: Lippincott Williams & Wilkins.

Reid, D. T., & Chiu, T. M. L. (2011). Research lessons learned: Occupational therapy with culturally diverse mothers of premature infants. *Canadian Journal of Occupational Therapy, 78*, 173–179. https://doi.org/10.2182/cjot.2011.78.3.5

Rentzou, K., Slutsky, R., Tuul, M., Gol-Guven, M., Kragh-Müller, G., Foerch, D. F., & Paz-Albo, J. (2019). Preschool teachers' conceptualizations and uses of play across eight countries. *Early Childhood Education Journal, 47*(1), 1–14. https://doi.org/10.1007/s10643-018-0910-1

Román-Oyola, R., Figueroa-Feliciano, V., Torres-Martínez, Y., Torres-Vélez, J., Encarnación-Pizarro, K., Fragoso-Pagán, S., & Torres-Colón, L. (2018). Play, playfulness, and self-efficacy: Parental experiences with children on the autism spectrum. *Occupational Therapy International*, Article ID 4636780. https://doi.org/10.1155/2018/4636780

Román-Oyola, R., Reynolds, S., Soto-Feliciano, I., Cabrera-Mercader, L., & Vega-Santana, J. (2017). Child's sensory profile and adult playfulness as predictors of parental self-efficacy. *American Journal of Occupational Therapy*, 71, 7102220010. https://doi.org/10.5014/ajot.2017.021097

Román-Oyola, R., Vazquez-Gual, C., Dasta-Valentin, I., Diaz-Lazzarini, G., Collazo-Aguilar, G., Yambo-Martinez, C., Bundy, A., Lane, S., & Bonilla-Rodriguez, V. (2019). Development of the Scale of Parental Playfulness Attitude (PaPA) during the co-occupation of play. *The American Journal of Occupational Therapy*, 73(4_Supplement_1). https://doi.org/10.5014/ajot.2019.73S1-PO8016

Ruble, L., McDuffie, A., King, A. S., & Lorenz, D. (2008). Caregiver responsiveness and social interaction behaviors of young children with autism. *Topics in Early Childhood Special Education*, 28, 158–170. https://doi.org/10.1177/0271121408323009

Runco, M. A. (2007). *Creativity theories and themes: Research, development, and practice*. San Diego, CA: Elsevier Academic Press.

Sapp, D. D. (1995). Creative problem-solving in art: A model for idea inception and image development. *Journal of Creative Behavior*, 29, 173–185. https://doi.org/10.1002/j.2162-6057.1995.tb00747.x

Schaefer, C. E., & Drewes, A. A. (2011). The therapeutic powers of play and play therapy. In C. E. Schaefer (Ed.), *Foundations of play therapy* (2nd ed., pp. 27–38). Hoboken, NJ: Wiley.

Schaefer, C., & Greenberg, R. (1997). Measurement of playfulness: A neglected therapist variable. *International Journal of Play Therapy*, 6(2), 21–31. https://doi.org/10.1037/h0089406

Schafer, G. E. (1994). Games of complexity: Reflections on play structure and play intervention. In J. Hellendoorn, R. van der Kooij, & B. Sutton-Smith (Eds.), *Play and intervention* (pp. 77–84). Albany: State University of New York Press.

Schlenz, K. C., Guthrie, M. R., & Dudgeon, B. (1995). Burnout in occupational therapists and physical therapists working in head injury rehabilitation. *American Journal of Occupational Therapy*, 49, 986–993. https://doi.org/10.5014/ajot.49.10.986

Schmid, T. (2004). Meanings of creativity within occupational therapy practice. *Australian Occupational Therapy Journal*, 51(2), 80–88. https://doi.org/10.1111/j.1440-1630.2004.00434.x

Schultz-Krohn, W. (2019). Competence and professional development. In B. A. Boyt Schell & G. Gillen (Eds.), *Willard & Spackman's occupational therapy* (32nd ed., pp. 1100–1115). Baltimore, MD: Lippincott Williams & Wilkins.

Schwartzberg, S. L. (1993). Therapeutic use of self. In H. L. Hopkins & H. D. Smith (Eds.), *Willard and Spackman's occupational therapy* (8th ed., pp. 269–274). Philadelphia, PA: Lippincott.

Sharma, K. A., & Clark, A. J. (2018, April 23). Empathy matters: The importance of imagination in occupational therapy. *OT Practice*, 7, 18–20.

Shen, X. S., Chick, G., & Zinn, H. (2014). Validating the Adult Playfulness Trait Scale (APTS): An examination of personality, behavior, attitude, and perception in the nomological network of playfulness. *American Journal of Play*, 6(3), 345–369.

Shine, S., & Acosta, T. Y. (1999). The effect of the physical and social environment on parent–child interactions: A qualitative analysis of pretend play in a children's museum. In S. Reifel (Ed.), *Play & culture studies: Vol. 2. Play contexts revisited* (pp. 123–139). Westport, CT: Ablex.

Shire, S. Y., Gulsrud, A., & Kasari, C. (2016). Increasing responsive parent–child interactions and joint engagement: Comparing the influence of parent-mediated intervention and parent psychoeducation. *Journal of Autism and Developmental Disorders*, 46(5), 1737–1747. https://doi.org/10.1007/s10803-016-2702-z

Shirk, S. R., Karver, M. S., & Brown, R. (2011). The alliance in child and adolescent psychotherapy. *Psychotherapy*, 48(1), 17–24.

Sivberg, B., Jakobsson U., & Lundqvist, P. (2019). Parent–infant interactions looking for instances of volitional social gaze versus reflexive gaze—an observational study. *Early Child Development and Care*, 189(11), 1737–1748, DOI: 10.1080/03004430.2017.1410479).

Skard, G., & Bundy, A. C. (2008). Test of playfulness. In L. D. Parham & L. S. Fazio (Eds.), *Play in occupational therapy for children* (2nd ed., pp. 71–93). St. Louis, MO: Mosby Elsevier.

Slade, A. (1987). A longitudinal study of maternal involvement and symbolic play during the toddler period. *Child Development*, 58, 367–375. https://doi.org/10.2307/1130513

Smith, R. L., Stagnitti, K., Lewis, A. J., & Pépin, G. (2015). The views of parents who experience intergenerational poverty on parenting and play: A qualitative analysis. *Child: Care, Health and Development*, 41(6), 873–881. https://doi.org/10.1111/cch.12268

Solman, B., & Clouston, T. (2016). Occupational therapy and the therapeutic use of self. *British Journal of Occupational Therapy*, 79(8), 514–516. https://doi.org/10.1177/0308022616638675

Sorce, J. F., & Emde, R. N. (1981). Mother's presence is not enough: Effect of emotional availability on infant exploration. *Developmental Psychology*, 17, 737–745. https://doi.org/10.1037/0012-1649.17.6.737

Spitzer, S. L. (2003a). Using participant observation to study the meaning of occupations of young children with autism and other developmental disabilities. *American Journal of Occupational Therapy*, 57(1), 66–76. https://doi.org/10.5014/ajot.57.1.66

Spitzer, S. L. (2003b). With and without words: Exploring occupation in relation to young children with autism. *Journal of Occupational Science*, 10(2), 67–79. https://doi.org/10.1080/14427591.2003.9686513

Spitzer, S. L. (2004). Common and uncommon daily activities in individuals with autism: Challenges and opportunities for supporting occupation. In H. Miller-Kuhaneck (Ed.), *Autism: A comprehensive occupational therapy approach* (2nd ed., pp. 83–106). Bethesda, MD: AOTA Press.

Spitzer, S. L. (2008). Play in children with autism: Structure and experience. In L. D. Parham & L. S. Fazio (Eds.), *Play in occupational therapy for children* (2nd ed., pp. 351–374). St. Louis, MO: Mosby Elsevier.

Steiner, A. M. (2011). A strength-based approach to parent education for children with autism. *Journal of Positive Behavior Interventions*, 13, 178–190. http://dx.doi.org/10.1177/1098300710384134

Sterman, J., Naughton, G., Froude, E., Villeneuve, M., Beetham, K., Wyver, S., & Bundy, A. (2016). Outdoor play decisions by caregivers of children with disabilities: A systematic review of qualitative studies. *Journal of Developmental and Physical Disabilities*, 28(6), 931–957. https://doi.org/10.1007/s10882-016-9517-x

Stern, D. N. (1974). Mother and infant at play: The dyadic interaction involving facial, vocal, and gaze behaviors. In M. Lewis & L. A. Rosenblum (Eds.), *The effect of the infant on its caregiver* (pp. 187–213). New York: John Wiley & Sons.

Stoffel, V. C. (2013). From heartfelt leadership to compassionate care (Inaugural Presidential Address). *American Journal of Occupational Therapy*, 67, 633–640. http://dx.doi.org/10.5014/ajot.2013.676001

Suizzo, M., & Bornstein, M. H. (2006). French and European American child–mother play: Culture and gender considerations. *International Journal of Behavioral Development*, 30, 498–508. https://doi.org/10.1177/0165025406071912

Tandon, P. S., Saelens, B. E., & Copeland, K. A. (2017). A comparison of parent and childcare provider's attitudes and perceptions about preschoolers' physical activity and outdoor time. *Child: Care, Health and Development*, 43(5), 679–686. https://doi.org/10.1111/cch.12429

Tasker, D., & Higgs, J. (2017). Constructing mindful dialogues in healthcare: A phenomenological study. In D. Tasker, J. Higgs, & S. Loftus (Eds.), *Community-based healthcare: The search for mindful dialogues* (pp. 11–24). Rotterdam, Netherlands: Sense Publishers.

Taylor, R., & Peloquin, S. M. (2008, April). Teaching the therapeutic use of self—the intentional relationship model. Presentation at the annual conference of the American Occupational Therapy Association, Long Beach, CA.

Taylor, R. R. (2008). *The intentional relationship: Occupational therapy and use of self*. Philadelphia, PA: F. A. Davis.

Taylor, R. R., Lee, S. W., Kielhofner, G., & Ketkar, M. (2009). Therapeutic use of self: A nationwide survey of practitioners' attitudes and experiences. *American Journal of Occupational Therapy*, 63, 198–207. https://doi.org/10.5014/ajot.63.2.198

Terr, L. C., Deeney, J. M., Drell, M., Dodson, J. W., Gaensbauer, T. J., Massie, H., et al. (2007). Playful "moments" in psychotherapy (Clinical Perspectives). *Journal of the American Academy of Child and Adolescent Psychiatry*, 45, 604–614.

Thomas, L., Howard, J., & Miles, G. (2006). The effectiveness of playful practice for learning in the early years. *The Psychology of Education Review*, 30, 52–58.

Thorne, B. (1993). *Gender play: Girls and boys in school*. New Brunswick, NJ: Rutgers University Press.

Tickle-Degnen, L. (2002). Client-centered practice, therapeutic relationship, and the use of research evidence. *American Journal of Occupational Therapy*, 56, 470–474.

Tietz, J., & Shine, S. (2001). The interaction of gender and play style in the development of gender segregation. In S. Reifel (Ed.), *Play & culture studies: Vol. 3. Theory in context and out* (pp. 131–146). Westport, CT: Ablex.

Todd, B. K., Fischer, R. A., Di Costa, S., Roestorf, A., Harbour, K., Hardiman, P., & Barry, J. A. (2018). Sex differences in children's toy preferences: A systematic review, meta-regression, and meta-analysis. *Infant and Child Development*, 27(2), e2064. https://doi.org/10.1002/icd.2064

Toomey, M. (2003). Creativity: Access to the spirit through occupation. In M. A. McColl (Ed.), *Spirituality and occupational therapy* (pp. 181–192). Ottawa, Ontario, Canada: Canadian Association of Occupational Therapists.

Tortora, S. (2006). *The dancing dialogue: Using the communicative power of movement with young children*. Baltimore, MD: Paul H. Brookes Publishing Co.

Trevarthen, C. (1980). The foundations of intersubjectivity: Development of interpersonal and cooperative understanding in infants. In D. R. Olson (Ed.), *The social foundations of language and thought* (pp. 316–342). New York: W. W. Norton.

U.S. Department of Health and Human Services, Health Resources and Services Administration, Maternal and Child Health Bureau. (2014). *The health and well-being of children: A portrait of states and the nation, 2011–2012*. Rockville, MD: U.S. Department of Health and Human Services. https://mchb.hrsa.gov/nsch/2011-12/health/index.html

Van keer, I., Ceulemans, E., Bodner, N., Vandesande, S., Van Leeuwen, K., & Maes, B. (2019). Parent–child interaction: A micro-level sequential approach in children with a significant cognitive and motor developmental delay. *Research in Developmental Disabilities*, 85, 172–186. https://doi.org/10.1016/j.ridd.2018.11.008

van Rheenen, D. (2001). Boys who play hopscotch: The historical divide of a gendered space. In S. Reifel (Ed.), *Play & culture studies: Vol. 3. Theory in context and out* (pp. 111–130). Westport, CT: Ablex.

van Tubbergen, M., Warschausky, S., Birnholz, J., & Baker, S. (2008). Choice beyond preference: Conceptualization and assessment of choice-making skills in children with significant impairments. *Rehabilitation Psychology*, 53(1), 93–100. https://doi.org/10.1037/0090-5550.53.1.93

Vegni, E., Mauri, E., D'Apice, M., & Moja, E.A. (2010). A quantitative approach to measure occupational therapist–client interactions: A pilot study, *Scandinavian Journal of Occupational Therapy*, 17(3), 217–224. https://doi.org/10.3109/11038120903147956

Vergeer, G., & MacRae, A. (1993). Therapeutic use of humor in occupational therapy. *American Journal of Occupational Therapy*, 47, 678–683. https://doi.org/10.5014/ajot.47.8.678

Wainwright, N., Goodway, J., Whitehead, M., Williams, A., & Kirk, D. (2019). Playful pedagogy for deeper learning: Exploring the implementation of the play-based foundation phase in Wales. *Early Child Development and Care*, 190(1), 43–53. https://doi.org/10.1080/03004430.2019.1653551adult

Waldman-Levi, A., Bundy, A., & Katz, N. (2015). Playfulness and interaction: An exploratory study of past and current exposure to domestic violence. *OTJR: Occupation, Participation and Health*, 35(2), 89–94. https://doi.org/10.1177/1539449214561762

Waldman-Levi, A., Grinion, S., & Olson, L. (2019). Effects of maternal views and support on childhood development through joint play. *The Open Journal of Occupational Therapy*, 7(4), 1–21. https://doi.org/10.15453/2168-6408.1613

Waldman-Levi, A., & Weintraub, N. (2015). Efficacy of a crisis intervention for improving mother–child interaction and the children's play functions. *The American Journal of Occupational Therapy*, 69(1), 1–11. https://doi.org/10.5014/ajot.2015.013375

Warren, S. F., & Brady, N. C. (2007). The role of maternal responsivity in the development of children with intellectual disabilities. *Mental Retardation and Developmental Disabilities Research Reviews*, 13, 330–338. https://doi.org/10.1002/mrdd.20177

Williams, D. (1992). *Nobody nowhere: The extraordinary autobiography of an autistic*. New York: Times Books.

Williams, E. I., Costall, A., & Reddy, V. (2018). Autism and triadic play: An object lesson in the mutuality of the social and material. *Ecological Psychology*, 30(2), 146–173. https://doi.org/10.1080/10407413.2018.1439140

Williams, S., & Paterson, M. (2009). A phenomenological study of the art of occupational therapy. *The Qualitative Report*, 14(4), 688–717.

Wing, L. (1995). Play is not the work of the child: Young children's perceptions of work and play. *Early Childhood Research Quarterly*, 10, 223–247. https://doi.org/10.1016/0885-2006(95)90005-5

Winters, C. (2016). Stress management techniques for occupational therapy practitioners. *SIS Quarterly Practice Connections, 1*(4), 14–16.

Wiseman, J. O., Davis, J. A., & Polatajko, H. J. (2005). Occupational development: Towards an understanding of children's doing. *Journal of Occupational Science, 12*(1), 26–35. https://doi.org/10.1080/14427591.2005.9686545

Wittman, P., & Velde, B. P. (2002). Attaining cultural competence, critical thinking, and intellectual development: A challenge for occupational therapists. *American Journal of Occupational Therapy, 56*(4), 454-456. https://doi.org/10.5014/ajot.41.7.454

Wong, C. (2013). A play and joint attention intervention for teachers of young children with autism: A randomized controlled pilot study. *Autism, 17,* 340–357. https://doi.org/10.1177/1362361312474723

Wright-St Clair, V. (2001). Caring: The moral motivation for good occupational therapy practice. *Australian Occupational Therapy Journal, 48*(4), 187–199.

Zango Martín, I., Flores Martos, J. A., Moruno Millares, P., & Björklund, A. (2015). Occupational therapy culture seen through the multifocal lens of fieldwork in diverse rural areas. *Scandinavian Journal of Occupational Therapy, 22*(2), 82–94. https://doi.org/ 10.3109/11038128.2014.965197

Zappaterra, T. (2018). The role of knowledgeable adults in children with disabilities' play: An exploratory research in Europe. *Today's Children: Tomorrow's Parents: An Interdisciplinary Journal, 47–48,* 74–85.

APPENDIX 6.1 Pediatric Occupational Therapy Communication Strategies Checklist

Child's Name: _____

Directions: Check the strategies you have used to communicate playfulness to the child. Then note the child's response in order to determine which strategies are most effective and which might be beneficial to utilize.

Communication Strategies	Have You Communicated Playfulness Through This Strategy*?	Child's Response[†] (Positive, Neutral, Negative)	Notes/Comments[¶]
Eyes *Look at the child* *Look between the child and a potential toy/play object*			
Face *Smile* *Exaggerate and hold positive emotional expressions* *Imitate the child's expression*			
Body *Turn and lean toward the child* *Imitate the child's actions* *Exaggerate and slow body movements such as head nodding, head wagging, or head cocking* *Hold out, manipulate, hide, or point to toys/objects*			

Communication Strategies	Have You Communicated Playfulness Through This Strategy*?	Child's Response† (Positive, Neutral, Negative)	Notes/Comments¶
Touch *To get attention* *To show toy, action*			
Voice (Vocalizations) *Use playful tone* *Vary pitch, loudness, rhythm* *Repeat sounds* *Imitate sounds and ways sounds are used by child*			
Language *Match language to child's development* *Use the words* play *and* choice *Minimize the word* work *and directing/correcting words* *Use language in song, melody, rhythm, or different voice (e.g., accent)*			
Imitate child's words *Use "kid play" words, phrases, and sounds* *Use humor, jokes, and mischievous tone* *Talk as if toys or body parts were alive and thinking*			

* These strategies must occur in a close enough space that the child can notice these actions.

† If the child's response is negative (e.g., agitation, destructiveness, withdrawal, pushing away, fussing, crying), it suggests that currently this is not an effective play communication strategy for him or her. If the child's response is positive (e.g., increased self-initiation, eye contact, affect/smiling, attention, orienting, leaning toward, participation, behavior modulation, vocalizations/communication), it suggests that this is an effective play communication strategy that should be continued for him or her. If the child's response is neutral (no observable response), the strategy cannot be discounted because he or she may respond later if the strategy is tried again.

¶ You may want to note specific details of the strategies and the child's response and/or your professional reasoning.

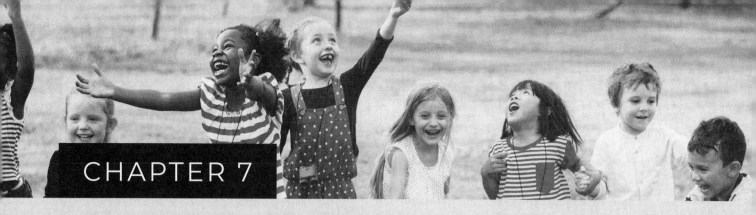

Selecting Play Activities Through Sound Professional Reasoning

Elissa Cunningham, OTD, OTR/L

Heather M. Kuhaneck, PhD, OTR/L, FAOTA

After reading this chapter, the reader will:

- Articulate sound professional reasoning for selecting appropriate play activities.
- Describe how occupational therapy models, pediatric frames of reference, activity analysis, and occupational analysis each contribute to play activity selection.
- Select play activities that are the "just-right-challenge" through sound professional reasoning.

It's the things we play with and the people who help us play that make a great difference in our lives.

—Fred Rogers

Occupational therapy practitioners must make a number of decisions to guide every clinical encounter with a child. In relation to play, the first decision is whether or not to use play, and then if play is chosen, the therapist must consider what to play, how to best engage the child in play, how much choice to allow, what materials to offer, how to interact with the child, and many more decisions, both small and large. Professional reasoning is the complex way of thinking involved in making these decisions. The reasoning is complex because occupational therapy practitioners select play activities both in terms of what will occur and how. The elements are selected for individual meaning and therapeutic value. The activity is crafted as it is selected to ensure that the play activity is experienced as an occupation.

Professional Reasoning for Play Selection

All aspects of occupational therapy practice require the use of professional reasoning. It has been defined as the way therapists plan, perform, and reflect on client care (Boyt, Schell, Gillen, & Scaffa, 2014; Márquez-Álvarez et al., 2019). Professional reasoning is actually made up of a variety of specific ways of thinking. Typically, in practice, occupational therapy practitioners use multiple forms of professional reasoning at once. These ways of thinking have been labeled scientific, diagnostic, pragmatic, management, procedural, interactive, collaborative, predictive, conditional, narrative, ethical, intuitive, propositional, and client-centered reasoning (Mattingly & Fleming, 1994; Schell & Schell, 2008; Unsworth, 2005). Each type of reasoning assists with different therapeutic decisions. As seen in **Table 7.1**, each type of professional reasoning

Table 7.1 Types of Professional Reasoning and Their Influence on Play Selection

Type of Reasoning	Description	Questions to Ask About an Activity Being Considered	Example of Influence on Play Experience Selection
Scientific	Making decisions based on evidence, clinical knowledge, and experience. Uses logical methods, including theory-based decision making, hypothesis testing, and statistical evidence.	Does this activity address the problem that I have hypothesized is an issue for this child? What is the scientific evidence regarding the effectiveness and safety of the activity?	Choose a specific play-based intervention approach based on the recent randomized controlled trial that showed it to be effective in improving pretense.
Pragmatic	Practical reality of a given situation—available materials, resources, and environmental supports as well as skills of the therapist. Pragmatic reasoning is about the factors not specific to the client but to the situation.	Can I do this activity in this setting safely? Is this activity appropriate for this setting? Do I have the proper space and materials to do this activity? Am I competent to use this activity?	Suggest a play activity different from the one a child preferred, because the materials or supplies for the preferred activity were not available. The therapist would try to make the available activity as similar as possible, given the limitations of the reality of the situation.
Procedural	Making decisions about specific therapeutic interventions for a specific condition. It may be based in science or established protocols or habit. This form of reasoning often is driven by diagnosis.	What activities are typically selected for individuals with this diagnosis?	Try games that work on basic imitation skills for a toddler just diagnosed with ASD because of knowledge that in ASD, imitation can be an area of difficulty. Start using button-operated toys with a toddler with cerebral palsy, knowing that the motor difficulties associated with the diagnosis can impact play access, and limited independence can lead to learned helplessness if not addressed.
Interactive	Focuses on a partnership with clients through the development of therapeutic relationships. Therapists seek to know and understand the interests of the client and what is perceived as meaningful or fun, seeking to find what motivates the client.	What is fun and meaningful for the child? What does this child like and enjoy? In what aspects of the activity is the child most interested?	Collaborate with the child to include play activities that the child prefers and considers fun, using what motivates the child in therapy.
Narrative	Consider the child within all of his or her varied roles and across the contexts of home, school, and community. Used in understanding the occupational profile of the child, enables the therapist to understand where the client came from, his or her history, present function, and future goals. Considers client's culture as well.	What activities are associated with the child's roles at home, at school, and in community? What are the goals identified by the child and the family?	Suggest including play or leisure activities in therapy that are important to the family, for example, helping the child be able to play football for the annual family game during Thanksgiving.

Type of Reasoning	Description	Questions to Ask About an Activity Being Considered	Example of Influence on Play Experience Selection
Ethical reasoning	Consider ethical dilemmas and implications. Weighs the risks and benefits of certain intervention choices or prioritizes service allocation.	What are the potential benefits of the activity? What are the "opportunity costs" of doing this activity as opposed to something else during the OT time? Am I using OT time and OT dollars wisely?	Choose an activity with the child that will provide the greatest benefit for the most areas. Carefully consider how the time of the therapy session is being used, and try not to engage in unnecessary power struggles that take away time from therapeutic activities. Always be ready and able to explain WHY you are doing what you are doing.
Conditional reasoning	Allows more experienced therapists to envision multiple possible outcomes and to look beyond the present, blending all forms of reasoning.	What is the possible future for this child, and could the activity help the child in that possible future?	Suggest play activities to specifically help prepare the child for future independence in areas that are likely to become difficult as the child gets older.

Data from Types of reasoning and descriptions are based on Bryze, K. C. (2008). Narrative contributions to the play history. In L. D. Parham & L. S. Fazio (Eds.), *Play in occupational therapy for children* (2nd ed., pp. 43–54). Mosby Elsevier; Mattingly, C., & Fleming, M. H. (1994). Interactive reasoning: Collaborating with the person. In C. Mattingly & M. H. Fleming (Eds.), *Clinical reasoning: Forms of inquiry in a therapeutic practice* (pp. 178–196). F. A. Davis; and Schell, B. B, & Schell, J. W. (2008). *Clinical and professional reasoning in occupational therapy.* Lippincott, Williams & Wilkins.

holds important considerations for successfully selecting play activities that comprehensively meet a child's interests and needs.

The Balancing Act of Play Selection

Occupational therapists leave their professional education programs with a wealth of knowledge that is both shared with other professions and unique to occupational therapy. Therapists use all this knowledge as a foundation for professional decision making; however, in the quest for client-centered practice, this knowledge must always be balanced with the information we have gathered from clients through evaluation and specific play assessment. When therapists get this right, sessions flow smoothly, and play happens easily. Imagine this balancing act of professional reasoning as a seesaw with two counterweights as depicted in **Figure 7.1**. On one side is the therapist's professional

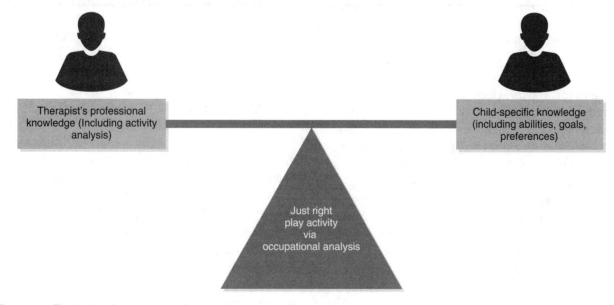

Therapist's professional knowledge (Including activity analysis)

Child-specific knowledge (including abilities, goals, preferences)

Just right play activity via occupational analysis

Figure 7.1 The balancing act of professional reasoning for play

knowledge and expertise in occupation. The other side of the seesaw holds the weight of the information that is unique and specific to that child, which is critical to make therapy client centered. The therapist balances both sides during professional reasoning through a tool specific to occupational therapy, occupational analysis, in order to create the just-right play activity.

Therapists' Professional Knowledge

Therapists must consider a variety of relevant knowledge in their decision making regarding play activities with clients. This knowledge, how we organize this knowledge, and how we think about this knowledge makes occupational therapists, OCCUPATIONAL therapists. There is a great deal of research as well as clinical experience to guide these decisions; however, there are also significant gaps in the evidence, which can limit its application. Therefore, to bridge this gap, we use unique guiding practice models and frames of reference to identify relevant evidence and organize its application for the diversity of individual children, families, schools, communities, and play dilemmas encountered in everyday practice.

Occupational Therapy Practice Models.

Occupational therapy practice models provide a basis for viewing and planning intervention and therapeutic activity selection through a uniquely occupation based lens (O'Brien & Kuhaneck, 2020). The models link research to clinical practice with specifically designed assessment methods and strategies for intervention associated with each. Occupational-centered practice models such as the Model of Human Occupation (MOHO), Occupational Adaptation (OA), and Person-Environment-Occupation-Performance (PEOP) provide overarching guiding principles for affecting change through therapeutic activities and methods. For example, the MOHO strategies for activity selection are based on the model's nine identified therapeutic methods (O'Brien & Kuhaneck, 2020). When using MOHO with pediatric clients, the therapist might focus on developing meaningful play activities because play is a child's primary occupation. If using this model, play choices might reflect a focus on developing patterns that foster occupational identity, internal locus of control, and thoughts and feelings of efficacy and validation (Taylor, 2017; O'Brien & Kuhaneck, 2020). The Occupational Adaptation model articulates concepts of participation with a goal of experiencing relative mastery (Grajo, 2017). Play selection using an occupational adaptation model would focus on

increasing adaptive capacity and feelings of effectiveness, efficiency, and satisfaction (Grajo, 2017). The use of play and playful activities can be powerful motivators towards the development of feelings and mastery when planning pediatric activities from this lens. The PEOP model postulates change through a dynamic interaction between the person, environment, and occupation (Bass, Baum, & Christiansen, 2017). This model relies heavily on the client narrative to drive activity selection and planning. Performance and environmental constraints and barriers are identified, and pediatric activities using this model focus on selecting playful activities that provide meaningful experiences to promote participation and occupational performance.

Occupational Therapy Frames of Reference.
In pediatric occupational therapy practice, models are used with frames of reference to guide evaluation and intervention (Kramer, Hinojosa, & Howe, 2019; Law, Missiuna, Pollock, & Stewart, 2005). Frames of reference are a more specific "set of interrelated internally consistent concepts, definitions and postulates that provide a systematic description of and prescription for a practitioner's interaction within a particular aspect of a profession's domain of concern" (Mosey, 1981, p. 129). Frames of reference relate theory to practice (Dunbar, 2007; Kramer et al., 2019). They are organizational structures for theory that provide more targeted information for problem identification and intervention options, as well as a common language to guide clinical practice decisions (Dunbar, 2007; Kramer et al., 2019). Many good resources are available that explain each frame of reference in depth for the reader who is unfamiliar (for example, Kramer et al., 2019). It is helpful to think of frames of reference as lenses through which you view a child's behavior and occupational performance. Just as one can put on and take off different glasses such as using reading or distance glasses at different times, one can use one or multiple frames of reference. These frames or lenses help in play selection by providing guidelines for what to focus on or prioritize (see **Table 7.2** for examples). Frames of reference may also lead a therapist to use one activity for many different reasons as exemplified in **Table 7.3**.

Activity Analysis.
Another aspect of the therapist's professional knowledge is the complex understanding of a large variety of activities gained through activity analysis. The process of activity analysis was detailed in Chapter 4, which emphasized its use as

Table 7.2 Applying Frames of Reference to Play Selection

Frame of Reference*	Play Selection Focus
Acquisition/behavior	Specific tasks identified as difficult for the child are the actual activities used in therapy. They are often broken down into steps or elements to target in part. Activities that target skill building for play are also used. Direct instruction, engagement, and repetition provided during play activities.
Ayres Sensory Integration (ASI)	Play is child directed and provides opportunities for varied and combined sensory inputs and challenges to improve praxis and regulation needed for play and other occupations.
Biomechanical	Play activities focus on strength, endurance, range of motion, or maintaining posture. Play activities may also use equipment or materials to provide external supports for positioning and postural control.
Cognitive behavioral	Play activities use cognitive strategies and/or reinforcement to shape successful performance.
Motor learning	Play activities focus on motor patterns used by the child in play, with practice, feedback, and repetition emphasized.
Neurodevelopmental treatment (NDT)	Play activities are set up to focus on postural control, movement patterns, and coordination but also emphasize motivation, environment, and function.

Data from Mosey, A. C. (1981). *Occupational therapy: Configuration of a profession*. Raven Press.
* See O'Brien and Kuhaneck (2020) for more information about frames of reference.

Table 7.3 Example of Different Reasons for Using the Same Activity

Activity	Reasons for Selecting Activity by Frame of Reference			
	Biomechanical	Sensory Integrative	NDT/Motor Control	Behavioral
Using therapy putty to create animals and pretending to feed the animals little balls of food	Therapy putty strengthens the fingers.	Therapy putty provides deep pressure input and proprioceptive input to the hands and fingers. Imitating or creating the animals and food provides motor planning challenges.	This is a bilateral activity that requires trunk control as the child pushes down onto the surface to roll, squish, and place the putty.	Making animals with therapy putty is a favorite activity and is being used as a reinforcer following completion of a less-favored task.

an assessment method. However, activity analysis is also an extremely important tool for determining the potential therapeutic uses of an activity, which is essential for activity selection (see **Box 7.1 for** details). For example, a therapist considering the activity of block building could complete the activity analysis format as provided in Chapter 4. This would allow the therapist to determine that block building could be used therapeutically for building a variety of visual-perceptual-motor, fine-motor, or praxis skills. It could also be used to improve pretend play, enhance creativity, or work on postural control depending on how the activity was designed, explained, and set up. See **Practice Example 7.1**, Tiffany's Options, for an example of possible play activities appropriate for one child.

Box 7.1 Questions to Aid Play Selection Using Activity Analysis*?

- What does this activity require for materials?
- Where is this activity usually performed?
- Who typically does this activity?
- How long does this activity typically take?
- What position is the activity typically done in?
- What are the motor, cognitive, sensory, perceptual, and social requirements of this activity?
- What might this activity be used for? How could it be used therapeutically?

*Please also refer back to Chapter 4 for more in-depth information on how to conduct an activity analysis.

PRACTICE EXAMPLE 7.1 Tiffany's Options

Tiffany is a 3½-year-old girl with a diagnosis of Down syndrome. As the occupational therapist for the preschool, you are in the classroom frequently. You have made the following observations of Tiffany during your evaluation and subsequent visits to her class:

Strengths: Tiffany is pleasant and sociable. She has friends in her classroom, and she enjoys being with and playing with her peers. She typically wants to do the same activities in the classroom that her peers are doing. She can match basic shapes. She enjoys movement. She is playful and silly and understands simple teasing and humor.

Difficulties: Tiffany can be strong willed. As is common with her diagnosis, she has low muscle tone and has difficulty maintaining an upright seated position for any period of time, often slumping in her chair. She has difficulty orienting clothing appropriately and often loses her balance during dressing tasks in the dress-up area. She has difficulty drawing shapes from memory. She has difficulty following multiple steps. She has demonstrated some evidence of tactile hyperresponsiveness and difficulty with crossing midline and using trunk rotation. She has delayed fine-motor control. Her motor and cognitive challenges sometimes interfere with her ability to play with her peers in the ways they are playing. This frustrates her, and she often gives up.

Tiffany's IEP goal areas are as follows:

- Copying prewriting shapes
- Buttoning large buttons
- Zipping backpack
- Cutting
- Dressing (donning coat, shoes)
- Sustaining play with peers
- Managing her frustration

Using activity analysis, you identify the following possible play activities that are each appropriate to work on one or more of her areas of need:

- Follow the leader
- Simon Says
- Crafts such as making puppets or simple faces
- Drawing, painting, coloring, tracing, maze, or dot-to-dot activities
- Making cereal or pasta necklaces
- Doll dress-up activities
- Costume dress-up activities
- Obstacle courses
- Small object construction games such as Legos or blocks
- Puzzles
- Memory matching games with shapes
- Marble maze games

Therapists should always have more than one possible play activity ready. Children may refuse something you suggest, or you may find a piece of equipment missing, a room unavailable, or any number of things that could create a need to change plans. Having multiple play activities ready allows the session to proceed successfully.

The Child-Specific Side of the Seesaw

Children each come to therapy with their own unique needs, desires, abilities, difficulties, and interests in relation to play. Through the evaluation process, we learn as much as we can about the child (see Chapters 3 and 4). This child-specific information allows the therapist to narrow the scope of potential play activities that might be appropriate out of the entire universe of play activities available. The resulting set of potential activities is more manageable for the therapist's pragmatic use.

Therapists select and construct activities that maximize the overlap between what the child wants to play, can play, and is actually able to gain access to play (see **Figure 7.2**). This may occur through expanding a child's preferences, perhaps through exposure to

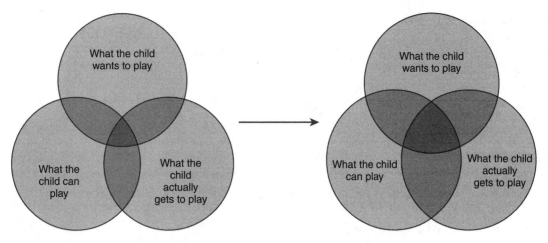

Figure 7.2 Maximizing the area of overlap between what the child wants to play, can play, and gets to play

new play experiences, thus increasing what the child *wants* to play. Or, it may occur through improving access to play through assistive technology or other modifications, thus altering what the child *can* play. Last, by adjusting the expectations or rules of important adults, or improving the opportunities the child has, the child can gain greater *access* to desired play.

Child Abilities. An important consideration in the selection of play activities is what the child can and cannot play, and why. The information from the evaluation process allows the therapist to consider the child's abilities in relation to the storehouse of knowledge of many possible activities to narrow the scope. For example, a therapist would be unlikely to attempt the activity of a 500-piece jigsaw puzzle for an adolescent who cannot match or discriminate any colors or complex shapes. The teen would likely require too much assistance or significant modifications in order to participate, and the activity could be too complicated to implement successfully. Jigsaw puzzles require finding the "right" piece in order to complete them and therefore could lead to frustration or feelings of failure for the teen. Instead, if the teen enjoyed fashion, the therapist might try an app or online game that dresses digital runway models with clothing, which could be used to work on goals of basic shape discrimination. The simple and familiar shapes of the clothing would likely be closer to the teen's ability. Also, the activity would have less possibility for "wrong" answers as within the realm of fashion, selecting unusual color combinations can be viewed as creative and thus provide a successful experience.

The therapist also may use knowledge of typical development in relation to the child's developmental level in the same way. For example, a therapist would

be unlikely to attempt dress-up and role-play activities with a toddler who is just beginning to pretend to talk on a toy cell phone because the developmental level of role play is much beyond the toddler's current developmental level in play. Instead, the therapist might try pretending to drive using a play steering wheel or pretending to feed a baby doll with a toy bottle because each are a better match for this toddler's developmental level. By eliminating activities whose demands require much higher abilities than the child possesses, which would be difficult to adapt, and focusing on those that are achievable, the therapist identifies a manageable subset of play activities specific to this child's abilities. The therapist considers those activities which require abilities at, below, or slightly above the child's level of abilities in alignment with the child's goals.

The therapist also must consider all the task requirements when selecting an activity to focus on one particular area. The higher the level of challenge in one demand, the greater the offset to other demands. For example, if the therapist significantly challenges a child's motor abilities, the rest of the activity demands should be easily within the child's capability. Likewise, if the therapist is challenging social skills, the motor demands should be easy enough for the child to engage in the social demands. If too many aspects of an activity are difficult, it could cause the activity to fail because the activity's overall difficulty level is just too great.

Child Goals. Another factor in considering possible activities is the child's goals. If the child has goals for peer play, the therapist would be unlikely to choose play activities that are isolated in nature and do not require interaction. If the child has goals for taking turns, the play selected must lend itself to turn-taking in some form. A card game like Solitaire would not suit that particular goal in its classic form unless modified to take turns in selecting each card. In contrast, turn-taking is an intrinsic part of a Go Fish card game. So, the therapist considers the child's goals in relation to the universe of play activities available and chooses those that can be used or adapted therapeutically to progress toward those goals.

Preferences. On the child side of the seesaw, there are also a variety of critical "preference" questions to answer as we select activities. What does the child want to be able to play? What do the child's caregivers want the child to be able to play? What do the child's peers or siblings want to play? Do all those preferences and desires match? Children may not be willing to engage in play activities that do not suit their preferences, or if they do engage, it may be with a halfhearted attempt or without real enjoyment. We try to select activities the child wants to play or activities that can be modified as such. If we seek to play with children, they should enjoy the experience from the activity we have crafted. Ideally, we select the play activity together and collaborate to make it both an enjoyable *and* therapeutic experience.

Occupational Analysis. While activity analysis provides the therapist with ideas of possible appropriate therapeutic activities, occupational analysis allows the therapist to specifically adjust and adapt to the specific child and situation in the moment based on all the concerns just mentioned (goals, preferences, abilities). Within a session, there is a constant and rapid shifting back and forth between activity analysis and occupational analysis.

Occupational analysis allows the therapist to collaborate with the child in relation to play activities. For example, a child might request a particular activity, and rather than saying no and getting into a potential power struggle, you may want to consider using it in that moment to support their motivation and autonomy. This requires flexible thinking. The therapist must quickly do activity analysis to determine if the demands of the activity match the child's needs and, if not, quickly determine if the activity can be adapted in a way to acquiesce to the child's request *and* use the activity therapeutically. The practice example of Tiffany highlights just such an occasion. Please see **Practice Example 7.2**, Tiffany's request for finger painting, for an illustration of professional reasoning through the use of activity and occupational analysis, and please also **see Figures 7.3** and **7.4** for the activity analysis of finger painting and **Figure 7.5** for a visual depiction of the professional reasoning process for Tiffany.

PRACTICE EXAMPLE 7.2 Tiffany's Request for Finger Painting

During this day in class, Tiffany has requested to engage in finger painting with her friends. You have the option of working with her in the classroom in the activity of finger painting, encouraging her to go to the dress-up area to work on dressing and clothing fasteners, or pulling her out to work on another activity you identified in Practice Example 7.1. After completing an activity analysis of finger painting (see Figures 7.3 and 7.4), you engage in a professional reasoning process to determine if you will select finger painting as a therapeutic intervention for Tiffany today. You use different aspects of professional reasoning when deciding if finger painting is an appropriate therapeutic activity (see **Table 7.4**). As part of this process, you also consider the child-specific factors including the classroom context, Tiffany's goals, and her current desire to participate in finger painting.

You agree to Tiffany's request for finger painting for several reasons. You know that you can work on at least one of her academic goal areas with this activity. Depending on how you set up the activity and the materials, you can also work on some of the client factors and skills that she typically has difficulty with such as cognition, postural control, and fine-motor control. And most important for you at this moment, selecting this activity allows Tiffany to participate and be included with her peers in a classroom activity that is playful and usually enjoyable for young children of her age.

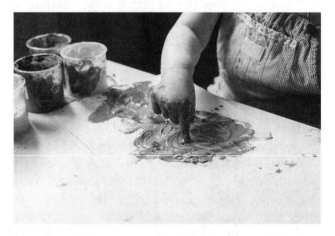

Figure 7.3 An occupational therapist does an activity analysis of the activity of finger painting without regard to a specific child

© Ievgeniia Shugaliia/Shutterstock.

Once the occupational therapist and child have agreed upon an activity, the therapist uses occupational analysis to prioritize which aspects of the activity demands will be emphasized to provide the

Name: Finger Painting Circles

Description: Child will paint circles on large paper placed on a table, using fingers rather than a paint brush.

Global Demands: Postural control for maintaining one's position and reaching for paint, isolating fingers, visual-perceptual motor skills and motor planning to imitate, copy, or draw a circle, depending on initial directions given.

Materials and Supplies Needed: Finger-paint, paper (preferably large), surface on which to paint, an easel could be helpful but not required, smock is also helpful but not required.

Safety Concerns: Finger-paint is nontoxic and safe, although children who frequently mouth their hands and fingers should be watched carefully to avoid unnecessary ingestion of paint. A child with balance issues could fall depending on how the child is positioned. There is potential for distress if the child has issues with tactile defensiveness or getting messy. A child with poor frustration tolerance could become upset with inability to complete the task.

Space Needed: This activity preferably requires an uncluttered and well-lit space on which to place the paper and paint. It can be done in a small or large room. It could be done on the floor in a prone position or standing, or sitting at a table. It does not require a large space.

Time Needed: The time required to paint a single circle may be merely seconds; however, the activity can be extended if multiple circles are drawn and perhaps colored in.

Steps or Processes to Complete the Activity
Step One: Extend index finger and flex other fingers
Step Two: Dip index finger in paint
Step Three: Place finger on paper
Step Four: Draw circle with paint
Repeat as desired

Movements Needed for Each Step
Step One: Extend index finger and flex other fingers- requires index finger extension, and finger flexion of all other fingers, uses full ROM in either flexion or extension depending on the digit, uses the PIP and DIP joints, uses the extensor indicis proprius, flexor digitorum, lumbricales muscles.

Step Two: Dip index finger in paint- requires shoulder flexion, elbow flexion and extension, wrist held in neutral or slight extension, with fingers held in prior placement, ROM is partial at the shoulder, elbow, and wrist, uses the pectoralis major, anterior deltoid, coracobrachialis, biceps brachii, brachioradialis, brachialis, triceps, extensor carpi radialis and ulnaris, extensor indicis proprius, flexor digitorum, lumbricales muscles.

Step Three: Place finger on paper- depending on the placement of the paper in relation to the body, requires shoulder flexion and extension, elbow extension, wrist extension, while maintaining the fingers in prior placement, uses the _pectoralis major, anterior deltoid, coracobrachialis, posterior deltoids, latissimus dorsi, triceps, extensor carpi radialis and ulnaris, extensor indicis proprius, flexor digitorum, lumbricales muscles.

Step Four: Draw circle with paint- requires shoulder flexion, ab and adduction, extension and horizontal flexion as the circle is formed, minimal elbow flexion and extension may also accompany shoulder motion depending on the body position in relation to the paper, fingers maintained in prior position, uses the pectoralis major, anterior deltoid, coracobrachialis, teres major and minor, medial deltoid, supraspinatus, posterior deltoid, latissimus dorsi, biceps brachii, brachioradialis, subscapularis, extensor indicis proprius, flexor digitorum, lumbricales muscles.

Figure 7.4 Activity analysis of finger painting

This activity requires little strength or endurance and it can be stopped at any time if the client fatigues. However, the shoulder flexors must hold the position against gravity while painting so repetitions could lead to shoulder fatigue. Lowering the arm to get more paint is assisted by gravity allowing some intermittent rest. Changing the position of the paper can also decrease the strength and endurance demand.

Praxis, Coordination, and Balance Needed: Requires minimal balance if seated, standing balance if standing, this is a unilateral activity, although could be bilateral if the paper needs to be held up on an easel with the non-dominant hand or if the finger paint container needs to be held by non-dominant hand, crossing midline is not required but could occur depending on the size of the circle made and the placement on the paper, need visual motor accuracy to target the finger to the paint and then the paper, timing is not a major issue with this activity, precise judgement of force is not required, although excessive force could rip the paper or push over an easel, forming the shape could be a novel movement and could require praxis.

Sensory Input Provided or Experienced: This activity will provide a tactile experience of the likely cold, wet feeling paint on the one finger, it will also provide a tactile experience of the finger dragging along the paper, and proprioceptive input as the finger presses on the paper. It will provide an experience of the impact of force used with the finger and the width of the line created or the depth of color created (lighter vs. heavier pressure leads to more or less color perhaps). There is also the visual experience of seeing the shape created by the movement that has been performed (what it feels like to form a circle). Requires depth perception for accurate reach and target to cup, spatial relations to place shape on paper, shape recognition, form and visual closure to complete shape on paper.

Thinking Skills Needed: Minimal sequencing to know when to get paint and then paint on paper. Minimal demands on attention span to follow through on drawing a circle.

Social Interaction Required: This activity can be done alone or cooperatively as a group sharing paper or space. It may require taking turns if paint is shared. Social requirements can vary greatly depending on how the activity is set up and who is in the area while the activity occurs.

Possible Emotional Responses or Associations: This activity can be structured, as in drawing a specific shape, or less structured, where the child can be creative and draw whatever he or she wants. In free drawing, there is much opportunity for success and productivity. If imitation and copying is required, there is the possibility for frustration and an impact on self-esteem.
This activity is a common childhood activity, usually of younger preschool-age children. The simplicity of the shape may be associated with the young child; however, the actual task of finger-painting can be enjoyed by any age. Individuals could associate the activity as "childish."

Figure 7.4 (Continued)

most therapeutic benefit at that moment. The therapist crafts the play activity to get the most out of it therapeutically while also attempting to maintain the child's enjoyment and experience of play. Read the next portion of the **Practice Example 7.3**, Tiffany, for an illustration of this aspect of practice.

Often, a selected activity is unsuccessful initially (See **Practice Example 7.4**). However, disappointing for therapist and child, an unsuccessful attempt provides further valuable information in adjusting activity selection. It informs ongoing professional reasoning in which the therapist decides quickly whether to adapt the activity to try to continue or to select an alternative activity. As therapists become more experienced, they are better able to quickly complete both activity analysis and occupational analysis in order to make these spontaneous activity decisions during a session. As Tiffany's case illustrates, just as important as activity selection and perhaps sometimes more important to the therapeutic process is activity adaptation. Activity adaptation utilizes similar professional reasoning processes as those required for activity selection and will be discussed further in the next chapter.

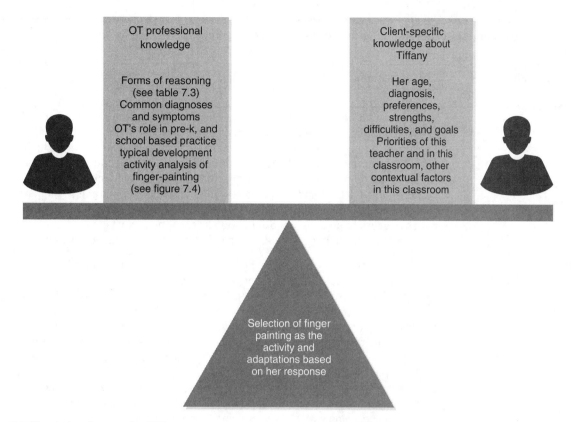

Figure 7.5 The balancing act for Tiffany

Table 7.4 Professional Reasoning Considerations for Selecting Finger Painting as an Activity for Tiffany

Type of Reasoning	Considerations
Scientific	From activity analysis of finger painting (Figure 7.4), you know this activity can be used to work on the perceptual and fine-motor skills that Tiffany has trouble with, as well as other areas of motor difficulties for which you have established goals. This activity could be appropriate to address these goals. There are few studies of finger painting as an intervention, and those available are not very rigorous (Basa, Sutarto, & Setiawan, 2020; Kurniawati, Hastuti, & Praherdhiono, 2018). However, you know from research that clients make greater improvements when they are invested in the activities you use in therapy. You know that some evidence suggests the importance of working with more skilled peers in elevating a child's performance. You also know that if finger painting is a regular activity in the classroom, then by focusing directly on finger painting in the classroom, you will not have to be concerned about generalization of skills to the natural environment.
Pragmatic	You are in Tiffany's classroom, and you have all the necessary equipment and materials to complete this activity. There is proper space and lighting. This is an educationally related activity that is already occurring in her classroom at this time, and it is therefore an appropriate choice.
Interactive	Tiffany has clearly indicated an interest in this activity. You also know that playing with her peers is very important to her. You are not certain which aspects of the activity might be most interesting to her at the moment, but based on your knowledge of Tiffany, you hypothesize it could be the social interaction with her peers.

(continues)

Table 7.4 Professional Reasoning Considerations for Selecting Finger Painting as an Activity for Tiffany

(continued)

Type of Reasoning	Considerations
Narrative	Tiffany's primary roles at this time are daughter, sibling, and student. Although this activity is not a necessary one for any of her current roles, you consider that this activity might be one she could engage in with her older sister or other members of her family. Additionally, you consider that this activity provides you with a fun way to work toward prewriting skills needed for her role as student. During your evaluation process, you determined from the family that they strongly emphasize Tiffany's full inclusion in all school and community events to the best of her ability. Finger painting is a common childhood and school activity. The family considers social interaction with her peers to be quite important and stresses the importance of her learning socially appropriate behaviors above specific fine-motor skills, for example.
Ethical	In this situation, no formal training is required to use finger painting, and there are no serious risks associated with this task. However, in choosing to spend a therapy session in this way you must consider if this is the most effective use of your time at this moment, or would another activity choice be better? If you refuse her request to participate in this activity, how will that influence her cooperation with you in whatever other activity to attempt? Will you get more out of the session if you select the activity that she already wishes to do? You know Tiffany's nature and can expect a serious "fight" if you refuse her and try to coax her into doing something else. From past experience, you know her strong-willed nature can lead to power struggles that last 15 minutes or more. It is better to get 15 minutes of "work" using this activity than spend it disagreeing with her about doing something else.
Conditional	Although, of course, the actual future for Tiffany is unknown, based on your experience with many other similar children and everything you know as a therapist and person, you hypothesize that Tiffany should be able to graduate high school and then perhaps live in a group home and have some form of employment. Although it may not be important in her future to be able to write more than her name, appropriate behaviors and social skills may be key to her ability to get and keep a job. If you had to balance working on specific motor skills or social skills, the social skill issues might be most important in the long term. Tiffany has many years of school ahead of her first, and the ability to demonstrate what has been learned in school often includes being able to write. This activity can be used to focus on both areas at once. You can practice prewriting skills while finger painting and also work on social interactions with peers at the same time. Agreeing to this activity with Tiffany also allows you to work in the classroom in an inclusive model of practice.

PRACTICE EXAMPLE 7.3 Crafting Specific Aspects of Tiffany's Selected Play

Based on what you know from the activity analysis, with finger painting, you could focus on cognitive demands, motor demands, and visual-perceptual demands as just a few of the areas to prioritize. Throughout the activity you can guide Tiffany toward any of those areas in the way you set up the activity or provide cuing and guidance.

Tiffany has goals for copying prewriting shapes and for dressing, and both of these can be addressed with this activity because she can make shapes with finger painting, and she will need to don her smock in preparation. You choose to begin with some of the cognitive and perceptual aspects of the task. You suggest that Tiffany gather the materials she needs. When you ask her what she needs in order to finger paint, Tiffany forgets her smock, but with reminders, she runs to the smock bin with a giggle. She is initially unable to orient the smock to place her arms and also loses her balance briefly when her shirt is over her head. She throws the shirt to the ground in frustration. You ask her to try again as you orient the shirt properly for her and provide cues and tactile prompts until she is able to succeed.

With the actual task of finger painting, she appears uncertain of the sequence of the steps to the activity and does not independently look to her peers for cues for where to begin. You consider ways to help her manage the two- to three-step activity sequence such as cueing her to watch and imitate her peers, modeling how to complete the activity, encouraging her to imitate your performance, providing only verbal cues without the model, or quickly creating a little song for her to repeat to herself to guide her movements. For example, using the tune of "This is the way we wash our clothes" (see https://www.youtube.com/watch?v=cRNaGwkEwB4), you might sing to her, "First we have to dip in paint, dip in paint, dip in paint, then we have to spread the paint all across the paper." You can encourage her to sing along with you as she does the movements to get the paint onto the paper. The next verse could be "Next we have to make a shape, make a shape, make a shape, then we have to make a shape, and I will make a circle." You then model making a circle in the finger paint and see if she will imitate. Not only does this made-up song address her sequencing, but it does so in a playful way, where other children are free to join in as well. Given your determination that her primary reason for wanting to do finger painting is to join other children, adding in play elements could make it more of a play experience.

PRACTICE EXAMPLE 7.4 Tiffany's Response

Once able to select a color of paint, place her hands and fingers in it, and then place it on the paper, she imitates the circles with you and smiles and engages with her peers, pleased with her circles. She also makes circles independently after imitating them.

Although you have focused on the cognitive and perceptual aspects of this activity for today, you note that Tiffany is unable to isolate individual fingers and instead uses her whole hand while painting. You also note that she winces and shakes her hand when it contacts the paint and becomes visibly upset when paint splashes onto her arm. When her peers begin to make more complex shapes on their paintings, Tiffany also wants to try these but becomes frustrated as she is unable to form the more complex shapes. You attempt to cue her to trace the shape you have drawn; but she refuses. When she asks to wash her hands and arms, complains of being tired, sits down on the floor, and refuses to participate further, you must decide whether to try to coax her to continue with finger painting in some way or select a new activity.

Based on your occupational analysis of Tiffany's performance with finger painting in the classroom, you make hypotheses about her performance in relation to your prior knowledge from her evaluation and your consideration of varied frames of reference (see **Table 7.5**). You begin to identify how you might alter this activity going forward or select a new activity based on what you have learned.

Because Tiffany also has goals to sustain play with peers and manage her frustration, you prioritize returning to the activity. You decide to try to coax her back by adapting the activity to decrease the demands that you feel are too challenging. You have decided the sensory aspects of the activity were distressing for her, and it was too difficult for her to meet the visual-perceptual-motor and praxis demands of forming the complex shapes her peers were forming. You quickly retrieve and then model for Tiffany how she could use shape stampers to paint complex pictures with her peers without having to touch the paint. However, as you do so, you have also decided that if she refuses, you will switch gears immediately and suggest a different activity to try to end on a successful note for the day.

Table 7.5 Use of Activity Analysis and Occupational Analysis of Finger Painting Within Different Frames of Reference to Guide Future Activity Choices

Frame of Reference	Activity Demands (from Activity Analysis)	Tiffany's Performance (Occupational Analysis)	Application to Future Activity Choices and Intervention Methods
Biomechanical	Finger painting requires postural control to sit at the table while reaching for materials and strength, range of motion, and endurance to maintain posture and reach for and manipulate materials.	Tiffany has difficulty maintaining an upright position in sitting, reaching and holding, and finger isolation.	■ Provide external supports or positioning during the activity to help maintain posture. ■ Choose and use materials and positions that will challenge and work on Tiffany's reaching, holding, and finger isolation within finger painting. ■ Consider activities outside of finger painting to build strength, endurance, and postural control.

(continues)

Table 7.5 Use of Activity Analysis and Occupational Analysis of Finger Painting Within Different Frames of Reference to Guide Future Activity Choices *(continued)*

Frame of Reference	Activity Demands (from Activity Analysis)	Tiffany's Performance (Occupational Analysis)	Application to Future Activity Choices and Intervention Methods
Cognitive	Finger painting requires an understanding of the sequence of the painting activity, the materials needed, and, in the case of forming shapes or letters, the direct steps or specific motor actions to form those shapes or letters.	Tiffany is uncertain of the materials needed and order of the steps for the activity. Tiffany is attempting to use strategies, including verbal mediation and singing, to draw shapes.	■ During finger painting, teach and use cognitive strategies for identifying and remembering steps and sequence of activity and materials needed. ■ Reinforce and give feedback regarding performance of motor tasks and use of strategy. ■ Follow with the use of the same strategies in similar tasks and activities that do not use finger paint.
NDT	Finger painting requires that she maintain an upright posture during painting, that she has adequate reach on and off her base of support, that she has adequate grasp and stroke patterns, and that she can cross midline with trunk rotation to reach all areas of the large paper.	Tiffany has difficulty remaining in an upright seated position. She has difficulty maintaining balance when putting on her smock. She also has difficulty isolating her finger when painting, and she does not cross midline with rotation but instead walks around the paper.	■ During activities, use therapeutic handling and motor practice in context with facilitation to address trunk strength and rotation when reaching, reaching on and off base of support, and proximal stability with finger isolation. ■ The activity of finger painting itself may or may not be used. ■ Any activity with those same necessary components will be acceptable.
ASI	Finger painting primarily provides tactile input in terms of the texture and feel of the paint and the temperature of the paint. In addition, this activity requires crossing midline on large paper, bilateral and unilateral hand use, motor planning for forming letters, and planning painting.	Tiffany has difficulty orienting the smock and placing her arms in. She becomes upset when paint touches her hands. She does not cross midline with rotation. Her motor planning for shape formation is poor.	■ Use deep touch pressure and proprioceptive activities to address tactile sensitivity. ■ Modify activities as necessary to change sensory input and demands for participation. ■ Develop and use a variety of activities to address motor planning. ■ It is likely, based on her reaction, that finger painting may be discouraged in the near term until she is better able to tolerate this type of input. Instead, other activities may be selected to work on the same goal areas. Over time, finger painting could be attempted again to judge progress.
Acquisitional approach with compensatory strategies	Finger painting requires maintenance of upright posture, joint mobility and strength to reach, finger isolation, endurance to complete tasks, vision, and cognitive demands such as sequencing.	Tiffany has decreased endurance for sitting, poor finger isolation, and limited balance when putting on clothes, and she is uncertain of the steps of task and the materials.	■ During finger painting, identify and use modifications for seating or position to decrease the demands on her postural control and endurance. ■ Tiffany could finger paint prone on the floor, at an easel, or sitting in a more supportive seat. ■ Create a visual material list or sequence of the activity for Tiffany to use. ■ A tool could be provided for her to use instead of her finger to get the paint, and she could paint using her whole hand if the desired outcome was for her to paint with her peers and engage in classroom activities.

Conclusion

Occupational therapy practitioners must continually select appropriate therapeutic activities and in a play-based approach, appropriate play activities. Selection occurs as the therapist uses professional reasoning to balance professional knowledge (theory, frames of reference, specific intervention approaches) with the knowledge of the client. Activity and occupational analyses enable selection of "just-right" play activities throughout each session. These decisions occur in collaboration with the child, based on sound professional reasoning using multiple forms of thinking simultaneously. Selecting pediatric play activities that are therapeutic, meaningful, and motivating exemplifies the fusion of art and science in occupational therapy. The right blend of professional reasoning and therapeutic use of self results in clinical choices that guide the child toward increased occupational performance and participation in play.

References

Basa, F. L., Sutarto, J., & Setiawan, D. (2020). Finger painting learning to stimulate motor development in early childhood. *Journal of Primary Education, 9*(2), 193–200.

Bass, J. D., Baum, C., & Christiansen, C. (2017). Person-environment-occupation-performance-model. In J. Hinojosa, P. Kramer, & C. B. Royeen (Eds.), *Perspectives on human occupation: Theories underlying practice* (2nd ed.). Philadelphia, PA: F. A. Davis.

Boyt Schell, B. A., Gillen, G., & Scaffa, M. (2014). Glossary. In B. A. Boyt Schell, G. Gillen, & M. Scaffa (Eds.), *Willard and Spackman's occupational therapy* (12th ed., p. 1231). Philadelphia, PA: Lippincott Williams & Wilkins.

Bryze, K. C. (2008). Narrative contributions to the play history. In L. D. Parham & L. S. Fazio (Eds.), *Play in occupational therapy for children* (2nd ed., pp. 43–54). St. Louis, MO: Mosby Elsevier.

Dunbar, S. (2007). *Occupational therapy models for intervention with children and families.* Thorofare, NJ: Slack

Grajo, L. C. (2017). Occupational adaptation. In J. Hinojosa, P. Kramer, & C. B. Royeen (Eds.), *Perspectives on human occupation* (2nd ed.). Philadelphia, PA: F.A. Davis.

Kramer, P., Hinojosa, J., & Howe, T. (2019). *Frames of reference for pediatric occupational therapy* (4th ed.). Baltimore, MD: Williams & Wilkins.

Kurniawati, A., Hastuti, W. D., & Praherdhiono, H. (2018). The effect of finger painting towards fine motor skill of intellectual disability. *Jurnal Penelitian dan Pengembangan Pendidikan Luar Biasa, 5*(1), 47–51. https://core.ac.uk/download/pdf/287323233.pdf

Law, M., Missiuna, C., Pollock, N., & Stewart, D. (2005). Foundations for occupational therapy practice with children. In J. Case-Smith (Ed.), *Occupational therapy for children* (pp. 53–87). St. Louis, MO: Mosby.

Márquez-Álvarez, L. J., Calvo-Arenillas, J. I., Talavera-Valverde, M. Á., & Moruno-Millares, P. (2019). Professional reasoning in occupational therapy: A scoping review. *Occupational Therapy International, 2019,* 6238245. https:// doi.org/10.1155 /2019/6238245

Mattingly, C., & Fleming, M. H. (1994). Interactive reasoning: Collaborating with the person. In C. Mattingly & M. H. Fleming (Eds.), *Clinical reasoning: Forms of inquiry in a therapeutic practice* (pp. 178–196). Philadelphia, PA: F. A. Davis.

Mosey, A. C. (1981). *Occupational therapy: Configuration of a profession.* New York: Raven Press.

O'Brien, J., & Kuhaneck, H. (2020). Using occupational therapy models and frames of reference with children and youth. In J. O'Brien & H. Kuhaneck (Eds.), *Case-Smith's Occupational therapy for children and adolescents* (8th ed., pp. 18–45). St. Louis, MO: Mosby.

Schell, B. B., & Schell, J. W. (2008). *Clinical and professional reasoning in occupational therapy.* Philadelphia, PA: Lippincott, Williams & Wilkins.

Taylor, R. R. (2017). *Kielhofner's model of human occupation* (5th ed.). Philadelphia, PA: Wolters Kluwer.

Unsworth, C. A. (2005). Using a head-mounted video camera to explore current conceptualizations of clinical reasoning in occupational therapy. *American Journal of Occupational Therapy, 59*(1), 31–40.

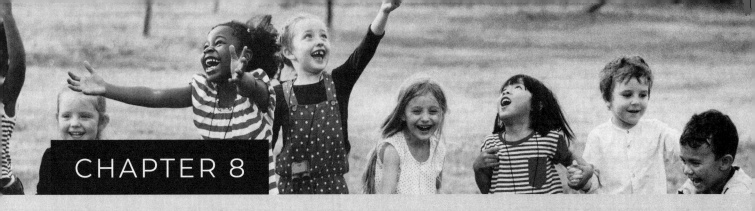

CHAPTER 8

Adapting Activities for Play and Therapy

Susan L. Spitzer, PhD, OTR/L

After reading this chapter, the reader will:

- Define and compare the terms *adaptation*, *modification*, and *grading* in relation to play.
- Articulate the distinct importance of both modifying and grading play activities in occupational therapy.
- Determine modifications and grading for various play demands for different clients.
- Differentiate play adaptations by frames of reference in occupational therapy.
- Select and implement adaptations fluidly to promote play based on professional reasoning.
- Adapt activities that the child is experiencing predominantly as "work" into more playful activities.

A child loves his play, not because it's easy, but because it's hard.

—Benjamin Spock

An activity often must be adapted if it is to be both play and the right fit for the child. Perhaps the child is not experiencing the measure of success necessary to continue without giving up. Or, perhaps the activity is so easy that there is no therapeutic benefit for the child. Maybe the therapist is still getting to know the child. Even experienced practitioners and children sometimes choose activities that end up being unsuitable as initially planned. Often the goals of therapy are *work* for the child, necessary activities the child needs to do but does not want to do. When these situations arise, occupational therapy practitioners combine activity analysis with their knowledge of the child to make targeted decisions on how best to alter the activity so that the child wants to participate and makes progress. To maintain the highest level of motivation and therapeutic benefit, therapists constantly adapt to make play just right for each individual.

Adapting for Play

Adaptation has endured as an essential quality of occupational therapy (Grajo, Boisselle, & DaLomba, 2018; Marshall, Myers, & Pierce, 2017). Adaptation is viewed as a transformation in and through occupations, enabling greater participation, both as a process and an outcome (Grajo et al., 2018). Occupational therapy practitioners value individuals' ability to adapt to changes such as aging, disability, and environmental factors. Acknowledgment of this human capacity forms the cornerstone for the use of adaptation as a tool of practice.

As an intervention, adaptation refers to changing the activity demands to better suit the person's individual factors and skills under a given circumstance (Marshall et al., 2017). The practitioner utilizes knowledge obtained previously from the activity analysis regarding demands and from the occupational analysis regarding how these demands intersect with the client (as described in Chapter 4). The occupational therapy practitioner adapts components of the activity based on whether each is a barrier or support for participation, often in collaboration with the child, family, and other team members. The specific function of each adaptation is intrinsic to its use because what is adaptive for one individual may not be adaptive or may even be disruptive for another individual or another context. The intent of adaptation is to decrease barriers and exploit strengths so that a child both can and wants to play. This just right challenge is determined by matching activity demands with the client's abilities and interests so that the child can successfully participate (Ayres, 1972, 2005; Burke, 1977; Mack, Lindquist, & Parham, 1982; Michelman, 1974; Robinson, 1977; Rogers, 1982; Tickle-Degnen & Coster, 1995). Occupational therapists' establishment of a just right challenge has strongly correlated with child engagement (Holland et al., 2018).

When the chosen activity is not within a child's current capabilities to participate, activity adaptation is necessary. Adapting may focus on one individual or multiple individuals within a group. Activity adaptations may be predominantly static in the form of modifications or dynamic in the form of grading, either or both of which may be used for each client.

Modifying for Play

Modifying is a specific type of occupational therapy intervention defined as "finding ways to revise the current context or activity demands to support performance . . . [which includes] compensatory techniques, including enhancing some features to provide cues, or reducing other features to reduce distractibility" according to the Occupational Therapy Practice Framework (AOTA, 2020) and Dunn, McClain, Brown, and Youngstrom (1998, p. 533). Modification of an activity requires altering a demand to allow a client to perform it at all or with less assistance. For example, for a child without any gross grasp who cannot hold a paintbrush to paint unless physically guided, but who has full active range of motion in the upper extremity, the activity of painting can be modified by placing a strap on the paintbrush. This modification removes the needs for grasp and assistance, allowing the child to participate by painting at an easel with his or her peers.

The occupational therapy practitioner modifies activities by considering alternative ways of how the activity could be performed in order to enable the child to participate (Spitzer, 2020). A modification is designed to be a relatively fixed or static element so that it can enable continued participation of the client, often in the absence of the therapist; however, ongoing monitoring and adjustments of modifications may be needed over

time to determine a workable modification and to adjust to a child's development. At a minimum, modifications remove barriers to make it easier for the child or adolescent to access play (see **Figure 8.1**). However, many clients also need modifications that support participation in play.

Modifications may include changes to the environment or the structure or form of the activity. For example, the occupational therapy practitioner might recommend turning off the television and electronic screens to decrease environmental distractors to social play (see Chapter 9 for extensive environmental play modifications). Or, in the case of the highly supported intervention of breaking down activities into steps (Missiuna et al., 2012; Steinbrenner et al., 2020; Wong et al., 2015), a therapist might modify the structure for assembly of an interlocking puzzle by providing a list of steps for the teen to follow. Or, the form may be altered by using adaptive equipment or assistive technology such as providing switch access so a child with a degenerative neuromotor disorder may play with a toy (Deitz & Swinth, 2008; Judge, Floyd, & Wood-Fields, 2010; Verver, Vervloed, & Steenbergen, 2019, 2020; Williams & Matesi, 1988). Many modifications are commercially available through therapy suppliers and toy manufacturers (for example: https://toyboxtools.hasbro.com/en-us/resources). However, many modifications must be customized for a specific child or individually determined to make sure the modification is right for a particular client.

Modifications may include adjustments to address client relevance and importance as well as other activity demands (see **Table 8.1** for examples of modifications for different kinds of activity demands). Modifications that balance the client's motivation with the activity's challenge

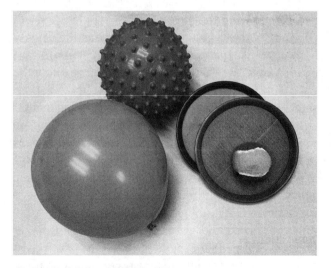

Figure 8.1 Object modifications such as a ball with knobs for gripping, a Velcro® mitt, and a balloon (clockwise from top) can increase access for playing ball
Courtesy of Susan L. Spitzer.

promote the just right challenge (Burke, 1977). In this way, modifications can also maximize client strengths to compensate (O'Brien & Soloman, 2013). To promote play and the child's intrinsic drive, the occupational therapy practitioner avoids stopping the child or saying no to his or her ideas, even when those ideas appear inconvenient or counter to therapeutic goals. Instead, the therapist immediately thinks of *how* to do what the child wants to do, how to modify the activity to make it happen while maintaining therapeutic benefit, as seen in the case of Benjamin (see **Practice Example 8.1**).

Grading for Play

Grading is used extensively as a core foundational tool in occupational therapy (Breines, 1986). Grading is the dynamic process of making demands easier or more difficult based on the client's performance so that the activity promotes progressive improvement in client performance, abilities, or skills. For example, grading the activity of throwing for a child could include gradually changing the distance or size of the target (see **Figure 8.2**). Grading play can mean the difference between a child feeling bored when an activity is too easy or frustrated when it is too hard, and a child being able to move forward and try a different activity or a different version of the current activity.

Grading often happens multiple times during an occupational therapy session, in the moment of activity performance to sustain the just right challenge (Ayres, 1979, 2005; O'Brien & Soloman, 2013). Activities are made easy enough for the client to participate in them and then gradually more difficult to build skills. The initial grading allows the child to gain practice and adapt to the activity, and the ongoing grading maximizes the therapeutic aspects of activities. As the child gains skills, activity supports are faded and challenges increased.

Activities can be graded to increase or decrease the challenge level in a variety of ways (Breines, 1986; Marshall et al., 2017; Neistadt et al., 1993; Piersol, 2014; Price & Miner, 2007). Selecting which way(s) to grade an activity for an individual should be based on the potential to create a successful challenge that promotes the child's skills. This just right challenge emerges from matching activity demands that address a client's needs with the client's abilities (Ayres, 1972, 2005; Burke, 1977; Mack, Lindquist, & Parham, 1982; Rogers, 1982; Tickle-Degnen & Coster, 1995). The therapist weighs various options and decides which activity demand(s) should be graded in order to meet therapeutic goals for an individual child's play (see **Table 8.1** for examples). The practitioner also determines the degree to which each demand is graded both in terms of incremental amount and frequency that an individual child needs and can tolerate. Similar acts of grading may occur at a faster or slower pace for different children.

PRACTICE EXAMPLE 8.1 Benjamin and Hospital Bed Modifications

Benjamin, a teenager, sustained multiple life-threatening injuries in a car accident. He had numerous surgeries and spent an extended stay in the local children's hospital. While in the hospital, he received occupational therapy to (1) increase his endurance for completion of daily activities and (2) regain function of his dominant left upper extremity (UE) for daily activities.

During one session, the occupational therapist brought in items for a board game. Benjamin expressed interest in the game, but just like most sessions, insisted on doing it while lying down in bed because he was tired. His occupational therapist recognized this common compensation for limited endurance, which was counterproductive for therapy because neither therapeutic goal could be addressed. The reasoning had been explained to Benjamin on multiple occasions, and he demonstrated clear memory and understanding of this need. After much coaxing, Benjamin usually acquiesced reluctantly. On this day, Benjamin was especially tired and resistant. The therapist was torn as to how to save the session and engage Benjamin—whether to insist on him sitting up and risk complete refusal or to allow him to lie down, which was counterproductive to his goals and might decrease arousal and visual attention.

Given that neither option was very promising, the occupational therapist began considering how to modify the game to play it lying down in bed, involving Benjamin in this problem solving. Benjamin was surprised at the therapist's own acquiescence in "round one," as they joked about who might win "round two" (the board game). He immediately became more alert and motivated as they problem-solved together how to modify the position of the board for him to reach and see. The board was propped up vertically against the bed rails on the right side so that he would need to reach with his left UE to play. Benjamin was facilitated in adding tape under each game marker so that it could stick to the vertical board. Benjamin was very engaged in the preparations and initiating the game. Shortly after, Benjamin expressed that he did not like playing the game this way and wanted to sit up, which was done for the remainder of the game.

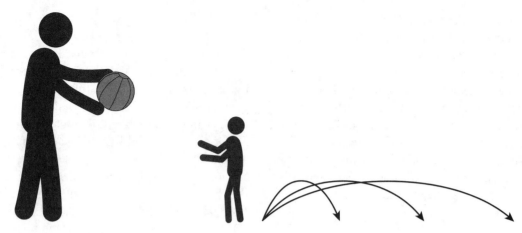

Figure 8.2 Catch can be graded for improving skill by gradually increasing the distance between players as skill grows

Table 8.1 Examples of Grading and Modifications for Play

Type of Demand*	Grading to Increase Skills/Function	Modification to Access Participation
Required body functions	■ Use toys with less resistance to decrease demand on strength and gradually increase resistance to increase demand on strength. ■ Increase the number of direct cues for a step to decrease demands for executive function; then gradually decrease the number and/or specificity of cues to increase executive function demands. ■ Decrease the sensory stimulation provided by an activity to decrease sensory demands and gradually increase the sensory stimulation to increase the sensory (tolerance/integration) demands. ■ Place objects to decrease range of motion needed and gradually adjust placement (direction or distance) to increase range of motion.	■ Increase visual contrast so that a child can trace. ■ Add a strap to a paintbrush for a child with involuntary hand movements. ■ Add switch adaptations to toys so that a child with limited range of motion and strength may access and play with them independently. ■ Reduce auditory and visual distractions. ■ Complete an activity in a different position from typical (such as seated) to accommodate for decreased respiratory function. ■ Provide supportive or padded seating for comfort. ■ Laminate pages of favorite book to prevent them from being torn due to uncontrolled heavy use of force.
Required body structures	■ N/A	■ Change games to be done with one hand, one eye, one foot, or different body parts. ■ Alter a bike so it can be pedaled with the arms rather than the legs.
Objects used and their properties	■ Use materials that are lighter to allow lifting and then gradually heavier to challenge strength. ■ Use toys that are bigger to aid manipulation or grasp and gradually decrease to challenge fine-motor skills. ■ Provide only a few objects at a time, and gradually increase the number to manage at once. ■ Gradually increase the number of pieces, decrease the size of pieces, and increase subtly among pieces in a puzzle.	■ String beads on pipe cleaners instead of laces so that a child can play independently. ■ Use stamps instead of crayons to create a picture. ■ Provide loop scissors to allow a child to participate in a craft activity.

Type of Demand*	Grading to Increase Skills/Function	Modification to Access Participation
Space demands	■ Make a wider and then gradually narrower pathway or remove and then gradually add obstacles to build navigation with a scooter, wheelchair, or bike. ■ Place pieces closer for reach and organization, and then gradually increase distance/location (such as in different drawers, shelves, cupboards).	■ Keep favorite toys in a bag on the side of the wheelchair or on lower shelves in the bedroom. ■ Remove obstacles to access a play area. ■ Add obstacles around a perimeter to create a smaller space to focus play. ■ Use signs, masking tape, chalk, furniture, etc. to mark a specific play area.
Social demands	■ Alter communication strategies to be easier (e.g., play game using only gestural/nonverbal cues), then gradually increase the number or type of communication strategies for greater complexity. ■ Gradually alter the number of individuals involved in a game (play games in pairs or teams). ■ Increase material availability to limit sharing demands and then gradually decrease materials to encourage sharing.	■ Use a communication device during game/activity to aid social interaction. ■ Advise peers to use a strategy (such as get close, tap arm, or show toy) to enable the child to attend to and understand the other child. ■ Use a turn-taking card to clarify when it is the child's turn vs. another's turn.
Required actions and performance skills	■ Gradually increase the challenge level of manipulative games by altering the manipulation strategy used such as which finger or fingers the child may use, the use of (non)dominant or both hands. ■ Increase stability of the surface and use of nonslip materials or rigid objects, then gradually decrease stability by using smooth, slick items to increase precision of motor demands. ■ Gradually increase the number and complexity of rules to build performance skills.	■ Use a keyboard (as opposed to writing) to create a story to compensate for poor fine-motor and organizational skills. ■ Change the rules of a game to allow increased success or participation. ■ Use a wait card to compensate for limited impulse control. ■ Use a card holder in a game for a teen with limited bilateral coordination.
Sequencing and timing	■ Decrease and then gradually increase the numbers of steps in a sequence. ■ Require the child to determine the steps with increasingly indirect cues. ■ Gradually decrease the amount of time allotted to complete a turn, step, or action in play such as by adding a timing criterion. ■ Gradually increase the duration of time playing one activity or waiting for a turn.	■ Extend time for play. ■ Provide pictures of each step for setting up a game or building. ■ Use timer to self-monitor timely completion or prepare for transition in an activity.
Relevance and importance to client	■ Gradually decrease the number or use of child's favorite toys, objects, and play themes to expand the child's interests into other play activities. ■ Include objects, actions, and play themes that are increasingly different from the child's interests to expand play repertoire.	■ Include child's favorite toys, objects, themes such as in a game of chase or pretending.

*Types of demands are from: AOTA, 2020. The practitioner identifies specific demands based on the activity analysis.
Note: For some demands, modification and grading may be similar; however, the intent of the adaptation and its temporal nature are what identifies it as either a modification or grading. If the primary intent is to allow maximal participation in context for an indefinite period of time, then this static adaptation is a modification. If the primary intent is to promote participation that progressively establishes, improves, or restores client skills and abilities, then this dynamic adaptation is considered grading.

Professional Reasoning for Adapting Play

Just as professional reasoning is used to select activities (see Chapter 7), it is used similarly to modify and grade activities once selected. Occupational therapy practitioners must select from a range of potential adaptations based on various considerations such as their anticipated impact on occupational performance, their feasibility, and the preferences and priorities of clients, family, and other stakeholders (Rigby, Trentham, & Letts, 2019; Weaver, 2018). Professional reasoning based on professional training is necessary to adapt play in alignment with scientific knowledge and frames of reference and in relation to the evolving dynamics of play.

Frames of Reference and Adapting Play

The occupational therapy practitioner often makes choices about how to adapt activities for therapeutic benefit according to the theoretical framework of a particular frame of reference. Considerations include the frame of reference's emphasis on modification or grading, on which activity demands to adapt, and on which outcomes of therapy can be expected, as seen in **Table 8.2**. For example, the neurodevelopmental treatment and sensory integration frames of reference place more emphasis on grading motor or sensory demands, with the outcome of intervention being a change in performance skills that leads to a change in participation in a variety of activities (Ayres, 2005; Michielsen,

Table 8.2 Activity Adaptations for Different Frames of Reference

Frames of Reference	Activity Adaptation Considerations
Acquisition/behavioral	<ul><li>Modify a new activity for learning by breaking it down into discrete sequenced steps.</li><li>Grade steps of a new activity over time to a larger number or greater complexity.</li><li>Modify environmental supports and barriers, whether antecedents or consequences, to increase the likelihood of positive participation (supports) and decrease the likelihood of participation challenges (barriers).</li><li>Grade positive reinforcers to fade after a task is learned.</li></ul>
Biomechanical	<ul><li>Modifications include orthoses and positioning to rest or compensate for physical limitations.</li><li>Grade stretch to increase ROM.</li><li>Grade duration, velocity resistance, and type of muscle contraction to increase strength and endurance.</li></ul>
Cognitive	<ul><li>Modification is directed by and occurs with the input of the child as he or she problem-solves strategies.</li><li>Grade process requirements to build a child's skill with making their own modifications and ability to use cognitive strategies.</li></ul>
Cognitive behavioral	<ul><li>Grade emotional and cognitive demands to increase a child's positive emotional reactions and motivation (i.e., positive self-talk, anger management, frustration tolerance) to engage in activities.</li></ul>
Motor learning	<ul><li>Modify movement constraints to provide active and successful participation in meaningful occupations that provide the child with repeated practice as well as intrinsic and extrinsic feedback.</li><li>Grade movement demands to require increased skill and variable adjustments within an activity.</li></ul>
Neurodevelopmental treatment	<ul><li>Grade activities for progressive improvement in the quality of movement to enhance the child's motor and postural skills.</li></ul>
Sensory integration	<ul><li>Grade combinations of sensory input and motor demands to provide the right level of challenge to enable the child to make an adaptive (more complex) response.</li><li>Recommend activity modification of sensory input in daily life to promote a healthy match for the child.</li></ul>

Vaughan-Graham, Holland, Magri, & Suzuki, 2019). In contrast, a cognitive frame of reference uses modification more extensively, specifically as a cognitive strategy for the child to apply (Chapparo, 2010; Dawson, McEwen, & Polatajko, 2017). When sensory integration and acquisition frames of reference are combined such as in school-based practice, both grading and modification may be used (AOTA,

2015). New factors may emerge necessitating adjustment of the frame(s) of reference to accommodate this clinical evidence (Spitzer, 2020). Knowing the tenets of the chosen frames of reference will support the reasoning needed to decide which frame(s) of reference to select and to guide decisions regarding which aspects of the activity are graded or modified for therapeutic benefit (see **Practice Example 8.2**).

PRACTICE EXAMPLE 8.2 Malia and Recess Adaptations

Malia was a second grader with Down syndrome who was fully included at school, where she received occupational therapy. One of her goals was to play cooperatively at recess. She often asked about recess and playing with her friends. She routinely went to the jump rope, hand ball, and four-square courts at recess. She stood in line for approximately 30 seconds and then went onto the court and tried to play, interrupting the game and annoying the other children, which often required adult intervention. The only time she waited longer was when she was standing next to her friend Jane, who held her hand and stroked her arm and back. When Malia did get a turn, she immediately missed the rope or ball, then yelled, "This is stupid," and took or kicked the ball or rope, bumping into children as she left, again disrupting play for the other children. After playing a game, she would immediately lie down. She did not consistently play—sometimes she just spent the recess either lying down, walking slowly while leaning on the fence, or sitting down by herself. The occupational therapy evaluation identified underlying challenges in the following areas: endurance, postural control, motor skills, process skills, emotional regulation, social interaction skills, tactile and proprioceptive hyporesponsivity, and problematic recess routines. The team understood that Malia's motor skills were common for children with Down syndrome; however, they were concerned that many of Malia's peers had started to say they did not want to play with her. Malia's occupational therapist considered possible adaptations based on different frames of reference as indicated in **Table 8.3**.

Table 8.3 Examples of Play Adaptations for Malia Based on Different Frames of Reference

Frames of Reference	Play Adaptations
Acquisition/behavioral	■ Modify playground games by breaking them down into discrete sequenced steps with numbers and pictures to follow (on a list or keyring), include step for what to do when her turn is over. ■ Modify rules for her, requiring her to select the game with the smallest line or follow Jane. ■ Provide frequent happy faces drawn as a positive reinforcer for each small success until she is able to follow all the steps for a game. Then reduce the frequency of happy faces.
Biomechanical	■ Grade jumping and ball activities for submaximal exertion and gradual increases in duration/repetition to increase endurance.
Cognitive	■ Grade activities and information to help Malia understand the consequences of her actions such selecting activities because different activities may have a shorter wait, be more fun/successful. ■ Grade activities to help her recognize and follow the steps, while providing choices as a modification to help her remember the steps. ■ Grade just enough information to help her identify what and how to adjust her body to improve motor performance. ■ Modify activities with a visual cue card about problem-solving different choices for handling anger (that is developed together with Malia) such as the following response choices: "Kick—no play. Yell—no play. Grab—no play. Play again. Play something different."

(continues)

Table 8.3 Examples of Play Adaptations for Malia Based on Different Frames of Reference   *(continued)*

Frames of Reference	Play Adaptations
Cognitive behavioral	■ Grade play activities with gradual increases in degree/frequency of errors (mistakes); with gradual increases in waiting time; with gradual decreases in preparation for missing, making errors, losing—starting with play activities that are a strength for her and later applying to challenging motor play. ■ Modify the activities by using a visual therapeutic script at the beginning to prepare and remind her to cognitively alter her behavior such as "Playing games can be tricky. Everybody makes mistakes sometimes. That's ok. We can try again." Or "My friends like it when I wait. I can watch my friends when I wait."
Motor learning	■ Modify jump rope by placing a piece of masking piece or chalk mark as a visual cue of where to stand as she learns how to jump rope. ■ Grade jump-rope demands by jumping initially over a stable rope laying on the ground, next a rope that is turned and kept on the ground until she jumps, then a slow-moving rope, and finally a gradually faster rope. ■ Modify ball activities by marking a line on the handball court wall for aiming; by substituting a balloon, soft grippable ball, large bean bag, hook-and-loop mitts. ■ Grade ball activities by throwing or bouncing the ball directly at her hands, gradually further from her center of gravity, and eventually requiring her to move her body to an increasing distance, and with gradually decreasing predictability. ■ Grade speed to gradually increase speed of the ball.
Neurodevelopmental treatment	■ Grade play activities for gradually increased postural demands.
Sensory integration	■ Modify recess with use of self-tickles on her arms to increase body awareness and positive state during recess. ■ Modify activities with heavy materials to increase proprioceptive feedback. ■ Grade demands for gradually refined use of force and tactile discrimination. ■ Modify jump rope by placing a piece of masking tape or chalk mark as a visual cue of where to stand to compensate for decreased somatosensation for body awareness in relation to the jump rope.

Integrating Layers of Reasoning for Adapting Play

An occupational therapy practitioner utilizes various forms of clinical reasoning based on professional training to adapt play. Scientific, pragmatic, interactive, narrative, and ethical reasoning are essential in determining adaptations. Each was described in the prior chapter in relation to activity selection, and here are applied to decisions regarding adaptation.

Scientific Reasoning

Scientific reasoning enables us to apply available scientific evidence in selecting adaptations. The occupational therapy practitioner utilizes modifications and grading, which are hypothesized to improve an individual child's participation based on available scientific evidence. For example, therapists commonly break down activities into steps and use visual strategies to modify activities for children with ASD because there is strong evidence to support these modifications will be effective (Missiuna et al., 2012; Steinbrenner et al., 2020; Wong et al., 2015).

Pragmatic Reasoning

Pragmatic considerations affect the occupational therapy practitioner's ability to adapt activities. Available materials, space, time, and other contextual factors influence which aspects of an activity can be changed and how. Theoretically, any factors can be adapted; however, some factors may be more feasible than others. Necessary materials or permission for an adaptation may not be present at the moment, and the therapist may need to determine the value and timeliness of obtaining them. Although at times a challenge, meeting pragmatic demands is one of the most rewarding creative endeavors in which occupational therapy practitioners engage and is highlighted in Chapter 9.

Interactive and Narrative Reasoning

Interactive and narrative reasoning are at the heart of establishing meaningful and playful interactions and activities for pediatric clients. Through these types of reasoning, play schemes and themes are developed and consistently adapted to establish and maintain a playful and motivating environment. This reasoning enables therapists to understand the daily routines and situations that the child may encounter and tailor therapeutic activities that best address the demands of those situations. The therapist suggests adaptations that suit the family, school, and cultural contexts. This reasoning helps the therapist grade activities playfully because he or she knows the child and family on an individually meaningful level. Grading activities in a playful manner contributes to a therapeutic narrative where the child is engaged as a successful player.

Interactive and narrative reasoning are relied upon heavily when managing the important social-emotional efficacy aspect of adapting an activity. Therapeutic use of self (see Chapter 6) is an important tool in this process. For example, an occupational therapist may take the blame for making an activity too easy or too hard. Statements like, "Oh my, I put that way too high, didn't I? I can barely reach it. Let me fix it and then we can try again" or "Wow, I made that as wide as a river, who can jump a whole river? Not me. I better make it smaller," can go a long way toward framing a child's perspective positively. Competition, if a child can handle it, can be useful when upgrading an activity. Interactive and narrative reasoning provide important information about what play themes may be fun and meaningful to the child, which can be used to make the level easier or harder or easing any anxiety the child may feel if he or she cannot accomplish a task as it was originally presented.

Ethical Reasoning

Ethical reasoning allows us to consider what will benefit the child and pose the least risk. Ethical reasoning is important when considering adaptation. The occupational therapist must weigh the value of different adaptations on occupational performance. For example, the therapist must consider whether to focus on the benefit of modifying an activity for immediate participation in play or the benefit of grading to build long-term adaptive skills to support a wider range of play. While both may be included, often one is emphasized at a time. If a child cannot participate in an activity without modifications, there may be significant developmental, social, and emotional risks of waiting for skills to develop. It is in these situations that we as occupational therapy practitioners can play an important role in using our expertise in activity analysis to find ways to modify aspects of the activity so that the child may engage and participate in it. Modifications may involve ethical considerations related to multiple stakeholders who are often involved in modifications such as rearranging items so that toys are stored on an accessible-level shelf or asking a family member or peer to be a playmate in a specific game. Some individuals are happy to help, and others find it burdensome. Weighing the benefits and risks of implementing or not implementing different modifications for the occupations of the child and others is essential to determine how strongly we should express and advocate for specific measures or present multiple options from which to select.

Determining Whether to Modify or Grade

Professional reasoning determines whether modifications or grading are selected. The occupational therapist considers the relationship of adaptations to an individual child's needs and the pragmatics of implementing those adaptations. Modifications that can be made easily given the social and physical environment are often selected to yield immediate increases in participation that can be carried over in the therapist's absence. Modifications are typically more compensatory in nature because they focus on adapting factors that are predominately external to the individual; but they also may build skills through allowing practice with new play activities over time. Nonetheless, this means that modifications often need to be changed as the child develops physically, emotionally, mentally, or spiritually and as the child needs or wants to engage in new play activities or in different physical and social environments. In contrast, grading tends to take more time to change performance because it primarily targets developing or restoring internal client factors; and grading requires a clinical judgment that reasonable progress in skills and abilities is achievable. Grading requires more ongoing effort from both the practitioner and client. Because grading is used for skill building, often these skills are adaptable across multiple activities and environments and provide a foundation for future skill development. Balancing the short-term and long-term needs given the constraints and opportunities within practice involves a combination of different forms of professional reasoning as seen in **Practice Example 8.3**.

Adapting in Unpredictable Moments to Promote Play

Occupational therapy is a dynamic process that entails ongoing assessment, analysis, and adaptation on a moment-by-moment basis, especially when focused on play. Preparation, attentive observations, and flexibility enable the therapist to be ready for

---

PRACTICE EXAMPLE 8.3 Malia: Professional Reasoning for Selecting Recess Adaptations

In order to select from the various possible adaptations identified for Malia (as listed in **Table 8.3**), the occupational therapist used professional reasoning to determine priorities given the school setting as well as her short-term and long-term needs. Clearly, the physical and sensory demands for Malia's play were critical because she did not have the skills to meet these demands. Pragmatically, it would be hard to modify these specific motor and social demands in a school setting because so many different adults and children would have to buy into the changes. At the same time, grading motor skills, postural control, sensory processing, and postural control would take time to yield results. Even the process skills might take longer in this case, given Malia's cognitive functioning. Interactive reasoning highlighted that recess was more work than play for Malia despite her having enough interest and knowledge to attempt the activities. The emerging narrative of disruptive behavior drove the therapist ethically to identify which modifications could be implemented immediately on the playground to meet these pressing needs. As a result, the occupational therapist opted to use cognitive and cognitive behavioral frames of reference to select modifications for process skills that offered positive social play outcomes in a relatively short period of time while safeguarding a supportive social context. Later, Malia's motor skills could be addressed to build her enjoyment and motivation to sustain engagement in recess play.

---

swift clinical analysis and action. The practitioner prepares by completing activity analyses beforehand to anticipate problem areas; maintaining a clear picture of the child's overall strengths, needs, and goals; and having a sound knowledge of play. Although the intervention plan is a guide for therapy, a variety of unanticipated events may occur in each treatment session. The therapist cannot predict the child's exact response to an activity or the opportunities that may emerge. Activities that are too hard can lead to frustration, anger, tantrums, and refusals to continue to participate. Activities that are too easy can lead to boredom, wandering attention, and eventual refusal to participate. Even a previously successful activity can become problematic, sometimes within the same session. The occupational therapy practitioner stays flexible to understand changes in the child's emotional state, needs, and desires and to carefully alter activities accordingly to continually motivate the child to engage and meet the next challenge. The actual methods for achieving therapy goals must be adaptable on a moment-by-moment basis to match where the child is at that point in time. Continual professional reasoning equips the occupational therapy practitioner to make immediate changes during an activity based in response to the real-time performance and reactions of the child (Spitzer, 2020), as illustrated in **Practice Example 8.4**.

PRACTICE EXAMPLE 8.4 Adjusting Adaptations in the Moment for Malia

Malia's occupational therapist also worked with her directly to build coordination and timing skills for successful participation in recess activities. The occupational therapist selected a motor learning frame of reference because of its focus on the skills that were judged most essential in building Malia's success.

During one session, the therapist suggested a game of balloon volley. Malia expressed excitement but constantly turned away and wandered off from the play area. The occupational therapist redirected Malia to return, but this did not change Malia's behavior, despite several repetitions. Given Malia's interest and knowledge of how to do the activity, the therapist considered what adaptation could be made so that Malia could play this activity and benefit therapeutically. The therapist mentally compared Malia's immediate performance with the evaluation findings and an activity analysis of balloon volley to create an occupational analysis and hypothesized that the most likely reason for Malia's leaving was poor sensory processing. Therefore, informed by a sensory integration frame of reference, the therapist placed a piece of masking tape to compensate as a visual modification for Malia to see where to stand. Malia immediately stayed on or near the masking tape X, which marked the treasure spot, ready to block the pirate balloon and safeguard the imagined "treasure."

The occupational therapist selected a red balloon as a modification. The balloon decreased the motor demands of volleyball because it moved slower and required less force to hit than a ball. The red color made it easier to see and track against the visual background of the playground. The therapist graded the activity by keeping a short distance and targeting the balloon directly at Malia's hands. However, no matter how much the therapist downgraded the distance, Malia could not hit the balloon toward the therapist, as she relied on a gross shoulder flexion motion causing the balloon to go over her head and behind her. Despite guidance and explanation, Malia continued to miss the balloon and was becoming increasingly frustrated. The therapist knew that this activity was neither play nor therapeutic; more adaptations were needed immediately in order to enable Malia to experience success before she decided to stop engaging altogether. Because the therapist wanted to facilitate more refined distal movements of her upper extremities, wanted to ensure success, and was concerned about Malia's fatigue, the therapist identified a modification that would address all these factors and suggested that they change to protect a different "treasure chest." This time, the therapist moved the masking tape X and had Malia sit across from her at a table and push the balloon to roll across the table. Although the masking tape was no longer needed as a visual modification, it was used to maintain play in the activity. The table constrained Malia's movements to be more successful, the rolling balloon was even easier to target than in the air, and the shift helped reenergize Malia's motivation to play. As Malia gained skill with this movement, the therapist gradually upgraded the activity by raising the distance of the balloon over the table. Malia was so excited with her success that she requested table balloon again next session, which was later upgraded by tying the balloon to the monkey bars for a constrained volleying before returning to the original activity.

As shown in **Figure 8.3**, once either the child or therapist has selected a play activity, the therapist continually attends to the child's performance to ascertain the child's level of participation. The occupational therapy practitioner skillfully observes the child's reactions to recognize both challenges and possibilities that emerge. The child's performance is analyzed in comparison with the activity demands to mentally update the occupational analysis. If the child is participating successfully and the demands are just right for sustaining play and meeting therapeutic goals, then the therapist need not intervene while continuing to monitor for changes in participation. If the child is participating successfully but the demands are inadequate for addressing therapeutic needs, then the therapist will need to upgrade activity demands to address

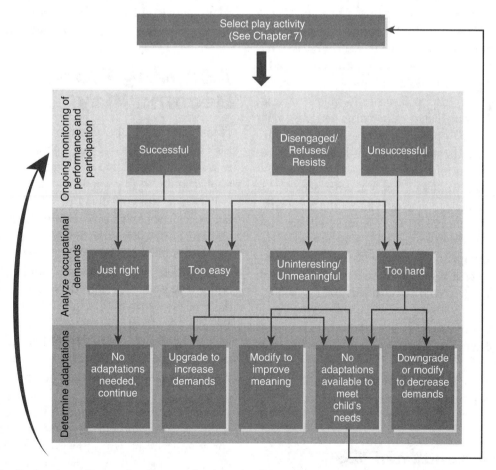

Figure 8.3 The Professional Reasoning Process for Adapting Play. After a play activity is selected, the occupational therapy practitioner continuously monitors the child's occupational performance. Based on these observations, the therapist assesses relevant demands to decide if and which adaptations are needed or if another activity selection is indicated

therapeutic goals. The therapist considers what aspects of the activity are too easy for the child, and how the activity can be made slightly more difficult to create an attainable challenge. The child may be having a very positive day and may be very agreeable and more playful than usual and be ready for increased demands.

If the child is unsuccessful or not participating, then the therapist will need to identify the mismatch in activity demands for the client based on the occupational analysis. The child may dislike all aspects or some part of the activity, and the therapist must modify the activity to ensure the demands are personally relevant and important enough to be experienced as play by the child. If a child is not participating because the activity demands are inadequate, then the therapist will need to upgrade the demands to engage the child's interest and motivation.

Commonly when a child is unsuccessful or not participating, the activity demands are too difficult. The child may be having a challenging day and may be tired, frustrated, or agitated. A playmate may be sick; a favorite toy may be missing, broken, or used by another; or construction workers may be creating different sounds, smells, sights, and dust. These instances are difficult to anticipate, but the therapist's skill during these moments can often "make or break" an intervention session. In this case, the therapist needs to determine which features are of immediate concern in disrupting participation in order to quickly adapt them to enable immediate ease of participation. What aspects of the environment can be adjusted? What aspects of the child's skills and client factors are currently hindering performance, and how can the activity be made easier to allow success? What aspects of the task are amenable to grading, and are the necessary materials and skills present? The therapist will have to judge how much to downgrade demands to ensure or gain client participation. More significant downgrading may be necessary for a client who is unengaged than for one who is participating unsuccessfully. When a client is not participating, it is often necessary to target those demands that increase clarity of what and how to do the activity to ensure the child understands what the activity offers and how to begin. If the activity cannot be graded and modified adequately, then the therapist must consider alternative activities or environments in which to engage the child.

Recognizing and Extending Opportunities for Play

In-the-moment professional reasoning enables the occupational therapy practitioner to promote new opportunities for play. A therapist cannot know everything, past and evolving, that is happening in a client's life. Therefore, the therapist must be open to new information, skills, and interests that provide new options for intervention and play.

By having a clear vision of what play is and focusing on the child's overall goals rather than just a specific planned activity, the occupational therapy practitioner is poised to adapt activities during the session to be playlike. Hints of play may occur briefly and unexpectedly, and the occupational therapy practitioner must be ready to seize these opportunities. It may be a comment, a sound, or a movement (Spitzer, 2008). It may be the first time the child does something new or more complicated (even if by chance). The child may merely glance at a person or object, or even suggest an idea. The therapist, then, can scaffold the child's play by grading just enough guidance or assistance for the child to initiate or continue a play activity (Baranek, Reinhartsen, & Wannamaker, 2001). If play is the goal, then to the greatest extent possible, the occupational therapy practitioner places the child's input foremost and then determines *how* to adapt to make it happen in the moment, as illustrated in the case of Thomas (see **Practice Example 8.5**).

Adapting Work to Become Play

One of the fortes of occupational therapy practice is the creative process of using a child's personal interest as a strength to change work into play. Not all of life is play, and not all of pediatric occupational therapy is play. The work involved in self-care, school work, and even friendships can be so important for a child. Children with disabilities often find a range of activities difficult, challenging, or otherwise frustrating. Current best practice in occupational therapy is to employ skill training and therapeutic practice within the context of occupations (Cahill & Beisbeir, 2020). Yet, often pediatric clients avoid participating in the very types of activities that would be most therapeutic for them. This complication is at the crux of why they need play-based occupational therapy. When addressing work activities, occupational therapy practitioners who have a strong understanding and valuing of play strive to move specific challenging activities on the continuum from work toward play. Although true play as occupation is not always achieved, adding play elements can still benefit a client's motivation, well-being, and participation. Play as a modality can make therapeutic work more playlike (see **Figure 8.4**). After

PRACTICE EXAMPLE 8.5 Thomas and an Unexpected Play Opportunity

Thomas was a bright first grader with ASD. He loved school work and preferred to do workbooks and read in his leisure time. He was receiving occupational therapy to increase his play skills, praxis, and postural control to engage in a variety of leisure activities, especially with other children. He preferred play themes related to categories of knowledge and information such as animals from different parts of the world along with their habitats and details of their behavior. He was not interested in pretend games of being the animals or in various topics in which his classmates were interested. He always read books at the beginning and end of each session in the waiting room. He often asked the therapist to read a book to him. She usually redirected him through such comments as "it is time to play." Reading was not a goal of therapy and seemed to be a detractor from therapy.

On one day when Thomas was a little more insistent, asking to take the book into the therapy room, his occupational therapist agreed to the request as long as he stood on a balance cushion to read it, and he agreed. When he finished, he put the book down and told her that he had another book to read, and before she could respond, he immediately held his hands together like a book and began a long stream of memorized words about a Spider-Man story. As soon as he paused, the occupational therapist offered, "Let's play Spider-Man!" "Okay," said Thomas. The occupational therapist stated that Thomas would *be* Spider-Man and began asking Thomas who the "bad guy, villains" were. Thomas gave her some names. They set up targets to be these named villains, and Thomas threw bean bag "spider-webs" at them with excitement at getting the bad guys. Thomas had accepted the Spider-Man role and expanded his play because his occupational therapist was flexible and adapted to Thomas's needs and desires in the moment.

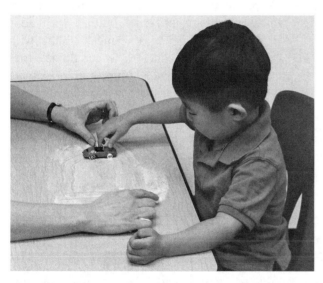

Figure 8.4 The use of a preferred play interest adapts the work of writing into play such as in the case of driving a toy car in shaving cream to form letters
Courtesy of David A. Morales.

all, research indicates that complete free choice is not necessary for children to experience an activity as play (King & Howard, 2014). There is moderate evidence to support use of play to address mental health, behavior, and social participation concerns of children and youth (Cahill, Egan, & Seber, 2020). Several studies have found play to be effective for increasing motor and other functional skills (Case-Smith, 2000; Case-Smith et al., 2013; Sakemiller & Nelson, 1998; Sparling, Walker, & Singdahlsen, 1984). Preliminary research has found that the use of play in therapy may increase the effectiveness of therapy for self-care and participation (McCoy et al., 2020). Without play, the

child can be resistive and even oppositional, but when work is transformed into play by a skillful therapist, it seems natural and playful. What a child wants to do and needs to do, coalesce.

Creating playful activities emanates from knowledge and professional reasoning. Occupational therapy practitioners transform work into play primarily by modifying features of the activity to increase client relevance and importance. The therapist must possess a strong knowledge of both activity analysis and play, in addition to knowledge of the child. Based on professional training, the occupational therapy practitioner conducts an occupational analysis and ongoing assessment that equip the therapist to create playful work activities. The therapist compares what the child likes (materials, themes) with what the child needs to do and weighs alternative possibilities of how the activity can be done (see **Appendix 8.1** for a worksheet to facilitate this process). The occupational therapy practitioner then combines elements of wants and needs into a unique therapeutic activity that the child enjoys. Interests are embedded into the work activity so that the activity becomes appealing and occupational (Kuhaneck, Spitzer, & Miller, 2010; Munier, Myers, & Pierce, 2008; Spitzer, 2008, 2010, 2017; Tomcheck & Koenig, 2016). The work activity is reframed into a play activity (Spitzer, 2003, 2004, 2008). In this way, the child engages in work that feels like play (D'Arrigo, Copley, Poulsen, & Ziviani, 2020). When children with and without disabilities participate in activities in which they can have fun and feel success with challenges, they report liking these activities (Miller & Kuhaneck, 2008), and they participate more (Heah, Case, McGuire, & Law, 2007). Research indicates that incorporating personal interests increases participation even in less-preferred activities for children with ASD (Gunn & Delafield-Butt, 2015; Leaf et al., 2012). Furthermore, several studies have found that incorporating personal interests is an effective intervention for improving skills for children and adolescents with ASD, including motor skills and school work (Carnahan, Musti-Rao, & Bailey, 2008; De Vries et al., 2015; Koegel, Singh, & Koegel, 2010; Kryzak & Jones, 2014; Lanou, Hough, & Powell, 2012; Winters-Messiers, 2007). By modifying the form of an activity with interests, occupational therapy practitioners can change the activity's meaning to be more playlike or create new play activities.

Infusing Play into ADLs

As children develop, they are expected to become more independent in activities of daily living (ADLs) and to tolerate these activities as a part of basic hygiene and as members of their social communities. Children may view self-care differently from adults and in diverse individual ways based on their own experiences of doing self-care with regard to social and physical contexts, perceived skill, and others' expectations (Chapparo & Hooper, 2005). For children with disabilities, many self-care activities may be perceived as work. The activities may be physically difficult, cognitively too demanding, or uncomfortable or painful because of sensory sensitivities. Occupational therapy practitioners may work on self-care skills or underlying abilities (motor control, bilateral coordination, sensory modulation, etc.) or make modifications that make self-care easier. A playful approach of adapting self-care activities into play can also be used to build skills, to grade the therapeutic challenge, and to increase the child's motivation to participate in therapy and in daily life. In this way, self-care intervention can also be tailored for individual child meaning (Chapparo & Hooper, 2005). Two studies have found toy and pretend play to be an effective modality for increasing mealtime participation for children with ASD (Ausderau, St. John, Kwaterski, Nieuwenhuis, & Bradley, 2019; Muesbeck, St. John, Kant, & Ausderau, 2018).

Dressing, toileting, and bathing cases are presented to help the reader visualize how play might be used in therapeutic sessions related to ADLs (see **Practice Examples 8.6–8.8**). Other ways of making self-care playful include dressing weighted animals and dolls, performing self-care routines with dolls or stuffed animals, helping a younger sibling with self-care, using a knife and fork to cut French fries or other unusual items, embedding songs in self-care (Kern, Wakeford, & Aldridge, 2007), playing button bingo (Stern, 2013), "tying-up" people or toys to practice tying shoelaces, tying string "legs" onto a paper octopus body, tying shoelaces in steps with a pirate story (Steese, 2009), and tying bows on a doll's hair or "gifts."

PRACTICE EXAMPLE 8.6 Eastlyn's Dressing, Modified and Graded for Play

Eastlyn was a 4-year-old with ASD. She had been receiving occupational therapy for a few months and was making consistent progress. Her mother asked the occupational therapist for help getting Eastlyn ready for an upcoming family trip to snow country. Her mother was concerned that her daughter would not be able to participate because she had not been able to get Eastlyn to tolerate wearing even socks or a jacket. Eastlyn also refused all other cold-weather clothes such as boots, mittens, heavy pants, and hat. The occupational therapist identified that Eastlyn's resistance was due primarily to her tactile hyperreactivity. The new clothes also required different motor skills than her familiar clothes with which she was independent. This meant she would have to follow directions more in order to build new skills with these new clothes. This was also a challenge because she really liked her routines and structure for doing things in the same way. This mismatch between what she needed to do and her abilities and interests was creating an experience of work for her and thus refusal. If Eastlyn could not tolerate appropriate clothing, given the cold climate for their vacation, her health would be jeopardized, or she would have to be inside all day with one parent while her brothers played outside with the other parent.

Eastlyn's mother wanted her to be included as part of the family. In preparation, her mother repeatedly brought out all the cold-weather clothes and had the whole family dress up, but Eastlyn was the only one to resist. It was getting closer to the trip, and Eastlyn was not getting any more comfortable with cold-weather dressing. The occupational therapist asked Eastlyn's mother to bring these cold-weather clothes to therapy. The occupational therapist wanted Eastlyn to (1) have positive feelings about the clothes so that she would be more willing to wear them and (2) have the proprioceptive-vestibular input that would help make the unfamiliar clothing textures more tolerable.

To change Eastlyn's experience of this dressing activity, the occupational therapist compared what she needed to do with her interests, abilities, and strengths in order to identify possible activity modifications (see **Table 8.4** for details). The occupational therapist planned to combine what Eastlyn needed to do (the winter clothes) with a playful sensory-motor activity that Eastlyn had consistently enjoyed. This play activity consisted of Eastlyn sitting in a swing, climbing backward up a ramp, lifting her feet to swing down the "mountain," and kicking a therapy ball placed on the floor. Eastlyn loved seeing the ball fly to the other end of the room. The role of clothes was graded to gradually increase use and sensory-motor demands. First, the occupational therapist began placing the clothes on top of the ball, telling Eastlyn they were going to pretend to "dress" the ball. The therapist asked Eastlyn which item to place next, eventually making a large pile of clothing on and around the ball. After the first time, when the clothing flew all over, Eastlyn laughed and became very interested, directing the therapist in which item to put next. After a few times, the occupational therapist announced that it was "Eastlyn's turn to get dressed." The occupational therapist gave her an option between two items, and Eastlyn picked a jumpsuit. Eastlyn allowed the therapist to help her put it on and then got back on the swing to continue the game. After a few times, the occupational therapist would suggest another item to wear, always giving Eastlyn a choice. They added mittens, a hat, boots, and a scarf until Eastlyn was covered in winter clothing (see **Figure 8.5**). The occupational therapist also took pictures, which were given to her family to review and discuss how fun it was to get dressed up for the snow. After this one session, Eastlyn was able to tolerate and practice snow dressing with her family at home and wear adequate cold-weather clothing to play in the snow on their family vacation.

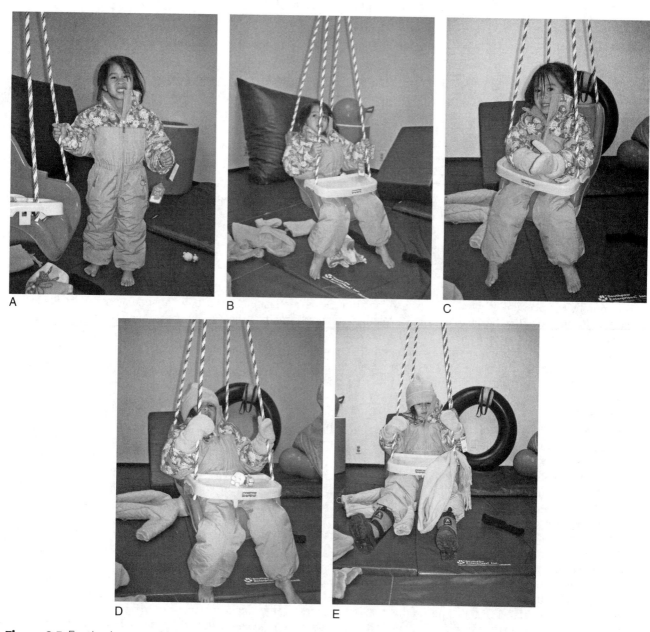

Figure 8.5 Eastlyn increased her tolerance for snow dressing during a graded playful therapy session. First was the jumpsuit (**A–B**), then the mittens (**C**), then the hat (**D**), and, finally, the scarf and boots (**E**)

Courtesy of Susan L. Spitzer.

Table 8.4 Professional Reasoning to Determine Possible Play Modifications for Eastlyn's Dressing

Activity Components	Demands ("Need to")	Child's Interest, Abilities, Strengths	Possible Modifications
Objects	▪ Heavy pants ▪ Jacket ▪ Hat ▪ Mittens/gloves ▪ Socks ▪ Boots ▪ Scarf	▪ Familiar clothes ▪ Character toys	▪ Use toys to model, direct, help
Sensory	▪ Tactile	▪ Vestibular	▪ Combine with a vestibular-based activity
Motor/action	▪ Bilateral coordination ▪ Hand use ▪ Motor Planning	▪ Independent dressing skills for familiar clothes ▪ Physical activity	▪ Combine with a physical activity
Social	▪ Follow direction	▪ Likes social interaction	▪ Increase social interaction
Cognitive	▪ Become independent	▪ Structure, routines	▪ Use an existing structure/routine

PRACTICE EXAMPLE 8.7 Devon and Toileting, Modified and Graded for Play

Devon was a 5-year-old with developmental delays and sensory modulation deficits. He was receiving school occupational therapy services. His preschool teacher was very concerned because Devon refused to go near the bathroom, let alone go in. Generally, he was very compliant and liked to help and please adults, but he became very upset when the staff insisted he use the bathroom. Occasionally, he had accidents and wet his clothing. He was very upset by this but still refused to go into the restroom. Next school year, the school days would be even longer, and Devon's refusal to use the restroom at school would likely interfere more with his educational program. His mother reported that he was independent with toileting at home but refused to use public restrooms in the community. The occupational therapist determined that Devon's resistance to toileting at school was likely due to his sensitivities to sound because the school restroom had old, loud plumbing that echoed in its large, tiled space.

The occupational therapist decided to schedule her sessions with Devon first thing in the morning, when the routine was for the class to use the restroom. First, she modified the routine and offered Devon interesting fine-motor games to play with outside the restroom door. This succeeded in getting Devon out from under the staircase, where he liked to wait, and next to the restroom as he waited for the other children, where he could become accustomed with the routine and be exposed to graded sensory stimuli. Once he was comfortable enough that he could really enjoy the toys, the occupational therapist upgraded the sensory and motor demands by having Devon be the restroom helper whose job was to push open the heavy door into the restroom. He was initially hesitant; the occupational therapist modeled opening the door first, and downgraded the demand by doing it together with him. In this way, the occupational therapist provided a way for Devon to take two steps into the restroom at a time when it was at its quietest (as the first student in), get heavy proprioceptive input to modulate his sensory sensitivities, and be in the helper role that he enjoyed. The occupational therapist gradually upgraded the door-opening demands by steadily decreasing physical assistance and slowing her movements until Devon was initiating and completing door opening on his own.

Getting Devon into the restroom for increasing lengths of time was the next step. This step was also modified as the occupational therapist suggested the toys be given a shower in the sink. First, the activity was downgraded to start with only one toy and then upgraded to increase the number of toys and consequently, the sensory demands over time. Eventually, Devon was able to spend most of the time giving the toys a "shower." Then the routine was modified as the therapist had him end by washing his hands. Later, the activity was modified to take the toys to "look in" the toilet stalls. By this time, on the days the occupational therapist was not there, Devon was consistently coming in with the class and washing his hands during toileting time. Eventually with continued modifications and grading, Devon began toileting at school.

PRACTICE EXAMPLE 8.8 Lucas and Play for Bathing

Lucas was a 9-year-old with mild intellectual disability, ADHD, and bipolar disorder. He seemed very aware that other children were able to do more than he was and did not like anything that made him feel like he stood out from other children his age. His parents wanted Lucas to be able to bathe himself adequately just like his younger brother was able to do. Lucas similarly desired competence and independence. Lucas was able to get in and out of the shower and turn the water on and off, but he barely wiped soap or a wash cloth on his body, finishing in 30 seconds without completely cleaning himself. When his parents gave him any directions or assistance, he became so angry that he stopped and refused to do any more. If they insisted, his negative behaviors would escalate into yelling, kicking, hitting, and throwing. They had tried a visual list of what to do, but this did not help either. After evaluating Lucas, the occupational therapist determined that Lucas's difficulties in bathing were due to sensitivity to touch, postural instability, poor sequencing, an impulsive and inattentive behavioral pattern, and dislike with being helped.

Part of the occupational therapy sessions focused on sensory processing and postural control to build underlying foundations for bathing, but Lucas also needed to establish an effective bathing routine. The occupational therapist suggested a "shower" obstacle course with a pretend bathroom, shower, soap, and water. Lucas liked the idea of a new game to play. The occupational therapist guided Lucas to establish rules together, starting from head to toe to make sure that all body parts were "washed" and counting to 10 for each body part to make sure each was washed completely. Lucas helped set up various obstacle courses with each step being a different part of the body to "wash." Lucas especially loved having the occupational therapist take a turn so that he could direct her to follow the rules (to remember what to do next and be sure she was thorough). In this way, showering was not a battle, but a fun play activity to which Lucas looked forward. The occupational therapist often engaged Lucas in building a narrative of how he was learning to bathe himself and how he could do this at home for real too, which he gradually did.

Infusing Play into Writing

A common reason that schoolchildren are referred to occupational therapy is for help with writing. Some children have trouble learning to write. Some have difficulty with forming letters correctly or legibly. Others have trouble with speed or sustaining endurance for writing assignments. Fine-motor skills, motor planning, and visual perception are common underlying challenges. However, currently strong research supports therapeutic practice over sensorimotor approaches for writing (Grajo, Candler, & Sarafian, 2020), so children need to participate in writing as part of therapy. Yet, children may perceive writing as a work activity, especially when directed by an adult (Breathnach, Danby, & O'Gorman, 2017). Although many children may want to write better, easier, and faster, they often hate the current overwhelming difficulty of writing and resist it or refuse to *work* on it. Making fun from the work of writing is quite a challenge, especially once children have had such negative experiences with it. Here we provide a number of examples of modifications we have used to incorporate meaning, abilities, and strengths to adapt writing to be more like play:

- Modify materials (such as soap foam, clay, markers, colored pencils, crayons, sand tray, paintbrush dipped in water with a chalkboard, body crayons to make "tattoos"; see **Figure 8.6**)

- Modify content (words)
    - Talk about or fill-in letters within words and sentences rather than isolated letters for children who can read or are more interested in this level despite not yet being able to write letters.
    - Write meaningful words that are
        - About the child's interests (car brands, foods, etc.)
        - About an upcoming event/holiday
        - Funny or socially "inappropriate" by adult standards (for ideas, see **Box 8.1**)
        - Silly made-up words (Many children find it fun to try to sound out words from random letters or hear the therapist do so. The therapist and child can even guess/make up a meaning for the "words.")
- Modify client relevance of writing:
    - Draw shapes and simple pictures first to get better visual-motor skill for using a pencil
    - Play tic-tac-toe with different letters or words instead of *X*'s and *O*'s
    - Play hangman
    - Guess the word (write dictated spelled words)
    - Incorporate writing into a play theme:
        - Hidden messages to pirates about hidden treasure or to monsters or ghosts
        - Banners or signs to use in "presentations" such as for a circus or store

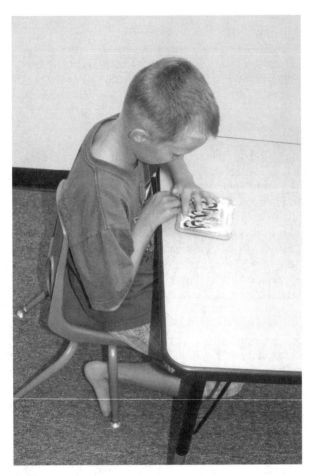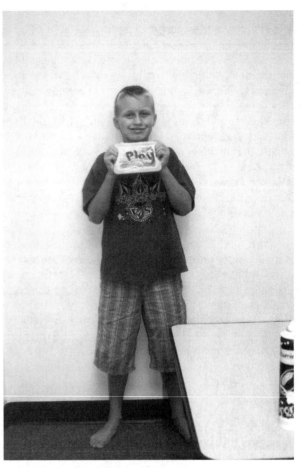

Figure 8.6 Modifying materials often can make the work of writing more like play

Courtesy of David A. Morales.

- Written score in a game with points (or make points up)
- Rules for an activity
- Board game with direction cards or written directions
- Card game with letters, numbers, or words to pick and write
- Letter tic-tac-toe

- Writing competitions—against self or others where neat letters get points for the child and messy ones are points for the therapist; upgrading by adding bonus points for neatness within a time frame
- Detective games—give clues that are written down by the "detective" on a notepad

Box 8.1 Examples of Words Children May Find More Interesting to Write

barf	gag	poop	spit	wahoo
belch	gas	potty	splat	wart
blah	gooey	pow	stinky	whoop
blast	gross	pus	toilet	yahoo
bonkers	horrifying	quack	trash	yawn
boogers	jabber	sewer	turd	yelp
burp	jeepers	slime	underpants	yuck
butt	jolt	slurp	vapor	zap
crash	ka-boom	smelly	venom	zany
crazy	magic	snarled	vermin	zillion
dodo	maniac	sneeze	vex	zip
fart	ooze	snore	vomit	zoom
flush	pee	snot	wacky	

Note: These words are presented as examples of what some children may prefer to write. They should be used with caution, in consideration of the child's sociocultural environment.

to then determine the answer to a mystery (similar to *Clue* game)

- Write a list of activities the child wants to do or has done
- Make a book about a topic that interests the child:
  - Occupational therapy memories—a picture and caption from each session
  - Jokes
  - Comic/cartoon—draw pictures or use stickers and then make talk balloons to write in the character comments
  - Favorite subjects such as cars, super heroes, planets, etc.
- Write a letter or word at the end of each pass through an obstacle course or scooter board path
- Keep a graph for the child to record his or her own performance on writing activities to track increasing performance and try to beat his or her previous score (points for amount of writing, speed, neatness, etc.)
- Make up own *MAD LIBS*
- Write a letter to someone real or made up
- Make a list of toys the child wants to get from a catalog
- Combine writing with another favorite interest:
  - For a child interested in geography, make a map of the country with names of all the states written
  - For a child interested in superheroes, when letters do not turn out well, put bad letters in "jail" (draw a square around them and put vertical lines through)
  - For a child interested in a particular character or object, use an appropriate colored pencil to do " writing" such as red for "Spider-Man" writing, black for "Darth Vader" writing, blue for "Cookie Monster" writing, etc.
  - Make a label for a food product (e.g., pizza box, soda can, candy bar, cereal box)

For children learning the prewriting skills of drawing lines and simple shapes, some of the aforementioned ideas can be graded for prewriting skills as well. However, you may also need to come up with unique modifications for children who find prewriting more work than play. For example, making intersecting lines for a railroad crossing sign can be less work for a child who is very interested in trains. But even using a pencil may be resisted by some children, and more creative playful approaches are needed such as presented in the Learning Without Tears (2021) readiness activities and illustrated in the case of Toni (see **Practice Example 8.9**). Unique ways of drawing can also be more playful. For example, faces can be drawn with washable markers and squirted with water to "melt" them, or they can be drawn on partially inflated balloons and then blown to "stretch the monster face" or "make a silly face."

PRACTICE EXAMPLE 8.9 Toni and Modified Prewriting

Toni was a 5-year-old with a seizure disorder and an anxiety disorder. She was very interactive socially and verbally but resisted all fine-motor and paper-and-pencil activities. She could make gross circular, vertical, and horizontal lines. The occupational therapy evaluation indicated difficulty with accuracy in reach, grasp, and release because of deficits in visual perception and motor control, which meant drawing and writing would require great effort. Toni's favorite activity was eating. She often talked about her favorite foods and loved to pretend she was eating. Her family wanted Toni to participate in academic-oriented paper-and-pencil activities such as writing.

To address this need, Toni's occupational therapist analyzed the activity demands for writing alongside her interests, abilities, and strengths to identify possible modifications to engage Toni (see **Table 8.5**, which summarizes this analysis). Because of Toni's resistance to using a pencil, the occupational therapist determined it was best to start by modifying prewriting activities to eliminate a pencil so that Toni would participate. She decided to use craft sticks to have Toni imitate making intersecting lines for a cross to embed the visual constructional aspects of prewriting. When presented with the craft sticks activity, Toni turned and walked away, refusing to come back.

For the next session, the occupational therapist planned additional modifications to increase personal meaning for Toni, an intervention that has been found to be effective in building motor control and motor learning (O'Brien & Lewin, 2008, 2009). The occupational therapist decided to capitalize on the fact that craft sticks are quite similar to sticks used in food items. She first held the sticks, pretended to lick one, and began banging the sticks on the table as she sang the beginning of the Lollipop song (Ross & Dixson, 1958). Toni smiled and watched the therapist, laughing as the therapist added an exclamatory "pop!" as she crossed her sticks together and put them on the table in this crossed position. Toni asked to play too, and they sang several rounds with Toni actively trying to place the craft sticks in a cross formation, a precursor to connecting lines for writing and drawing. With a foundation of engagement in social play, further upgrading and modifications could be made to build Toni's skills and eventually apply these with writing.

Table 8.5 Professional Reasoning to Determine Play Modifications for Toni's Writing

Activity Components	Demands ("Need to")	Child's Interest, Abilities, Strengths	Possible Modifications
Objects	■ Paper ■ Pencil	■ Food and eating	■ Paper/pencil alternatives ■ Food items/themes
Sensory	■ Somatosensory processing—praxis ■ Visual attention and perception	■ Good visual attention to people's faces and whole-body actions ■ Good language processing	■ Full body actions, done at or near face ■ Language directions to match her motor control and compensate for visual perception ■ Larger items with contrasting/bold colors
Motor/action	■ Fine-motor ■ Visual-motor ■ Sedentary	■ Able to sit at table for extended periods of time for eating and social interaction	■ Larger items
Social	■ Responding to follow direction	■ Likes social interaction, talking ■ Good social skills	■ Increase social interaction
Cognitive	■ Sequencing ■ Become independent	■ Likes novelty and dramatic play	■ Make the actions playful ■ Focus the activity more on process than outcome
Location/space	■ Table	■ Comfortable at table	■ N/A

Infusing Play into Cutting

Cutting with scissors is another common referral concern for pediatric occupational therapy practitioners. Typically, the child has significant challenges in developing this skill and thus perceives it as more work than play. This contrasts with the reaction of typical children who may show great pride in their developing cutting skills. For the child who is uninterested in or resistive to using scissors, modifying objects, their use, and client relevance may help in transforming cutting into a playful activity as seen with Viviana (see **Practice Example 8.10**). Additional suggestions for playful cutting modifications include

- Use scissors as puppet mouths to "talk" to each other
- Use scissors as mouths to "eat" paper
- Snip small pieces of paper as cargo to load a truck/train, as food for a character, or as raindrops to fall
- Make a path on paper with stamps/stickers of monsters or dinosaurs and then "chase"/"eat" them with the scissors

- Place a sticker at the beginning and end of the line, such as a dog at the beginning and a bone at the end or a car at one end and a house at the other
- Cut different materials, such as play-dough and straws
- Cut a small amount at the end of each pass through an obstacle course or scooter board path
- Cut through a "ribbon" of paper to start each round of an obstacle course like a ribbon-cutting ceremony.
- Cut items that can be used as props in play:
  - Costumes out of paper and tape—color, cut, and tape things onto clothes or skin (clowns with red circles on cheeks, spots on a dog or leopard, red nose for "Rudolph")
  - Trace, color, and cut large numbers to make a sports jersey
  - Cut items to make paper dolls, dogs, super heroes, etc.

Minimizing the Work in "Play" Activities

A young client may pick up a toy, smile, explore it, and hand it to the therapist. From here, the occupational

PRACTICE EXAMPLE 8.10 Viviana and Cutting Modified and Graded

Viviana, was a 5-year-old with ASD, who resisted visual motor activities. When presented with scissors, she screamed in protest and pulled her arm away, refusing to touch the scissors. Clearly, scissors had taken on negative meaning, but the occupational therapist's inquiries could not identify any specific occurrences where she or anyone else was cut with scissors. Different kinds of scissors were tried but the reaction was the same as she consistently resisted this work.

Given the negative reactions to scissors and the need to develop some motor skills to experience success, the occupational therapist decided first to work on related activities that did not use scissors and asked her teacher to try to put a temporary hold on scissors for Viviana. The occupational therapist decided to use a scissor-type tongs to allow Viviana to build up needed skills while creating a different meaning (see **Figure 8.7**). First the "bunny" tongs were used just to hold and move in various different activities like any other toy. Once Viviana was comfortable with the bunny tongs, the use was upgraded by having her slip her fingers inside the handles to get comfortable with the tactile sensation. Then the activity was upgraded again to use the bunny tongs to grab something, specifically her favorite snack item. Initially, the therapist physically guided the process for immediate success. Further grading involved slowing the speed of assistance for Viviana to tolerate the work and time delay to getting the snack, lessening the use of her second hand on the tongs, and then gradually providing less physical assistance from the therapist. Once she could open the tongs by herself using one hand, Viviana had the motor skills needed for self-opening scissors. The activity then was modified with self-opening scissors to cut her favorite snack food into pieces to eat. Because of the history of positive playful experiences created with the bunny tongs, Viviana was willing to participate in this new use of scissors. Initially, she was physically guided for success and quick access to the snack, but the activity was graded to gradually decrease therapist assistance as Viviana began to apply her skills. Later, the activity was modified to add paper strips, which were alternated with snack items.

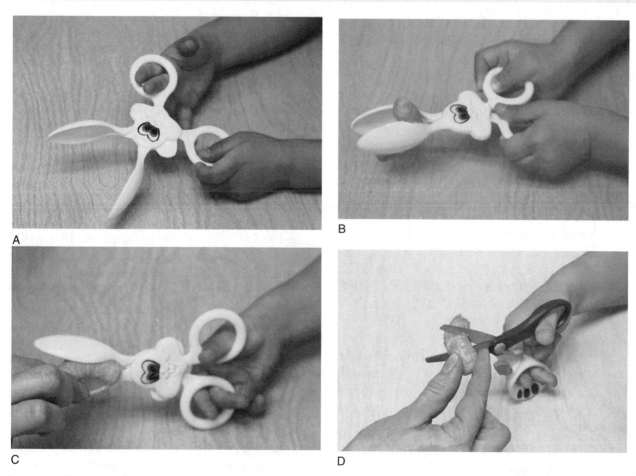

Figure 8.7 The use of "bunny" tongs was downgraded to object play initially to engage Viviana. Then it was gradually upgraded to holding the handles (**A**), using the bunny tongs to hold her favorite snack item (**B**), and using one hand on the handles (**C**). After skills were built, the activity was modified with self-opening scissors to cut her favorite snack food into pieces that she could eat (**D**)

therapy practitioner can suggest a playful way of holding or placing the toy to address therapeutic goals. An older child may reach for a rope offered by the therapist and respond, "Hey, I'm a cowboy!" From here, the occupational therapy practitioner and client build a story line around this idea, with the therapist suggesting materials or actions to work on therapeutic goals that are consistent with this story line. This is the ideal, and it is a beautiful, wondrous process when it occurs.

Unfortunately, the reality is that many of our clients do not possess such a playful approach or the ability to adapt their play ideas with therapeutic goals. Even activities that are commonly called play and seen as play by other children in the general society may not be experienced as play by individual pediatric clients. For example, some children are not interested in any of the play that the other children are doing at recess or in their neighborhoods. Thus, the children play by themselves. This is problematic when the child wants to have friends or needs to develop social interaction skills. A common option is building skills so that the child can join successfully in the activities the children are playing, which in turn can increase the experience of play. However, even with foundational skills, some children will not be motivated to play what other children are playing. Another possibility is offering other play activities (such as board games at recess) or getting other children to play what the client wants to play. But this option too may be inadequate as other children may not share the client's interest or may lack in-depth knowledge to play games based on the client's interest (such as detailed knowledge about how solar systems are created or all the countries and capitals of the world). In such cases, adapting the game into play for a particular client is needed. Research supports that including a child's interests can be effective for promoting play participation, especially for children with ASD (i.e., Baker, 2000; DiCarlo, Schepis, & Flynn, 2009; Jung & Sainato, 2015; Koegel et al., 2012; Kryzak et al., 2013; Owens et al., 2008; Porter, 2012; Reinhartsen, Garfinkle, & Wolery, 2002; Vismara & Lyons, 2007; Wimpory, Hobson, & Nash, 2007). If the client can perceive it as play, he or she will be more motivated to participate in the activity. The gap between the interests of a client and the play context can be bridged with occupational analysis and evaluation of the child to guide modifications, as in the case of Zach (see **Practice Example 8.11**).

Conclusion

Adapting play is a specialized intervention skill that rests on the serious work of professional reasoning

PRACTICE EXAMPLE 8.11 Zach and Recess

Zach was a 9-year-old with ADHD and highly gifted intelligence, also described as twice exceptional or 2E. Zach liked other people and had a strong desire for social interaction with all ages of children and adults. At recess, however, he mostly played by himself, enacting elaborate make-believe stories of kind animals that play together and avoid attacks by "mean" animals. The other children played soccer during recess. When asked if he wanted to play with the other children, Zach responded "yes," but said that he did not want to play soccer because "it is mean and you get hurt." Although some other activities were available, the other children still wanted to play soccer. If Zach was going to play with the other children, he would need to be able to play soccer, he would need to be willing to participate in soccer, and ideally he would want to *play* soccer.

The occupational therapist decided to modify soccer into a game that interested Zach by adding Zach's interest in make-believe animal stories. The therapist relied heavily on narrative analysis to negotiate a story with Zach as described by Price and Miner (2007). Together in their sessions, they created a storybook about horses and wolves kicking rocks, in a manner supported by research studies (Keeling, Smith Myles, Gagnon, & Simpson, 2003; Spencer, Simpson, Day, & Buster, 2008), which is provided in **Appendix 8.2**. Then, Zach was willing to try playing soccer as he could use his imaginative strength to transform it into play.

in order to be both occupation focused and client centered. The occupational therapy practitioner grades and modifies activities to match the individual client's interests and needs. Modifications are aimed at immediate participation by enabling access and ensuring client meaning and motivation. Although a child may experience a range of daily activities as work, through occupational therapy, the work can be modified into play or play-like experiences. Grading sustains play as well as builds a child's skills by incrementally increasing and decreasing activity demands to present achievable challenges. The spontaneous and dynamic aspects of play are difficult to plan adaptations with certainty. However, with a strong foundation in activity analysis, knowledge of play, and awareness of the child's interests, occupational therapy practitioners are well positioned for this formidable and rewarding aspect of practice and are ready to seize spontaneous opportunities to create just right play in the moment.

References

American Occupational Therapy Association (AOTA). (2015). Occupational therapy for children and youth using sensory integration theory and methods in school-based practice. *American Journal of Occupational Therapy, 69*(Suppl. 3), 6913410040. https://doi.org/10.5014/ajot.2015.696S04

American Occupational Therapy Association (AOTA). (2020). Occupational therapy practice framework: Domain & process (4th ed.). *American Journal of Occupational Therapy, 74* (Supplement 2), 7412410010. https://doi.org/10.5014/ajot.2020.74S2001

Ausderau, K. K., St. John, B., Kwaterski, K. N., Nieuwenhuis, B., & Bradley, E. (2019). Parents' strategies to support mealtime participation of their children with autism spectrum disorder. *American Journal of Occupational Therapy, 73*(1), 301205070p1–7301205070p107. https://doi.org/10.5014/ajot.2019.024612

Ayres, A. J. (1972). *Sensory integration and learning disorders.* Los Angeles, CA: Western Psychological Services.

Ayres, A. J. (1979). *Sensory integration and the child.* Los Angeles, CA: Western Psychological Services.

Ayres, A. J. (2005). *Sensory integration and the child: 25th* anniversary edition. Los Angeles, CA: Western Psychological Services.

Baker, M. J. (2000). Incorporating the thematic ritualistic behaviors of children with autism into games: Increasing social play interactions with siblings. *Journal of Positive Behavior Interventions, 2*(2), 66–84. https://doi.org/10.1177/109830070000200201

Baranek, G. T., Reinhartsen, D. B., & Wannamaker, S. W. (2001). Play: Engaging young children with autism. In R. A. Huebner (Ed.), *Autism: A sensorimotor approach to management* (pp. 313–351). Gaithersburg, MD: Aspen.

Breathnach, H., Danby, S., & O'Gorman, L. (2017). "Are you working or playing?" Investigating young children's perspectives of classroom activities. *International Journal of Early Years Education, 25*(4), 439–454. https://doi.org/10.1080/09669760.2017.1316241

Breines, E. (1986). *Origins and adaptations: A philosophy of practice.* Lebanon, NJ: Geri-Rehab, Inc.

Burke, J. P. (1977). A clinical perspective on motivation: Pawn versus origin. *American Journal of Occupational Therapy, 31*(4), 254–258.

Cahill, S. M., & Beisbeir, S. (2020). Practice guidelines— Occupational therapy practice guidelines for children and youth ages 5–21 years. *American Journal of Occupational Therapy, 74,* 7404397010. https://doi.org/10.5014/ajot.2020.744001

Cahill, S. M., Egan, B. E., & Seber, J. (2020). Activity- and occupation-based interventions to support mental health, positive behavior, and social participation for children and youth: A systematic review. *American Journal of Occupational Therapy, 74*(2), 402180020p1–7402180020p287. https://doi.org/10.5014/ajot.2020.038687

Carnahan, C., Musti-Rao, S., & Bailey, J. (2008). Promoting active engagement in small group learning experiences for students with autism and significant learning needs. *Education and Treatment of Children, 32,* 37–61. https://doi.org/10.1353/etc.0.0047

Case-Smith, J. (2000). Effects of occupational therapy services on fine motor and functional performance in preschool children. *American Journal of Occupational Therapy, 54,* 372–380. https://doi.org/10.5014/ajot.54.4.372

Case-Smith, J., Frolek Clark, G. J., & Schlabach, T. L. (2013). Systematic review of interventions used in occupational therapy to promote motor performance for children ages birth–5 years. *American Journal of Occupational Therapy, 67,* 413–424. http://dx.doi.org/10.5014/ajot.2013.005959

Chapparo, C. (2010). Perceive, recall, plan and perform: Occupational centred task-analysis and intervention system. In S. Rodger (Ed.), *Occupation centred practice with children: A practical guide for occupational therapist* (pp. 183–202). Hoboken, NJ: Wiley-Blackwell.

Chapparo, C. J., & Hooper, E. (2005). Self-care at school: Perceptions of 6-year-old children. *American Journal of Occupational Therapy, 59*(1), 67–77. https://doi.org/10.5014/ajot.59.1.67

D'Arrigo, R. G., Copley, J. A., Poulsen, A. A., & Ziviani, J. (2020). The engaged child in occupational therapy. *Canadian Journal of Occupational Therapy, 87*(2), 127–136. https://doi.org/10.1177/0008417420905708

Dawson, D., McEwen, S., & Polatajko, H. (Eds.). (2017). *Cognitive orientation to daily occupational performance in occupational therapy: Using the CO–OP approach to enable participation across the lifespan.* Bethesda, MD: AOTA Press.

Deitz, J. C., & Swinth, Y. (2008). Accessing play through assistive technology. In L. D. Parham & L. S. Fazio (Eds.), *Play in occupational therapy for children* (2nd ed., pp. 395–412). St. Louis, MO: Mosby Elsevier.

De Vries, D., Beck, T., Stacey, B., Winslow, K., & Meines, K. (2015). Music as a therapeutic intervention with autism: A systematic review of the literature. *Therapeutic Recreation Journal, 49,* 220–237.

DiCarlo, C. F., Schepis, M. M., & Flynn, L. (2009). Embedding sensory preference into toys to enhance toy play in toddlers with disabilities. *Infants & Young Children, 22*(3), 188–200. https://doi.org/10.1097/IYC.0b013e3181abe1a1

Dunn, W., McClain, L. H., Brown, C., & Youngstrom, M. J. (1998). The ecology of human performance. In M. E. Neistadt & E. B. Crepeau (Eds.), *Willard & Spackman's occupational therapy* (9th ed., pp. 525–535). Philadelphia, PA: Lippincott Williams & Wilkins.

Grajo, L., Boisselle, A., & DaLomba, E. (2018). Occupational adaptation as a construct: A scoping review of literature. *The Open Journal of Occupational Therapy, 6*(1), 2. https://doi.org/10.15453/2168-6408.1400

Grajo, L. C., Candler, C., & Sarafian, A. (2020). Interventions within the scope of occupational therapy to improve children's academic participation: A systematic review. *American Journal of Occupational Therapy, 74,* 7402180030. https://doi.org/10.5014/ajot.2020.039016

Gunn, K. C. M., & Delafield-Butt, J. T. (2015). teaching children with autism spectrum disorder with restricted interests: A review of evidence for best practice. *Review of Educational Research.* https://doi.org/10.3102/0034654315604027

Heah, T., Case, T., McGuire, B., & Law, M. (2007). Successful participation: The lived experience among children with disabilities. *Canadian Journal of Occupational Therapy, 74*(1), 38–47. https://doi.org/10.2182/cjot.06.10

Holland, C., Yay, O., Gallini, G., Blanche, E., & Thompson, B. (2018). Relationships between therapist and client actions during sensory integration therapy for young children with autism. *American Journal of Occupational Therapy*, 72(4, Supplement 1), 7211515250. https://doi.org/10.5014/ajot.2018.72S1-PO4034

Judge, S., Floyd, K., & Wood-Fields, C. (2010). Creating a technology-rich learning environment for infants and toddlers with disabilities. *Infants & Young Children*, 23(2), 84–92. https://doi.org/10.1097/IYC.0b013e3181d29b14

Jung, S., & Sainato, D. M. (2015). Teaching games to young children with autism spectrum disorder using special interests and video modelling. *Journal of Intellectual & Developmental Disability*, 40(2), 198. http://dx.doi.org/10.3109/13668250.2015.1027674

Keeling, K., Smith Myles, B., Gagnon, E., & Simpson, R. (2003). Using the power card strategy to teach sportsmanship skills to a child with autism. *Focus on Autism and Other Developmental Disabilities*, 18, 103–109. https://doi.org/10.1177/10883576030180020

Kern, P., Wakeford, L., & Aldridge, D. (2007). Improving the performance of a young child with autism during self-care tasks using embedded song interventions: A case study. *Music Therapy Perspectives*, 25(1), 43–51, https://doi.org/10.1093/mtp/25.1.43

King, P., & Howard, J. (2014). Factors influencing children's perceptions of choice within their free play activity: The impact of functional, structural and social affordances. *Journal of Playwork Practice*, 1(2), 173–190. https://doi.org/10.1332/205316214X14114616128010

Koegel, L., Matos-Freden, R., Lang, R., & Koegel, R. (2012). Interventions for children with autism spectrum disorders in inclusive school settings. *Cognitive and Behavioral Practice*, 19(3), 401–412.

Koegel, L. K., Singh, A. K., & Koegel, R. L. (2010). Improving motivation for academics in children with autism. *Journal of Autism and Developmental Disorders*, 40(9), 1057–1066. https://doi.org/10.1007/s10803-010-0962-6

Kryzak, L. A., Bauer, S., Jones, E. A., & Sturmey, P. (2013). Increasing responding to others' joint attention directives using circumscribed interests. *Journal of Applied Behavior Analysis*, 46(3), 674–679. https://doi.org/10.1002/jaba.73

Kryzak, L. A., & Jones, E. A. (2014). The effect of prompts within embedded circumscribed interests to teach initiating joint attention in children with autism spectrum disorders. *Journal of Developmental and Physical Disabilities*, 27, 265–284. https://doi.org/10.1007/s10882-014-9414-0

Kuhaneck, H., Spitzer, S., & Miller, E. (2010). *Activity analysis, creativity and playfulness in pediatric occupational therapy: Making play just right*. Sudbury, MA: Jones & Bartlett Learning.

Lanou, A., Hough, L., & Powell, E. (2012). Case studies on using strengths and interests to address the needs of students with autism spectrum disorders. *Intervention in School and Clinic*, 47, 175–182. https://doi.org/10.1177/1053451211423819

Leaf, J. B., Oppenheim-Leaf, M. L., Leaf, R., Courtemanche, A. B., Taubman, M., McEachin, J., …

Learning Without Tears. (2021). *Readiness & Writing*. Gaithersburg, MD: Learning Without Tears.

Mack, W., Lindquist, J. E., & Parham, L. D. (1982). A synthesis of occupational behavior and sensory integration concepts in theory and practice, Part 1. Theoretical foundations. *American Journal of Occupational Therapy*, 36(6), 365–374.

Marshall, A., Myers, C., & Pierce, D. (2017). Centennial topics—A century of therapeutic use of the physical environment. *American Journal of Occupational Therapy*, 71, 7101100030. https://doi.org/10.5014/ajot.2017.023960

McCoy, S. W., Palisano, R., Avery, L., Jeffries, L., Laforme Fiss, A., Chiarello, L., & Hanna, S. (2020). Physical, occupational, and speech therapy for children with cerebral palsy. *Developmental Medicine and Child Neurology*, 62(1), 140–146. https://doi.org/10.1111/dmcn.14325.

Michelman, S. S. (1974). Play and the deficit child. In M. Reilly (Ed.), *Play as exploratory learning* (pp. 157–207). Beverly Hills, CA: SAGE Publications, Incorporated.

Michielsen, M., Vaughan-Graham, J., Holland, A., Magri, A., & Suzuki, M. (2019). The Bobath concept—a model to illustrate clinical practice. *Disability and Rehabilitation*, 41 (17), 2080–2092. https://doi.org/10.1080/09638288.2017.1417496

Miller, E., & Kuhaneck, H. (2008). Children's perceptions of play experiences and play preferences: A qualitative study. *American Journal of Occupational Therapy*, 62, 407–415. https://doi.org/10.5014/ajot.62.4.407

Missiuna, C. A., Pollock, N. A., Levac, D. E., Campbell, W. N., Whalen, S. D. S., Bennett, S. M., … Russell, D. J. (2012). Partnering for change: An innovative school-based occupational therapy service delivery model for children with developmental coordination disorder. *Canadian Journal of Occupational Therapy*, 79(1), 41–50. https://doi.org/10.2182/cjot.2012.79.1.6

Muesbeck, J., St. John, B. M., Kant, S., & Ausderau, K. K. (2018). Use of props during mealtime for children with autism spectrum disorders: Self-regulation and reinforcement. *OTJR: Occupation, Participation and Health*, 38(4), 254–260. doi:10.1177/1539449218778558

Munier, V., Myers, C. T., & Pierce, D. (2008). Power of object play for infants and toddlers. In L. D. Parham & L. S. Fazio (Eds.), *Play in occupational therapy for children* (2nd ed., pp. 219–249). St. Louis, MO: Mosby Elsevier.

Neistadt, M. E., McAuley, D., Zecha, D., & Shannon, R. (1993). An analysis of a board game as a treatment activity. *American Journal of Occupational Therapy*, 47(2), 154–160. https://doi.org/10.5014/ajot.47.2.154

O'Brien, J., & Lewin, J. E. (2008, November). Part 1: Translating motor control and motor learning theory into occupational therapy practice for children and youth (continuing education article), *OT Practice*, 13(21), E1–CE8.

O'Brien, J., & Lewin, J. E. (2009, January). Part 2: Translating motor control and motor learning theory into occupational therapy practice for children and youth (continuing education article), *OT Practice*, 14(1), CE1–CE8.

O'Brien, J. C., & Soloman, J. W. (2013). *Occupational analysis and group process*. St. Louis, MO: Elsevier.

Owens, G., Granader, Y., Humphrey, A., & Baron-Cohen, S. (2008). LEGO® therapy and the social use of language programme: An evaluation of two social skills interventions for children with high functioning autism and Asperger syndrome. *Journal of Autism and Developmental Disorders*, 38(10), 1944.

Piersol, C. V. (2014). Occupational therapy: Selection, gradation, analysis, and adaptation. In M. V. Radomski & C. A. Trombly Latham (Eds.), *Occupational therapy for physical dysfunction* (7th ed., pp. 360–393). Philadelphia, PA: Lippincott Williams & Wilkins.

Porter, E. (2012). Spotlight on: Autism speaks and finding a voice for all children with an ASD. *Children's Legal Rights Journal, 32*, 76.

Price, P., & Miner, S. (2007). Occupation emerges in the process of therapy. *American Journal of Occupational Therapy, 61*(4), 441–450. https://doi.org/10.5014/ajot.61.4.441

Reinhartsen, D. B., Garfinkle, A. N., & Wolery, M. (2002). Engagement with toys in two-year-old children with autism: Teacher selection versus child choice. *Research and Practice for Persons with Severe Disabilities, 27*(3), 175–187.

Rigby, P. J., Trentham, B., & Letts, L. (2019). Modifying performance contexts. In B. A. Boyt Schell & G. Gillen (Eds.), *Willard & Spackman's occupational therapy* (13th ed., pp. 460–479). Baltimore, MD: Lippincott Williams & Wilkins.

Robinson, A. L. (1977). Play: The arena for acquisition of rules for competent behavior. *American Journal of Occupational Therapy, 31*(4), 248–253.

Rogers, J.C. (1982). The spirit of independence: The evolution of a philosophy. *American Journal of Occupational Therapy, 36*(11), 709-715.

Ross, B., & Dixson, J. (1958). Lollipop. Recorded by The Chordettes. Cadence Records.

Sakemiller, L. M., & Nelson, D. L. (1998). Eliciting functional extension in prone through the use of a game. *American Journal of Occupational Therapy, 52*(2), 150–157. https://doi.org/10.5014/ajot.52.2.150

Sherman, J. A. (2012). Observational effects on the preferences of children with autism. *Journal of Applied Behavior Analysis, 45*(3), 473–483. http://doi.org/10.1901/jaba.2012.45-473

Sparling, J. W., Walker, D. F., & Singdahlsen, J. (1984). Play techniques with neurologically impaired preschoolers. *American Journal of Occupational Therapy, 38*, 603–612. https://doi.org/10.5014/ajot.38.9.603

Spencer, V. G., Simpson, C. G., Day, M., & Buster, E. (2008). Using the power card strategy to teach social skills to a child with autism. *TEACHING Exceptional Children Plus, 5*(1), Article 2. http://escholarship.bc.edu/education/tecplus/vol5/iss1/art2

Spitzer, S. L. (2003). With and without words: Exploring occupation in relation to young children with autism. *Journal of Occupational Science, 10*(2), 67–79. https://doi.org/10.1080/14427591.2003.9686513

Spitzer, S. L. (2004). Common and uncommon daily activities in individuals with autism: Challenges and opportunities for supporting occupation. In H. Miller-Kuhaneck (Ed.), *Autism: A comprehensive occupational therapy approach* (2nd ed., pp. 83–106). Bethesda, MD: AOTA Press.

Spitzer, S. L. (2008). Play in children with autism: Structure and experience. In L. D. Parham & L. S. Fazio (Eds.), *Play in occupational therapy for children* (2nd ed., pp. 351–374). St. Louis, MO: Mosby Elsevier.

Spitzer, S. L. (2010). Common and uncommon daily activities in children with an autism spectrum disorder: Challenges and opportunities for supporting occupation. In H. Miller Kuhaneck & R. Watling (Eds.), *Autism: A comprehensive occupational therapy approach* (3rd ed., pp. 203–233). Bethesda, MD: American Occupational Therapy Association.

Spitzer, S. L. (2017). *Making play out of work: Engaging children. Web-based continuing education.* Seattle, WA: Medbridge. https://www.medbridgeeducation.com/course-catalog/details/making-play-out-of-work-engaging-children-susan-spitzer-occupational-therapy/

Spitzer, S. L. (2020). Observational assessment and activity analysis. In J. O'Brien and H. Kuhaneck (Eds.), *Case-Smith's occupational therapy for children* (8th ed., pp. 135–157). St. Louis, MO: Elsevier.

Steese, B. (2009). Pirates of the CariBOOTin': Following the map to shoe tying success. *ADVANCE for Occupational Therapy Practitioners, 25*(7), 29–30.

Steinbrenner, J. R., Hume, K., Odom, S. L., Morin, K. L., Nowell, S. W., Tomaszewski, B., … Savage, M. N. (2020). *Evidence-based practices for children, youth, and young adults with autism.* Chapel Hill: The University of North Carolina at Chapel Hill, Frank Porter Graham Child Development Institute, National Clearinghouse on Autism Evidence and Practice Review Team.

Stern, B. Z. (2013, February 11). Button bingo: A fun addition to the occupational therapy toolbox. *OT Practice,* 7–8.

Tickle-Degnen, L., & Coster, W. (1995). Therapeutic interaction and the management of challenge during the beginning minutes of sensory integration treatment. *The Occupational Therapy Journal of Research, 15*(2), 122-141.

Tomchek, S. D., & Koenig, K. P. (2016). *Occupational therapy practice guidelines for individuals with autism spectrum disorder.* Bethesda, MD: AOTA Press.

Verver, S. H., Vervloed, M. P., & Steenbergen, B. (2019). The use of augmented toys to facilitate play in school-aged children with visual impairments. *Research in Developmental Disabilities, 85*, 70–81. https://doi.org/10.1016/j.ridd.2018.11.006

Verver, S. H., Vervloed, M. P., & Steenbergen, B. (2020). Facilitating play and social interaction between children with visual impairments and sighted peers by means of augmented toys. *Journal of Developmental and Physical Disabilities, 32*, 93–111. https://doi.org/10.1007/s10882-019-09680-6

Vismara, L. A., & Lyons, G. L. (2007). Using perseverative interests to elicit joint attention behaviors in young children with autism: Theoretical and clinical implications for understanding motivation. *Journal of Positive Behavior Interventions, 9*(4), 214–228.

Weaver, L. L. (2018). Participation in ADLs for individuals with ASD. In R. Watling & S. L. Spitzer (Eds.), *Autism across the lifespan: A comprehensive occupational therapy approach* (4th. ed., pp. 269–285). Bethesda, MD: AOTA Press..

Williams, S. E., & Matesi, D. V. (1988). Therapeutic intervention with an adapted toy. *American Journal of Occupational Therapy, 42*, 673–676.

Wimpory, D. C., Hobson, R. P., & Nash, S. (2007). What facilitates social engagement in preschool children with autism? *Journal of Autism and Developmental Disorders, 37*(3), 564–573.

Winter-Messiers, M. (2007). From tarantulas to toilet brushes: Understanding the special interest areas of children and youth with Asperger's syndrome. *Remedial and Special Education, 28*, 140–152. https://doi.org/10.1177/07419325070280030301

Wong, C., Odom, S. L., Hume, K. A., Cox, C. W., Fettig, A., Kurcharczyk, S., et al. (2015). Evidence-based practices for children, youth, and young adults with autism spectrum disorder: A comprehensive review. *Journal of Autism and Developmental Disorders. 45*(7), 1951–1966. https://doi.org/10.1007/s10803-014-2351-z

APPENDIX 8.1 Modifying Work into Play: Worksheet

Child's Name:	
Activity Child Needs to Do:	

<u>Directions</u>: Note core activity demands the child needs to do (from the activity analysis) as well as the child's preferences and skills. Compare these two columns to identify ways of modifying the activity to include what the child can and wants to do. Then, try modifications to determine child's level of acceptance, resistance, or interest.

Activity Components*	Activity Demands	Child's Interests, Abilities, Strengths	Analysis: Possible Modifications
Objects Used (toys, materials, shape, color, size, etc.)			
Sensory Features (visual, auditory, tactile, vestibular, proprioceptive)			
Motor/Action Features (eyes, posture, hand use, movements, motor skill/ coordination, etc.)			
Cognitive Features (sequencing, problem solving, construction, imagination, etc.)			
Social Features (interaction with people)			
Location & Space			

* Activity components are based on AOTA (2020) and applied for most common use in pediatrics. However, therapists are urged to modify as needed to best suit individual practice settings.

APPENDIX 8.2 Zach's Story from Occupational Therapy: Modifying Soccer to Be Play

Horses vs. Wolves
The horses lived on one side of the forest and wolves lived on the other side.

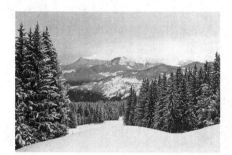

© Dmitry Naumov/Shutterstock.

1

One day, they woke up. The horses tried to kick a big rock to knock down the wolves' den made out of rocks. The wolves tried to kick the big rock to knock down the horses' house made of wood. Sometimes, the wolves hit the horses' house and sometimes the horses hit the wolves' den. Each time, it hurt their home and they tried to get even with the other side. Sometimes, the wolves blocked the horses' rock and kicked it back at their house. Sometimes, the horses blocked the wolves' rock and kicked it back at their den.

2

Sometimes a horse or wolf got hit by the rock. They didn't get hurt. They just got a little dizzy and they got up and kept kicking.

3

Sometimes one horse was blocked by the wolves so it kicked the rock to another horse who could kick it at the wolves' den. Sometimes one wolf was blocked by the horses so it kicked the rock to another wolf who could kick it at the horses' house.

4

They kept kicking and kicking until the afternoon. The moon started coming up and they got tired. They dropped the rock and fell on the ground and went to sleep.
zzzzzzzzzzzzzzzzzzzz

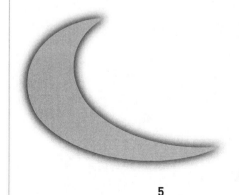

5

The next morning, they got up and started kicking again.

6

Then suddenly, the horses and wolves became friends.

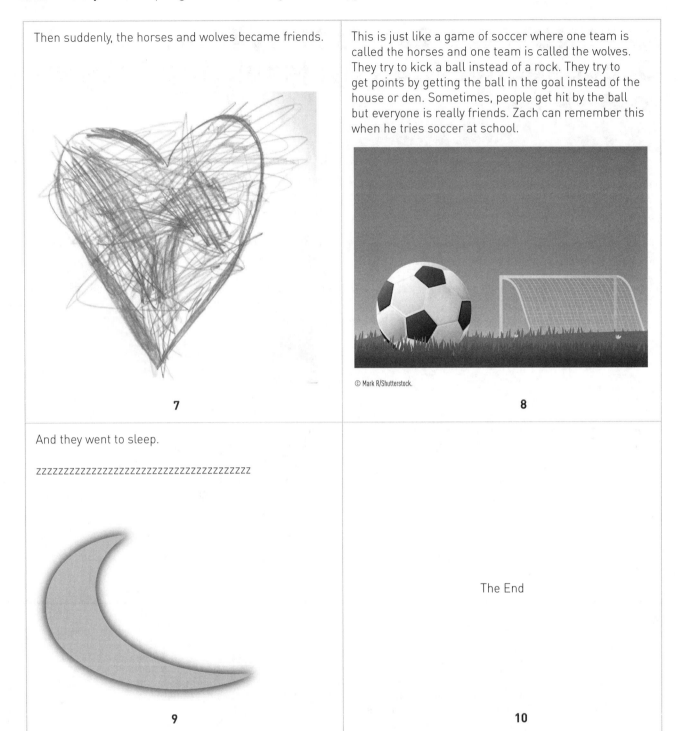

7

This is just like a game of soccer where one team is called the horses and one team is called the wolves. They try to kick a ball instead of a rock. They try to get points by getting the ball in the goal instead of the house or den. Sometimes, people get hit by the ball but everyone is really friends. Zach can remember this when he tries soccer at school.

© Mark R/Shutterstock.

8

And they went to sleep.

zzzzzzzzzzzzzzzzzzzzzzzzzzzzzzzzzzzzzzzzzzz

9

The End

10

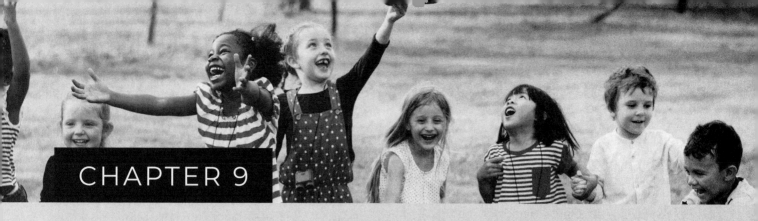

CHAPTER 9

Playful Play Spaces

Susan L. Spitzer, PhD, OTR/L

Alexia E. Metz, PhD, OTR/L

Heather M. Kuhaneck, PhD, OTR/L, FAOTA

After reading this chapter, the reader will:

- Describe the importance of environmental context for occupational therapy practice related to play.
- Determine the affordances and barriers of play environments and objects.
- Discuss the advantages of targeting the environment to promote play.
- Select appropriate play spaces and materials.
- Use play spaces and materials therapeutically.
- Adapt play environments and objects to improve play using the concept of person-environment fit.

Good play environments have magical qualities that transcend the here and now, the humdrum and the typical. They have flow qualities—qualities that take the child to other places and other times. They are permeated with awe and wonder, both in rarity and in imaginative qualities.

—Joe Frost

Alongside other professional fields and with a wealth of well-established research, occupational therapy has adopted a transactional model of performance that recognizes that the environment is inseparable from human function (American Occupational Therapy Association [AOTA], 2020; Law et al., 1996). For children's play spaces, occupational therapy practitioners seek to create a person–environment fit for play by attending to the affordances offered by play environments and objects (Aziz & Said, 2015). Children's preferred play spaces provide an array of affordances for play, while balancing familiarity and novelty to promote exploration (Robinson, 1977). They are safe and accessible, allowing independent mobility and

engagement (Castonguay & Jutras, 2009). Although theoretically any space can become a space for play to occur, certain spaces are more conducive for play than others. For a child with a disability, some spaces can present significant barriers to play. In these cases, occupational therapy practitioners promote the development of play spaces that foster and encourage play, through specific environmental modifications as well as training of key adults or peers. Occupational therapy practitioners address the physical environment's safety, usability, and spatial arrangement and the personal relevance of specific environments and objects in them, as well as the influence of the social environment, to promote inclusive opportunities to play. Using direct and indirect interventions, practitioners apply their knowledge to help families, children, and others select playful play spaces, adapt play spaces to become more apt to promote play, and advocate for policy changes that promote greater access to playful spaces. In this chapter, we will highlight very specific strategies to promote play through explicit attention to many aspects of the environment for play.

Promoting Play Through the Environment

Occupational therapy's attention to the features of environmental context is supported by research. Environmental supportiveness has been linked to playfulness and participation for children with and without developmental disabilities (Bundy, Waugh, & Brentnall, 2009; Hamm, 2006; Rosenberg, Bart, Ratzon, & Jarus, 2013; Waldman-Levi & Erez, 2015). In contrast, environmental barriers may reduce participation for children and youth with disabilities such as lack of community programs, parental attitudes, social attitudes, physical design or accessibility, geographic location, transportation, financial resources, and temporal elements (Anaby, Law, Teplicky, & Turner, 2015; Kang, Hsieh, Liao, & Hwang, 2017). In consideration of the myriad ways in which the environment can support or hinder play, occupational therapy practitioners often use models that consider both affordances and person–environment fit.

Affordances

In typical development, children play in many different spaces (Lynch & Stanley, 2018), and being a part of varied environments can be important for a child's social interaction and community inclusion. The physical parameters, social features, and objects in the environment are tangible components of a play activity. The environment may provide opportunities such as inviting movement, engaging in shared activities with others, or enjoying a nice space in which to be (King, Rigby, & Batorowicz, 2013). These opportunities are widely referred to as "affordances" in the literature about play environments.

Affordances were first explored as a theoretical concept by Gibson (1977) in relation to human perception and are a prominent construct of ecological psychology (Scaratino, 2003). Affordances refer to the properties of objects and the environment that invite a specific type of use or method of interaction (May-Benson & Cermak, 2007). As such, they may be considered as a positive aspect of an environment. However, it is important to note that affordances may be either positive or negative. Positive affordances invite positive opportunities for action, whereas negative ones provide potential threats (Scaratino, 2003).

Affordances are not actualized until both perceived by and acted upon by a child. Each child may be both a "perceiver" of the possibilities and an "actor" in an environment. But importantly, the physical environment provides the affordance, whether or not the child perceives it. Affordances exist because of physical properties of an object or environment; however, they may or may not be acted upon by any particular child or individual (Scaratino, 2003). In addressing the environment, occupational therapy practitioners promote environmental features that afford engagement and its perception.

Affordances are of two types, respectively termed goals and happenings. Goal affordances are environmental or object properties that are "do-able" with the intention of a doer, such as climbable or catchable (see **Figures 9.1** and **9.2**). Happening affordances are properties of environments or objects that can occur unintentionally to an individual such as getting burned by something that is hot, falling off a cliff, or having a door open inward and being hit by it. In occupational therapy, both intentional and unintentional properties are weighed by therapists in promoting participation and ensuring safety in play.

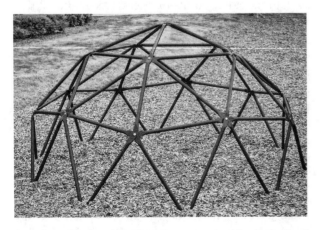
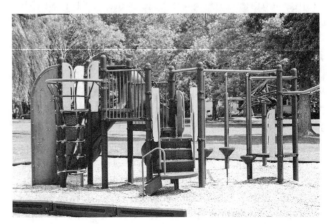

Figure 9.1 These objects and spaces provide goal affordances for climbing

Left: © Ronan Odonohoe/Shutterstock; Right: © Chris Bradshaw/Shutterstock.

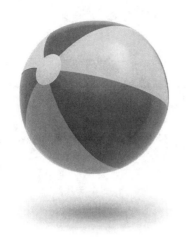

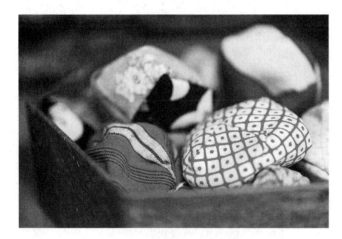

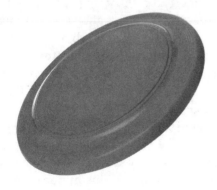

Figure 9.2 These objects provide goal affordances for catching

Top: © Chones/Shutterstock; Middle: © Tack-Ma/Shutterstock; Bottom: © New Africa/Shutterstock.

Person–Environment Fit

While the opportunity to play is a necessary prerequisite, it does not guarantee play will occur, as environmental opportunities interact with other factors (King et al., 2013). Participation for children and adolescents with disabilities is based on the interdependence between personal factors and environmental ones (Humphry & Wakeford, 2006; Rosenberg et al., 2013; Gibson, King, et al., 2017). The individual must be able to perceive and utilize the affordances offered. If the environmental affordances do not fit the individual, they may actually become barriers such as causing anxiety if the affordances are unattainable and boredom if too easy (Rigby, Trentham, & Letts, 2019; Skard & Bundy, 2008). This research supports the importance of person–environment "fit."

Person–environment fit theories are built on three basic hypotheses (van Vianen, 2018). First, the match or fit between a person and the environment is a better predictor of outcomes than either person or environment alone. Second, outcomes are believed to be best when the characteristics of the person and the environment are compatible, regardless of whether a person has high or low levels of a specific characteristic. Last, in situations where there is not "fit," positive outcomes are reduced. This lack of fit can occur when there is either too little or too much of some particular attribute. These theories suggest that the fit between the child's characteristics and the play environment would be of utmost importance in predicting play; however, more research testing them in relation to play outcomes is needed (Aziz & Said, 2015). Some of the many aspects of a play space that could influence fit and thus the play that occurs include the amount of space, the type of space, the things in the space, the arrangement of materials, potential play partners, the amount of adult assistance or interference, and the quantity and type of toys. Each of these could interact differently with a child's gender identity, age, developmental level, physical abilities, and other child characteristics (see **Figure 9.3**).

Of importance is that the affordances of a play space can either invite or repel a child (Heft, 1988). A child has agency and will, and although the environment provides the affordances, the child makes decisions about which will be "actualized" (Prieske, Withagen, Smith, & Zaal, 2015). Therefore, it is important to understand which affordances most invite children to play and how those affordances interact with the capabilities of a child. Occupational therapy practitioners can use this knowledge to maximize features of environments that are more likely to foster play performance.

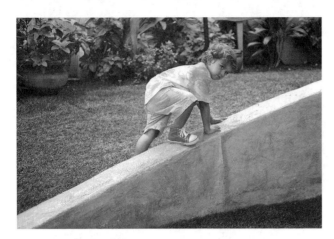 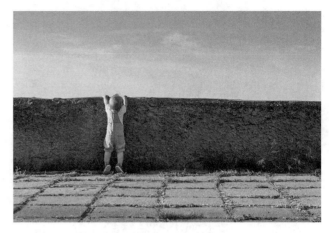

Figure 9.3 Aspects of the environment interact with child characteristics to create person–environment fit, or lack of fit. In the first photo, the child is tall enough and the wall is short enough that he is able to climb, whereas in the second, the child may be unsuccessful in climbing

Left: © glenda/Shutterstock; Right: © Yehor Milohrodskyi/Shutterstock.

Targeting the Physical Play Environment

Ensuring Safety in Play Environments

Any play environment must be safe and comfortable for the child and others who may be present (Lane & Mistrett, 2008; Rigby & Huggins, 2003; Skard & Bundy, 2008). Safety is a critical consideration of families and other caregivers for children and adolescents with intellectual disabilities who may be vulnerable due to limitations in safety awareness and problem solving (Venema, Vlaskamp, & Otten, 2017). The child and caregiver should feel relaxed, enabling freedom to explore and take risks (Robinson, 1977).

The occupational therapy practitioner must consider the risks for injury with alternatives that allow the child to play. Children with disabilities, especially those with emotional and behavioral challenges, are at higher risk of injury (Sinclair & Xiang, 2008). The environment should therefore be safeguarded from potential dangers. For example, the occupational therapy practitioner must guard against potential injury from tripping/falling hazards, electrical equipment and outlets, sharp items, toxic materials, and small objects on which the child can choke. This may involve altering the environment itself or being

prepared to intervene to protect the child. Carpeting, floor mats, or blankets may be added to provide cushioning to a floor when falling is anticipated (Isbell & Isbell, 2007).

Outdoor spaces have other potential hazards. The occupational therapy practitioner may use such opportunities to help the child learn about safety in the environment, such as cars in parking lots or children swinging on the playground. Basic first aid supplies should be available to ensure appropriate assistance if an injury occurs. Soft surfaces and adequate fencing provide playground safety measures that children and their families value (Nasar & Holloman, 2013). A safe temperature and adequate shade for sun protection are necessary (Olsen, Kennedy, & Vanos, 2019). Anticipating potential hazards in the environment allows the occupational therapy practitioner to be ready to respond immediately in an effective and sympathetic manner if necessary. Sometimes, using a different park or other space can help as in the case of Daniel (see **Practice Example 9.1**).

Another aspect of safety is cleanliness. The environment must be clean and sanitary. Supplies and strategies for ensuring sanitation between and during use must be available. Institutional policies and procedures to ensure health should be developed and followed.

PRACTICE EXAMPLE 9.1 Daniel: Adapting Safe Space for Play

Daniel was a 10-year-old with learning disabilities and ADHD who always wanted to do stunts, such as flying flips from the monkey bars, for which his safety was at risk. Therefore, his occupational therapist consulted with Daniel's mother to encourage a gymnastics class focused on trapeze acts. Daniel became a very good trapeze artist and looked forward to these special opportunities for physically extreme play.

Whether a play environment is safe for a specific child depends on the interaction of the environment and the individual client's factors. In assessing safety, the occupational therapist must anticipate which affordances the client may use or may happen to them to determine if there are any potential threats to safety (see **Box 9.1**). For example, regardless of age, a child may enjoy throwing or licking items. For such a child, adaptations must be determined for all items that afford throwing or licking to ensure safety to the child and others and minimize damage. This may mean relocation of throwable and lickable items or adult supervision to potentially intervene. Similarly, a child with an intellectual disability or visual-perceptual weaknesses may not notice that he or she has entered the path of a child swinging or car moving when chasing after a ball. In this case, the occupational therapist may consider physical barriers, visual markers, or adult supervision to safeguard or alert this child to adjust to potential dangers. For a child with a motor impairment, therapists place themselves on the side of weakness or danger in order to decrease reaction time and injury. Although physical adaptations and adult supervision are both effective for safety, occupational therapists typically prioritize physical adaptations because these facilitate play better than adult intervention of stopping and redirecting children, which tends to interrupt and restrict play.

Box 9.1 Environmental Safety Considerations Tailored for Each Child

- Cleanliness adequate for child's medical conditions and health status
- Adequate cleaning and sanitation options
- Safe temperature
- Adequate shade for sun protection
- Tripping and falling hazards such as changes in surface height and objects
- Hardness of surfaces child may fall on or against
- Electrical equipment and outlets
- Sharp items
- Toxic materials
- Allergens
- First aid supplies
- Safety of objects that may be thrown, kicked, or mouthed
- Actions of others that may knock into, bump, or distract (such as cars, running children, dogs jumping)
- Sounds, visual sensations, or other factors that may distract or frighten

---

Determining Safety of Play Materials

Safety of toys and objects used in play is fundamental. Though toys can be delightfully engaging objects, if they are not well made or carefully matched to the abilities of the client, they can be a source of great tragedy. Children likely rarely think about safety, but parents consider it as one of their most important factors in toy selection (Al Kurdi, 2017; All things Toys, 2018; Christensen & Stockdale, 1991; Fallon & Harris, 1989).

The Consumer Product Safety Commission (CPSC) is a U.S. federal regulatory agency that aims to reduce risk or danger of injury and death resulting from unsafe products, including toys. They report more than 200,000 injuries and upward of a dozen deaths in children each year related to toys. For children under age 3, the most common accidents involve choking on small parts. For older children, falls and crashes involving ride-on toys (including collisions with motor vehicles) are the most common. Some incidents result from children drowning while playing with toys in or near open water. Other common toy-related injuries include lacerations, contusions and abrasions, sprains and strains, fractures, asphyxiation, poisoning, and internal injuries from ingestion of hazardous parts such as batteries and magnets. The CPSC works to reduce toy-related injury and death by setting safety standards, recommending product recalls, and educating the public.

Oral contact is one of the greatest risks of danger that toys present to children. The principal danger is asphyxiation by choking. Toys with small parts (diameter of 1.75 inches or smaller), balloons, and marbles must be labeled for use only by children age 3 years and older. Small, round, elastic objects are a particular choking hazard, such as rubber balls, because they can easily slip into and lodge within the airway but compress and expand during maneuvers to remove them. In addition to choking, swallowing small toy parts can be dangerous. Toys with strong magnets are to be labeled for use only by children age 14 and older.

Children with disabilities may be more susceptible to injury (Fraser, Doan, Lundy, Bevill, & Aceros, 2019). Therefore, it becomes extremely important for occupational therapy practitioners to consider the safety of all play materials independently (see **Table 9.1** for a list of common safety considerations). Determining if a play object is safe for a child involves a realistic consideration of what that specific child may do with the object. Will the

Table 9.1 Common Safety Concerns for Toys and Other Play Objects

Object Features	Safety Concerns
Sharp points	■ Can cause puncture wounds or cuts.
Heating elements	■ Can cause burns. ■ Should only be used with adult supervision and be safely discarded if damaged.
Electrically operated	■ Can cause electrical shock. ■ Must be manufactured with safety features and have warning labels (in the U.S.). ■ Should only be used with adult supervision and be safely discarded if damaged. ■ Should not be used in or near water.
Strings or cords	■ Can cause strangulation.
Makes loud noises	■ Can damage hearing (Mahboubi et al., 2013).
Propels objects	■ Can cause eye injuries.
Lasers	■ Can cause eye injuries (Raoof et al., 2014).
Hinges	■ Can pinch or cause impingement injuries.
Strong magnetic or electrical fields	■ Can interfere with shunts, pacemakers, and implanted medication delivery systems (American Heart Association, 2016, Huh & Roldan, 2016, Zuzak, Balmer, Schmidig, Boltshauser, & Grotzer, 2009).
Ride-on	■ Can be involved in fall and collision accidents. ■ Should only be used with appropriate supervision, in safe areas (away from stairs, traffic, and open water). ■ Should be used with protective equipment, such as helmets and knee/elbow pads.

child use the item in its intended way? Is the object durable enough to withstand the force the child may use considering the child's kinesthetic functioning, ability to grade force, frustration tolerance, anger management, and so on? Will the child try to mouth it, break it open, stand on it, or throw it? If the object may reasonably be expected to break, will the pieces have sharp edges or create other hazards? Misuse of toys is one of the most common safety hazards of toys (Yu & Schwebel, 2018), so how the toy is likely to be used is an essential consideration. Two primary ways to reduce the risk of toy-related injury and death are to select and modify objects (1) to minimize physical hazards and (2) to be appropriate for the child's age and developmental status. A determination of safety for play materials is not an elimination of risk as much as a weighing of risks to minimize hazards and danger (see **Practice Example 9.2**).

Minimizing Physical Hazard in Play Materials. Basic toy safety is determined by manufacturers, but their guidelines and practices do not always ensure safety, especially for children with disabilities (Fraser et al., 2019; Kulak & Stein, 2016). Under the guidance of the U.S. Consumer Product

Safety Commission (CPSC), toy labeling practices aim to assist consumers. Therapists must be aware that the CPSC's regulatory oversight does not encompass objects not manufactured or sold as toys. The CPSC specifies labeling for some risks. Additionally, therapists must minimize risk by inspecting and maintaining the physical condition of toys, considering their clients' ability to play safely, modifying toys or play to reduce danger, and providing appropriate supervision. Beyond following specific guidelines, the CPSC further recommends securely storing toys that may represent any risk of injury in order to prevent unsupervised play. Be aware that toys later determined to be unsafe may be recalled; however, not all unsafe toys are successfully recalled (Yu & Schwebel, 2018).

When addressing their clients' therapy goals, occupational therapy practitioners may select toys that have risky features like small parts, unsecured battery compartments, or unknown composition for clients' therapy sessions. For example, a travel version of a popular game or a miniature doll may be chosen because their small parts present the opportunity to build fine-motor skills. When selecting toys like this, therapists must be vigilant. With children under age 3 or clients with a tendency to

PRACTICE EXAMPLE 9.2 Leyla's Play with Unsafe Objects

Leyla was a 9-year-old who sustained a head injury when hit by a car last year. As part of a home evaluation, an occupational therapist observed Leyla playing while holding an unused scented dryer sheet, which she repeatedly smelled. The therapist asked the father if this was common, and he explained that since the accident, the dryer sheets had become a favorite play item. Although Leyla was clearly enjoying the dryer sheet, the occupational therapist was concerned about the chemicals contained in fragranced dryer sheets (Potera, 2011), especially because Leyla was exposing herself to chemicals at a higher level and in a more direct manner than likely anticipated by the manufacturer. In order to respect and understand the family's context, the occupational therapist asked, "What do you think about this?" The father then shared that he was concerned that this was abnormal behavior and had tried to keep the dryer sheets away from Leyla, but she would find them and cry and be upset for the rest of the day if the dryer sheet was removed.

Despite sharing the father's concern about the dryer sheets albeit for different reasons, the occupational therapist also wanted to be respectful of Leyla's play interests. Given the disruption of removal of the scented dryer sheets, the occupational therapist considered other options for adapting this play object and asked if the family had tried unscented dryer sheets. The family reported they were unaware of unscented dryer sheets. The therapist also explained the safety concerns and recommended that the family consult the poison control hotline or physician who could provide expertise on the safety of continuing to use fragranced dryer sheets in her play. The family decided to substitute unscented dryer sheets immediately, and Leyla quickly stopped using them in her play. The therapist then worked with Leyla and her family to identify and provide her with alternate sensory-rich play objects to expand her play such as through various forms of water play.

put objects in their mouths, practitioners must provide constant direct supervision—remaining within reach and able to prevent the client from putting any toy parts in their mouths. Small parts should be counted before play and recounted afterward to ensure all items are returned to safe storage. Therapists must prevent clients from accessing batteries, perhaps taping over compartments that are not secured. After play with objects not manufactured or sold as toys, children should wash their hands. Toys for oral motor play must be too large to entirely fit into the client's mouth, sturdy enough to withstand biting and chewing, and labeled as chemically safe for oral use. The Food and Drug Administration suggests that even when oral toys are considered generally safe, children should not mouth/chew them unsupervised and that such toys should be thrown away when they show any wear.

Adjusting Safety for Development. When considering safety, occupational therapy practitioners should choose toys that are developmentally appropriate for their clients. Age-appropriate labeling of toys is not required by law. When it does appear, it has been applied to a toy's packaging by the manufacturer through consultation with a third-party laboratory that has been certified by the CPSC (Kulak & Stein, 2016). Assessors follow guidelines set forth in 2002 by the CPSC that include safety guidelines (Therrell, 2002); developmental stages, based on Piaget's writings and normative developmental milestones; categories of play, such as exploratory play, construction

play, and role play; and toy characteristics, such as number/shape/size of parts, colors, materials, motor skills required, sensory elements, and realism. They also assess toys' durability through use and abuse testing, and assess their reference to popular media, such as television shows and book characters. The starting point for assessing a toy's developmental labeling is the manufacturer's intended audience for advertising, promotion, and marketing. Toys must meet all the guidelines for the youngest age group to which they are targeted.

While developmental labeling may help parents and other caregivers select appropriate toys for children in the general public, therapists must understand that age-appropriate labeling guidelines reflect normative development and social expectations. Therefore, therapists must evaluate toys based on individual clients' abilities and interests. For example, a toy marketed as being for "ages 6 and up" may have media references and pretend play elements that appeal to a therapist's 10-year-old client with muscular dystrophy but require motor skills that present an overly difficult challenge for him/her, introducing risk of injury. On the other hand, toys suitable for play by a 19-month-old toddler may be safer and more easily manipulated by the client, but the colors and themes may seem too juvenile to him/her. The therapist must take the age-appropriate labeling as only the starting point in selecting toys and then consider modifying toys or play to help a client engage richly but safely. And given that therapists frequently encounter toys without labeling in schools, centers, and homes, occupational therapy practitioners must become proficient with matching toys to the complete developmental profiles of individual clients.

When recommending toys for home or center use, therapists must counsel families to consider the safety of all children in the environment. Toys not suitable for play by some children in that location must be securely stored. Families may need education about which objects require supervision.

Establishing Accessibility and Usability for Play

A play space is accessible when the environment fits the individual's body functions and structures (Rigby et al., 2019). Aspects of the environment that do not fit the child create barriers to play. Often families avoid places to play because of challenges with accessibility (Hinojosa & Kramer, 2008). The Americans with Disabilities Act (ADA, 1990) provides a legal mandate for accessibility and has helped promote accessibility in public spaces, transportation, schools, and playgrounds. For example, curb cuts and ramps allow clients who use wheelchairs and others with differences in mobility to access swings, climbing structures, and sports fields (see **Figure 9.4**). The U.S. government has developed detailed guidelines for accessible playgrounds (U.S. Access Board, 2005). As new spaces are being developed and older spaces being renovated, key accessibility elements are being included. For example, wide and flat pathways and grab bars are more typically included. Playgrounds also now often include rest areas, shade, different sensory features (such as textures, sounds, spinning items to watch), and equipment that can be used in multiple positions (such as standing, sitting, laying down, or with a wheelchair). This has resulted in increased knowledge and availability of products to enhance accessibility in homes too. Accessibility is critical to supporting the right of inclusion in play across settings for all children (Rigby et al., 2019).

Developers who use principles of universal design are creating spaces that can be used easily and safely by the greatest number of people possible (Rigby et al., 2019; Young, 2013). Principles of universal design are commonly used in pediatric occupational therapy clinics. Such environments offer inclusive play opportunities because individuals with disabilities need not use separate play materials or be in a separate area but instead can use the same materials in the same space. Occupational therapy practitioners have much to contribute in designing play environments that are accessible to diverse children. Despite these recent achievements, many homes, schools, playgrounds, and community sites have environmental barriers that prevent an individual child from accessing play. Even universal design cannot anticipate the needs of all individuals and also is inconsistently implemented in play spaces (Lynch, Moore, & Prellwitz, 2018).

When the environment is not accessible or usable by a child, the occupational therapist determines how the environment can be modified to what the child can already do (Rigby et al., 2019). For example, the addition of a ramp, grab bars, handles, or step stool may enable a child access to different heights where

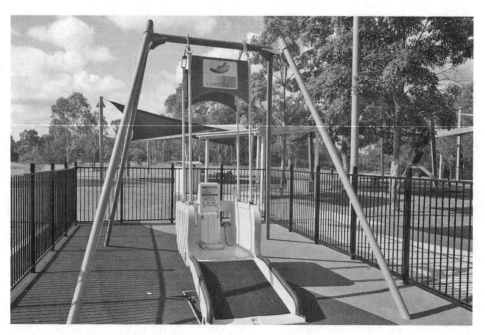

Figure 9.4 A ramp to this swing allows wheelchair access
© POC/Shutterstock.

play occurs (Stout, 1988). Children themselves may have ideas of what can be "built" to increase their access (Wenger, Schulze, Lundström, & Prellwitz, 2020). Open spaces have been found to be very important for play (Bundy & Du Toit, 2019), so the therapist may recommend rearrangement of furniture or other items to create adequate space for play. Adding a texture to increase grip on knobs and handles, seating surfaces, or floors can decrease slipping. Moving toys and play materials to an open shelf or higher or lower surface can enable a child to reach their own toys (Morozini, 2015; Pierce, 2000). Brighter lighting in a specific area may increase visibility of a surface change or a falling hazard, whereas softer light can provide necessary calm for a child. For children and adolescents with ASD and sensory processing differences, modifications of noise, light, and space can enhance access and security for participation (Krieger et al., 2018; Silverman & Tyszka, 2017). Technology can even allow a child to be transported virtually to an environment the child cannot otherwise access (AOTA, 2015), perhaps due to a compromised immune system or limited neighborhood resources. To individualize environmental adaptations for a child, the occupational therapy practitioner's professional reasoning focuses on the possibility of play for each child, determining what the child would play if only the space and materials were different.

Implementing identified adaptations depends on the type of setting and the nature of the adaptation. At times, especially in clinical settings, the therapist may have the power to modify the environment instantly. In natural settings, occupational therapists often use expert consultation, such as landscape architects, and advocacy with stakeholders to implement identified environmental adaptations (AOTA, 2015; Anaby et al., 2015; Rigby & Huggins, 2003; Rigby & Rodger, 2006). The occupational therapy practitioner often must take the time to explain to the person in authority (parent or other caregiver, teacher, principal, municipality, etc.) the professional reasoning for why and how this would benefit a child as well as the importance of play in order to get permission or resources allocated for the modification. With adaptation, others who use the environment must be considered, including their personal factors and the impact of environmental adaptations for their occupations as well (Rigby et al., 2019). Some families may welcome the idea of moving a chair out of the way and putting sofa cushions on the floor for play, and others may reject such a suggestion as disruptive to function or aesthetics. In natural environments, the occupational therapy practitioner generally has less control over the

environment than in a clinic and must be ready to adapt the environment and treatment activities. When venturing into new environments, more planning and onsite clinical reasoning are required to ensure the client's safety and success.

Play objects and their properties must be useable given the child's unique makeup so that play is possible. Toys that meet universal design principles such as ease, clarity, and adjustability increase the likelihood of use for a greater number of children with different abilities without the time and expense of adaptation (Lane & Mistrett, 2008; Ray-Kaeser et al., 2018; Ruffino et al., 2006). The object needs to be easy enough to use in intended and desired ways so the child can be successful without creating so much effort that play is lost (Lane & Mistrett, 2008; Ruffino et al., 2006). The way to play with the toy or other materials needs to be clear so the child can determine what to do with it without causing boredom or frustration that derails play (Lane & Mistrett, 2008). The more adjustable an object, the more it can be played with by multiple children (Lane & Mistrett, 2008; Ruffino et al., 2006). When the play items complement the child's abilities, the focus of engagement is on play without distraction from incompatible features. If the available play objects are not functional for a specific child, then the occupational therapy practitioner will modify them to be usable for play (see **Table 9.2** for examples). Although the research on modifying play objects has focused on its use as an intervention tool rather than play per se, it has been found effective for supporting therapeutic outcomes in children with ASD and cerebral palsy (Besion, 2018; dos Santos Nunes, da Conceição Júnior, Santos, Pereira, & de Faria Borges, 2017). Toys augmented with radio frequencies have been effective for increasing exploratory and parallel play for children with visual impairments (Verver et al., 2019, 2020). Parent–child play with animated toys has been found to facilitate creative play, cognitive development, and communication similarly to stuffed animals (Sung, 2018).

Selecting Spaces and Features That Promote Play

Occupational therapy practitioners select and utilize physical characteristics that have been found to promote play. First and foremost, a space that promotes play must have opportunities for what the child wants to play (King & Howard, 2014; Lynch, 2018). Ideally, the space should allow movement of bodies and materials to create and adapt for play. Such environments allow for the necessary choice children need to enable play

Table 9.2 Common Factors in Selecting and Modifying Play Objects for Usability

Object Traits	Selection Considerations	Common Modifications
Number of pieces	■ Easy enough to assemble.	■ Reduce the number of pieces available at a time. ■ Provide pictures or guides of models, steps, or directions. ■ Keep pieces together in a box, box top, bag, hula hoop, or other container to locate and reach. ■ Organize the pieces into separate categories/containers. ■ Add hook & loop fasteners or magnets to connect pieces.
Sounds	■ Volume control. ■ Corresponding lights, vibration, or other signals. ■ Verbal messages should be accompanied by written ones.	■ Add bells, hook & loop tape, or other sound-enhancing material. ■ Muffle volume with material or removing batteries. ■ Provide written or pictorial guidance/rules.
Visual	■ Bright and high-contrast colors. ■ Other sensory stimuli such as sounds, vibration, textures, or movement to substitute or complement visual features. ■ Parts should have texture, light, contrasting color, or be large enough to distinguish from other parts.	■ Provide a contrasting color surface. ■ Highlight parts with colored tape, permanent markers, paint, etc. ■ Add bells, hook & loop tape, radiofrequency technology, or other sound-enhancing materials. ■ Add hook & loop tape, wax-coated string, puffy paint/glue, felt, or other textured material to distinguish objects or parts.
Weight, size, shape, durability	■ Light enough to manipulate, carry, etc. ■ Large enough to grasp. ■ Have places where child can hold and carry. ■ Be small enough to reach around and carry if needed. ■ Have a secure base to prevent it from being knocked over accidentally. ■ Be heavy enough to provide sensory feedback. ■ Objects must be durable enough to withstand the child's force and actions without causing frustration, stress, or anger that derails play.	■ Add strap or string to aid lifting, pulling. ■ Add rubber bands or other anti-slip material to aid grasp and decrease dropping. ■ Place on carpet square, rollers, etc. to increase ease of moving the item. ■ Add padding to heavy items to decrease painful impact. ■ Place on a nonslip surface. ■ Secure objects with hook & loop tape, clips, or magnetic tape to keep stable. ■ Add weights, bag of sand/dry goods, hook & loop tape, magnets, etc. to increase weight or resistance. ■ Reinforce/cover loose/weak parts with packaging tape. ■ Remove loose, weak, easily breakable parts. ■ Protect from client's liquid secretions by covering such as with a plastic bag.
Movement of parts	■ Knobs, pieces, buttons, switches, etc. must be large enough to grasp. ■ Must be easy enough to move (limited force to depress, rotate, connect, slide, etc.).	■ Extend or enlarge knobs, handles, etc. with clay, foam, craft sticks, etc. ■ Add switch access to mechanical items. ■ Change position of objects to increase access. ■ Add rubber bands or anti-slip tape to sustain grasp on parts.

Data from Blanche, E. I. (2008). Play in children with cerebral palsy: Doing with—not doing to. In L. D. Parham & L. S. Fazio (Eds.), *Play in occupational therapy for children* (2nd ed., pp. 375–393). Mosby Elsevier; Bracegirdle, H. (1992). The use of play in occupational therapy for children: How the therapist can help. *British Journal of Occupational Therapy, 55,* 201–202; Ferland, F. (2005). *The Ludic model: Play, children with physical disabilities and occupational therapy* (2nd ed.). Canadian Association of Occupational Therapists; Deitz, J. C., & Swinth, Y. (2008). Accessing play through assistive technology. In L. D. Parham & L. S. Fazio (Eds.), *Play in occupational therapy for children* (2nd ed., pp. 395–412). Mosby Elsevier; Costa, M., Périno, O., & Ray-Kaeser, S. (2018). *TUET: Toys & Games Usability Evaluation Tool manual, questionnaire and development Process.* AIJU, Technological Institute for Children's Products & Leisure; Verver, S. H., Vervloed, M. P., & Steenbergen, B. (2019). The use of augmented toys to facilitate play in school-aged children with visual impairments. *Research in Developmental Disabilities, 85,* 70–81. https://doi.org/10.1016/j.ridd.2018.11.006; and Williams, S. E., & Matesi, D. V. (1988). Therapeutic intervention with an adapted toy. *American Journal of Occupational Therapy, 42,* 673–676.

(King, Batorowicz, Rigby, McMain-Klein, et al., 2014; King, Gibson, et al., 2014; King, Rigby, et al., 2014; King, Rigby, & Avery, 2016; Skard & Bundy, 2008). Given that tabletop activities tend to indicate work for children, simply moving to the floor or inside a "fort" can help promote play. Diversity of opportunities such as different heights and surfaces can promote development in other areas such as motor learning (Isbell & Isbell, 2007). Outdoor environments for play tend to offer large space, flexibility, and an unstructured social agenda (Blake et al., 2018; Ideishi, Ideishi, Gandhi, & Yuen, 2006; Miller & Kuhaneck, 2008). Natural environments such as fields and forests allow for more complex and creative play (Herrington & Brussoni, 2015; Luchs & Fikus, 2013) and longer play episodes (Luchs & Fikus, 2013), in part because of their increased affordances for play (Refshauge et al., 2013). Research indicates that outdoor play spaces are optimized for play by having views; pathways to connect areas; different and separate spaces; natural elements such as mud, vegetation, and insects; and physical challenges (Brussoni, Ishikawa, Brunelle, & Herrington, 2017; Herrington & Lesmeister, 2006; Kuh, Ponte, & Chau, 2013). Time in outdoor play itself has been associated with lower traffic volumes, yard access, and increased neighborhood greenness (Lambert, Vlaar, Herrington, & Brussoni, 2019). Children with disabilities have expressed a desire to connect with the natural environment more in their play (Harding et al., 2009).

Aesthetics and other pleasurable sensory features have also been associated with engaging environments for youth with and without disabilities (King, Rigby, et al., 2014; King, Rigby, & Avery, 2016). Green and blue colors tend to be most preferred by both healthy children and pediatric patients, while white is least favored; however, individuals may vary dramatically (Park, 2009). Natural lighting is often preferable, and fluorescent lighting can be uncomfortable for children who are sensitive to its subtle flickering (Isbell, Jones, Schmid, & Woodbury, 2014). Noise may be more distracting or bothersome for some children with disabilities but can be muffled with rugs or pillows (Isbell et al., 2014). Specifically, if children play in an area with the TV on, the background sounds and visuals can shorten play episodes (Courage, Murphy, Goulding, & Setliff, 2010; Masur, Flynn, & Olson, 2015).

Adapting Physical Elements for Play

When the space does not adequately support play, adaptations ensure that children have an environment in which to play (AOTA, 2008; Ideishi et al., 2006).

The occupational therapy practitioner may target the environment through direct services to facilitate play during therapy or in consultation and by advocating to adapt the natural daily living environments to promote the child's play (AOTA, 2015, 2017; Marshall, Myers, & Pierce, 2017). Targeting the environment has been found to be an effective aspect of pediatric interventions (Kreider, Bendixen, Huang, & Lim, 2014; Waldman-Levi & Erez, 2015). Environmental adaptations can be especially important for children with visual impairments (Retting, 1994) and with physical disabilities, particularly mobility limitations (Novak & Honan, 2019; Skar, 2002).

Occupational therapy practitioners adapt the environment in such a way that each client has opportunities to play with minimal, if any, therapist or caregiver direction and guidance. The focus is on physical and social environmental cues, on which the research shows children rely to shape their experience of whether the activity is play (Chapparo & Hooper, 2002; Goodhall & Atkinson, 2017; Howard, 2002; King & Howard, 2014). For example, King and Howard's (2014) research identified that a critical factor for promoting an experience of play is the amount of choice the child has based on various environmental features or affordances. To promote the richness of play, environmental adaptations prioritize choice over adult direction and prompting. With adaptations to promote play, the practitioner and caregivers can use fewer directions to "do this" (for example "climb the ladder") and fewer rules to limit behavior ("no climbing up the slide") because the guidance is implicit in the environmental affordances, if they match the child's ability to perceive the affordance. Research supports that new habits can be maintained through contextual cues, which tend to trigger a behavior automatically without people having to rely on their own effortful control or external rewards (Neal, Wood, Labrecque, & Lally, 2012; Quinn, Pascoe, Wood, & Neal, 2010; Wood & Neal, 2016). When the environment affords play that the child perceives and supports person-environment fit, the adults intervene less because the environment encourages the child to play, suggests to the child what can be played, indicates how it can be played, and offers others with whom to play.

Arranging the Play Space

To promote therapeutic or developmental gains, the space should be arranged to allow the child easy access to those materials that the practitioner, parent, or other caregiver wants the child to explore and reduce access to materials that interfere with play (Florey &

Greene, 2008; Hinojosa & Kramer, 2008). Likewise, materials that require supervision may be placed out of reach but should be easily accessible by the therapist or caregiver when needed. There must be enough playthings to build the child's skills and allow choice (Florey & Greene, 2008; Hyndman, 2015; Lally & Stewart, 1990). However, there should not be so many materials that social interaction is discouraged or that the child becomes disorganized or distracted (Burke, 2010; Frost, Shinn, & Jacobs, 1998; Lane & Mistrett, 2008; Ray-Kaeser et al., 2018). Studies have shown that children play more when 3–4 toys are available in comparison with 12–21 toys (Bjorkland & Bjorkland, 1979; Dauch, Imwalle, Ocasio, & Metz, 2018). The number of items may be graded for a child to rely on fewer physical materials in play or be able to manage a greater number of objects in play. For example, gradually removing objects from play activities was effective in increasing symbolic play for children with autism spectrum disorder (ASD) (Lee, Qu, Hu, Jin, & Huang, 2020). For another child, the therapist may opt to remove a particular object on which the child is overly focused or that causes anxiety or negative behaviors. Organizing materials has also been found to increase young children's participation in challenging activities (Waldman-Levi & Erez, 2015). Florey and Greene (2008) recommended setting up activities in advance for children with behavioral and emotional problems who may have trouble waiting and focusing during setup. Such factors can be maximized in a therapeutic environment where the occupational therapy practitioner has a high level of control and can adapt the environment directly. In natural environments, a therapist may suggest spaces within a setting that are more conducive or collaborate with others to adapt spaces to better support an individual's play.

Selecting and Adapting Play Objects

Play items or objects represent and set a frame for play (Duncan, 2015). Simply having toys does not necessarily mean a child will play. Play objects must have a variety of compatible features to encourage and enable a child to play. They must also have specific properties that allow them to be used therapeutically. Play objects must be relevant to and meaningful for the child, appealing, flexible, available, and they must "fit" the child's age, developmental level, and social abilities.

Relevancy. Materials must be compatible with the child's functioning and of interest to the child (Ray-Kaeser et al., 2018). Play objects also need to be used

in ways that are personally important and relevant to the child. Occupational therapy practitioners select and adapt play objects in the environment based on how the features match to a client's ability, interests, and therapeutic goals. The occupational therapist carefully considers the properties of materials (Knox, 1993) and how they might be used (Ferland, 2005; Gibson, 1988) through activity analysis and evaluation of the child. The affordances of the items must fit both the child's interests and abilities (Rigby & Huggins, 2003). For example, object features such as color and type can impact how children play with them (Fulcher & Hayes, 2018). The occupational therapy practitioner relies on a client-specific occupational analysis to determine if the objects need to be adapted to better match a client's interests, strengths, and needs.

Appeal. Play objects should be appealing and invite the child to participate. The materials may be appealing because of their aesthetic qualities (Heljakka, 2018; Lane & Mistrett, 2008) or because of the child's particular interest. Bright colors are usually appealing (Blanche, 2008; Deitz & Swinth, 2008). A toy may also be appealing if it is responsive to the child's actions, such as making a noise or movement when the child interacts with it (Blanche, 2008; Deitz & Swinth, 2008) (see **Figure 9.5**). Toys with multisensory and multimodal experiences appeal to a variety of children with and without disabilities (Lane

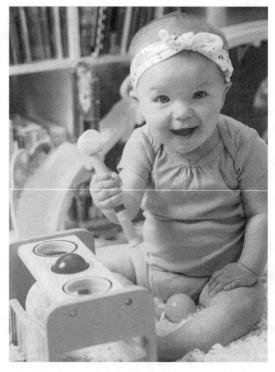

Figure 9.5 Appealing toys are often colorful and invite action
Courtesy of Kyle O'Brien.

& Mistrett, 2008). Adapting a toy to match a child's sensory preferences can increase play with that toy as well as increase independent functional toy play (DiCarlo, Schepis, & Flynn, 2009). A toy must also be easy enough to use that it is fun to play with (Blanche, 2008; Lane & Mistrett, 2008).

Using toys or props with a narrative theme related to favorite television shows, movies, books, or video games or that have another emotional connection for the child encourages their use in play (Heljakka, 2018). Incorporating objects related to special interests is considered best practice specifically for children with ASD (Tomchek & Koenig, 2016). These valued features of a toy or play object afford the child personal agency and promote play as occupation (Heljakka, 2018; Lynch, 2018), as illustrated in the case of Allison (see **Practice Example 9.3**).

While there are some items with which many children like to play, all items do not impact play in the same way for all children. For example, the same toy has been found to vary significantly in its impact on play quality depending on the gender, socioeconomic status, and ethnicity of the child playing with it (Trawick-Smith, Wolff, Koschel, & Vallarelli, 2015).

Flexibility. Play objects should also be flexible. Generally, adaptable features allow for more creative play possibilities, without clear right and wrong ways to play, and thus are more motivating for a variety of children (Blanche, 2008; Lane & Mistrett, 2008; Ruffino, Mistrett, Tomita, & Hajare, 2006). For example, toys and materials that can be used in a wide variety of ways include building blocks, playdough, water, bubbles, dolls, cups, cars, sand, and swings (Blanche, 2008; Trawick-Smith et al., 2015). Such flexible toys have been found to generate the highest quality of play for preschoolers (Trawick-Smith et al., 2015). Materials that have flexible uses can allow for more affordances for both play and therapeutic gains. Clinical environments are full of materials whose intended use often is more therapeutic than playful (Blanche, 2008). Often these activities must be used in unintended, playful ways in order to make them both therapeutic and play.

Social Fit. Because children are part of a social context and because social play is often a goal for children with disabilities, the social properties of the materials are also important. Toys and other objects can support shared play (Kultti & Pramling, 2015) or, in the case of children with ASD, can disrupt social interaction (Williams, Costall, & Reddy, 2018). Toys that support independent play may interfere with social play (Verver, Vervloed, & Steenbergen, 2019, 2020). Based on activity and occupational analyses, the occupational therapist considers how well the properties of the materials are suited for social play (Baranek, Reinhartsen, & Wannamaker, 2001; Quilitch & Risley, 1973). Again, this is an intersection between the affordances of the objects and their actual use by a child and their social network. The availability of, and interest in, play materials among the child's playmates must be considered. For example, what are the preferred activities of children of this age? Are computer games available in this child's everyday context? Is there safe playground equipment available?

Some children with disabilities prefer materials that are uncommonly used by others or prefer to use their play objects in unconventional ways.

PRACTICE EXAMPLE 9.3 Allison and a New Play Opportunity

Allison was a preschooler with ASD and limited speech. One of her occupational therapy goals was to initiate (select) play activities. She was just beginning to initiate activities and spontaneous language. Her speech-language therapist recommended that adults try to respond contingently to her language because she often said words that seemed to lack meaning in the current situation. By responding accurately to the words, it was reasoned, Allison would begin to understand the meaning of the words.

During this session, Allison had selected a swing. Her occupational therapist was asking her what she wanted to throw. The therapist and Allison's mother were giving ideas when suddenly Allison said, "Triangle." There was no obvious triangle visible in the room, and this seemed like a random, possibly meaningless word. Thus, Allison's mother explained, "You can't throw a triangle. There's no triangle." Although Allison's mother was correct, the occupational therapist wanted to seize on Allison's rare initiation and offered, "If you want a triangle, you can throw *to* a triangle." To adapt to Allison's idea, her occupational therapist quickly cut a triangle out of colored construction paper and taped it to the floor for Allison to throw bean bags to it. Whether Allison's comment was an intentional idea for the activity is unclear, but her occupational therapist's valuing and integrating it are clear.

If the child wants to play with materials that are not of interest to other children, the occupational therapist may use these materials in new ways to bridge the gap between the child and peers (Kuhaneck, Spitzer, & Miller, 2010; Spitzer, 2008, 1010). For example, a child who likes to hold a favorite toy might learn to play catch or tag with that toy with another child or other children. The occupational therapy practitioner may use materials of interest to the child in combination with materials that are of interest to the child's peers. For example, a child interested in DVD cases might learn to transport them in a wagon or give them a ride on toy cars. This social mediation of play objects is based on their physical affordances as well as emotional properties for the players, connecting children to their peers and the social world (Kibele, 2008; Williams et al., 2018). Including preferred play items can be effective in promoting social play for children and adolescents especially those with ASD (Boyd, et al., 2007; Dunst, et al., 2012; Gunn & Delafield-Butt, 2015; Kaboski et al., 2014; Koegel et al., 2012; Koegel, Kim, Koegel, & Schwartzman, 2013; Kryzak, Bauer, Jones, & Sturmey, 2013; Kryzak & Jones, 2014; Lindsay, et al., 2017; Vismara & Lyons, 2007; Watkins, O'Reilly, Kuhn, & Ledbetter-Cho, 2019; Wimpory, Hobson, & Nash, 2007).

Availability. Selecting toys that are both commonly available and accessible to children with disabilities is important (Lane & Mistrett, 2008). The occupational therapy practitioner may want to avoid selecting specialized materials and instead select items that are available to the child in their everyday environments in order for therapeutic experiences to be generalized outside of occupational therapy sessions. Florey and Greene (2008) recommended using crafts and games to which the children are otherwise commonly exposed because this allows the child to build skills for activities in which they can participate outside therapy. However, commonly available toys may not be of interest to or accessible to children with disabilities. So therapists find themselves balancing what is natural in the child's environment, forging paths to adapt the natural environment, and grading materials from specialized to common.

Age and Developmental Fit. Age appropriateness should also be considered in selecting materials (Blanche, 2008). Age appropriateness involves considerations of both the child's developmental and chronological age. If materials are appropriate for the child's chronological age, this can help the child be included in the general community. However, such standards for age appropriateness are culturally determined and may not match the child's interests or abilities. For example, some typically developing adults play with toys such as dioramas and character toys (Heljakka & Harviainen, 2019). If a child's developmental age is significantly lower than his or her chronological age, he or she may not have the interest or ability to engage in age-appropriate activities, and the self-selected developmentally matched play activities are more likely to be occupational (O'Connor, Butler, & Lynch, 2020). Regardless of developmental age, the child may have an interest that is most common in children who are older or younger. In these cases of mismatched age-appropriateness, the occupational therapist may consider activities that promote a higher play stage (Lane & Mistrett, 2008); consider computer-based activities, which are often interesting to a wide age range of children (Deitz & Swinth, 2008); or consider how to select and adapt activities to address developmental and chronological age needs. Sharing the clinician's professional reasoning on this matter can be very helpful in building parent, teacher, and caregiver support for the child's play. It is important to balance external and internal valuations of play when selecting and adapting age appropriateness of play materials, or we run the risk of devaluing the child's play and unintentionally removing the child's agency and personal meaning (see **Practice Example 9.4**).

Therapeutic Affordances. Various properties are given careful thought to select objects for play that also address a child's needs and therapeutic goals. For example, heavy toys may help provide stability for a child with tremors, increase strength in a child recovering from an injury or illness, or give feedback in a child with poor kinesthetic awareness. Adding novelty in materials or how they are used can be exciting and promote play (Parham, 1992; Trawick-Smith et al., 2015); however, novelty often must be graded so as not to be too overstimulating (Robinson, 1977). Durability of items may be downgraded over time to promote greater calibration, precision, or frustration tolerance.

Making Something from "Nothing"

The potential world of objects and environments are always circumscribed to some degree by the

PRACTICE EXAMPLE 9.4 Charlie: Adapting Age-Appropriate Play

Charlie was a 16-year-old and diagnosed with an intellectual disability. The school psychologist determined that most of his cognitive abilities were at the 2- to 4-year-old level of functioning. A key transition goal that was identified by the team was independent leisure, but there had been no progress in this area. Charlie constantly requested someone else's help to do leisure activities and keep him occupied except for using his tablet computer, which he used to look at music videos online. The team did not want to allow unlimited use of the tablet computer because (1) they wanted it to remain a salient reinforcer for other activities and (2) they wanted Charlie to develop more active forms of leisure for cognitive stimulation, development, and physical health. The occupational therapist identified a number of strengths that supported Charlie's participation, including his social interest; enjoyment of many adult-led activities; ability to find routinely used objects at home, at school, and in his backpack; better processing of visual and concrete information; and greatest independence with routine features of activities. The team also reported that Charlie did enjoy looking through young children's books, playing in a sandbox, and riding the park swings by himself, but the team discouraged these as inappropriately juvenile play. In sum, Charlie's interests for leisure activities were developmentally appropriate, but not age appropriate and thus not a good fit with the social context.

When the occupational therapist asked about other options for Charlie to play on his own, the team explained they had filled an activity box with various craft and other small items for him to use constructively at his desk. When directed to get the activity box, Charlie did not start using the items until initiated by an adult. He was given a stack of construction paper and told to pick a piece. Instead, he put all the papers in stacks on the floor by color. Looking at the other items in the bin, the occupational therapist quickly determined that the remaining items were not a good fit for Charlie's abilities based on activity analysis coupled with assessment of Charlie's motor, cognitive, and sensory impairments. Charlie could not perceive or act on the affordances of these objects.

To recognize the team's strength, the occupational therapist commended the team on their idea of creating a leisure activity box and suggested that occupational therapy could focus on using this box for independence by adapting it. The occupational therapist planned to prepare a list with pictures and labels of free-time activities that Charlie could do on his own that could be affixed to the top of the activity box. This list would be developed over time, starting with some matching "games." For example, the therapist presented Charlie with a deck of "cards" and, with minimal assistance to initiate, he immediately began matching the cards on the table. The category of card games was age-appropriate and acceptable to the team. The game's modified "rules" fit Charlie's abilities and interests. Charlie was able to perceive and act on these affordances. Charlie now had his first true play activity for his leisure activity box.

immediate setting. It may be that a child's favorite, desired, or best-suited toy is not available or allowed. In other cases, few toys, games, or objects in general may be available. Even space may be very limited such as in crowded housing. Factors such as poverty, war, systemic racism, or institutionalization are often at work when resources are severely limited. Lack of resources can deprive children of play (King & Howard, 2014; Leadley & Hocking, 2017; Nolan & Pells, 2020). In these circumstances, the occupational therapy practitioner often participates in advocacy as well as creative adaptation to ensure that play is not impoverished.

Although a lack of objects can be a constraint, a therapist's professional reasoning and a child's imagination can identify and adapt existing materials, no matter how sparse, to maximize play. Children do not need specific toys but can use generic items to substitute for many different items in play, especially if the general shape is similar to the intended one (Burns-Nader, Scofield, & Jones, 2019). Common toys or household objects such as towels, blankets, pillows, furniture, and food items may be used in playful ways (Hinojosa & Kramer, 2008; Nwokah, Hsu, & Gulker, 2013). For example, young children often enjoy pots, pans, and utensils to bang, stack, sort, and scoop in object play (see **Figure 9.6**). Using alternate items such as bricks and pieces of wood in constructive play may actually improve spatial thinking and creativity (Ness & Farenga, 2016). Sod, dirt, plants, bugs, water, and other natural items can inspire children's play (Puhakka et al., 2019). Recyclable items and trash such as plastic containers, egg cartons, newspaper, magazines, scrap paper, and cardboard boxes can often be transformed in play (Engelen et al., 2018; see **Figure 9.7**). The occupational therapist may make or instruct parents and other caregivers in how to make inexpensive toys (Esdaile & Sanderson, 1987; see **Figure 9.8**). Toys and objects may not even be needed in play activities if the therapist

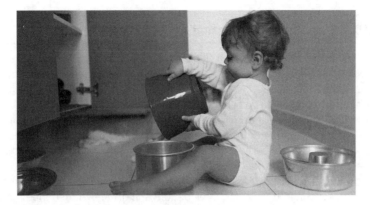

Figure 9.6 Children can play with household objects when toys are unavailable or limited
© Bricolage/Shutterstock.

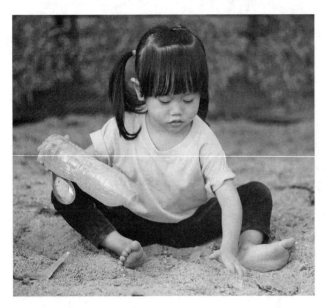

Figure 9.7 Safe and cleaned recyclable or trash items can also become playthings
© GOLFX/Shutterstock.

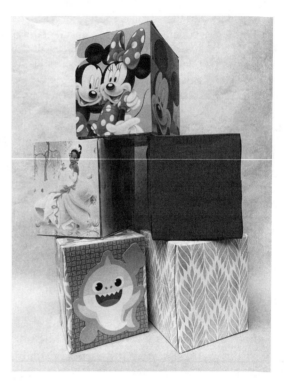

Figure 9.8 Used tissue boxes are repurposed into building blocks that afford constructional play and bilateral coordination for a toddler as long as they are determined to be safe. When modified with paint; pictures cut from old books, magazines, or greeting cards or other decoration, the box blocks can include a child's preferred play interests to promote play as occupation
Courtesy of Susan L. Spitzer.

and child use their bodies and ideas to invent sensorimotor or pretend games (Hinojosa & Kramer, 2008). Sometimes, occupational therapists may bring their own items to use or lend during home visits, but they tend to rely more heavily on what is present in the environment, even if that is limited (Nwokah et al., 2013).

With limited resources, it is essential that the occupational therapy practitioner, child, and others not be constrained by an object's socially sanctioned purpose. Instead, the therapist considers all affordances of available items and how they intersect with the play interests and desires at hand. Based on creative professional reasoning, the same objects can be utilized in dramatically different play activities to address the therapeutic needs of diverse clients. Certainly when using objects for unintended purposes, occupational therapists must assess safety more thoroughly.

Research supports that play can be used as an effective intervention for various developmental and behavioral outcomes for those with limited resources (Cochran & Cochran, 2017; Knauer et al., 2016; Milteer, Ginsburg, & Mulligan, 2012; Worku et al., 2018). Even when children lack play spaces in their neighborhoods, when cities agree, shutting down streets has been an effective modification to increase outdoor, active, and physical play opportunities, even if only on a temporary or intermittent basis (Cortinez-O'Ryan, Albagli, Sadarangani, & Aguilar-Farias, 2017; Umstattd Meyer, Bridges, Schmid, Hecht, & Pollack Porter, 2019). Families may be referred to toy lending libraries, sometimes hosted by public libraries (Bastiansen & Wharton, 2013) or, specifically for adaptive toys, hospitals and not-for-profits—Lekotek, for example. The gathering of "junk material," as in programs of loose parts play, is another way to enhance play spaces and encourage creative play with easily gathered materials that are typically low cost (Daly & Beloglovsky, 2014; Flannigan & Dietze, 2017; Gibson, Cornell, & Gill, 2017).

Ensuring Representation, Diversity, and Inclusion in Play Spaces

Environments and playthings are imbued with social meaning. They can reflect historical and contemporary cultural imagery. This can include representation of stereotypes (Coyne, Linder, Rasmussen, Nelson, & Birkbeck, 2016; Coyne, Linder, Rasmussen, Nelson, & Collier, 2014; Sherman & Zurbriggen, 2014) and exclusion by absence. Children detect and apply symbolism in toys (Martin, Eisenbud, & Rose 1995; Saha et al. 2014). If toys and environments do not represent the children and do not include what is important in a positive manner, then children may experience stigma about culture, gender, disability, or other factors. Public stigma can lead to self-stigma (Vogle, Bitman, Hammer, & Wade, 2013). Inclusive play spaces provide a diversity of play objects with toys that are representative of the children who will be playing with them, without biased divisions.

Therapists should avoid toys that depict or reinforce derogatory stereotypes. Most toys available in the commercial market reflect an aesthetic that represents Western cultures, Anglo/Caucasian beauty standards, slender body shapes, typical development, traditional gender roles, and heteronormative family structure (Almeida, 2017), with many fewer toys representing diversity factors. Not seeing oneself reflected in play materials may lead to feelings of being an outsider or having poor self-worth. There is an emerging trend toward manufacturing diverse and inclusive toys. Play with toys representing diversity can reduce anxiety toward peers (O'Neill, McDonald, & Jones, 2018) and may help children embrace their own differences.

Therapists should try to have a variety of toys across diversity factors in their practice settings (Smith, 2013), particularly including toys that depict disability (O'Neill et al., 2018). The nonprofit organization #toylikeme (toylikeme.org) advocates for disability-inclusive toys, linking to toy sellers whose dolls, stuffed animals, and toys depict disability positively.

Occupational therapy practitioners must minimize unintentional divisions in play spaces. Play spaces often are arranged in thematic areas, for example, a center for block play and a center for pretend play. This may appeal to children's preferences in play, in this case constructive and fantasy play. It may also help a therapist create structured opportunities for play that targets desired skills such as motor coordination or ideation. On the other hand, this segregation may inadvertently deter play across diversity factors such as gender, when boys engage primarily in constructive play areas and girls primarily in fantasy play areas. Removing physical barriers between these areas can allow children to blend elements of play together, contributing to a climate of acceptance and encouragement of a variety of play experiences (Isenberg & Jalongo, 2003). Using gender-neutral and cultural-neutral themes in play centers can also encourage exploration of novel play materials (Isenberg & Jalongo, 2003). By decreasing gender and cultural divisions, the child may experience greater internal control to play in new ways.

Intervening with the Social Environment

A safe and accessible physical environment is not enough to ensure social inclusion for physical activity (Knibbe, Biddiss Gladstone, & McPherson, 2016). Social rules must allow play (Morozini, 2015; Pierce, 2000), and intervention also may require adapting aspects of the social environment that support or impede play (Chien, Branjerdporn, Rodger, & Copley, 2017; Humphry & Wakeford, 2006; Rigby & Huggins, 2003; Skard & Bundy, 2008; Sturgess, 2003). For example, a family environment (support, rules, and habits) can be more important than the physical environment for increasing children's outside play (Remmers et al., 2014).

Rules for play must be achievable by all the players or else some players are excluded by the rules. For example, most ball games have rules about the number of bounces, holding, hitting, etc., but the rules can always be changed in a group to allow sitting in a ball game, more than one bounce in tennis, more tries to hit in baseball, closer proximity for hitting/catching/serving, a larger area for the ball to be in, and points for hitting regardless of aim (Braga, Tracy, & Taliaferro, 2015).

Attitudes about perceived limitations or needs and other social practices can create barriers for play. Social expectations about appropriate play may reduce opportunities for child-directed play if it is perceived as immature or abnormal behavior (Blake et al., 2018; Brodin, 2018). In contrast, when the social environment is welcoming, children are free to participate (Anaby et al., 2015).

Enhancing social environments for activities is likely to increase children's participation and development of skills (Arbesman, Bazyk, & Nochajski, 2013; Batorowicz, King, Mishra, & Missiuna, 2016; Waldman-Levi & Erez, 2015). Children with disabilities sometimes negotiate their own play environments (Harding et al., 2009). When building supportiveness of the social environment for play, occupational therapy practitioners may adapt the composition of the social environment

as well as educate and train children and others in the environment.

Providing Play Partners

The occupational therapy practitioner, through therapeutic use of self, creates a therapeutic social environment that promotes play (see Chapter 6 for details). Furthermore, the occupational therapist considers who is or might be involved in play in daily life as well as in therapy sessions. As primary play partners, family members may be included in therapy sessions. Peers may be primary play partners or may be desired future play partners. Play partners who are resourceful support play activities, and those who are empowering support play occupations (O'Connor et al., 2020).

Children prefer to play with other children over playing with adults (Miller & Kuhaneck, 2008). The therapist may want to have peers or siblings present to support a playful environment and/or to build play skills (Allodi & Zappaterra, 2017; Baranek et al., 2001; Florey & Greene, 2008; see **Figure 9.9**). For example, peers may encourage more pretense, higher level play, and more prosocial behaviors (Rubenstein & Howes, 1976). Even children who

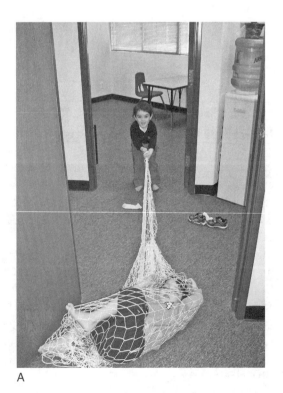
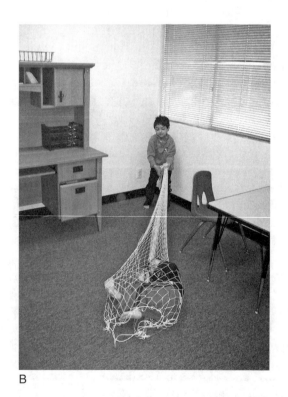

A   B

Figure 9.9 Play can be promoted by including other social play partners. Two brothers work on cooperative play by taking turns with one playing the lion and the other playing the lion catcher (A); and then switching roles (B)
Courtesy of Susan L. Spitzer.

do not have the skills to socially interact on their own may enjoy having other children present or watching other children (Blake et al., 2018). The therapist may need to create a new social environment such as developing an interest group in a high school for students to enjoy music together (Anaby et al., 2015). Research indicates that play is increased with familiar children but decreased with unknown children, adults, and large numbers of children who crowd the space (King & Howard, 2014). Therefore, the therapist considers the number of play partners that will support the child as well as their familiarity to the child. Many children with disabilities do best initially in a smaller social environment that can be expanded later for complexity as well as increasing social interest (Humphry & Wakeford, 2006).

A range of personal characteristics may make some potential play partners a better match than others for an individual. Developmentally, some children do better with younger children and simpler interaction strategies, some benefit from similar-aged peer modeling, and others from older children who may be more patient and/or provide more guidance (see **Figure 9.10**). Other characteristics to consider include loudness, physicality, humor, affect, kindness, ideas, skills, and interests. However, research indicates that merely finding a play partner may be more important than finding the one with particular characteristics, as peers will also learn to play with the child (Kent, Cordier, Joosten, Wilkes-Gillan, & Bundy, 2020).

By creating a match between players instead of focusing on the disability, the occupational therapy practitioner promotes play, especially social play. Such peer-mediated approaches to increasing play skills have been well established as an effective intervention, especially for children with ASD (Hatzenbuhler, Molteni, & Axe, 2019; Lory, Rispoli, & Gregori, 2018; Whalon, Conroy, Martinez, & Werch, 2015); however, periodic monitoring and troubleshooting may be needed over time to sustain this form of intervention (Collins, Hawkins, & Flowers, 2018).

When suitable playmates cannot be found, computer-based options may provide a substitute. Therapists or other adults work behind the scenes to operate interactive robotics or avatars that appear to children as playmates. For example, Kory-Westlund and Breazeal (2019) created a robot to be a playmate. The robot, "Green," had an expressive face and joint attention gaze ability (smart phone), had a child-like voice, and was referred to in a gender-neutral way. When the robot behaved like a friend by matching its language ability to the children's, children learned more new words and mirrored Green's language style more. This is an example of a study that helps define a characteristic of a good play partner, and it also provides support for the use of technology to provide playmates for children.

Promoting Playful Environments Through Educating Others

The attitudes, knowledge, and skills of family members, peers, teachers, and others may be supports or barriers for play. To maximize these supports and minimize these barriers, occupational therapy practitioners often educate and train others. Sharing AOTA's handouts on

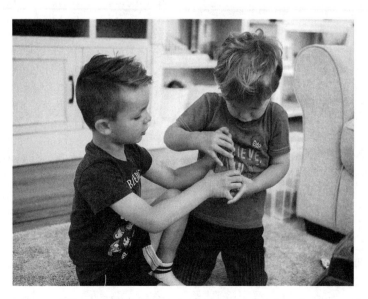

Figure 9.10 Finding a play partner at the appropriate developmental level enhances play and provides opportunities for peer guidance

Courtesy of Kyle O'Brien.

Box 9.2 Suggestions to Help Others Select Appropriate Toys*

1. Look for toys that do not tell the child what to do or direct the way the play occurs.
2. Look for toys that allow creativity and do not ask a child to supply one thing or one answer.
3. Look for toys that build imagination such as those that can be taken apart and put together in multiple ways.
4. Look for toys that encourage social interaction.

Data from Hirsh-Pasek, K., A., & Golinkoff, R. M. (2006). How to choose toys for your baby. In S. Ettus (Ed.), *The experts' guide to the baby years* (pp. 246–248). Clarkson Potter. https://kathyhirshpasek.com/wp-content/uploads/sites/9/2015/08/PLAY_toys_for_your_baby.pdf

selecting toys and promoting play may provide a start for helping a family or other caregiver understand the importance of play and general ways to support it (AOTA, 2011a, 2011b). Also see **Box 9.2** for more suggestions for helping others select appropriate toys. More specific education and training involves enhanced understanding of an individual child's abilities and desires for play, adjusting interactions to fit a specific child's play, balancing control in play, and building equitable relationships.

The occupational therapy practitioner may need to help family members and peers adapt their interactions to create a playful experience (Hinojosa & Kramer, 2008; Lally & Stewart, 1990; Lane & Mistrett, 2008; Skard & Bundy, 2008). Occupational therapists may want to encourage the specific parental and teacher behaviors that have been found to enhance child play such as being responsive and nurturing to the child (Fiese, 1990; Mahoney & Solomon, 2016; Tamis-LeMonda, Damast, Baumwell, & Bornstein, 1996). Encouraging parents and other caregivers to pause and give the child time to respond has also been included in effective social environmental interventions (Waldman-Levi & Erez, 2015). Helping other players to facilitate play involves teaching them many of the same particular skills that the therapist uses to help the child play. Family and peers may need to recognize and respond to small initiations or uncommon play interests to reinforce and build on the child's efforts. The occupational therapy practitioner may note, "Did you see/hear how the child did _____ to show _____?" By explaining why the therapist is doing what he or she is doing, by modeling strategies, by coaching and encouraging the family member or peer, and by noting the child's actual or potential response, the occupational therapist helps the

family and peers develop skills for playing with the particular child. Explicit guidance is often needed because the therapist's strategies and child's cues can be too subtle for some players to recognize as they disappear into play.

Just like new occupational therapy practitioners, parents, other caregivers, and peers may need assistance to share power and promote choice. They may struggle with determining how much direction to give and how much control to exert. Adult support is often necessary to ensure children have opportunities to play (Hyndman, 2015). Certainly, adult structure such as identifying locations for different play, leading activities, and providing games/sports equipment/objects can be effective for increasing children's play (Hyndman, 2015). However, too much adult structure such as an excess of rules can function to prohibit many forms of play. Children must be allowed to exercise choices and have a level of control in order to play (King, Batorowicz, Rigby, McMain-Klein, et al., 2014; King, Gibson, et al., 2014; King, Rigby, & Avery, 2016; King, Rigby, Batorowicz, et al., 2014; Skard & Bundy, 2008).

Research indicates that environments that support participation provide a sense of social belonging and equitable interactions among all children and adolescents, regardless of disability status (Edwards, Cameron, King, & McPherson, 2019; King, Batorowicz, Rigby, McMain-Klein, et al., 2014; King, Batorowicz, Rigby, Pinto, et al., 2014; King, Rigby, & Avery, 2016; King, Rigby, Batorowicz, et al., 2014; Knibbe et al., 2016; Krieger, Piskur, Schulze, Jakobs, Beurskens & Moser, 2018; Smart et al., 2018). When power is equalized so that children do not dominate and are not dominated by others, play is possible for all (Skard & Bundy, 2008). Parents are more willing to allow children and adolescents freedom to engage in such a safe environment, which alleviates parent concerns about the risk of abuse and neglect (Robinson & Graham, 2019). Therapists may educate, coach, model, or collaborate to adapt a more supportive level of choice and control, in order to allow the child to have a balance of freedom and essential structure to play as illustrated with Mateo (see **Practice Example 9.5**). In some cases, occupational therapists work with a group or institution such as an entire school to implement an antibullying program that has been found to be an effective intervention (Arbesman et al., 2013). The research of King and colleagues indicates that the more an inclusive community is created, the more participation by children and adolescents with very diverse disabilities (King, Curran, & McPherson, 2013; King et al., 2016; Smart et al., 2018).

PRACTICE EXAMPLE 9.5 Mateo: Getting in the Game

Mateo was a third grader with cerebral palsy who used an AAC program on a tablet computer to communicate. Although his learning disabilities resulted in delayed academic skills, Mateo was included in a regular education classroom with an assistant. His parents had repeatedly stated that their top goal for Mateo was to be part of the class so that he could have friends and learn to be with other people for a full and meaningful life. And Mateo himself showed a strong interest in his peers.

The teacher requested the occupational therapist come during math games. Math games were used several times a week so that the children could help each other learn and practice new math skills. The teacher said that they did not know what to do with Mateo because he was behind in math and could not keep up with the other students in the games. The occupational therapist observed the class playing two math games, one using dice and the other using tile pieces. Each group of students pushed into a rough circle, with Mateo behind the circle with his assistant. All the students were very focused on the math concepts and seemed to be enjoying the games except Mateo, whose affect was flat. Mateo's only action was to enter what his assistant said into his tablet. The occupational therapist noted that Mateo was physically separate from the other students as well as uninvolved in their interactive play. The occupational therapist determined that the "games" for Mateo had been focused on the labor-intensive process of getting his work done. He had no control, choice, or opportunities to engage in the play.

The occupational therapist then suggested several modifications designed to promote play opportunities for Mateo:

- The addition of a plastic cup in the dice game so that Mateo could take an equal turn in rolling the dice
- Offering Mateo opportunities to hand out materials such as math tiles to give him a role in the group
- Use of screen shots of answers in his AAC program to be used as his work so that he could use his AAC program for communication
- Tape on the floor to mark a large enough space for Mateo to fit into the same space as his peers (with his assistant behind/outside the circle)
- Assistant's role to be assisting with screen shots and encouraging him to initiate and respond to the comments of other students about the math games
- Consider establishing a role of student scribe, who rotates in recording math problems and answers.

After a few weeks, the occupational therapist observed Mateo physically, verbally, and emotionally engaged in the math games.

Conclusion

Proper selection and adaptations of the play space, play objects, and social play environment provide greater opportunities for children to play and are therefore important aspects of occupational therapy intervention. Occupational therapy practitioners select and modify physical environments and objects to minimize barriers and ensure individual children have safe access to use the affordances within a play space, maximizing even severely restricted resources. They select, arrange, and adapt physical elements to ensure choice as well as personal meaning and relevance. When the environment provides the just right "fit" for the child, it invites play, children need less adult directing of their actions, and they can experience more fun. Occupational therapy practitioners help structure the social world of play partners and educate and train others to understand and interact through play. As a result, children and adolescents with a diversity of abilities are included together in play.

References

Al Kurdi, B. (2017). *Investigating the factors influencing parent toy purchase decisions: Reasoning and consequences.* International Business Research, 10(4), 104–116. https://doi.org/10.5539/ibr.v10n4p104

All things toys. (2018). *Toy study by field agent.* https://info.fieldagent.net/all-things-toys-download

Allodi, M. W., & Zappaterra, T. (2017). *Users' needs on play for children with disabilities.* Presentation, Conference: Disability, Recognition and "Community living." Diversity of practices and plurality of values. At: Lausanne. European Society for Disability Research. https://doi.org/10.13140/RG.2.2.13038.51528

Almeida, D. B. L. D. (2017). On diversity, representation and inclusion: New perspectives on the discourse of toy campaigns. *Linguagem em (Dis) curso, 17*(2), 257–270. https://dx.doi.org/10.1590/1982-4017-170206-6216

American Heart Association. (2016). *Devices that may interfere with ICDs and pacemakers.* https://www.heart.org/en/health-topics/arrhythmia/prevention--treatment-of-arrhythmia/devices-that-may-interfere-with-icds-and-pacemakers

American Occupational Therapy Association (AOTA). (2008). Societal statement on play. *American Journal of Occupational Therapy, 62,* 707–708. https://doi.org/10.5014/ajot.62.6.707

American Occupational Therapy Association (AOTA). (2011a). Building play skills for healthy children & families. *American Occupational Therapy Association.* www.aota.org/playtips

American Occupational Therapy Association (AOTA). (2011b). How to pick a toy: Checklist for toy shopping. *American Occupational Therapy Association.* https://www.aota.org/~/media/Corporate/Files/AboutOT/consumers/Youth/Play/Toys%20tip%20sheet.pdf

American Occupational Therapy Association (AOTA). (2015). Occupational therapy's perspective on the use of environments and contexts to facilitate health, well-being, and participation in occupations. *American Journal of Occupational Therapy, 69* (Suppl. 3), 6913410050. http://dx.doi.org/10.5014/ajot.2015.696S05

American Occupational Therapy Association. (2017). Guidelines for occupational therapy services in early intervention and schools. *American Journal of Occupational Therapy, 71*(Suppl. 2), 7112410010p1–7112410010p10. https://doi.org/10.5014/ajot.2017.716S01

American Occupational Therapy Association (AOTA). (2020). Occupational therapy practice framework: Domain & process (4th ed.). *American Journal of Occupational Therapy, 74* (Supplement 2).

Americans With Disabilities Act of 1990, 42 U.S.C. § 12101 et seq. (1990).

Anaby, D., Law, M., Teplicky, R., & Turner, L. (2015). Focusing on the environment to improve youth participation: Experiences and perspectives of occupational therapists. *International Journal of Environmental Research and Public Health, 12,* 13388–13398. https://doi.org/10.3390/ijerph121013388

Arbesman, M., Bazyk, S., & Nochajski, S. M. (2013). Systematic review of occupational therapy and mental health promotion, prevention, and intervention for children and youth. *American Journal of Occupational Therapy, 67,* e120–e130. http://dx.doi.org/10.5014/ajot.2013.008359

Aziz, N. F., & Said, I. (2015). Outdoor environments as children's play spaces: Playground affordances. *Play, Recreation, Health, and Well Being, 1*–22. https://doi.org/10.1007/978-981-4585-96-5

Baranek, G. T., Reinhartsen, D. B., & Wannamaker, S. W. (2001). Play: Engaging young children with autism. In R. A. Huebner (Ed.), *Autism: A sensorimotor approach to management* (pp. 313–351). Gaithersburg, MD: Aspen.

Bastiansen, C., & Wharton, J., (2013). Getting ready for play! Toy collections in public libraries. *Children and Libraries, Winter 2015,* 13–29.

Batorowicz, B., King, G., Mishra, L., & Missiuna, C. (2016). An integrated model of social environment and social context

for pediatric rehabilitation. *Disability and Rehabilitation, 38*(12), 1204–1215. http://dx.doi.org/10.3109/09638288.2015.1076070

Besion, S. (2018). Supporting play for the sake of play in children with disabilities. *Today's Children: Tomorrow's Parents: An Interdisciplinary Journal, 47*–48, 7–17.

Bjorklund, G., & Bjorklund, R. (1979). An exploratory study of toddlers' satisfaction with their toy environments. *NA—Advances in Consumer Research, 6,* 400–406.

Blake, A., Sexton, J., Lynch, H., Moore, A., & Coughlan, M. (2018). An exploration of the outdoor play experiences of preschool children with autism spectrum disorder in an Irish preschool setting. *Today's Children: Tomorrow's Parents: An Interdisciplinary Journal, 47*–48, 100–119.

Blanche, E. I. (2008). Play in children with cerebral palsy: Doing with—not doing to. In L. D. Parham & L. S. Fazio (Eds.), *Play in occupational therapy for children* (2nd ed., pp. 375–393). St. Louis, MO: Mosby Elsevier.

Boyd, B. A., Conroy, M. A., Mancil, G. R., Nakao, T., & Alter, P. J. (2007). Effects of circumscribed interests on the social behaviors of children with autism spectrum disorders. *Journal of Autism and Developmental Disorders, 37,* 1550–1561. https://doi.org/10.1007/s10803-006-0286-8

Bracegirdle, H. (1992). The use of play in occupational therapy for children: How the therapist can help. *British Journal of Occupational Therapy, 55,* 201–202.

Braga, L., Tracy, J. F., & Taliaferro, A. R. (2015). Physical activity programs in higher education: Modifying net/wall games to include individuals with disabilities. *Journal of Physical Education, Recreation & Dance, 86*(1), 16–22. https://doi.org/10.1080/07303084.2014.978417

Brodin, J. (2018). "It takes two to play": Reflections on play in children with multiple disabilities. *Today's Children: Tomorrow's Parents: An Interdisciplinary Journal, 47*–48, 28–39.

Brussoni, M., Ishikawa, T., Brunelle, S., & Herrington, S. (2017). Landscapes for play: Effects of an intervention to promote nature-based risky play in early childhood centres. *Journal of Environmental Psychology, 54,* 139–150. https://doi.org/10.1016/j.jenvp.2017.11.001

Bundy, A., & Du Toit, S. H. J. (2019). Play and leisure. In B. A. Boyt Schell & G. Gillen (Eds.), *Willard & Spackman's occupational therapy* (13th ed., pp. 805–827). Baltimore, MD: Lippincott Williams & Wilkins.

Bundy, A. C., Waugh, K., & Brentnall, J. (2009). Developing assessments that account for the role of the environment: An example using the test of playfulness and test of environmental supportiveness: Occupation, participation and health occupation, participation and health. *OTJR: Occupation, Participation, and Health, 29*(3), 135–143. https://doi.org/10.3928/15394492-20090611-06

Burke, J. P. (2010). What's going on here? Deconstructing the interactive encounter (Eleanor Clarke Slagle Lecture). *American Journal of Occupational Therapy, 64,* 855–868. https://doi.org/10.5014/ajot.2010.64604

Burns-Nader, S., Scofield, J., & Jones, C. (2019). The role of shape and specificity in young children's object substitution. *Infant Child Development, 28*(2), e2124. https://doi.org/10.1002/icd.2124

Castonguay, G., & Jutras, S. (2009). Children's appreciation of outdoor places in a poor neighborhood. *Journal of*

Environmental Psychology, *29*(1), 101–109 https://doi .org/10.1016/j.jenvp.2008.05.002

Chapparo, C. J., & Hooper, E. (2002). When is it work? Perceptions of six year old children. *Work*, *19*(3), 291–302.

Chien, C. W., Branjerdporn, G., Rodger, S., & Copley, J. (2017). Exploring environmental restrictions on everyday life participation of children with developmental disability. *Journal of Intellectual & Developmental Disability*, *42*(1), 61–73.

Christensen, K. E., & Stockdale, D. F. (1991). Predictors of toy selection criteria of preschool children's parents. *Children's Environments Quarterly*, *8*(1), 25–36.

Cochran, J. L., & Cochran, N. H. (2017). Effects of child-centered play therapy for students with highly-disruptive behavior in high-poverty schools. *International Journal of Play Therapy*, *26*(2), 59.https://doi.org/10.1037/pla0000052

Collins, T. A., Hawkins, R. O., & Flowers, E. M. (2018). Peer-mediated interventions: A practical guide to utilizing students as change agents. *Contemporary School Psychology*, *22*(3), 213–219. DOI 10.1007/s40688-017-0120-7

Cortinez-O'Ryan, A., Albagli, A., Sadarangani, K. P., & Aguilar-Farias, N. (2017). Reclaiming streets for outdoor play: A process and impact evaluation of "Juega en tu Barrio" (Play in your Neighborhood), an intervention to increase physical activity and opportunities for play. *PLoS ONE*, *12*(7): e0180172. https://doi.org/10.1371/journal.pone.0180172

Costa, M., Périno, O., & Ray-Kaeser, S. (2018). *TUET: Toys & Games Usability Evaluation Tool manual, questionnaire and development Process*. Ibi (Alicante), Spain: AIJU, Technological Institute for children's products & leisure.

Courage, M. L., Murphy, A. N., Goulding, S., & Setliff, A. E. (2010). When the television is on: The impact of infant-directed video on 6- and 18-month olds' attention during toy play and on parent–infant interaction. *Infant Behavior and Development*, *33*(2), 176–188. https://doi.org/10.1016/j .infbeh.2009.12.012

Coyne, S. M., Linder, J. R., Rasmussen, E. E., Nelson, D. A., & Birkbeck, V. (2016). Pretty as a princess: Longitudinal effects of engagement with Disney princesses on gender stereotypes, body esteem, and prosocial behavior in children. *Child Development*, *87*(6), 1909–1925.

Coyne, S. M., Linder, J. R., Rasmussen, E. E., Nelson, D. A., & Collier, K. M. (2014). It's a bird! It's a plane! It's a gender stereotype!: Longitudinal associations between superhero viewing and gender stereotyped play. *Sex Roles*, *70*(9), 416–430.

Daly, L., & Beloglovsky, M. (2014). *Loose parts: Inspiring play in young children* (Vol. *1*). St Paul, MN: Redleaf Press.

Dauch, C., Imwalle, M., Ocasio, B., & Metz, A. E. (2018). The influence of the number of toys in the environment on toddlers' play. *Infant Behavior and Development*, *50*, 78–87. https://doi.org/10.1016/j.infbeh.2017.11.005

Deitz, J. C., & Swinth, Y. (2008). Accessing play through assistive technology. In L. D. Parham & L. S. Fazio (Eds.), *Play in occupational therapy for children* (2nd ed., pp. 395–412). St. Louis, MO: Mosby Elsevier.

DiCarlo, C. F., Schepis, M. M., & Flynn, L. (2009). Embedding sensory preference into toys to enhance toy play in toddlers with disabilities. *Infants & Young Children*, *22*(3), 188–200. https://doi.org/10.1097/IYC.0b013e3181abe1a1

dos Santos Nunes, E. P., da Conceição Júnior, V. A., Santos, L. V. G., Pereira, M. F. L., & de Faria Borges, L. C. (2017). Inclusive toys for rehabilitation of children with disability: A systematic review. In M. Antona & C. Stephanidis C. (Eds.), *Universal access in human–computer interaction. Design and development approaches and methods*. UAHCI 2017. Lecture Notes in Computer Science, 10277, 503–514. Cham: Springer. https:// doi.org/10.1007/978-3-319-58706-6_41

Duncan, P. A. (2015). Pigs, planes, and Play-Doh: Children's perspectives on play as revealed through their drawings. *American Journal of Play*, *8*(1), 50–73.

Dunst, C. J., Trivette, C. M., & Hamby, D. W. (2012). Effect of interest-based interventions on the social-communicative behavior of young children with autism spectrum disorders. *Center for Early Literacy Learning*, *5*(6), 1–10.

Edwards, B. M., Cameron, D., King, G., & McPherson, A. C. (2019). Contextual strategies to support social inclusion for children with and without disabilities in recreation. *Disability and Rehabilitation*, *43*(11), 01615–1625. https://doi.org/10.10 80/09638288.2019.1668972

Engelen, L., Wyver, S., Perry, G., Bundy, A., Chan, T. K. Y., Ragen, J., Bauman A., & Naughton, G. (2018). Spying on children during a school playground intervention using a novel method for direct observation of activities during outdoor play. *Journal of Adventure Education and Outdoor Learning*, *18*(1), 86–95. https://doi.org/10.1080/14729679.2017.1347048

Esdaile, S., & Sanderson, A. (1987). Teaching parents toy making: A practical guide to early intervention. *British Journal of Occupational Therapy*, *50*, 266–271.

Fallon, M. A., & Harris, M. B. (1989). Factors influencing the selection of toys for handicapped and normally developing preschool children. *The Journal of Genetic Psychology*, *150*(2), 125–134. https://doi.org/10.1080/00221325.1989.9914584

Ferland, F. (2005). *The Ludic model: Play, children with physical disabilities and occupational therapy* (2nd ed.). Ottawa, Ontario: Canadian Association of Occupational Therapists.

Fiese, B. H. (1990). Playful relationships: A contextual analysis of mother-toddler interaction and symbolic play. *Child Development*, *61*(5), 1648–1656. https://doi .org/10.1111/j.1467-8624.1990.tb02891.x

Flannigan, C., & Dietze, B. (2017). Children, outdoor play, and loose parts. *Journal of Childhood Studies*, 53–60.

Florey, L. L., & Greene, S. (2008). Play in middle childhood. In L. D. Parham & L. S. Fazio (Eds.), *Play in occupational therapy for children* (2nd ed., pp. 279–299). St. Louis, MO: Mosby Elsevier.

Fraser, A., Doan, D., Lundy, M., Bevill, G., & Aceros, J. (2019). Pediatric safety: Review of the susceptibility of children with disabilities to injuries involving movement related events. *Injury Epidemiology*, *6*(1), 1–9. http://dx.doi.org/10.1186 /s40621-019-0189-8

Frost, J. L., Shin, D., & Jacobs, P. J. (1998). Physical environments and children's play. In O. N. Saracho & B. Spodek (Eds.), *Multiple perspectives on play in early childhood education* (pp. 255–294). Albany: State University of New York Press.

Fulcher, M., & Hayes, A. R. (2018). Building a pink dinosaur: The effects of gendered construction toys on girls' and boys' play. *Sex Roles*, *79*, 273–284 https://doi.org/10.1007/s11199-017 -0806-3

Gibson, B. E., King, G., Teachman, G., Mistry, B., & Hamdani, Y. (2017). Assembling activity/setting participation with disabled young people. *Sociology of Health & Illness*, *39*(4), 497–512. https://doi.org/10.1111/1467-9566.12496

Gibson, E. J. (1988). Exploratory behavior in the development of perceiving, acting, and the acquiring of knowledge. *Annual Review of Psychology, 39*(1), 1–42.

Gibson, J. J. (1977). The theory of affordances. In R. Shaw & J. Bransford (Eds.), *Perceiving, acting and knowing: Toward an ecological psychology* (pp. 67–82). Hillsdale, NJ: Erlbaum.

Gibson, J. L., Cornell, M., & Gill, T. (2017). A systematic review of research into the impact of loose parts play on children's cognitive, social and emotional development. *School Mental Health, 9*(4), 295–309.

Goodhall, N., & Atkinson, C. (2017). How do children distinguish between "play" and "work"? Conclusions from the literature. *Early Child Development and Care, 189*(10), 1695–1708.

Gunn, K. C., & Delafield-Butt, J. T. (2015). Teaching Children With Autism Spectrum Disorder With Restricted Interests. *Review of Educational Research, 86*(2), 408–430. https://doi.org/10.3102/0034654315604027

Hamm, E. M. (2006). Playfulness and the environmental support of play in children with and without developmental disabilities. *OTJR: Occupation, Participation and Health, 26*(3), 88–96. https://doi.org/10.1177/153944920602600302

Harding, J., Harding, K., Jamieson, P., Mullally, M., Politi, C., Wong-Sing, E., Law, M., & Petrenchik, T. M. (2009). Children with disabilities' perceptions of activity participation and environments: A pilot study. *Canadian Journal of Occupational Therapy, 76*(3), 133–144.

Hatzenbuhler, E. G., Molteni, J. D., & Axe, J. B. (2019). Increasing play skills in children with autism spectrum disorder via peer-mediated matrix training. *Education and Treatment of Children, 42*(3), 295–319. https://doi.org/10.1353/etc.2019.0014

Heft, H. (1988). Affordances of children's environments: A functional approach to environmental description. *Children's Environments Quarterly, 5,* 29e37. https://doi.org/10.1006/jevp.2001.0249

Heljakka, K. (2018). Toy design universals for the 21st century: Designing play value in toys for children, adults, and transgenerational players. In *Collection of articles of the 2nd International Conference on Play Culture in Modern Childhood,* Moscow, Russia, NAIR.

Heljakka, K., & Harviainen, J. T. (2019). From displays and dioramas to doll dramas: Adult world building and world playing with toys. *American Journal of Play, 11*(3), 351–378. https://trepo.tuni.fi/bitstream/handle/10024/116158/From%20Displays%20and%20Dioramas_2019.pdf?sequence=2

Herrington, S., & Brussoni, M. (2015). Beyond physical activity: The importance of play and nature-based play spaces for children's health and development. *Current Obesity Reports, 4*(4), 477–483. https://doi.org/10.1007/s13679-015-0179-2

Herrington, S., & Lesmeister, C. (2006). The design of landscapes at child-care centres: Seven Cs. *Landscape Research, 31*(1), 63–82. https://doi.org/10.1080/01426390500448575

Hinojosa, J., & Kramer, P. (2008). Integrating children with disabilities into family play. In L. D. Parham & L. S. Fazio (Eds.), *Play in occupational therapy for children* (2nd ed., pp. 321–334). St. Louis, MO: Mosby Elsevier.

Hirsh-Pasek, K., A., & Golinkoff, R. M. (2006). How to choose toys for your baby. In S. Ettus (Ed.), *The experts' guide to the baby years* (pp. 246–248). New York, NY: Clarkson Potter. https://kathyhirshpasek.com/wp-content/uploads/sites/9/2015/08/PLAY_toys_for_your_baby.pdf

Howard, J. (2002). Eliciting young children's perceptions of play, work and learning using the activity apperception story procedure. *Early Child Development and Care, 172,* 489–502. https://doi.org/10.1080/03004430214548

Huh, B., & Roldan, C. J. (2016). Magnetic fields and intrathecal pump malfunction. *The American Journal of Emergency Medicine, 34*(1), 115e5–115e61. http://dx.doi.org/10.1016/j.ajem.2015.04.084

Humphry, R., & Wakeford, L. (2006). An occupation-centered discussion of development and implications for practice. *American Journal of Occupational Therapy, 60,* 258–267. https://doi.org/10.5014/ajot.60.3.258

Hyndman, B. (2015). Where to next for school playground interventions to encourage active play? An exploration of structured and unstructured school playground strategies. *Journal of Occupational Therapy, Schools, & Early Intervention, 8*(1), 56–67. http://dx.doi.org/10.1080/19411243.2015.1014956

Ideishi, S. K., Ideishi, R. I., Gandhi, T., & Yuen, L. (2006). Inclusive preschool outdoor play environments. *School System Special Interest Section Quarterly, 13*(2), 1–4.

Isbell, C., & Isbell, R. T. (2007). On the move: Environments that stimulate motor and cognitive development in infants. *Dimensions of Early Childhood, 35*(3), 30. http://www.grecs.org/wp-content/uploads/2015/01/On-the-Move.pdf

Isbell, C., Jones, K., Schmid, R., & Woodbury, R. (2014). Environments in outpatient pediatric occupational therapy clinics. *OT Practice, 19*(10), 19–20. https://www.aota.org/~/media/Corporate/Files/Secure/Publications/OTP/2014/OTP%20Vol%2019%20Issue%2019.pdf

Isenberg, J. P., & Jalongo, M. R. (Eds.). (2003). *Major trends and issues in early childhood education: Challenges, controversies, and insights.* New York: Teachers College Press.

Kaboski, J. R., Diehl, J. J., Beriont, J., Crowell, C. R., Villano, M., Wier, K., & Tang, K. (2014). Brief report: A pilot summer robotics camp to reduce social anxiety and improve social/vocational skills in adolescents with ASD. *Journal of Autism and Developmental Disorders, 45,* 3862–3869. https://doi.org/10.1007/s10803-014-2153-3

Kang, L. J., Hsieh, M. C., Liao, H. F., & Hwang, A. W. (2017). Environmental barriers to participation of preschool children with and without physical disabilities. *International Journal of Environmental Research and Public Health, 14*(5), 518. https://doi.org/10.3390/ijerph14050518

Kent, C., Cordier, R., Joosten, A., Wilkes-Gillan, S., & Bundy, A. (2020). Can we play together? A closer look at the peers of a peer-mediated intervention to improve play in children with autism spectrum disorder. *Journal of Autism and Developmental Disorders,* 1–14. https://doi.org/10.1007/s10803-020-04387-6

Kibele, A. (2008). *Meaning in action: Toys and other objects in early childhood.* Presentation at the annual conference of the American Occupational Therapy Association, Long Beach, CA.

King, G., Batorowicz, B., Rigby, P., McMain-Klein, M., Thompson, L., & Pinto, M. (2014). Development of a measure to assess youth self-reported experiences of activity settings (SEAS). *International Journal of Disability, Development and Education, 61*(1), 44–66. http://dx.doi.org/10.1080/1034912X.2014.878542

King, G., Batorowicz, B., Rigby, P., Pinto, M., Thompson, L., & Goh, F. (2014). The leisure activity settings and experiences of youth with severe disabilities. *Developmental Neurorehabilitation*, *17*(4), 259–269. https://doi.org/10.3109/17518423.2013.799244

King, G., Curran, C. J., & McPherson, A. (2013). A four-part ecological model of community-focused therapeutic recreation and life skills services for children and youth with disabilities. *Child: Care, Health and Development*, *39*(3), 325–336. https://doi.org/10.1111/j.1365-2214.2012.01390.x

King, G., Gibson, B. E., Mistry, B., Pinto, M., Goh, F., Teachman, G., & Thompson, L. (2014). An integrated methods study of the experiences of youth with severe disabilities in leisure activity settings: The importance of belonging, fun, and control and choice. *Disability and Rehabilitation*, *36*(19), 1626–1635. https://doi.org/10.3109/09638288.2013.863389

King, G., Kingsnorth, S., Sheffe, S., Vine, R., Crossman, S., Pinto, M., Curran, C. J., & Savage, D. (2016). An inclusive arts-mediated program for children with and without disabilities: Establishing community and an environment for child development through the arts. *Children's Health Care*, *45*(2), 204–226, https://doi.org/10.1080/02739615.2014.996885

King, G., Rigby, P., & Avery, L. (2016). Revised Measure of Environmental Qualities of Activity Settings (MEQAS) for youth leisure and life skills activity settings. *Disability and Rehabilitation*, *38*(15), 1509–1520, https://doi.org/10.3109/09638288.2015.1103792

King, G., Rigby, P., & Batorowicz, B. (2013). Conceptualizing participation in context for children and youth with disabilities: An activity setting perspective. *Disability and Rehabilitation*, *35*(18), 1578.1585. https://doi.org/10.3109/09638288.2012.748836

King, G., Rigby, P., Batorowicz, B., McMain-Klein, M., Petrenchik, T., Thompson, L., & Gibson, M. (2014). Development of a direct observation Measure of Environmental Qualities of Activity Settings. *Developmental Medicine & Child Neurology*, *56*(8), 763–769. https://doi.org/10.1111/dmcn.12400

King, P., & Howard, J. (2014). Factors influencing children's perceptions of choice within their free play activity: The impact of functional, structural and social affordances. *Journal of Playwork Practice*, *1*(2), 173–190. https://doi.org/10.1332/205316214X14114616128010

Knauer, H. A., Kagawa, R. M., Garcia-Guerra, A., Schnaas, L., Neufeld, L. M., & Fernald, L. C. (2016). Pathways to improved development for children living in poverty: A randomized effectiveness trial in rural Mexico. *International Journal of Behavioral Development*, *40*(6), 492–499. https://doi.org/10.1177/0165025416652248

Knibbe, T. J., Biddiss, E., Gladstone, B., & McPherson, A. C. (2016). Characterizing socially supportive environments relating to physical activity participation for young people with physical disabilities. *Developmental Neurorehabilitation*, *20*(5), 294–300. https://doi.org/10.1080/17518423.2016.1211190

Knox, S. H. (1993). Play and leisure. In H. L. Hopkins & H. D. Smith (Eds.), *Willard and Spackman's occupational therapy* (8th ed., pp. 260–268). Philadelphia: Lippincott.

Koegel, R., Fredeen, R., Kim, S., Danial, J., Rubinstein, D., & Koegel, L. (2012). Using Perseverative Interests to Improve Interactions Between Adolescents with Autism and their Typical Peers in School Settings. *Journal of Positive Behavior Interventions*, *14*(3), 133–141. http://doi.org/10.1177/1098300712437043

Koegel, R., Kim, S., Koegel, L., & Schwartzman, B. (2013). Improving socialization for high school students with ASD by using their preferred interests. *Journal of Autism and Developmental Disorders*, *43*(9), 2121–2134.

Kory-Westlund, J. M., & Breazeal, C. (2019). A long-term study of young children's rapport, social emulation, and language learning with a peer-like robot playmate in preschool. *Frontiers in Robotics and AI*, *6*, 81.

Kreider, C. M., Bendixen, R. M., Huang, Y. Y., & Lim, Y. (2014). Centennial vision—Review of occupational therapy intervention research in the practice area of children and youth 2009–2013. *American Journal of Occupational Therapy*, *68*, e61–e73. http://dx.doi.org/10.5014/ajot.2014.011114

Krieger, B., Piskur, B., Schulze, C., Jakobs, U., Beurskens, A., & Moser, A. (2018). Supporting and hindering environments for participation of adolescents diagnosed with autism spectrum disorder: A scoping review. *PLoS ONE*, *13*(8): e0202071. https://doi.org/10.1371/journal.pone.0202071

Kryzak, L. A., Bauer, S., Jones, E. A., & Sturmey, P. (2013). Increasing responding to others' joint attention directives using circumscribed interests. *Journal of Applied Behavior Analysis*, *46*(3), 674-679. https://doi.org/10.1002/jaba.73

Kryzak, L. A., & Jones, E. A. (2014). The effect of prompts within embedded circumscribed interests to teach initiating joint attention in children with autism spectrum disorders. *Journal of Developmental and Physical Disabilities*, *27*, 265–284. https://doi.org/10.1007/s10882-014-9414-0

Kuh, L. P. Ponte, I., & Chau, C. (2013). The impact of a natural playscape installation on young children's play behaviors. *Children, Youth and Environments*, *23*(2), 49. https://doi.org/10.7721/chilyoutenvi.23.2.0049

Kuhaneck, H.M., Spitzer, S. L., & Miller, E. (2010). *Activity Analysis, Creativity, and Playfulness in Pediatric Occupational Therapy: Making Play Just Right*. Boston, MA: Jones and Bartlett Publishers, LLC.

Kulak, S., & Stein, R. E. K. (2016). Toy age-labeling: An overview for pediatricians of how toys receive their age safety and developmental designations. *Pediatrics*, *138*(1). http://dx.doi.org/10.1542/peds.2015-1803

Kultti, A., & Pramling, N. (2015). Bring your own toy: Socialisation of two-year-olds through tool-mediated activities in an Australian early childhood education context. *Early Childhood Education Journal*, *43*, 367–376. https://doi.org/10.1007/s10643-014-0662-5

Lally, J. R., & Stewart, J. (1990). *Infant/toddler caregiving: A guide to setting up environments*. Sacramento, CA: California Department of Education.

Lambert, A., Vlaar, J., Herrington, S., & Brussoni, M. (2019). What is the relationship between the neighbourhood built environment and time spent in outdoor play? A systematic review. *International Journal of Environmental Research and Public Health*, *16*(20), 3840. https://doi.org/10.3390/ijerph16203840

Lane, S. J., & Mistrett, S. (2008). Facilitating play in early intervention. In L. D. Parham & L. S. Fazio (Eds.), *Play in occupational therapy for children* (2nd ed., pp. 413–425). St. Louis, MO: Mosby Elsevier.

Law, M., Cooper, B., Strong, S., Stewart, D., Rigby, P., & Letts, L. (1996). The person-environment-occupation model: A transactive approach to occupational performance. *Canadian Journal of Occupational Therapy, 63*(1), 9–23. https://doi.org/10.1177/000841749606300103

Leadley, S., & Hocking, C. (2017). An occupational perspective of childhood poverty. *New Zealand Journal of Occupational Therapy, 64*(1), 23–31. Availability: <https://search.informit.com.au/documentSummary;dn=743435363990857;res=IELNZC>ISSN: 1171-0462.

Lee, G. T., Qu, K., Hu, X., Jin, N., & Huang, J. (2020). Arranging play activities with missing items to increase object-substitution symbolic play in children with autism spectrum disorder. *Disability and Rehabilitation*, 1–13. https://doi.org/10.1080/09638288.2020.1734107

Lindsay, S., Hounsell, K.G., & Cassiani, C. (2017). A scoping review of the role of LEGO® therapy for improving inclusion and social skills among children and youth with autism. *Disability Health Journal, 10*(2), 173–182. https://doi.org/10.1016/j.dhjo.2016.10.010.

Lory, C., Rispoli, M., & Gregori, E. (2018). Play interventions involving children with autism spectrum disorder and typically developing peers: A review of research quality. *Review Journal of Autism and Developmental Disorders, 5*, 78–89. https://doi.org/10.1007/s40489-017-0124-2

Luchs, A., & Fikus, M. (2013). A comparative study of active play on differently designed playgrounds. *Journal of Adventure Education and Outdoor Learning 13*(3), 206–222. https://doi.org/10.1080/14729679.2013.778784

Lynch, H. (2018). Which playspaces are appropriate for our children? In P. Encarnação, S. Ray-Kaeser, & N. Bianquin (Eds.), *Guidelines for supporting children with disabilities' play: Methodologies, tools, and contexts* (pp. 98–108). Berlin: Sciendo.

Lynch, H., Moore, A., & Prellwitz, M. (2018). From policy to play provision: Universal design and the challenges of inclusive play. *Children, Youth and Environments, 28*(2), 12–34. https://doi.org/10.7721/chilyoutenvi.28.2.0012

Lynch, H., & Stanley, M. (2018). Beyond words: Using qualitative video methods for researching occupation with young children. *OTJR: Occupation, Participation and Health, 38*(1), 56–66. https://doi.org/10.1177/1539449217718504

Mahboubi, H., Oliaei, S., Badran, K. W., Ziai, K., Chang, J., Zardouz, S., ... Djalilian, H. R. (2013). Systematic assessment of noise amplitude generated by toys intended for young children. *Otolaryngology–Head and Neck Surgery, 148*(6), 1043–1047. https://doi.org/10.1177/0194599813482293

Mahoney, G., & Solomon, R. (2016). Mechanism of developmental change in the PLAY project home consultation program: Evidence from a randomized control trial. *Journal of Autism and Developmental Disorders, 46*(5), 1860–1871.

Marshall, A., Myers, C., & Pierce, D. (2017). Centennial topics—A century of therapeutic use of the physical environment. *American Journal of Occupational Therapy, 71*, 7101100030. https://doi.org/10.5014/ajot.2017.023960

Martin, C. L., Eisenbud, L., & Rose, H. (1995). Children's gender-based reasoning about toys. *Child Development, 66*, 1453–1471.

Masur, E. F., Flynn, V., & Olson, J. (2015). The presence of background television during young children's play in American homes. *Journal of Children and Media, 9*(3), 349–367. https://doi.org/10.1080/17482798.2015.1056818

May-Benson, T. A., & Cermak, S. A. (2007). Development of an assessment for ideational praxis. *American Journal of Occupational Therapy, 61*(2), 148–153. https://doi.org/10.5014/ajot.61.2.148

Miller, E., & Kuhaneck, H. (2008). Children's perceptions of play experiences and play preferences: A qualitative study. *American Journal of Occupational Therapy, 62*, 407–415. https://doi.org/10.5014/ajot.62.4.407

Milteer, R. M., Ginsburg, K. R., & Mulligan, D. A. (2012). The importance of play in promoting healthy child development and maintaining strong parent–child bond: Focus on children in poverty. *Pediatrics, 129*(1), e204–e213. https://doi.org/10.1542/peds.2011-2953.

Morozini, M. (2015). Exploring the engagement of parents in the co-occupation of parent–child play: An occupational science's perspective. *International Journal of Prevention and Treatment, 4*(2A), 11–28.

Nasar, J. L., & Holloman, C. H. (2013). Playground characteristics to encourage children to visit and play. *Journal of Physical Activity & Health, 10*(8), 1201–1208. Retrieved from https://search.proquest.com/docview/1464891218?accountid=143111

Neal, D. T., Wood, W., Labrecque, J., & Lally, P. (2012). How do habits guide behavior? Perceived and actual triggers of habits in daily life. *Journal of Experimental Social Psychology, 48*. 492–498. https://doi.org/10.1016/j.jesp.2011.10.011

Ness, D., & Farenga, S. J. (2016). Blocks, bricks, and planks: Relationships between affordance and visuo-spatial constructive play objects. *American Journal of Play, 8*(2), 201–227.

Nolan, A., & Pells, K. (2020). Children's economic and social rights and child poverty: The state of play. *The International Journal of Children's Rights, 28*(1), 111–132. https://doi.org/10.1163/15718182-02801006

Novak, I., & Honan, I. (2019). Effectiveness of paediatric occupational therapy for children with disabilities: A systematic review. *Australian Occupational Therapy Journal, 66*(3), 258–273. https://doi.org/10.1111/1440-1630.12573

Nwokah, E., Hsu, H. C., & Gulker, H. (2013). The use of play materials in early intervention: The dilemma of poverty. *American Journal of Play, 5*(2), 187–218.

O'Brien, J., Boatwright, T., Chaplin, J., Geckler, C., Gosnell, D., Holcombe, J., et al. (1998). The impact of positioning equipment on play skills of physically impaired children. In M. Carlisle Duncan, G. Chick, & A. Aycock (Eds.), *Play & culture studies: Volume 1*. Diversions and divergences in fields of play (pp. 149–160). Greenwich, CT: Ablex.

O'Connor, D., Butler, A., & Lynch, H. (2020). Partners in play: Exploring "playing with" children living with severe physical and intellectual disabilities. *British Journal of Occupational Therapy*, 0308022620967293.

Olsen, H., Kennedy, E., & Vanos, J. (2019). Shade provision in public playgrounds for thermal safety and sun protection: A case study across 100 play spaces in the United States. *Landscape and Urban Planning, 189*, 200–211. https://doi.org/10.1016/j.landurbplan.2019.04.003

O'Neill, D., McDonald, D., & Jones, S. (2018). Toying with inclusivity. *BMJ, 2018*; 363: k5193. https://doi.org/10.1136/bmj.k5193

Parham, L. D. (1992). Strategies for maintaining a playful atmosphere during therapy. *Sensory Integration Special Interest Section Newsletter, 15*(1), 2–3.

Park, J. G. (2009). Color perception in pediatric patient room design: Healthy children vs. pediatric patients. *HERD: Health Environments Research & Design Journal*, 2(3), 6–28. https://doi.org/10.1177/193758671300600402

Pierce, D. (2000). Maternal management of the home as a developmental play space for infants and toddlers. *American Journal of Occupational Therapy*, 54, 290–299. https://doi.org/10.5014/ajot.54.3.290

Potera, C. (2011). Indoor air quality: Scented products emit a bouquet of VOCs. *Environmental Health Perspectives*, 119(1). https://doi.org/10.1289/ehp.119-a16

Prieske, B., Withagen, R., Smith, J., & Zaal, F. T. J. M. (2015). Affordances in a simple playscape: Are children attracted to challenging affordances? *Journal of Environmental Psychology*, 41, 101–111. https://doi.org/10.1016/j.jenvp.2014.11.011

Puhakka, R., Rantala, O., Roslund, M. I., Rajaniemi, J., Laitinen, O. H., Sinkkonen, A., & ADELE Research Group. (2019). Greening of daycare yards with biodiverse materials affords well-being, play and environmental relationships. *International Journal of Environmental Research and Public Health*, 16(16), 2948. https://doi.org/10.3390/ijerph16162948

Quilitch, H. R., & Risley, T. R. (1973). The effects of play materials on social play. *Journal of Applied Behavior Analysis*, 6, 573–578. https://doi.org/10.1901/jaba.1973.6-573

Quinn, J. M., Pascoe, A. T., Wood, W., & Neal, D. T. (2010). Can't control yourself? Monitor those bad habits. *Personality and Social Psychology Bulletin*, 36, 499–511. https://doi.org/10.1177/0146167209360665

Raoof, N., Chan, T. K. J., Rogers, N. K., Abdullah, W., Haq, I., Kelly, S. P., & Quhill, F. M. (2014)."Toy" laser macular burns in children. *Eye*, 28(2), 231–234. https://doi.org/10.1038/eye.2013.315

Ray-Kaeser, S., Perino, O., Costa, M., Schneider, E., Kindler, V., & Bonarini, A. (2018). Which toys and games are appropriate for our children? In P. Encarnação, S. Ray-Kaeser, & N. Bianquin (Eds.), *Guidelines for supporting children with disabilities' play: Methodologies, tools, and contexts* (pp. 67–84). Berlin: Sciendo.

Refshauge, A. D., Stigsdotter, U. K., Lamm, B., et al. (2013). Evidence-based playground design: Lessons learned from theory to practice. *Landscape Research*, 40(2), 226–246. https://doi.org/10.1080/01426397.2013.824073

Remmers, T., Broeren, S. M., Renders, C. M., Hirasing, R. A., van Grieken, A., & Raat, H. (2014). A longitudinal study of children's outside play using family environment and perceived physical environment as predictors. *International Journal of Behavioral Nutrition and Physical Activity*, 11(1), 76. https://doi.org/10.1186/1479-5868-11-76

Retting, M. (1994). The play of young children with visual impairments: Characteristics and interventions. *Journal of Visual Impairment & Blindness*, 88, 410–420.

Rigby, P., & Huggins, L. (2003). Enabling young children to play by creating supportive play environments. In L. Letts, P. Rigby, & D. Stewart (Eds.), *Using environments to enable occupational performance* (pp. 155–176). Thorofare, NJ: Slack.

Rigby, P., & Rodger, S. A. (2006). Developing as a player. In S. Rodger & J. Ziviani (Eds.), *Occupational therapy with children: Understanding children's occupations and enabling participation* (pp. 177–199). Oxford, UK: Blackwell.

Rigby, P. J., Trentham, B., & Letts, L. (2019). Modifying performance contexts. In B. A. Boyt Schell & G. Gillen (Eds.), *Willard & Spackman's occupational therapy* (13th ed., pp. 460–479). Baltimore, MD: Lippincott Williams & Wilkins.

Robinson, A. L. (1977). Play: The arena for acquisition of rules for competent behavior. *American Journal of Occupational Therapy*, 31(4), 248–253.

Robinson, S., & Graham, A. (2019). Promoting the safety of children and young people with intellectual disability: Perspectives and actions of families and professionals. *Children and Youth Services Review*, 104, 104404. https://doi.org/10.1016/j.childyouth.2019.104404

Rosenberg, L., Bart, O., Ratzon, N. Z., & Jarus, T. (2013). Personal and environmental factors predict participation of children with and without mild developmental disabilities. *Journal of Child and Family Studies*, 22(5), 658–671. http://dx.doi.org/10.1007/s10826-012-9619-8

Rubenstein, J., & Howes, C. (1976). The effects of peers on toddler interaction with mother and toys. *Child Development*, 597–605.

Ruffino, A. G., Mistrett, S. G., Tomita, M., & Hajare, P. (2006). The Universal Design for Play Tool: Establishing validity & reliability. *Journal of Special Education Technology*, 21(4), 25–38. https://doi.org/10.1177/016264340602100404

Saha, S., Doran, E., Osann, K. E., Hom, C., Movsesyan, N., Rosa, D. D., ... Lott, I. T. (2014). Self-concept in children with Down syndrome. *American Journal of Medical Genetics, Part A*, 164(8), 1891–1898. DOI 10.1002/ajmg.a.36597

Scarantino, A. (2003). Affordances explained. *Philosophy of Science*, 70(5), 949–961.

Sherman, A. M., & Zurbriggen, E. L. (2014)."Boys can be anything": Effect of Barbie play on girls' career cognitions. *Sex Roles*, 70(5), 195–208.

Silverman, F., & Tyszka, A. C. (2017). Centennial topics—Supporting participation for children with sensory processing needs and their families: Community-based action research. *American Journal of Occupational Therapy*, 71, 7104100010. https://doi.org/10.5014/ajot.2017.025544

Sinclair, S. A., & Xiang, H. (2008). Injuries among US children with different types of disabilities. *American Journal of Public Health*, 98(8), 1510–1516. https://doi.org/10.2105/AJPH.2006.097097

Skar, L. (2002). Disabled children's perceptions of technical aids, assistance and peers in play situations. *Scandinavian Journal of Caring Sciences*, 16(1), 27–33. https://doi.org/10.1046/j.1471-6712.2002.00047.x

Skard, G., & Bundy, A. C. (2008). Test of playfulness. In L. D. Parham & L. S. Fazio (Eds.), *Play in occupational therapy for children* (2nd ed., pp. 71–93). St. Louis, MO: Mosby Elsevier.

Smart, E., Edwards, B., Kingsnorth, S., Sheffe, S., Curran, C. J., Pinto, M., Crossman, S., & King, G. (2018). Creating an inclusive leisure space: Strategies used to engage children with and without disabilities in the arts-mediated program Spiral Garden. *Disability and Rehabilitation*, 40(2), 199–207. https://doi.org/10.1080/09638288.2016.1250122

Smith, C. (2013). Using personal dolls to learn empathy, unlearn prejudice: Personal doll training. South Africa. *The International Journal of Diversity in Education*, 12(3).

Spitzer, S. L. (2008). Play in children with autism: Structure and experience. In L. D. Parham & L. S. Fazio (Eds.), *Play in Occupational Therapy for Children* (2nd ed., pp. 351–374). St. Louis, MO: Mosby Elsevier.

Spitzer, S. L. (2010). Common and Uncommon Daily Activities in Children with an Autism Spectrum Disorder: Challenges and Opportunities for Supporting Occupation. In H. Miller Kuhaneck & R. Watling (Eds.), *Autism: A Comprehensive Occupational Therapy Approach* (3rd ed., pp. 203–233). Bethesda, MD: American Occupational Therapy Association.

Stout, J. (1988). Planning playgrounds for children with disabilities. *American Journal of Occupational Therapy*, 42, 653–657. https://doi.org/10.5014/ajot.42.10.653

Sturgess, J. (2003). A model describing play as a child-chosen activity—is this still valid in contemporary Australia? *Australian Occupational Therapy Journal*, 50, 104–108. https://doi.org/10.1046/j.1440-1630.2003.00362.x

Sung, J. (2018). How young children and their mothers experience two different types of toys: A Traditional stuffed toy versus an animated digital toy. *Child Youth Care Forum*, 47, 233–257. https://doi.org/10.1007/s10566-017-9428-8

Tamis-LeMonda, C. S., Damast, A. M., Baumwell, L., & Bornstein, M. H. (1996). Sensitivity in parenting interactions across the first two years: Influences on children's language and play. *Infant Behavior and Development*, 19, 230. https://doi.org/10.1016/s0163-6383(96)90284-2

Therrell, J. A. (2002). *Age determination guidelines: Relating children's ages to toy characteristics and play behavior.* Washington, DC: U.S. Consumer Product Safety Commission (CPSC).

Tomchek, S. D., & Koenig, K. P. (2016). *Occupational therapy practice guidelines for individuals with autism spectrum disorder.* Bethesda, MD: AOTA Press.

Trawick-Smith, J., Wolff, J., Koschel, M., & Vallarelli, J. (2015). Effects of toys on the play quality of preschool children: Influence of gender, ethnicity, and socioeconomic status. *Early Childhood Education Journal*, 43(4), 249–256. https://doi.org/10.1007/s10643-014-0644-7

Umstattd Meyer, M. R., Bridges, C. N., Schmid, T. L., Hecht, A. E., & Pollack Porter, K. M. (2019). Systematic review of how Play Streets impact opportunities for active play, physical activity, neighborhoods, and communities. *BMC Public Health*, 19, 335. https://doi.org/10.1186/s12889-019-6609-4

U.S. Access Board. (2005). *Accessible play areas: A summary of accessibility guidelines for play areas.* Washington, DC. https://www.access-board.gov/attachments/article/1369/play-guide.pdf

van Vianen, A. E. M. (2018). Person–environment fit: A review of its basic tenets. *Annual Review of Organizational Psychology and Organizational Behavior*, 5(1), 75–101. https://doi.org/10.1146/annurev-orgpsych-032117-104702

Venema, E., Vlaskamp, C., & Otten, S. (2017). Safety first! The topic of safety in reversed integration of people with intellectual disabilities. *Journal of Policy and Practice in Intellectual Disabilities*, 14(2), 146–153. https://doi.org/10.1111/jppi.12179

Verver, S. H., Vervloed, M. P., & Steenbergen, B. (2019). The use of augmented toys to facilitate play in school-aged children with visual impairments. *Research in Developmental Disabilities*, 85, 70–81. https://doi.org/10.1016/j.ridd.2018.11.006

Verver, S. H., Vervloed, M. P., & Steenbergen, B. (2020). Facilitating play and social interaction between children with visual impairments and sighted peers by means of augmented toys. *Journal of Developmental and Physical Disabilities*, 32, 93–111. https://doi.org/10.1007/s10882-019-09680-6

Vismara, L. A., & Lyons, G. L. (2007). Using perseverative interests to elicit joint attention behaviors in young children with autism: Theoretical and clinical implications for understanding motivation. *Journal of Positive Behavior Interventions*, 9(4), 214–228.

Vogle, D. L., Bitman, R. L., Hammer, J. H., & Wade, J. G. (2013). Is stigma internalized? The longitudinal impact of public stigma on self-stigma. *Journal of Counseling Psychology*, 60(2), 311–316.

Waldman-Levi, A., & Erez, A. B. H. (2015). Will environmental interventions affect the level of mastery motivation among children with disabilities? A preliminary study. *Occupational Therapy International*, 22(1), 19–27. https://doi.org/10.1002/oti.1380

Watkins, L., O'Reilly, M., Kuhn, M., & Ledbetter-Cho, K. (2019). An interest-based intervention package to increase peer social interaction in young children with autism spectrum disorder. *Journal of Applied Behavior Analysis*, 52(1), 132–149. https://doi.org/10.1002/jaba.514.

Wenger, I., Schulze, C., Lundström, U., & Prellwitz, M. (2020). Children's perceptions of playing on inclusive playgrounds: A qualitative study. *Scandinavian Journal of Occupational Therapy*, 28(2), 136–146. https://doi.org/10.1080/11038128.2020.1810768

Whalon, K. J., Conroy, M. A., Martinez, J. R., & Werch, B. L. (2015). School-based peer-related social competence interventions for children with autism spectrum disorder: A meta-analysis and descriptive review of single case research design studies. *Journal of Autism and Developmental Disorders*, 45(6), 1513–1531. http://dx.doi.org/10.1007/s10803-015-2373-1

Williams, E. I., Costall, A., & Reddy, V. (2018). Autism and triadic play: An object lesson in the mutuality of the social and material. *Ecological Psychology*, 30(2), 146–173. https://doi.org/10.1080/10407413.2018.1439140

Williams, S. E., & Matesi, D. V. (1988). Therapeutic intervention with an adapted toy. *American Journal of Occupational Therapy*, 42, 673–676.

Wimpory, D., Hobson, R.P., & Nash, S. (2007). What Facilitates Social Engagement in Preschool Children with Autism? *Journal of Autism and Developmental Disorders*, 37, 564–573.

Wood, W., & Neal, D. T. (2016). Healthy through habit: Interventions for initiating & maintaining health behavior change. *Behavioral Science & Policy*, 2(1), 71–83. 10.1353/bsp.2016.0008

Worku, B. N., Abessa, T. G., Wondafrash, M., Lemmens, J., Valy, J., Bruckers, L., Kolsteren, P., & Granitzer, M. (2018). Effects of home-based play-assisted stimulation on developmental performances of children living in extreme poverty: A randomized single-blind controlled trial. *BMC Pediatrics*, 18, 29. https://doi.org/10.1186/s12887-018-1023-0

Young, D. (2013). Universal design and livable communities. *Home & Community Health Special Interest Section Quarterly*, 20(1), 1–4.

Yu, X., & Schwebel, D. C. (2018). The public health challenge of consumer non-compliance to toy product recalls and proposed solutions. *International Journal of Environmental Research and Public Health*, 15(3), 540. http://dx.doi.org/10.3390/ijerph15030540

Zuzak, T. J., Balmer, B., Schmidig, D., Boltshauser, E., & Grotzer, M. A. (2009). Magnetic toys forbidden for pediatric patients with certain programmable shunt valves? *Child's Nervous System*, 25(2), 161. https://doi.org/10.1007/s00381-008-0770-x

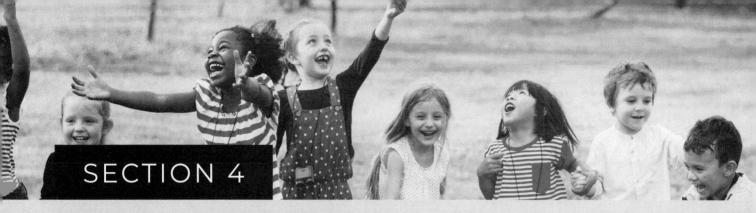

SECTION 4

Play Applications in Varied Contexts

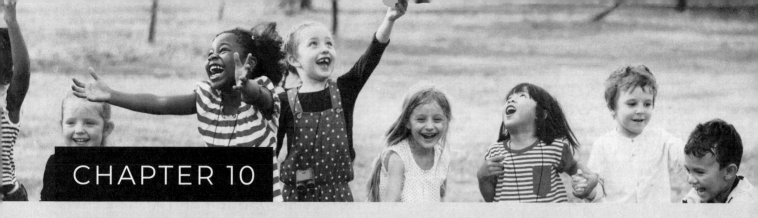

CHAPTER 10

Play in School-Based Occupational Therapy

Amy Y. Burton, OTD, OTR/L

Heather M. Kuhaneck, PhD, OTR/L, FAOTA

After reading this chapter, the reader will:

- Justify a focus on play in school-based occupational therapy.
- Describe the value of recess.
- Identify ways to use play as a tool to promote learning and educational goal attainment.
- Articulate appropriate methods of advocacy to increase play in schools.

Do not … keep children to their studies by compulsion but by play.

—Plato

Occupational therapy practitioners in educational settings promote access to all aspects of the school environment and the curriculum (American Occupational Therapy Association [AOTA], 2017). Our primary goal in this setting is to enable students to function in their role as a student, which includes learning, socializing, engaging in school activities, and participating in recess, physical education, and extracurricular activities. Despite the importance of play in occupational therapy and its value for education, play typically has not been a primary focus of occupational therapy intervention in the schools. The need to address play is becoming more pressing as play is becoming less commonplace in schools, even in the grades with younger-age children. There now are many barriers to play in schools, barriers that occupational therapy practitioners are well poised to diminish. Although

much of our work in school-based practice is with students with disabilities, the evolution of educational and disability law enables occupational therapy practitioners to promote play for all students. This chapter will provide strategies for doing so.

The Context of School-Based Practice and Play

Unlike some of the other contexts in which occupational therapists practice, multiple laws impact occupational therapy provision in school. There are laws that provide for education, laws that limit discrimination, and laws that promote access. Some laws are specific to children with disabilities receiving special education, while others are for children in the general education environment. Each of the laws influences occupational therapy practice in slightly different ways and these influences suggest varied ways of promoting play for students.

The Relationship of Legal Mandates with Play

Special Education Law

Before 1975, children with disabilities were not entitled to attend school, nor receive occupational therapy in the schools. The Education for All Handicapped Children Act (EHA; P.L. 94-142), passed in 1975, ensured that children with disabilities had a right to attend school and to receive the services necessary to allow them to learn and participate. Most children who now receive services in the schools do so because of this law, revised as the Individuals with Disabilities Education Act (IDEA) in 1990 and reauthorized most recently in 2004 (2004; P.L. 108-446). Children with disabilities must be provided with a free appropriate public education (FAPE) in the least restrictive environment (LRE). An individualized education program (IEP) for special education and related services for children with disabilities from 3 to 21 years of age must be provided, if an educational team deems the child requires these services to benefit from the public education provided (§ 300.17). Occupational therapy is provided as part of an IEP as a related service, which is defined as the "developmental, corrective, and other supportive services as are required to assist a child with a disability to benefit from special education …" (IDEA 2004, Final Regulations, § 300.34, 2006). Special education law also supports participation and services for extracurricular activities outside the school day (IDEA, 2017; U.S. Department of Education, 2013).

Through this legislation, school-based occupational therapy practitioners are mandated to help children with disabilities get the most out of their specially designed instruction (special education). Occupational therapy practitioners assist children with disabilities to engage in their role as students and to develop their ability to participate in all school occupations. School-based occupational therapy in special education can promote play in many ways. Our interventions may use play to address academic skills or social skill development, may occur during play activities in recess and physical education, and may address social participation with playful extracurricular activities. Extracurricular activities may include before- and after-school programs (e.g., social and leisure groups, sports, and clubs) as a part of out-of-school-time (OST) (Centers for Disease Control [CDC], 2019). Many of these play and leisure activities may need to be adapted to include students with special education needs, an area of occupational therapy expertise. As the law also specifically mentions the importance of students with disabilities to graduate from school with the ability to live independently and have economic self-sufficiency, it is important that occupational therapy practitioners also understand the research linking play to creativity and work performance to support the importance of play as a focus in the schools.

Nondiscrimination and Access Laws

Occupational therapy may also be provided in the school under the laws of either the Rehabilitation Act of 1973 or the Americans with Disabilities Act, both of which promote access and ensure nondiscrimination. These laws, meant to enhance educational access and reduce discrimination for those with disabilities, have over time integrated varied forms of occupational therapy in the schools (Ball, 2018, Chan, Dennis, Kim, & Jankowski, 2017; Colman, 1988; Coutinho, & Hunter, 1988; Dunn, 1988; Ottenbacher, 1982). Through these laws, occupational therapy practitioners can provide support to enhance inclusion in play activities throughout the school day. Therapists can analyze activities, student performance, and environments to facilitate participation and access for students with disabilities regardless of eligibility for special education. Collaboration and program development with school teams are another integral piece to supporting access to play under these laws.

General Education Laws

Occupational therapy in the schools is also supported under general education laws such as the Elementary and Secondary Education Act (ESEA) of 1965. This law, which was amended and reauthorized as No Child Left Behind (NCLB) (P.L. 107-110), and then replaced in 2015, by the Every Student Succeeds Act (ESSA) (Pub.L. No. 114-95), provides for occupational therapy as a "specialized instructional support." Multitiered systems of support (MTSS) is an education initiative that is a part of ESSA (ESSA, 2015) and includes both Response to Intervention (RtI) and positive behavioral interventions and supports (PBIS), processes designed to identify and intervene with students who are struggling. ESSA allows occupational therapy practitioners to assist children in the general education population.

With the evolution of federal law meant to ensure success for all students, occupational therapy provision in the schools should be broad and address schoolwide initiatives to promote student achievement and health (Ball, 2018). Occupational therapy practitioners work with groups, populations, and systems to promote the health, well-being, and participation of all individuals (AOTA, 2020). They work to help prevent disparities influenced by socioeconomic status, obesity, and other risk factors that can impact play and learning for students. Therefore, occupational therapy practitioners have a role in promoting play with all children in school settings, regardless of an identified disability (AOTA, 2017). This includes using play to support health and well-being, as well as to promote academic achievement and encourage eventual employment.

The Importance of Play for Learning

In addition to the evidence provided in Chapters 1 and 2 about the importance of play, there is growing evidence that play is critical to the type of learning today's students need to succeed in life (Parker & Thompson, 2019; Zosh et al., 2017). Rote memorization and learning material that is easy to regurgitate for standardized tests is not what is needed for many of the jobs of the 21st century, and because of this, there has been a recent push for education reform, including the use of more play and game-based learning (see **Figure 10.1**) (Hamari et al., 2016; Parker & Thompson, 2019; Qian & Clark, 2016). Research shows that play helps children learn, and therefore, participation in this occupation can and should be an integral aspect of students' education. However, there can be barriers to this type of service provision in the schools that must be surmounted.

Barriers to Address in Implementing Play in the Schools

Although play can be incredibly important and was historically an activity available to children at school, there are now many barriers for occupational therapy practitioners who wish to engage in play with their clients in this context. These include the recent push to enhance academic performance even for very young schoolchildren, differing ideas about professional role boundaries, and aspects of the school context that limit availability of time and space for play. Therapists must fully understand these barriers in order to address them.

Academic Priorities

Because school-based occupational therapy is a related service that supports education, it is influenced by academic standards. Play has a limited presence in the academic curriculum beyond preschool, and therefore it is sometimes overlooked in the planning process for students. Because professional resources and student learning time are constrained by the parameters of the school day, the team may question if play skills are a priority, especially if there are additional student needs that more directly relate to the curriculum. Often educational team members may need therapists to clarify the relationship of play to education so that it can be brought to the forefront of discussions for program planning.

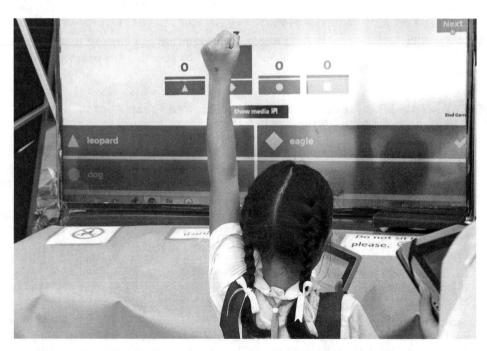

Figure 10.1 Game-based and playful education may promote learning as well as enjoyment
© Hi-Point/Shutterstock.

Team Roles and Boundaries

Occupational therapy practitioners may also need to inform others about the role of their profession (AOTA, 2017), particularly in relation to play. Other team members may not understand that the breadth of occupational therapy practice includes play as a major occupation. Other professionals on the team may mistakenly believe play falls exclusively under their purview and is not part of the occupational therapy role. Therapists report that in practice, it is common for other professionals, such as the special education teacher, to evaluate and target play (Kuhaneck et al., 2013). This role overlap can create a barrier if misunderstood but an opportunity for team collaboration if clarified.

Limited Opportunity

In addition to the misperceptions that educational law and professional scope somehow disallows our focus on play, another barrier to occupational therapy practitioners' inclusion of play in school settings is merely a lack of time for play. Occupational therapy practitioners do report time as a barrier to address play skills within the schools (Couch et al., 1998, Kuhaneck et al., 2013).

As more school time is devoted to curriculum "work," there is less available for play. Access to play during school through school breaks, recess, gym, sports, and art programs have decreased over time (Ginsburg, 2007; Hyndman, 2017b). In the 1960s, children often started school at age 6 or 7, spent a good portion of the school day at play and engaging in physical activity, and had a lengthy lunch period (Gray, 2014). Now, children start school at younger ages and participate in greater academic content earlier in their school careers (Bassok et al., 2016; Keskin, 2018).

Children spend a majority of their day either in school or in structured after-school activities. Opportunities for free play are limited for all students, but especially for individuals with disabilities in the educational setting. For individuals with disabilities, there may be even fewer recreational opportunities with peers and more solitary and passive activities (Buttimer & Tierney, 2005; Solish et al., 2010). Occupational therapists can be instrumental in creating opportunities to play despite the time barrier by inserting play into other activities and by investigating and incorporating the student's preferences throughout their participation in academic activities (Maciver et al., 2019).

Student Age

With older elementary, middle school, or high school students, it can be more difficult to introduce and encourage play, and it is less likely to be a part of the school day or classroom activities (Conklin, 2014; Fine, 2014; Wolk, 2017). Although play/leisure can be important for youths' social engagement and participation and can be critical for learning skills that prepare them for later employment, youth working on these areas in therapy may not enjoy time away from their peers or may see therapy as a disruption (Kelly, Strauss, Arnold, & Stride, 2020; Papp, Classen, & Judge, 2021). Youth may also be embarrassed by the need for support or be fearful of the possibility of embarrassing themselves (Payne, Ward, Turner, Taylor, & Bark, 2013; Shimmell, Gorter, Jackson, Wright, & Galuppi, 2013). Youth play for those with disabilities can be seen as highly restricted and overly influenced by adults (Brockman et al., 2011; Glenn et al., 2013). However, having fun in therapy may improve youth engagement somewhat (King et al., 2020; see **Practice Example 10.1**). Focusing on personal

---

PRACTICE EXAMPLE 10.1 Alexander and a Play-Inspired Fresh Approach

Alexander, a teenager attending a specialized school focused on social and emotional development, had received occupational therapy services for as long as he could remember. He disliked occupational therapy sessions because he had services for many years and therefore deemed it "for babies." Although he would participate and was congenial during therapy sessions, his occupational therapy practitioner did not feel that he was fully invested in the process. This was an issue, as he was getting older and the team felt he needed to take some ownership of his progress at school.

To better address his current needs, his therapist began to conduct informal interviews on Alexander's interests in general and related to his therapy. He expressed that he loved technology and wished he could do more of his education on the computer because he hoped to work in a technology field one day.

Based on this new information, the occupational therapy practitioner decided to explore different apps and games that worked on his specific IEP goals. Social-emotional learning, self-regulation, and meditation apps were his favorite ones to use. Many of these were video game–based and had a feature that awarded his continued participation and success. This transformed his negative perception of school work into something that was more motivating and playful. He liked the idea that he could use his phone to track his emotions and arousal throughout the day. His parents also loved that he could report progress by showing the data he took independently. Once this was introduced into his session, Alexander's demeanor shifted. After his interests were acknowledged and age-appropriate play was introduced into his sessions, Alexander was more receptive to participate and learn.

interests, playfulness, and humor as play are also appropriate for older children and adolescents (see Chapter 16 for detailed strategies).

Natural Contexts for Play in the Schools

There are a few natural environments in the schools that lend themselves most easily to focusing on play. While many of the playful practices described throughout this book could perhaps be put into place by the school-based occupational therapy practitioner in classroom or academic areas, it is most practical and seamless to do so on the playground during recess. However, recess is not the only place where occupational therapy practitioners can make a difference in the play of children at school. Therapists are encouraged to think outside of the (sand)box and venture into other aspects of the school day where our skills and perspective about play also can be influential. Indoor play times, whether for free time or for indoor recess, are additional opportunities for the occupational therapy practitioner in schools. After-school activities, extracurricular programs, and schoolwide play promotion/prevention support also provide opportunities for occupational therapy practitioners to become involved in play for students. It is important that therapists understand these contextual demands in order to intervene appropriately.

Recess

Recess is defined by the CDC (n.d.) as "a regularly scheduled period in the school day for physical activity and play that is monitored by trained staff or volunteers" and has been described as "a necessary break in the day for optimizing a child's social, emotional, physical, and cognitive development" (American Academy of Pediatrics [AAP], 2013, p. 186). Although children in preschool and kindergarten may have some free play time as part of their classroom experience, as they enter the higher grades, recess is the only free play time available. This free time during the school day has important benefits for education and society.

Benefits of Recess. The AAP (Council on School Health et al., 2013) cites four primary positive outcomes that may be achieved with recess: (1) improved fitness due to more physical activity (see **Figure 10.2**), (2) better attentiveness, (3) improved learning, and (4) the ability to practice social-emotional skills. Some of these benefits have been discussed in the literature for years, while others have been a more

recent addition. For example, Pellegrini (Pellegrini & Bjorklund, 1997; Pellegrini & Davis, 1993; Pellegrini, Huberty, & Jones, 1995) has been arguing for the importance of recess for learning since the 1990s. His research suggests that it enhances academic performance by allowing a break between difficult tasks requiring persistent attention in children who have not yet developed the capacity for lengthy attention spans. His studies and others suggest that students are more attentive when they have recess. The longer recess was delayed, the more inattentive children became and the more active they were once allowed to have recess (Jarrett et al., 1998; Pellegrini & Davis, 1993; Pellegrini et al., 1995).

Current evidence supports all the benefits mentioned earlier (Council on School Health et al., 2013; Jarrett, 2019; Pellegrini, 2008; Pellegrini & Bohn, 2005; Ramstetter & Murray, 2017; Waite-Stupiansky & Findlay, 2002). Large-scale studies have found that teachers report better behavior in students who have a recess each day of 15 minutes or more (Barros, Silver, & Stein, 2009). Studies of both exercise and learning and the impact of recess suggest that vigorous movement and physical activity promotes improved academic performance and achievement (Michael et al., 2015), as well as better attention to task in the classroom (Mahar, 2011; Martin, Farrell, Gray, & Clark, 2018; Stapp & Karr, 2018) (see **Figures 10.3** and **10.4**) and executive control (Hillman et al., 2014).

Recently, the Let's Inspire Innovation 'N Kids (LiiNK) project has produced a wealth of evidence supporting the role of recess in producing better classroom behavior, greater student attention and listening skills, and a host of other benefits, while not sacrificing academic performance (Bauml, Patton, & Rhea, 2020; Clark & Rhea, 2017; Rhea & Bauml, 2018; Rhea & Rivchun, 2018). This project started in Texas, based on the educational methods and successes noted in Finland. Schools in the LiiNK program train their teachers and administrators and provide 15-minute outdoor recess breaks four times every day. Impressive results have been attained across 24 schools (Texas Christian University, n.d.; see https://liinkproject.tcu.edu/results/).

Changes in Recess over Time. Given the current evidence, one might assume that recess would be commonplace, highly valued, and considered a priority in today's schools. However, this is not always the case. Ironically, recess was actually heavily valued in earlier times. The amount of recess students receive and the value placed on that portion of the school day has fluctuated over the last 100 years or so.

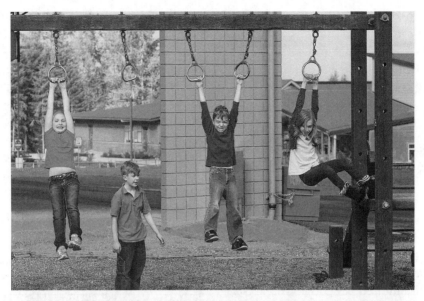

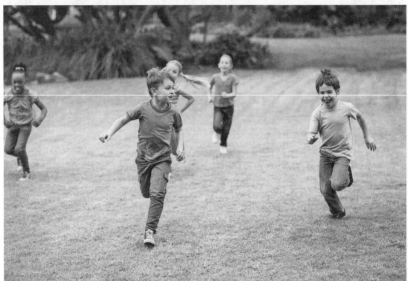

Figure 10.2 Recess allows for greater physical activity, an important benefit

Top: © MPH Photos/Shutterstock; Bottom: © wavebreakmedia/Shutterstock.

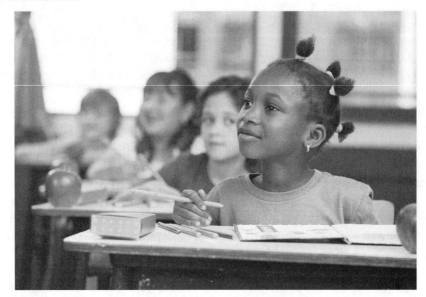

Figure 10.3 Recess may allow children to attend better

© GagliardiPhotography/Shutterstock.

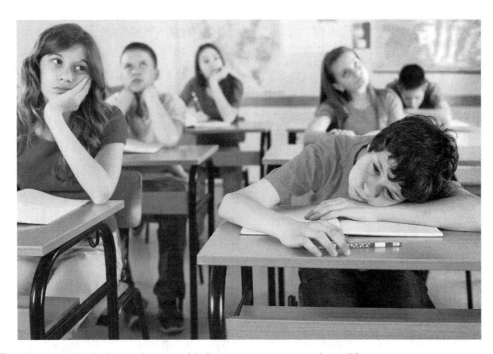

Figure 10.4 Recess may also help teachers avoid classroom scenes such as this
© SaMBa/Shutterstock.

Development and Growth of Recess Initially as recess became a part of education in America, it did so with the support and encouragement of a variety of individuals who strongly believed in its importance for children's growth and development. These individuals, primarily teachers and school administrators, understood play as integral to learning, and movement and physical activity as integral to children's ability to attend. From the late 1800s through the late 1900s, recess enjoyed a prominent role in the average student's school day.

Recess advanced across the United States hand in hand with kindergarten in the latter half of the 1800s (Frost & Sutterby, 2017; Saporo, 1989). The very first public kindergarten opened in the United States in St. Louis in 1873, and its creation, as well as access to public kindergartens across the United States, can be traced in large part to Susan Blow (Moore & Sabo-Risely, 2018). These early programs likely took many of their ideas from Froebel, who began the very first kindergarten and coined the term, and who had implemented the first sand gardens for children. Froebel stressed the importance of nature for learning and the role of the outdoor garden area for games, for young children to enhance their development (Frost & Sutterby, 2017; Moore & Sabo-Risley, 2018). However, the real beginning of recess at school in the United States is likely due to Amos Branson Alcott, a teacher who began each school day with an hour of outdoor play and socialization in the yard, which was called gymnastics (Alcott, 1861; Sanborn & Harris, 1893). Through the growth of kindergartens, playgrounds,

and educational reforms in the early 1900s, recess, as a designated time and place to play, became a highly valued and common practice for children during the school day (Ramstetter & Murray, 2017).

Recess as an Endangered Activity About 100 years later, there came a push for improved educational performance, with more time devoted to academics and less to recess (Jarrett, 2019; Pellegrini, 2008; Ramstetter & Murray, 2017). While in 1989, a survey documented that 90% of schools held recess at least once per day (Pellegrini, 1995), across much of the United States, recess time has declined since (Ramstetter & Murray, 2017). Significant decreases in the percentage of schools that provide recess after lunch were noted between 2006 and 2014 (Ramstetter & Murray, 2017). Now, only 82.8% of elementary schools provide any daily recess (CDC, 2015). Even for those schools that do provide recess, since the early 2000s the number of minutes of recess provided to children has been reduced as well (Ramstetter & Murray, 2017). One recent study of 500 teachers suggested that their students now average 25 minutes per day for recess (Voice of Play, 2018); however, the CDC reports that the average is 27 minutes (CDC, 2015). It is also quite easy, however, to find individual parents reporting anecdotally on the Internet that their child gets only 10 minutes of recess per day IF all of the children have behaved (Campbell, 2019).

Recess is not universally provided to all students, so not every child gets the same amount of recess per day. There are disparities in the number of minutes of recess reported by city schools and rural schools (Ramstetter & Murray, 2017), and recess varies by grade and age. Recess is more common for those in fifth grade or below. Recess access drops substantially between fifth and sixth grades, with sixth graders only getting recess in 34.9% of schools (CDC, 2015).

Some children get no recess because they are often in trouble. Teachers frequently use recess as a reward or punishment, and 86% of surveyed teachers reported having taken recess away at some point in time (Voice of Play, 2018). Although children report that they can understand why teachers do this, they do not perceive it to be a helpful strategy (Fink & Ramstetter, 2018). Even the teachers who use recess as a reward/punishment report they understand the benefits of recess and worry that this discipline strategy is weak (Ramstetter & Fink, 2019). However, they use it in response to behavioral concerns, work not being completed, or the need for additional academic intervention.

Even with the restrictions on recess in the schools of late, recess remains one of the most readily available play opportunities for school-based occupational therapy practitioners and one that is a natural context for peer interaction, movement, pretense, and more. As will be discussed later, there are many strategies for promoting play in the schools that can all be used at recess. Additionally, occupational therapy practitioners, armed with knowledge regarding the importance of recess, can be strong advocates for its continued inclusion and perhaps even expansion.

Playing Indoors

Schools may require students to play indoors due to inclement weather, playground construction or inaccessibility, for short classroom breaks, or for other planned or unforeseen circumstances. Therefore, occupational therapy practitioners may need to or wish to address play within the indoor environment. The context of recess, indoor vs. outdoor, changes the type of play that occurs. For example, indoor recess provides less opportunity for active physical play, particularly for girls, unless it is specifically structured, for example, by providing opportunities for dance or restricting access to cell phones (Erwin, Koufoudakis, & Beighle, 2013; Pawlowski, Nielsen, & Schmidt, 2021; Scudieri & Schwager, 2017; Tran, Clark, & Racette, 2013). The adequacy of indoor recess as a play opportunity may be supported or limited by the materials available, the space provided, and the training of the teachers (Lodewyk & McNamara, 2019; Novak, 2000; Segura-Martínez et al., 2020; Verstraete, Cardon, De Clercq, & De Bourdeaudhuij, 2006; see **Figure 10.5**).

Extracurricular Activities

Extracurricular activities also provide a natural avenue for play and can provide needed opportunities for students with disabilities to practice social skills and experience social inclusion (Brooks, Floyd, Robins, & Chan, 2015). Although extracurricular activities often are not specifically part of the IEP or used to work on IEP goals (Agran, Dymond, Rooney-Kron, & Martin,

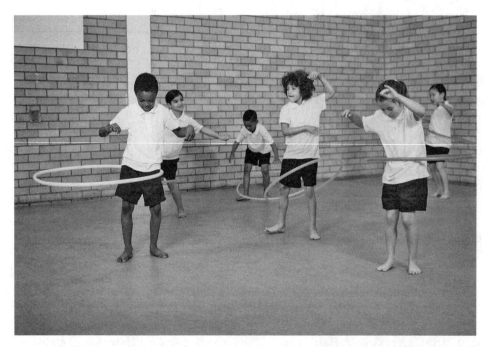

Figure 10.5 Indoor recess can be made more active if materials are provided and activities are structured properly
© wavebreakmedia/Shutterstock.

2020), these experiences may in fact improve social and educational outcomes (Bills, 2020; Mahoney, Cairns, & Farmer, 2003; Palmer, Elliott, & Cheatham, 2017), reduce the likelihood of being bullied (Haegele, Aigner, & Healy, 2020), and impact well-being (Oberle et al., 2019). However, few students with disabilities participate in these experiences (Agran et al., 2017). Participation may be somewhat related to the needs for student support and the use of specific communication devices (Dymond, Rooney-Kron, Burke, & Agran, 2020).

Embracing Our Full Role: Practices and Strategies for Promoting Play in Schools

Occupational therapy practitioners may address play as a primary occupation in school-based settings or use play as part of an intervention to achieve educationally related goals. Play can be introduced into a student's program by identifying developmental concerns, selecting appropriate play-based assessments that inform the team, and creating appropriate play goals and objectives (Ray-Kaeser & Lynch, 2017; Swinth & Tanta, 2008). Occupational therapy practitioners collaborate with the team to develop interventions that help the child achieve meaningful outcomes, including play and socializing with peers. Occupational therapy practitioners should focus on each individual's strengths and interests when exploring and developing play (Bundy, 1993; Tanta & Kuhaneck, 2020) to enhance engagement and support the play experience.

Play can be integrated into all aspects of occupational therapy in the schools. Therapy should not always look like a continuation of class time. While play may at times be used as a reward or a way to encourage compliance during an occupational therapy session, that should not be the only use of play. Although occupational therapy sessions may require a level of structure in order to meet goals set forth in the IEP, activities should still be fun and inviting for the child, and the course of therapy should feel fluid, creative, and playful (Tanta & Kuhaneck, 2020). The therapist should encourage meaningfulness and engagement by analyzing play and providing the just-right challenge during sessions. The occupational therapy practitioner should be present and supportive but not overly intrusive.

Many of the practices described throughout this text also can encourage and increase opportunities for play in occupational therapy in the schools (AOTA, 2020). These include recommendations for assessing and planning for play, creating play-based goals and objectives, promoting greater access to play, using natural contexts, including peers in play, embracing a playful style, encouraging new interests, ensuring safety, allowing choice, and focusing on generalization.

Assessing and Planning for Play at School

The value of assessing play at school is twofold. First, play skills, inclusion, and peer social interactions may be a direct concern. Second, assessment of play helps to establish an understanding of a child's participation within the school environment (Tanta & Kuhaneck, 2020). Play-based assessment creates a more vivid illustration of the student's complete performance skills and inclusion within the schools. In addition, it presents an opportunity to discover how the child has adapted thus far in order to get involved and succeed and their strengths.

Play assessment at school may involve an evaluation of the physical and social environment, the activity demands, and the students' abilities. To begin this process, occupational therapists can observe play as it naturally occurs. In school settings, observation of play allows for a unique opportunity to have an immediate comparison to typical peers and environmental demands. This offers insight and analysis of contextual fit. Ideally, play observation is nonfacilitated and has minimal adult direction (Kelly-Vance & Ryalls, 2020). Often, therapists will need to observe a child several times in a variety of settings and with different play partners, as performance may fluctuate from day to day and between peers (Kelly-Vance & Ryalls, 2020; Tanta & Kuhaneck, 2020). For example, an occupational therapist can observe structured play during a physical education class, free-play in the classroom, and recess outdoors on the playground. Occupational therapists can view children's choices and capabilities, then examine how functional and satisfied they are with them (Bundy, 1993; Richardson, 2019).

Occupational therapists can interview parents, teachers, paraprofessionals, and recess aides to understand what games are played, what materials are available, what the space looks like, and the social dynamics of play within the schools. Structured questionnaires and informal interviews are appropriate methods to gather this information. In addition, formal instruments can guide practitioners in analyzing occupational and environmental barriers and supports in the schools. See Chapters 4 and 5 for detailed information about specific play assessment tools that may be indicated.

Assessment information on occupational performance, strengths, interests, the environmental and activity demands, and play participation drives the program planning process to make occupational therapy more individualized, client centered, and motivating for the student. These are necessary aspects to a comprehensive and strengths-based play assessment in the schools, which can then lead to the development of appropriate, play-based goals.

School Play Goals

IEP goals can focus on various components of play, such as improving physical skills, social interaction, or self-regulation needed for play. Goals can also emphasize aspects of playfulness and characteristics of play such as a student's initiation, engagement, motivation, and attention for play. In addition, goals can focus on overall play participation (Ray-Kaeser & Lynch, 2017). Occupational therapists should collaborate with the team to create IEP goals that, when achieved, will foster real play. They should know what type of play is appropriate for the child's age or stage, what types of play and materials are available, and for how long play should be expected to last. For example, an objective could be written to increase a student's time engaged in play activities to match the actual duration of recess or the length of a typical game played during free time in the classroom.

Goals should always be specific and individualized. Therefore, it is important to think about the child's strengths, needs, and the contextual demands to determine what skills must be prioritized. Be sure to add in degree statements to indicate challenging, yet attainable frequency or trials, duration of engagement, accuracy, etc. You should also consider the conditions that detail the specific environmental, temporal, and social contexts, materials used, and level of prompting. When developing an appropriate intervention plan, consider the criteria for mastery of objectives, such as whether demonstration of a certain skill will be in the therapy room or in the general education environment, in simulated or natural play, and with peers or alone. This will influence the context for data collection, who captures the data, and how often it is collected. For play-based goal ideas, please see **Box 10.1**.

Play Intervention in School

With the various barriers discussed earlier, school-based occupational therapy practitioners may struggle

---

Box 10.1 Sample Play-Related IEP Goals

- Student will initiate a play activity with a peer.
- Student will attend to a game with peers for 10 minutes.
- Student will engage in cooperative play with peers.
- Student will work with peers toward mutual team goals during a playground game.
- Student will play with peers for the duration of outdoor recess requiring no adult support.
- Student will successfully share toys with a peer.
- Student will select (or choose) a play activity from a visual array of three.
- Student will attempt to play with five new games or toys.
- Student will independently complete X skill (fine motor, gross motor, postural, social, communication, behavioral, etc.) during a specific play activity.
- Student will manipulate X items or objects demonstrating efficient, accurate, and timely movements during a play activity.
- Student will play on the playground for 20 minutes, demonstrating no signs of fatigue.
- Student will participate in a play activity (on the playground, in classroom, gym, etc.) following all school or classroom rules.
- Student will demonstrate a specific number of verbal exchanges or physical interactions with a peer during play.
- Student will engage in a new adapted play activity with peers.
- Student will independently access at least two classroom toys (play environments, activities, etc.) during indoor recess.
- Student will request help when requiring (physical, social, emotional, cognitive, executive functioning, etc.) support during play activities.

---

with how and when to support this play in their intervention plans (Couch et al., 1998; Kuhaneck et al., 2013), defaulting to educational "work." But despite threats to recess and the narrow interpretation of educational law, there are incredible opportunities for play intervention that can impart a lasting and meaningful effect on children and school systems. Some are presented here to inspire your own creativity and ingenuity in addressing play in school-based practice.

Improving Access to Play

Students with special needs have unique challenges that can be problematic when accessing play with and without typical peers. They may differ in their performance of certain skills, play preferences and behaviors, choice of play objects, and modes of play (Besio &

Amelina, 2017; Case-Smith & Kuhaneck, 2008; Clifford & Bundy, 1989; Desha et al., 2003; Dominguez et al., 2006). In addition, individuals with disabilities have limited access to and engagement in play due to social, activity, and environmental barriers (Imms, 2008; King et al., 2009; Majnemer et al., 2008).

Therapists can help teachers and administrators in the selection of appropriate play-based materials and activities that encourage participation of all students. They can also review aspects of the curriculum to make recommendations for playful instruction based on the specific lessons taught in class as seen in **Practice Example 10.2**. Adding play within the classroom ensures that all children will have opportunities to engage in more structured play with peers. Ideally, play repertoires developed in the classroom will be generalized to all settings within the school.

Occupational therapy practitioners can support access to meaningful play through adapting and modifying activities and the environment within the classroom or playground (see **Figure 10.6**). This may include changing criteria for participation or creating new and playful ways to demonstrate success and understanding. Some examples of this are altering the rules of a game, using special equipment, or reducing the expectations for play. Also, eliminating waiting or "down time" or adding additional breaks, depending on the needs of the child, may be important to increase inclusion.

In addition, occupational therapy practitioners can make suggestions for less-structured, accessible play outside the classroom. One way to do this is by helping teachers and school administrators make playgrounds more accessible. The Playable Space

---

PRACTICE EXAMPLE 10.2 Increasing Play in Educational Activities Through Occupational Therapy

Carla, an occupational therapy practitioner in a general education elementary school, knew the importance of play and wanted to promote access for all students, especially those with special needs. Due to her large caseload, however, she felt she didn't have enough time to assess and create these opportunities for each student. To address this, she worked with the kindergarten teachers during grade-level meetings on a monthly basis to review lesson plans for the upcoming weeks. She then collaborated to develop playful instructional methods to teach their lessons.

For the first section of the curriculum, the kindergarten teachers planned to introduce the concept of "seasons." Carla researched seasonal music and dance videos to be used on the interactive whiteboards. She organized a scavenger hunt for seasonal items within the classroom. Fall leaves, gourds, corn stalks, and scarecrows were hidden around the room. Students worked together to find a specific object given verbal directions from the teacher. In addition to learning new vocabulary, these creative teaching methods also reinforced the underlying skills of following directions and teamwork. Carla also created an obstacle course that included seasonal themes and items in the hallway, which the students rotated through during "centers" time. Using equipment from the OT room, such as a balance beam and scooter boards, along with some painters' tape and contact paper stickers, she designed a sensory pathway. Artificial, decorative leaves were sprinkled with seasonal essential oils and tacked to the floor so that students could walk or hop over them. Small hay bales were used as obstacles instead of cones. Not only did the students enjoy this special experience, but the parents did too. With the permission of the principal, Carla recruited parent volunteers to oversee the hallway station.

During these weeks, Carla had the students on her caseload work separately to develop skills for navigating classroom spaces, searching for items, and negotiating the various aspects of the hallway obstacle course. This preteaching prepared her students for more natural play and interactions with peers in the classroom, as some of the adaptations and modifications were introduced and practiced beforehand during therapy sessions. This enhanced student confidence and self-efficacy. The children looked forward to therapy sessions and even strived harder to grasp concepts and movements more independently, knowing that they would be doing these again in class. Some students had play-based goals that worked seamlessly with this direct type of intervention. However, Carla used these activities for all of her students, to prepare them for higher-level precision and occupational performance.

The teachers appreciated the ideas and support for designing play spaces and activities. They reported that students were more engaged and focused and displayed less disruptive behaviors during instructional time. The students who received occupational therapy services benefited because they were able to address real occupational performance barriers and have objectives reinforced throughout the week. And Carla saw value in this because the time that went into planning was offset by the team's investment in obtaining therapeutic materials and helping set up therapy spaces. As time progressed, teams of teachers, administrators, and parents became more involved in the process. Carla found that it became more of a collaborative effort enabling her to allocate less time to prepare for it each month.

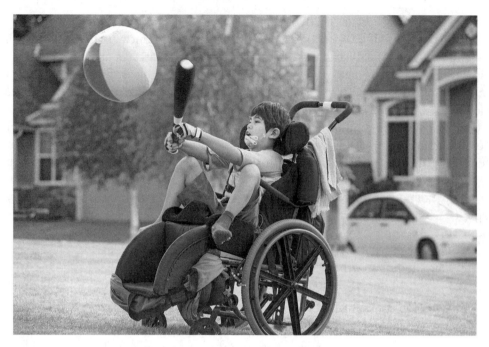

Figure 10.6 Modifying activities may allow students with disabilities to play. This boy needed a larger and lighter ball and bat in order to engage in "baseball" with peers
© Jaren Jai Wicklund/Shutterstock.

Quality Assessment Tool (Play England, 2009) can help identify design principles that promote access to individuals with disabilities, so that they can play with and alongside their nondisabled peers. Modifications could include safety matting for potential falls, wheelchair-accessible equipment and ramps, and high-back swings for trunk support (see **Figure 10.7**; Greutman, 2016).

Including Peers in Play

Because play does not always occur in isolation or with adults, occupational therapy practitioners should consider including peers and providing group therapy when addressing play (Swinth & Tanta, 2008). Depending on the individualized needs of the child in accordance with the IEP, and if allowed by

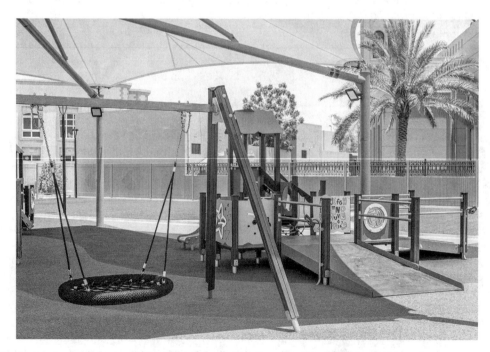

Figure 10.7 Playground equipment can be adapted or built to be wheelchair accessible
© Bojani/Shutterstock.

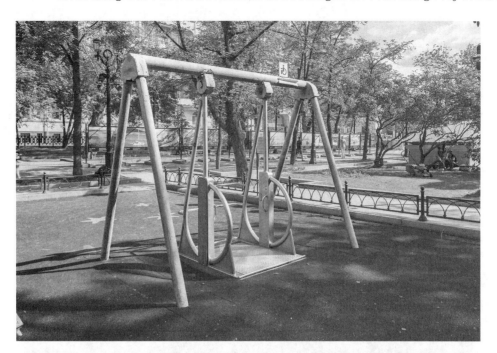

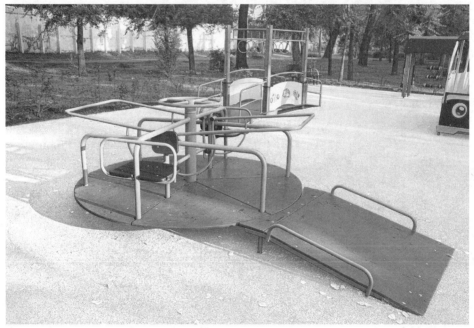

Figure 10.7 (Continued)

Top: © Studio MDF/Shutterstock; Bottom: © Beyger/Shutterstock.

district policy, typical peers may be added to sessions or brought into therapeutic play activities during naturally occurring events, such as recess. Likewise, students with special needs who have similar or associated occupational therapy goals can be grouped together to enhance play interactions.

In addition to being motivating and self-reinforcing, providing group therapy that focuses on play can help children deal with real-life contextual challenges (Brady, 2019). Group therapy allows for peer modeling, which is an important strategy to promote new learning (Egel et al., 1981; Werts et al., 1996).

In addition, students grow an appreciation for each other's needs and can support one another both in and outside therapy time. They can be each other's cheerleader when in occupational therapy sessions and each other's advocate in the classroom and on the playground. Please see **Figures 10.8** and **10.9** for illustrations of students with disabilities playing with nondisabled peers.

During naturally occurring play times, the therapist can encourage games with peers that are fun, yet accessible for the student. For example, the occupational therapy practitioner may bring in a special piece of

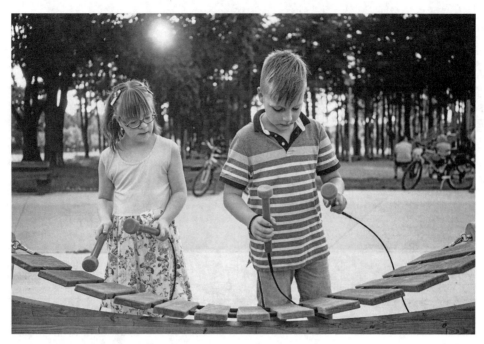

Figure 10.8 Typical peers can provide a model during play activities

© Vesnaandjic/E+/Getty Images.

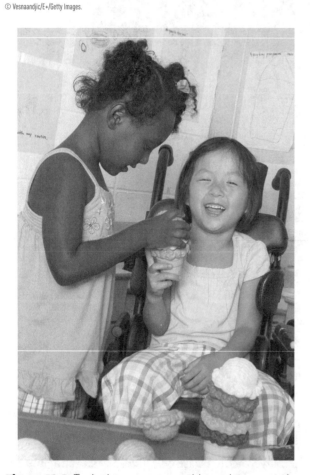

Figure 10.9 Typical peers can provide assistance and support for play

© ktaylorg/E+/Getty Images.

equipment or toy that other peers may find interesting. The therapist or child can recruit friends to participate and encourage the game to continue after the therapist leaves. For example, during a therapy session, the occupational therapist can begin a game of "four-square," during recess time and recruit others that want to play. That way, the focus of the play can be with peers while the occupational therapy practitioner supports the skills of the child and facilitates the group. It is important to let others, especially their typically developing peers, see the child's strengths shine through. It is also beneficial to let the other children in the classroom see how adaptations to play can be just as fun.

Taking On a Playful Style

While occupational therapy practitioners' interactive style during therapy in a school setting may involve a more directive role at times, it is important to try to elicit student independence, playfulness, and authentic responses through engagement in a real play experience (Cabrera et al., 2017; Tanta & Kuhaneck, 2020). You can demonstrate skills and foster imitation by being fun, playful, and encouraging. Model appropriate reactions that are typical consequences of various play scenarios. For example, when a student with a developmental coordination disorder struggles with how to move efficiently in a scooter board activity, do not be afraid to say, "I don't know, what should we do?" Laugh with the child and model a healthy response when a mistake is made and say, "Oops, oh, well! Get back on, and let's go!"

In promoting individualized and self-directed play, occupational therapy practitioners must consider their various roles with the child. This includes acknowledging the influence of adult presence, using an appropriate therapeutic style to engage children, and fostering a good "fit" in the therapeutic interaction (Glenn et al., 2013; Trawick-Smith & Dziurgot, 2011; Tsai, 2015). The therapist must be playful, yet establish boundaries for rules and behavior. You will need to choose, and be flexible with, the specific interpersonal modes that can support ongoing learning and enhance the therapeutic relationship with the child (Taylor, 2008). Please also see Chapter 6 for more specific information on this topic.

Encouraging New Play Interests

While supporting access to existing play activities, occupational therapy practitioners can also begin to encourage new interests. The introduction of novel, yet accessible activities helps to expand the child's play repertoire and potential social connections. After analyzing the performance, social, and contextual aspects of various activities, the therapist may explore creative ways to engage the child. The occupational therapy practitioner can generate new aspects of play or develop new play activities based on activity analysis, ongoing assessment of the child's skills, and creating the "just-right challenge" as depicted in **Practice Example 10.3**. However, it is important to collaborate on the development of these ideas, as differences may exist between therapist-developed play activities and existing modes or rules of play recognized by peers. Deviations that stray too far from typical peer games might impact a child's willingness to participate. Therefore, the occupational therapy practitioner must be sure to include the child's interests and preferences

when exposing students to and developing new play repertoires (Imms et al., 2009). Please also see Chapter 16 for more on this topic.

Ensuring Safety

When considering the match between a child and the various play activities available, one must ensure the safety of the child. Occupational therapy practitioners must acknowledge that children may want to engage in self-directed play that is not feasible or reasonably safe for them. This is particularly an issue at school, as there is the potential for peer pressure and threats to social status. It is important to find a balance between what a student chooses and what is safe. If the occupational therapy practitioner identifies limitations that exist, then modifications and adaptations can be implemented with safety in mind. Rules may need to be established around safe play, should the therapist identify a mismatch between the activity, the environment, and the child's choices, interests, and abilities (Richardson, 2019). Guidance regarding safe play can be instituted class- or schoolwide to universally protect all students, regardless of a disability. However, there must be a balance between ensuring safety and avoiding significant injury, and removing all risk and choice from a child's play.

Allowing Choice

By allowing some level of choice throughout the therapy session, you can enhance the playful aspect of therapy. Let the child choose between activities (or

---

PRACTICE EXAMPLE 10.3 Matching Play Interests and Needs at School

Emily, a new occupational therapy practitioner, started a job in a general education elementary school. Upon receiving her caseload in the beginning of the year, she realized that she had several fourth- and fifth-grade students with various physical and social-emotional needs. Emily enthusiastically began developing intervention plans, eagerly incorporating play into each of her activities.

Emily developed a modified game of soccer, which would allow for her students to participate and achieve a level of mastery. She introduced the idea to a small group of her students, but quickly discovered that there was some resistance to participation. The students argued that this was not the way soccer is played on the playground and that no one would want to change the rules. Emily encouraged the students to participate despite their complaints, certain that the skills that they would learn in therapy would carry over to real play. She reasoned that by learning to play with modifications, the students' skills would improve so that they could better access recess with their peers. However, the students quickly became disengaged, and Emily found it difficult to establish therapeutic rapport.

Emily then decided to create a completely different game that addressed her students' needs and was accessible to them. She designed a modified Quidditch game (a fictional sport from the *Harry Potter* series), which could be introduced to her students and, eventually, brought to the playground. This novel game, while applying some of the same skills used in her modified soccer game, had different rules and materials. Emily figured that this would present a new opportunity for play that their peers might accept on the playground. Her students loved the idea, were excited for therapy sessions, and could not wait to teach the other kids at recess how to play. Emily was able to help her students achieve their therapeutic objectives and established a lasting and meaningful bond with them.

parts of an activity) and then expand on their choices to tailor their choice toward the goals you wish to work on. This can offer you an opportunity to assess or intervene in something new with the student. It also provides a sense of control for the child in the play experience. Choice can be embedded in therapy sessions by allowing students to pick between play options, elaborate in the activity, or decide when certain aspects of the play should terminate.

Promoting Generalization of Play Skills

Occupational therapy practitioners must consider the practicality of play skills that are emphasized in therapy and how these skills can be generalized to a child's real play outside of therapy. Occupational therapy practitioners teach skills and strategies to improve participation. However, once children leave the occupational therapy session, they ultimately must be able to use these techniques and skills independently with peers or with other supports.

To promote generalization, occupational therapy practitioners should attempt to use the same play equipment, rules, and terminology that exists in the child's world. Taking advantage of those opportunities will help the child apply skills and techniques outside of occupational therapy sessions (Clark & Hollenbeck, 2019).

It is important that therapists recognize the applicability of certain strategies and ensure that they do not create unnecessary dependence on others, particularly adults (Swinth & Tanta, 2008). This could inhibit natural play or reflect poorly on the child in the eyes of peers. To enhance generalization of skills, occupational therapy practitioners should also focus on educating the team members on this concept. Those that interact with the child can be coached on the appropriate level of support without being overly prescriptive, accommodating, or invasive. Ultimately, time spent in collaboration with the team will enhance carryover and teacher satisfaction and improve student outcomes (Sayers, 2008).

Using Natural School Contexts for Play

As described previously, recess, indoor play, and extracurricular activities provide natural contexts in which play can occur. Often these are missed opportunities for play. Addressing the range of natural play contexts is an important tool for countering limited opportunities for play in school and in school-based occupational therapy.

Although individual circumstances and IEP objectives may lead to an intervention plan that requires treatment using both real and simulated play within a designated therapy space, working in the natural context is ideal (AOTA, 2017; Anaby et al., 2019). Occupational therapy services in the natural school context may be provided as a "push-in" service within the classroom, recess, or other play opportunities during the school day. It allows the therapist to create strategies and provide support as the need arises. Working in natural environments also allows for ongoing assessment and may ignite new ideas for play. The occupational therapy practitioner can observe real games, rules, and roles played by peers and help establish new ones that include the student. Providing services in the natural environment also gives the occupational therapy practitioner an opportunity to engage peers in play with the child.

Intervening for Play During Recess.

Recess is a primary vehicle of play in the schools and represents the natural environment where the therapist can take on a playful approach; consider the balance between safety, risks, and choice; and promote generalization of occupational therapy into naturally occurring play with peers. Although recess is a perfect location for occupational therapy services for many children, it is also a portion of the school day that is threatened and declining despite its many benefits.

There is limited research on occupational therapy intervention during recess with the exception of the Sydney Playground Project (Bundy et al., 2011, 2017), which includes both child-based and adult-based interventions on student's physical activity, social skills, and play. This 13-week program consists of the introduction of unstructured play materials on the playground for children to use (such as car tires, milk crates, and cardboard boxes) and a parent and teacher workgroup focusing on their perceptions of play and reframing the concept of children's healthy risk taking. Results indicated increases in the amount and duration of physical activity, along with reduced sedentary activity.

Bundy et al. (2008) described these "loose parts or scrounge" play materials as readily available, nonconventional play items. Access to these objects on the playground led to reports of more social, creative, active, and resilient children. In addition, the team found a significant increase in playfulness. In this study, creativity, rather than physical ability, was highlighted, making this quite appealing for schools. Individuals with disabilities were able to access and be included in this play during recess, just like their typically developing peers. The researchers recognized these outcomes as a demonstration of the potential role of occupational therapists in providing intervention during recess.

Loose parts play programs have also been attempted in schools in the United States, but data collection has been limited to date (Borges et al., 2020; Hoover, Qu, & Wilkinson, 2019). In these small-scale programs, however, the play of the children on the playground became more creative, active, and interactive. This is an area of potential growth for occupational therapy in the schools, but one that needs more research.

Intervening During Indoor Play.
The variety and availability of toys, games, and other materials within the classroom are important to analyze (Wachs, 1985). Therapists can do an inventory of what types of toys each classroom has and promote sharing between rooms, depending on the profile of students in each room. They can also advocate for the purchase of new materials, should the availability of accessible toys be limited. Having appropriate materials for indoor recess can improve physical activity and engagement (Novak, 2000; Segura-Martínez et al., 2020; Verstraete et al., 2006).

Therapists can also help remove barriers to navigating the smaller, and possibly more cluttered, environment to create play spaces that promote imagination and creativity. Movement and physical activity may be limited or restricted during indoor play (Tran et al., 2013). However, if outdoor play is not possible, this may be students' only opportunity for physical activity. Occupational therapy practitioners can support teachers by providing materials, resources, and activities to enhance movement during indoor play and breaks (Erwin et al., 2013; Khorana et al., 2019; Lodewyk & McNamara, 2019; Novak, 2000; Pawlowski et al., 2021; Scudieri & Schwager, 2017; Verstraete et al., 2006). Children's yoga, hula hoop, and dance activities may be a fun way to incorporate movement without using too much space. Occupational therapy practitioners have insight that can be shared with teachers to make indoor play more appropriate, accessible, and meaningful to students.

Intervening During Extracurricular Activities.
Occupational therapy practitioners can provide feedback on extracurricular program goals and lesson plans, observe the space and materials, and talk with program directors regarding possible barriers to participation. If the child is already enrolled and attending, and depending on district policies, the occupational therapy practitioner can observe performance within these programs to help provide more targeted support. While occupational therapy services may not extend beyond the school day, skills developed in therapy and the provision of environmental modifications and strategies can enhance participation in OST and help districts meet legal mandates for access and inclusion in these programs.

Providing Schoolwide Supports.
Through the MTSS framework, occupational therapy practitioners play a role in providing system supports to districts, schools, and classrooms as a whole. Team collaborations may include planning for and providing high-quality instruction within the classroom, universal screening, progress monitoring, and data-informed decision making following a system of tiers (Cahill, 2019). Under MTSS, Tier 1 focuses on schoolwide and whole classroom supports. This may involve educating teams about play development (Kelly-Vance & Ryalls, 2020). Enrichment and promotion of play skills at Tier 1 can include providing evidence-based resources to the team, purchasing materials, problem solving, establishing and scheduling appropriate times for play, aid in home carryover, and helping with designing accessible playgrounds. Occupational therapists can be part of creating a schoolwide peer-to-peer program (Ziegler, Matthews, Mayberry, Owen-DeSchryver, & Carter, 2020) that, although primarily meant to foster inclusion, can also be a vehicle for promoting play between younger peers and leisure for older students. The staff who form these programs identify possible activities such as school clubs, field trips, or other school events that students with and without disabilities can participate in together on a regular basis. If selected properly, the activities can also foster play.

Social and emotional learning (SEL) is a process that complements and refines the MTSS and PBIS frameworks (CASEL, 2018). It is a schoolwide, systematic approach that integrates social and emotional skill development into all aspects of instruction in the schools. Engagement in play reinforces the foundational aspects of SEL, which include self-awareness, self-management, responsible decision making, relationship skills, and social awareness. Occupational therapy practitioners can support schools by promoting accessible play as a means to integrate and practice SEL and enhance equitable outcomes for all.

Advocating for Play at School

Although academic priorities, limited opportunities, and reductions in recess time create obstacles that can hinder occupational therapy practitioners in fully embracing play at school, these barriers are not insurmountable. When occupational therapy providers take on their roles as advocates, they can make meaningful changes in improving the quality of practice and opportunities for play. By providing education and team collaboration, occupational therapy practitioners can promote play on a systems level, reaching as many children as possible. In this way, school occupational therapy practitioners become ambassadors of play and may even take on policy change beyond the school walls (see Chapter 2 for more information on Becoming a Play Ambassador).

Promoting Inclusive Play at School.

Occupational therapy practitioners can advocate for change by informing others about the significance of play both as an end and a means (Swinth & Tanta, 2008). This includes educating specific stakeholders such as school administrators, general and special education teachers, paraprofessionals, parents/caretakers, and other IEP team members. You can communicate the importance of play in the schools by sharing resources and research related to how it impacts cognition, language, social-emotional skills, and executive functioning (Council on School Health et al., 2013; Yogman et al., 2018). You can educate them on the areas of advanced knowledge and life skills developed in play, such as the art of negotiation, tolerance, and the foundation of democracy (Hyndman, 2017a). You might include information about modern teaching methods that capitalize on play to create learning environments that move beyond content and emphasize innovation, critical thinking, and communication (Golinkoff & Hirsh-Pasek, 2016; Yogman et al., 2018). Also, you can also provide current literature and initiatives on the benefits of recess and physical activity (Council on School Health et al., 2013; Richardson, 2019). When schools understand the relationship of play to academics, they are more likely to prioritize play as well.

Advocacy also can happen in larger forums to address a greater number of people at once. You can ask the school administrator for permission to provide an in-service during after-school parent groups and at staff meetings. If time is limited during these meetings, you can do a series of mini-workshops across time. And if those forums are not available, you can provide teacher handouts and tip sheets on the benefits and development of play that they can read on their own (see **Box 10.2** for resources). Peruse local parent and teacher groups on social media to determine if these platforms are appropriate for sharing resources related to play. In addition, the occupational therapy practitioner can provide workshops on play to families after school hours.

Box 10.2 Resources for Play Advocacy

AOTA. (2011). *Building Play Skills for Healthy Children & Families*.

- https://www.aota.org/-/media/Corporate/Files/AboutOT/consumers/Youth/Play/Building%20Play%20Skills%20Tip%20Sheet%20Final.pdf
- AOTA. (2012). *Learning Through Play*. https://www.aota.org/~/media/Corporate/Files/Practice/Children/Browse/Play/Learning%20Through%20Play%20tip%20sheet.pdf
- CDC. (2017). *Strategies for Recess in Schools*. https://www.cdc.gov/healthyschools/physicalactivity/pdf/2016_12_16_schoolrecessstrategies_508.pdf
- CDC. (2014). *State Indicator Report on Physical Activity*. https://www.cdc.gov/physicalactivity/downloads/PA_State_Indicator_Report_2014.pdf
- CDC. (2020a). *Developmental Milestones*. https://www.cdc.gov/ncbddd/actearly/milestones/index.html
- CDC. (2020b). *Overweight and Obesity*. https://www.cdc.gov/obesity/index.html
- Project Zero—the Pedagogy of Play. Pedagogy of Play | Project Zero (harvard.edu)
- Blog about Playful Learning. The Pedagogy of Play blog (popatplay.org)
- U.S. Play Coalition. (2020). https://usplaycoalition.org/
- LiiNK Project. https://liinkproject.tcu.edu/
- Playworks. https://www.playworks.org/
- Peaceful Playgrounds. https://peacefulplaygrounds.com/
- *Guide to Indoor Recess*. https://www.playworks.org/resource/recess-rain-snow/

This will reinforce the importance of play and the breadth of the occupational therapy profession. By educating families, in time, you may find that conversations about play are more common and program planning in the schools includes more discussion about play.

Advocate for Additional Play Options and Opportunities.

Occupational therapy practitioners can recommend possible ways to incorporate opportunities for play throughout the school day in various contexts. You can work with administrators and teachers to brainstorm scheduled play breaks. You can also help educators identify alternatives to removing outdoor play and recess as a behavioral or academic consequence (Bento & Dias, 2017; Council on School Health et al., 2013).

Occupational therapy practitioners can support students by advocating with the team for adapting and modifying schoolwide play activities, materials, and the environment. For example, you might help to identify alternative options for play at recess, such as board games for children who lack gross motor skills. You can teach the teams how to incorporate universal design and accessible play in their classrooms. Additionally, you can work with the school administrator to assess the environment and identify barriers imposed by the current playground space and equipment. Because playground designers often lack knowledge of the needs of children with disabilities and how to create accessible spaces (Woolley, 2013), occupational therapy practitioners can be consultants on the development of inclusive and accessible playgrounds at school. You can help seek funding through grants or budgets with the town parks and recreation departments. Once the green light is given, occupational therapy practitioners can help schools purchase appropriate equipment that promotes play for students with and without disabilities so that everyone can play together.

Advocate for Changes to Internal Policies.
Occupational therapists can also advocate for the alteration of policies and rules that restrict free play opportunities for the greater ease of behavior management or in the quest for student safety by reducing all risk. For example, many young children seek movement opportunities such as hanging upside down, going down slides head first, or climbing up the slides. These activities are typically forbidden at recess. However, the occupational therapist could advocate for safe ways to incorporate these types of activities at certain times or with certain types of active adult guidance. The therapist might also advocate for changes to the playground to improve safety, thereby allowing students more freedom to move in their desired ways during free play at recess.

Promoting Play Through External Policy Change.
Advocacy can extend beyond the walls of the school. Occupational therapy practitioners can consider policy change within their local communities and statewide. First, you can identify which person, system, and organizations are influential. Are there already existing groups that are involved in the conversation? Are there people who could create some leverage and possibly assist in gaining access to funding, grants, or policy change? Stay connected to specific legislation that supports recess, access to physical activity, and childhood obesity initiatives. If there are specific bills that support play in schools, ask your legislators to support them. You can visit your local and state politicians' websites to see if they have already shown support of the bill. And do not

forget to leave your name and contact information so that you can be a resource to them.

You can also work with your state occupational therapy organizations and their lobbyists to express concern with access to play, recess, and outdoor time; spread interest; gain insight to emerging policies and barriers; and possibly start a task force that promotes play in schools. In addition, you can align policy strategies with community health priorities (Hyndman, 2017c). Do not be afraid to work with communities, legislators, and organizations, share the role of occupational therapy, and target specific ways in which play can be enhanced for all children and youth.

Advocacy Through Modeling.
The best way to advocate for change is to practice what you preach. Therefore, it is important that occupational therapy practitioners have a foundation in play theory, development, and practice. When a therapist offers informed support within the classroom, teachers and other team members will recognize the value of those strategies (Schefkind, 2019). Teams will become familiar with play as an occupation and area of our expertise once occupational therapy practitioners make it a part of the discussion and program (see **Practice Example 10.4**). In order to be a visionary and influence a shift in practice, occupational therapy practitioners need to prepare to be good advocates of play. A clear starting point is self-educating on integrating play in practice. It is important to attend courses on play, examine appropriate play assessment tools, and seek mentorship from more experienced therapists in play (Couch et al., 1998; Kuhaneck et al., 2013; Tanta & Kuhaneck, 2020).

Conclusion

Occupational therapy practitioners consider students' participation in all actual and possible contexts of play within the schools. In order for students to expand their play, occupational therapy practitioners assess, plan, provide various levels of direct intervention, and offer suggestions for promoting accessible and individualized play so that children can engage as freely as possible. Therapists can seize missed opportunities for play at school through addressing recess, indoor play, and extracurricular activities. To overcome powerful institutional barriers to incorporating play in the school setting, advocacy is prioritized. By embracing our full role with play in schools, occupational therapy practitioners help students engage and enjoy learning and promote the skills and abilities they will need for their future.

PRACTICE EXAMPLE 10.4 Educating About Play Through Doing Play

Regan is an occupational therapy practitioner who works in a specialized school providing intensive support to individuals with intellectual disabilities. On her caseload is Paul, a nonverbal, 6-year-old diagnosed with autism spectrum disorder, intellectual disability, and a seizure disorder.

Due to unforeseen circumstances, Regan was charged to deliver school-based, telehealth services for a duration of time. She saw this as a chance for his team to assess how play is incorporated at home. During their first virtual therapy session, Regan saw that Paul's mother was visibly distressed and struggling to get her son to sit down in front of the computer. She complained, "Everything is a fight with him. He only wants to do his own thing." This was a clear opportunity to educate his mother on the importance of play and getting down into the child's world. Regan calmed Paul's mother by letting her know that "it's okay" and asked if she could bring the computer screen to the floor where he played. Regan had worked with Paul for several months and knew that she could reach him by imitating his actions and letting him lead. It was important that they connected with him by being a part of his natural play and interests so that they could eventually expand on them. While Paul played with cars, so did Regan. They sang, made noises, and laughed together. Regan found that exaggerated noises and facial expressions also helped to engage Paul through the computer screen. She shared with his mother that it is okay that he doesn't sit at a table for therapy sessions. It's more important that he learns and is engaged.

Within the first couple of telehealth therapy sessions, Regan and Paul's mother completed an interest and toy inventory of the household via interview to examine what would be appropriate for his skill level and to encourage variety in play. Through that process, Regan found that the family's dog was highly motivating and comforting to Paul. Their dog was able to be used during sessions, emphasizing how play can be used therapeutically. Regan began to discuss how to use play to address his IEP objectives of using "gentle hands," taking turns, increasing duration of appropriate play, and using his communication device. She urged his mother to highlight and reinforce these concepts and skills more authentically while he's playing. Regan suggested that she could teach "gentle hands" by petting their dog softly and recognizing the positive response of the dog such as commenting on how the dog likes gentle hands. She could guide Paul to use his communication device to ask for help, request a turn, and label items. Also, she could present alternative actions and materials to expand his play repertoire. This coaching model helped empower Paul's mother. She expressed how relieved she felt having had this knowledge, after feeling ashamed for so many years for not being able to "control" her child. Educating families on the importance of play can help them feel powerful in the therapeutic process and as part of the educational team.

References

Agran, M., Dymond, S., Rooney-Kron, M., & Martin, J. (2020). Examining whether student participation in school-sponsored extracurricular activities is represented in IEPs. *Intellectual and Developmental Disabilities*, 58(6), 472–485.

Agran, M., Wojcik, A., Cain, I., Thoma, C., Achola, E., Austin, K. M., … Tamura, R. B. (2017). Participation of students with intellectual and developmental disabilities in extracurricular activities: Does inclusion end at 3:00? *Education and Training in Autism and Developmental Disabilities*, 52(1), 3–12.

Alcott, A. B. (1861). *Superintendent's report of the Concord Schools to the school committee, for the year 1860–61.* https://concordlibrary.org/CFPL/anteBellumDocs/reports/pages/1861/schoolSuperReport/page_21.html

American Occupational Therapy Association (AOTA). (2011). *Building play skills for healthy children & families.* https://www.aota.org/About-Occupational-Therapy/Patients-Clients/ChildrenAndYouth/Building-Play-Skills-Healthy.aspx?gclid=Cj0KCQjw5auGBhDEARIsAFyNm9FI2lzDcJ7i2QHEkp8F-ozWJeTw4DoGsNGXIw29WK6ExK1m2yreF3caApxzEALw_wcB

American Occupational Therapy Association (AOTA). (2012). *Learning through play.* https://www.aota.org/About-Occupational-Therapy/Patients-Clients/ChildrenAndYouth/Play.aspx

American Occupational Therapy Association (AOTA). (2017). Guidelines for occupational therapy services in early intervention and schools. *American Journal of Occupational Therapy*, 71(Suppl. 2), 7112410010. https://doi.org/10.5014/ajot.2017.716S01

American Occupational Therapy Association (AOTA). (2020). Occupational therapy practice framework: Domain and process (4th ed.). *American Journal of Occupational Therapy*, 74. https://doi.org/10.5014/ajot.2020.74S2001

Anaby, D. R., Campbell, W. N., Missiuna, C., Shaw, S. R., Bennett, S., Khan, S.,… & GOLDs (Group for Optimizing Leadership and Delivering Services). (2019). Recommended practices to organize and deliver school-based services for children with disabilities: A scoping review. *Child: Care, Health, and Development*, 45(1), 15–27.

Ball, M. A. (2018). Revitalizing the OT role in school-based practice: Promoting success for all students. *Journal of Occupational Therapy, Schools, & Early Intervention*, 11(3), 263–272. https://doi.org/10.1080/19411243.1445059

Barros, R. M., Silver, E. J., & Stein, R. E. (2009). School recess and group classroom behavior. *Pediatrics*, 123(2), 431–436. https://doi.org/10.1542/peds.2007-2825

Bassok, D., Latham, S., & Rorem, A. (2016). Is kindergarten the new first grade? *Aera Open*, 2(1), 1–31. https://doi.org/10.1177/2332858415616358

Bauml, M., Patton, M. M., & Rhea, D. (2020). A qualitative study of teachers' perceptions of increased recess time on teaching, learning, and behavior. *Journal of Research in Childhood Education*, 1–15. https://doi.org/10.1080/02568543.2020.1718808

Bento, G., & Dias, G. (2017). The importance of outdoor play for young children's healthy development. *Porto Biomedical Journal*, 2(5), 157–160. http://dx.doi.org/10.1016/j.pbj.2017.03.003

Besio, S., & Amelina, N. (2017). Play in children with physical impairment. In S. Besio, D. Bulgarelli, & V. Stancheva-Popkostadinova (Eds.), *Play development in children with disabilities* (pp. 120–136). Warsaw: De Gruyter.

Bills, K. L. (2020). The direct relationship between bullying rates and extracurricular activities among adolescents and teenagers with disabilities. *Journal of Evidence-Based Social Work*, 17(2), 191–202.

Borges, K., Denny, G., Desai, R., Donato, L., Funaro, R., Wilkinson, K., & Miller Kuhaneck, H. (2020). Reimagining recess. ConnOTA Annual Conference. https://www.researchgate.net/profile/Heather-Miller-Kuhaneck

Brady, E. (2019). Best practices in providing group interventions to support participation. In G. F. Clark, J. E. Rioux, & B. E. Chandler (Eds.), *Best practices for occupational therapy in schools* (2nd ed., pp. 349–355). Bethesda, MD: AOTA Press.

Brockman, R., Jago, R., & Fox, K. R. (2011). Children's active play: Self-reported motivators, barriers, and facilitators. *MBC Public Health*, 11(461), 1–7. https://doi.org/10.1186/147-2458-11-461

Brooks, B. A., Floyd, F., Robins, D. L., & Chan, W. Y. (2015). Extracurricular activities and the development of social skills in children with intellectual and specific learning disabilities. *Journal of Intellectual Disability Research*, 59(7), 678–687.

Bundy, A. (1993). Assessment of play and leisure: Delineation of the problem. *American Journal of Occupational Therapy*, 47(3), 217–222. https://doi.org/10.5014/ajot.47.3.217

Bundy, A., Engelen, L., Wyver, S., Tranter, P., Ragen, J., Bauman, A., … Naughton, G. (2017). Sydney playground project: A cluster-randomized trial to increase physical activity, play, and social skills. *Journal of School Health*, 87(10), 751–759. https://doi.org/10.1111/josh.12550

Bundy, A. C., Luckett, T. Naughton, G. A., Tranter, P. J., Wyver, S. R., Ragen, J., … Spies, G. (2008). Playful interaction: Occupational therapy for all children on the school playground. *American Journal of Occupational Therapy*, 62, 522–527. https://doi.org/10.5014/ajot.62.5.522

Bundy, A. C., Naughton, G., Tranter, P., Wyver, S., Baur, L., Schiller, W., … Brentnall, J. (2011). The Sydney playground project: Popping the bubblewrap—unleashing the power of play: A cluster randomized controlled trial of a primary school playground-based intervention aiming to increase children's physical activity and social skills. *BMC Public Health*, 11, 680. https://doi.org//10.1186/1471-2458-11-680

Buttimer, J., & Tierney, E. (2005). Patterns of leisure participation among adolescents with a mild intellectual disability. *Journal of Intellectual Disabilities*, 9(1), 25–42. https://doi.org/10.1177/1744629505049728

Cabrera, N. J., Karberg, E., & Malin, J. L. (2017). The magic of play: Low-income mothers' and fathers' playfulness and children's emotion regulation and vocabulary skills. *Infant Mental Health Journal*, 36(6), 1–14. https://doi.org/10.1002/imhj.21682

Cahill, S. M. (2019). Best practices in multi-tiered systems of support. In G. F. Clark, J. E. Rioux, & B. E. Chandler (Eds.), *Best practices for occupational therapy in schools* (2nd ed., pp. 211–217). Bethesda, MD: AOTA Press.

Campbell, L. (2019). Teachers withholding recess as punishment does more harm than good. *Healthline Parenthood*. https://www.healthline.com/health-news/why-are-teachers-punishing-kids-with-adhd-by-taking-away-recess

CASEL. (2018). Connecting schoolwide SEL with other school-based frameworks. https://schoolguide.casel.org/uploads/2019/01/SEL_MTSS-and-PBIS.pdf

Case-Smith, J., & Kuhaneck, H. M. (2008). Play preferences of typically developing children and children with developmental delays between ages 3 and 7 years. *Occupation, Participation, and Health*, 28(1), 19–29. https://doi.org/10.3928/15394492-20080101-01

Centers for Disease Control and Prevention (CDC). (2014). *State indicator report on physical activity*. https://www.cdc.gov/physicalactivity/downloads/PA_State_Indicator_Report_2014.pdf

Centers for Disease Control and Prevention (CDC). (2015). *Results from the school health policies and practices study 2014*. https://www.cdc.gov/healthyyouth/data/shpps/pdf/shpps-508-final_101315.pdf

Centers for Disease Control (CDC). (2017). *Strategies for recess in schools*. https://www.cdc.gov/healthyschools/physicalactivity/pdf/2016_12_16_schoolrecessstrategies_508.pdf

Centers for Disease Control and Prevention (CDC). (2019). *Out of school time supports student health and learning*. https://www.cdc.gov/healthyschools/ost.htm#:~:text=Out%20of%20School%20Time%20(OST,j275school%20is%20not%20in%20session

Centers for Disease Control and Prevention (CDC). (2020a). CDC's developmental milestones. https://www.cdc.gov/ncbddd/actearly/milestones/index.html

Centers for Disease Control and Prevention (CDC). (2020b). Overweight & obesity. https://www.cdc.gov/obesity/index.html

Centers for Disease Control and Prevention (CDC). (n.d.). *Recess*. https://www.cdc.gov/healthyschools/physicalactivity/recess.htm

Chan, C., Dennis, D., Kim, S. J., & Jankowski, J. (2017). An integrative review of school-based mental health interventions for elementary students: Implications for occupational therapy. *Occupational Therapy in Mental Health*, 33(1), 81–101. https://www.researchgate.net/deref/http%3A%2F%2Fdx.doi.org%2F10.1080%2F0164212X.2016.1202804

Clark, G. F., & Hollenbeck, J. (2019). Best practices in school occupational therapy interventions to support participation. In G. F. Clark, J. E. Rioux, & B. E. Chandler (Eds.), *Best practices for occupational therapy in schools* (2nd ed., pp. 341–348). Bethesda, MD: AOTA Press.

Clark, L. E., & Rhea, D. J. (2017). The LiiNK Project®: Comparisons of recess, physical activity, and positive emotional states in grades K–2 children. *International Journal of Child Health and Nutrition*, 6(2), 54–61. http://dx.doi.org/10.6000/1929-4247.2017.06.02.1

Clifford, J. M., & Bundy, A. C. (1989). Play preference and play performance in normal boys and boys with sensory integrative dysfunction. *Occupational Therapy Journal of Research*, 9(4), 202–217. https://doi.org/10.1177/153944928900900402

Colman, W. (1988). The evolution of occupational therapy in the public schools: The laws mandating practice. *American*

Journal of Occupational Therapy, *42*(11), 701–705. https://doi.org/10.5014/ajot.42.11.701

Conklin, H. G. (2014). Student learning in the middle school social studies classroom: The role of differing teacher preparation. *The Elementary School Journal*, *114*(4), 455–478.

Couch, K., Deitz, J. C., & Kanny, E. M. (1998). The role of play in pediatric occupational therapy. *American Journal of Occupational Therapy*, *52*, 111–117. https://doi.org/10.5014/ajot.52.2.111

Council on School Health, Murray, R., Ramstetter, C., Devore, C., Allison, M., Ancona, R., … & Young, T. (2013). The crucial role of recess in school. *Pediatrics*, *131*(1), 183–188. https://doi.org/10.1542/peds.2012-2993

Coutinho, M. J., & Hunter, D. L. (1988). Special education and occupational therapy: Making the relationship work. *American Journal of Occupational Therapy*, *42*(11), 706–712. https://doi.org/10.1177/153944928900900402

Desha, L. N., Ziviani, J., & Rodger, S. (2003). Play preferences and behavior of preschool children with autistic spectrum disorder in the clinical environment. *Physical & Occupational Therapy in Pediatrics*, *23*(1), 21–42. https://doi.org/10.1080/J006v23n01_03

Dominguez, A., Ziviani, J., & Rodger, S. (2006). Play behaviours and play object preferences of young children with autistic disorder in a clinical play environment. *Autism*, *10*(1), 53–69. https://doi.org/10.1177/1362361306062010

Dunn, W. (1988). Models of occupational therapy service provision in the school system. *American Journal of Occupational Therapy*, *42*(11), 718–723. https://doi.org/10.5014/ajot.42.11.718

Dymond, S. K., Rooney-Kron, M., Burke, M. M., & Agran, M. (2020). Characteristics of secondary age students with intellectual disability who participate in school-sponsored extracurricular activities. *The Journal of Special Education*, *54*(1), 51–62.

Egel, A. L., Richman, G. S., & Koegel, R. L. (1981). Normal peer models and autistic children's learning. *Journal of Applied Behavioral Analysis*, *14*(1), 3–12. https://doi.org/10.1901/jaba.1981.14-3

Erwin, H., Koufoudakis, R., & Beighle, A. (2013). Children's physical activity levels during indoor recess dance videos. *Journal of School Health*, *83*(5), 322–327.

Every Student Succeeds Act (ESSA). (2015). *20 U.S.C. § 6301, Pub. L. 114-95, Stat. 1802, S. 1177*. https://www.congress.gov/114/plaws/publ95/PLAW-114publ95.pdf

Fink, D. B., & Ramstetter, C. L. (2018). "Even if they're being bad, maybe they need a chance to run around": What children think about recess. *Journal of School Health*, *88*(12), 928–935.

Frost, J., & Sutterby, J. A. (2017). Our proud heritage: Outdoor play is essential to whole child development. *Young Children*, *72*(3), 82–85. https://www.naeyc.org/resources/pubs/yc/jul2017/outdoor-play-child-development

Ginsburg, K. (2007). The importance of play in promoting healthy child development and maintaining strong parent-child bonds. *Pediatrics*, *119*(1), 182–191. https://doi.org/10.1542/peds.2006-2697

Glenn, N. M., Knight, C. J., Holt, N. L., & Spence, J. C. (2013). Meanings of play among children. *Childhood*, *20*(2), 185–199. https://doi.org/10.1177/0907568212454751

Golinkoff, R. M., & Hirsh-Pasek, K. (2016). *Becoming brilliant: What science tells us about raising successful children*. Washington, DC: APA Press. https://doi.org/10.1037/14917-000

Gray, P. (2014). *Free to learn: Why unleashing the instinct to play will make our children happier, more self-reliant, and better students for life*. New York: Basic Books.

Greutman, H. (2016). *Modification ideas of playground play for children. Growing hands-on kids*. https://www.growinghandsonkids.com/modification-ideas-playground-play-for-children.html

Haegele, J. A., Aigner, C., & Healy, S. (2020). Extracurricular activities and bullying among children and adolescents with disabilities. *Maternal and Child Health Journal*, *24*(3), 310–318.

Hamari, J., Shernoff, D. J., Rowe, E., Coller, B., Asbell-Clarke, J., & Edwards, T. (2016). Challenging games help students learn: An empirical study on engagement, flow and immersion in game-based learning. *Computers in Human Behavior*, *54*, 170–179. https://www.researchgate.net/deref/http%3A%2F%2Fdx.doi.org%2F10.1016%2Fj.chb.2015.07.045

Hoover, M., Qu, A., & Wilkinson, K. (2019). Reimagining recess! Retrieved from https://digitalcommons.ithaca.edu/cgi/viewcontent.cgi?article=1686&context=whalen

Hyndman, B. (2017a). School playgrounds as a place of learning. In B. Hyndman (Ed.), *Contemporary school playground strategies for healthy students* (pp. 23–36). Singapore: Springer.

Hyndman, B. (2017b). The state of playgrounds in Australian schools. In B. Hyndman (Ed.), *Contemporary school playground strategies for healthy students* (pp. 23–36). Singapore: Springer.

Hyndman, B. (2017c). Policy influences on students within school playgrounds. In B. Hyndman (Ed.), *Contemporary school playground strategies for healthy students* (pp. 85–91). Singapore: Springer.

Imms, C. (2008). Children with cerebral palsy participate: A review of the literature. *Disability and Rehabilitation*, *30*(24), 1867–1884. https://doi.org/10.1080/09638280701673542

Imms, C., Reilly, S., Carlin, J., & Dodd, K. J. (2009). Characteristics influencing participation of Australian children with cerebral palsy. *Disability and Rehabilitation*, *31*(26), 2204–2215. https://doi.org/10.3109/0963828090297106

Individuals with Disabilities Education Act (IDEA). (2004). *Final Regulations, § 300.34, (2006)*.

Individuals with Disabilities Education Act (IDEA). (2017). *§ 300.117 Non-academic settings*. Ed.gov. https://sites.ed.gov/idea/regs/b/b/300.117

Jarrett, O. (2013). *A research-based case for recess*. Clemson, SC: US Play Coalition.

Jarrett, O. S., Maxwell, D. M., Dickerson, C., Hoge, P., Davies, G., & Yetley, A. (1998). The impact of recess on classroom behavior: Group effects and individual differences. *Journal of Education Research*, *92*(2), 121–126. https://psycnet.apa.org/doi/10.1080/00220679809597584

Kelly-Vance, L., & Ryalls, B. O. (2020). Best practices in play assessment and intervention. In A. Thomas & J. Grimes (Eds.), *Best practices in school psychology V* (5th ed., pp. 549–560). Bethesda, MD: NASP. http://citeseerx.ist.psu.edu/viewdoc/download?doi=10.1.1.530.2447&rep=rep1&type=pdf

Kelly, C. M., Strauss, K., Arnold, J., & Stride, C. (2020). The relationship between leisure activities and psychological resources that support a sustainable career: The role of leisure seriousness and work-leisure similarity. *Journal of Vocational Behavior*, *117*, 103340.

Keskin, B. (2018). The myth of the well-known "solution" of push-down academics. *Journal of Family Strengths*, *18*(1), 10.

Khorana, P., Koch, P. A., Trent, R., Gray, H. L., Wolf, R. L., & Contento, I. R. (2019). The effects of wellness in the schools (WITS) on physical activity during recess in New York City public schools. *Physical Activity and Health*, *3*(1).

King, G., Petrenchik, T., Law, M., & Hurley, P. (2009). The enjoyment of formal and informal recreation and leisure activities: A comparison of school-aged children with and without physical disabilities. *International Journal of Disability, Development, and Education*, *56*(2), 109–130. https://doi .org/10.1080/10349120902868558

King, G., Chiarello, L. A., Ideishi, R., D'Arrigo, R., Smart, E., Ziviani, J., & Pinto, M. (2020). The nature, value, and experience of engagement in pediatric rehabilitation: perspectives of youth, caregivers, and service providers. *Developmental neurorehabilitation*, *23*(1), 18–30.

Kuhaneck, H. M., Spitzer, S. L., & Miller, E. (2010). *Activity analysis, creativity, and playfulness in pediatric occupational therapy: Making play just right*. Sudbury, MA: Jones & Bartlett Learning.

Kuhaneck, H. M., Tanta, K. J., Coombs, A. K., & Pannone, H. (2013). A survey of pediatric occupational therapists' use of play. *Journal of Occupational Therapy, Schools, and Early Intervention*, *6*(3), 213–227. https://doi.org/10.1080/194112 43.2013.850940

Lodewyk, K., & McNamara, L. (2019). Recess enjoyment, affect, and preferences by gender and developmental level in elementary school. *Journal of Teaching in Physical Education*, *39*(3), 360–373.

Maciver, D., Rutherford, M., Arakelyan, S., Kramer, J. M., Richmond, J., Todorova, L.,... & Forsyth, K. (2019). Participation of children with disabilities in school: A realist systematic review of psychosocial and environmental factors. *PloS One*, *14*(1), e0210511.

Mahar, M. T. (2011). Impact of short bouts of physical activity on attention-to-task in elementary school children. *Preventive Medicine*, *52*, S60–S64. https://doi.org/10.1016/j .ypmed.2011.01.026

Mahoney, J. L., Cairns, B. D., & Farmer, T. W. (2003). Promoting interpersonal competence and educational success through extracurricular activity participation. *Journal of Educational Psychology*, *95*(2), 409–418. https://doi.org/10.1037/0022 -0663.95.2.409

Majnemer, A., Shevell, M., Law, M., Birnbaum, R., Chilingaryan, G., Rosenbaum, P., & Poulin, C. (2008). Participation and enjoyment of leisure activities in school-aged children with cerebral palsy. *Developmental Medicine and Child Neurology*, *50*(10), 751–758. https://doi.org/10.1111/j.1469 -8749.2008.03068.x

Martin, H., Farrell, A., Gray, J., & Clark, T. B. (2018). Perceptions of the effect of recess on kindergartners. *Physical Educator*, *75*(2), 245–254. https://doi.org/10.18666/TPE-2018-V75-I2-7740

Michael, S. L., Merlo, C. L., Basch, C. E., Wentzel, K. R., & Wechsler, H. (2015). Critical connections: Health and academics. *Journal of School Health*, *85*(11), 740–758. https:// doi.org/10.1111/josh.12309

Moore, M., & Sabo-Risley, C. (2018). Our proud heritage: Sowing the seeds of hope for today: Remembering the life and work of Susan Blow. *Young Children*, *73*(5). https://www .naeyc.org/resources/pubs/yc/nov2018/remembering-life -work-susan-blow

Novak, D. E. (2000). *Help! It's an indoor recess day*. Thousand Oaks, CA: Corwin Press.

Oberle, E., Ji, X. R., Magee, C., Guhn, M., Schonert-Reichl, K. A., & Gadermann, A. M. (2019). Extracurricular activity profiles and wellbeing in middle childhood: A population-level study. *PLoS One*, *14*(7), e0218488.

Ottenbacher, K. (1982). Occupational therapy and special education: Some issues and concerns related to Public Law 94-142. *American Journal of Occupational Therapy*, *36*(2), 81– 84. https://doi.org/10.5014/ajot.36.2.81

Palmer, A. N., Elliott III, W., & Cheatham, G. A. (2017). Effects of extracurricular activities on postsecondary completion for students with disabilities. *The Journal of Educational Research*, *110*(2), 151–158.

Parker, R., & Thomsen, B. S. (2019). *Learning through play at school. A study of playful integrated pedagogies that foster children's holistic skills development in the primary school classroom*. [White paper]. Billund, Denmark: The LEGO Foundation, 75.

Pawlowski, C. S., Nielsen, J. V., & Schmidt, T. (2021). A ban on smartphone usage during recess increased children's physical activity. *International Journal of Environmental Research and Public Health*, *18*(4), 1907.

Payne, S., Ward, G., Turner, A., Taylor, M. C., & Bark, C. (2013). The social impact of living with developmental coordination disorder as a 13-year-old. *British Journal of Occupational Therapy*, *76*(8), 362–369.

Peaceful Playgrounds. (n.d.). *Peaceful playgrounds*. Retrieved from https://peacefulplaygrounds.com/

Pellegrini, A. D. (1995). *School recess and playground behavior*. Albany: State University of New York. ED 379 095.

Pellegrini, A. D. (2008). The recess debate: A disjuncture between educational policy and scientific research. *American Journal of Play*, *1*(2), 181–191. https://psycnet.apa.org/doi/10.1007/978 -1-4939-0623-9_12

Pellegrini, A. D., & Bjorklund, D. F. (1997). The role of recess in children's cognitive performance. *Educational Psychologist*, *32*(1), 35–40. https://www.researchgate.net/deref/http %3A%2F%2Fdx.doi.org%2F10.1207%2Fs15326985ep3201 _3https://doi.org/10.1207/s15326985ep3201_3

Pellegrini, A. D., & Bohn, C. M. (2005). The role of recess in children's cognitive performance and school adjustment. *Educational Researcher*, *34*(1), 13–19. https://www .researchgate.net/deref/http%3A%2F%2Fdx.doi.org%2F10.3 102%2F0013189X034001013

Pellegrini, A. D., & Davis, P. L. (1993). Relations between children's playground and classroom behaviour. *British Journal of Educational Psychology*, *63*(1), 88–95. https://doi .org/10.1111/j.2044-8279.1993.tb01043.x

Pellegrini, A. D., Huberty, P. D., & Jones, I. (1995). The effects of recess timing on children's playground and classroom behaviors. *American Educational Research Journal*, *32*(4), 845–864. EJ 520 960. https://www.researchgate.net/deref /http%3A%2F%2Fdx.doi.org%2F10.2307%2F1163338

Play England. (2009). *Playable space quality assessment tool*. http://www.playengland.org.uk/media/211694/quality-assessment-tool.pdf

Playworks. (n.d.). Playworks.org. https://www.playworks.org/

Qian, M., & Clark, K. R. (2016). Game-based learning and 21st century skills: A review of recent research. *Computers in Human Behavior*, 63, 50–58. https://www.researchgate.net/deref/http%3A%2F%2Fdx.doi.org%2F10.1016%2Fj.chb.2016.05.023

Ramstetter, C. L., & Fink, D. B. (2019). Ready for recess? The elementary school teacher's perspective. *American Educator*, 42(4), 34–37.

Ramstetter, C., & Murray, R. (2017). Time to play: Recognizing the benefits of recess. *American Educator*, 41(1), 17. https://www.aft.org/ae/spring2017/ramstetter_and_murray

Ray-Kaeser, S., & Lynch, H. (2017). Occupational therapy perspective on play for the sake of play. In S. Besio, D. Bulgarelli, & V. Stancheva-Popkostadinova (Eds.), *Play development in children with disabilities* (pp. 155–165). Warsaw: De Gruyter.

Rhea, D., & Bauml, M. (2018). An innovative whole child approach to learning: The LiiNK Project®. *Childhood Education*, 94(2), 56–63.

Rhea, D. J., & Rivchun, A. P. (2018). The LiiNK Project®: Effects of multiple recesses and character curriculum on classroom behaviors and listening skills in grades K–2 children. *Frontiers in Education*, 3, 9.

Richardson, E. (2019). Best practices in play, leisure, and extracurricular skills to enhance participation. In G. F. Clark, J. E. Rioux, & B. E. Chandler (Eds.), *Best practices for occupational therapy in schools* (2nd ed., pp. 429–436). Bethesda, MD: AOTA Press.

Sanborn, F., & Harris W. T (1893). *A. Bronson Alcott: His life and philosophy* (Vol. 2). Cambridge, MA: University Press. https://babel.hathitrust.org/cgi/pt?id=mdp.39015037048538&view=1up&seq=13

Saporo, A. V. (1989). Joseph Lee. In H. Ibrahim (Ed.), *Pioneers in leisure and recreation* (pp. 65–76). Reston, VA: American Alliance for Health, Physical Education, Recreation and Dance. https://files.eric.ed.gov/fulltext/ED308157.pdf

Sayers, B. R. (2008). Collaboration in school settings: A critical appraisal of the topic. *Journal of Occupational Therapy, Schools, and Early Intervention*, 1(2), 170–179. https://doi.org/10.1080/19411240802384318

Schefkind, S. (2019). Best leadership practices through everyday advocacy. In G. F. Clark, J. E. Rioux, & B. E. Chandler (Eds.), *Best practices for occupational therapy in schools* (2nd ed., pp. 71–76). Bethesda, MD: AOTA Press.

Scudieri, D., & Schwager, S. (2017). Structured recess: Finding a way to make it work. *Journal of Physical Education, Recreation & Dance*, 88(4), 34–39.

Segura-Martínez, P., Molina-García, J., Queralt, A., del Mar Bernabé-Villodre, M., Martínez-Bello, D. A., & Martínez-Bello, V. E. (2020). An indoor physical activity area for increasing physical activity in the early childhood education classroom: An experience for enhancing young children's movement. *Early Childhood Education Journal*, 1–15.

Solish, A., Perry, A., & Minnes, P. (2010). Participation of children with and without disabilities in social, recreational, and leisure activities. *Journal of Applied Research in Intellectual Disabilities*, 23(3), 226–236. https://doi.org/10.1111/j.1468-3148.2009.00525.x

Stapp, A. C., & Karr, J. K. (2018). Effect of recess on fifth grade students' time on-task in an elementary classroom. *International Electronic Journal of Elementary Education*, 10(4), 449–456. https://doi.org/10.26822/iejee.2018438135

Swinth, Y., & Tanta, K. (2008). Play, leisure, and social participation in educational settings. In L. D. Parham & L. S. Fazio (Eds.), *Play in occupational therapy for children* (2nd ed., pp. 299–317). St. Louis, MO: Mosby Elsevier.

Tanta, K. J., & Kuhaneck, H. (2020). Assessment and treatment of play. In J. C. O'Brien & H. Kuhaneck (Eds.), *Case-Smith's occupational therapy for children and adolescents* (8th ed., pp. 239–266). St. Louis, MO: Elsevier.

Taylor, R. R. (2008). *The intentional relationship: Occupational therapy and use of self*. Philadelphia, PA: F. A. Davis.

Texas Christian University. (n.d.). *LiiNK*. https://liinkproject.tcu.edu/

Tran, I., Clark, B. R., & Racette, S. B. (2013). Physical activity during recess outdoors and indoors among urban public school students, St. Louis, Missouri, 2010–2011. *Preventing Chronic Disease*, 10, E196.

Trawick-Smith, J., & Dziurgot, T. (2011). "Good-fit" teacher–child play interactions and the subsequent autonomous play of preschool children. *Early Childhood Research Quarterly*, 26(1), 110–123. https://doi.org/10.1016/j.ecresq.2010.04.005

Tsai, C. Y. (2015). Am I interfering? Preschool teacher participation in children play. *Universal Journal of Educational Research*, 3(12), 1028–1033. https://doi.org/10.13189/ujer.2015.031212

U.S. Department of Education. (2013). *U. S. Department of Education clarifies schools' obligation to provide equal opportunity to students with disabilities to participate in extracurricular athletics*. https://www.ed.gov/news/press-releases/us-department-education-clarifies-schools-obligation-provide-equal-opportunity-s

U.S. Play Coalition. (n.d.). Usplaycoalition.org. https://usplaycoalition.org/

Verstraete, S. J., Cardon, G. M., De Clercq, D. L., & De Bourdeaudhuij, I. M. (2006). Increasing children's physical activity levels during recess periods in elementary schools: The effects of providing game equipment. *European Journal of Public Health*, 16(4), 415–419.

Voice of Play. (2018). 2018 Survey on recess. https://voiceofplay.org/2018-survey-recess/

Wachs, T. D. (1985). Toys as an aspect of the physical environment: Constraints and nature of relationship to development. *Topics in Early Childhood Special Education*, 5(3), 31–46. https://doi.org/10.1177/027112148500500304

Waite-Stupiansky, S., & Findlay, M. (2002). The fourth R: Recess and its link to learning. *The Educational Forum*, 66(1), 16–25. https://doi.org/10.1080/00131720108984795

Werts, M. G., Caldwell, N. K., & Wolery, M. (1996). Peer modeling of response chains: Observational learning by students with disabilities. *Journal of Applied Behavior Analysis*, 29(1), 53–66. https://psycnet.apa.org/doi/10.1901/jaba.1996.29-53

Woolley, H. (2013). Now being social: The barrier of designing outdoor play spaces for disabled children. *Children & Society*, 27(6), 448–458. https://doi.org/10.1111/j.1099-0860.2012.00464.x

Yogman, M., Garner, A., Hutchinson, J., Hirsh-Pasek, K., & Golinkoff, R. M. (2018). The power of play: A pediatric role in enhancing development in young children. *Pediatrics*, 142(3). https://doi.org/10.1542/peds.2018-2058

Ziegler, M., Matthews, A., Mayberry, M., Owen-DeSchryver, J., & Carter, E. W. (2020). From barriers to belonging: Promoting inclusion and relationships through the peer to peer program. *TEACHING Exceptional Children*, 52(6), 426–434.

Zosh, J. M., Hopkins, E. J., Jensen, H., Liu, C., Neale, D., Hirsh-Pasek, K., ... Whitebread, D. (2017). *Learning through play: A review of the evidence. [White paper]*. Billund, Denmark: The Lego Foundation. https://doi.org/10.13140/RG.2.2.16823.01447

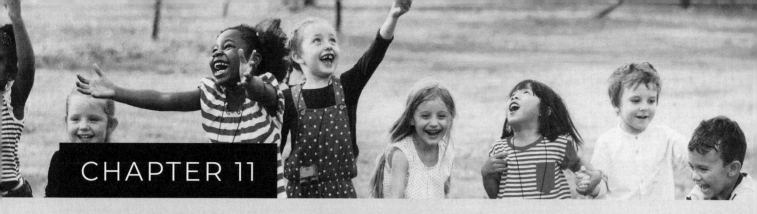

CHAPTER 11

Parent–Child Play and Attachment: Promoting Play Within Families

Amiya Waldman-Levi, PhD OTR/L

After reading this chapter, the reader will:

- Identify attachment theory's main concepts and their relevance to occupational therapy practice with families.
- Describe the connections between parent–child play and attachment.
- Communicate the value of parent–child relationships to children's development and well-being.
- Assess and determine areas for intervention regarding parent–child play.
- Apply professional reasoning to guide parent–child play-based intervention to promote joint play.

Let kids be kids; just let them be Princesses, pirates; let the bath be the sea! … Let them build castles, do cartwheels, and find shells in the sand.
If they need a little help, then please give them a hand!
—Jennifer Caldwell

The essence of human relationships stems from, as well as depends on, primary relationships with parents. Parent–child play is one of the most fundamental co-occupations parents can share with their children (Waldman-Levi & Bundy, 2016). Parent–child relationships and attachment patterns shape and influence the play experience. Attachment supports exploration and play, and the extensive research on attachment clarifies how the parent–child bond sets the foundation for children's future relationships and ability to develop emotionally, socially, and cognitively. Factors such as a child's disability, parental mental illness, trauma, and poverty can disrupt attachment and create barriers for adult–child play. Hence, understanding attachment and its impact on the parent–child play experience can deepen occupational therapy practice with children and their families. This chapter introduces attachment theory and its connection to the parent–child play experience, provides measures to assess parent–child play, and suggests ways to promote play in families.

Throughout this chapter, I will use the term *parent–child play* and discuss attachment patterns between parents and their children because most of the research in attachment and parent–child play has been done with parents, mostly mothers. However, we do know that many times the primary caregiver may be someone other than the parent and expect this information to be similarly relevant.

Attachment

Attachment is an innate motivational force of seeking and maintaining contact with significant others. It was first described as a psychological connectedness between individuals (Bowlby, 1969). Attachment develops over time and is considered as enhancing survival within an evolutionary perspective (Draper & Beisky, 1990). The attachment system consists of human response to basic and relational needs and stressors (attachment style), mental capacity, and behaviors in the context of intimate relations (i.e., close friendship, spousal, family, and parenting). An infant's attachment style formation is the outcome of a relational-developmental process that depends on the parental care provided to the infant. Attachment theory describes the course of this process, the outcomes of the process in terms of attachment styles, and the impact these styles have on all aspects of future intimate relationships.

The Progression of Attachment Theory

Attachment theory, originally developed by John Bowlby in the 1950s and 60s, provides a framework for understanding the responses of infants when separated from their parents and/or experiencing neglect in the course of their upbringing (Belsky, 1999a). Bowlby's observations of parent–infant relations led him to conclude that the root of human relations is in the need for protection and proximity. He conceptualized attachment theory to explain the infant's primary bond with mothers to fulfill their need for survival. Decades following its development, attachment theory has expanded and flourished with ample empirical and intervention studies, yielding an entire approach that psychologists use when treating adults, couples, and families, as well as young children. In occupational therapy practice, understanding attachment provides us with a lens for viewing, assessing, and treating within the family relationship, and specifically addressing parent–child play.

Development of Attachment

Attachment develops during the first months of an infant's life and then is further shaped and organized to support human relations throughout life (Bowlby, 1988). The development of attachment is a process that occurs in stages and has varied impacts across different developmental stages of an individual's life.

A Process

Attachment develops through an intricate interconnection between an infant's behavior and a parental response. Bowlby noticed that when infants are distressed, they signal this to their parent (see **Figure 11.1**). Their signals are initially sensory and motor in nature, for instance, heightened muscle tone, eye opening, a shift of gaze, and varied forms of cry (Bowlby, 1988). These signals are meant to elicit the parent's response.

Infants signal their needs for protection against fear in general and particularly fear of loss. Infants require care and protection from their parents to survive; the parent's response to the infant's survival signals shapes their attachment system. An infant's experience of fear during everyday encounters triggers their need for protection and proximity. For example, an infant may fear having clothes removed while their body is exposed to a lower temperature, dipping in tub water, or loud or unfamiliar sounds and voices.

Figure 11.1 Infants have many ways to signal their distress to their primary caregivers, including facial expressions, cries, and body positioning
© Slavomir Durej/Shutterstock.

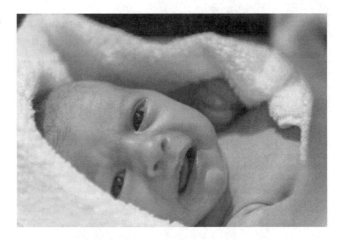

Attachment is a product of how well children signal as well as adjust to their parents' response. For example, one infant may learn he or she needs to cry loud and long to elicit a parental response, while another infant's soft signs of discomfort or distress are responded to immediately and consistently. Attachment offers a safe haven, a buffer against the effects of stress and uncertainty as well as a secure base. The sense of secure base allows infants to explore their world and most adaptively respond to their environment. Hence, secure dependency complements autonomy.

Parental emotional availability and responsiveness are building blocks for secure attachment (see **Figure 11.2**). Any response is better than no emotional response. Fear and uncertainty activate attachment needs, but if these needs fail in eliciting a comforting response from attachment figures, then this leads to a process of protest, clinging, depression, and despair, eventually resulting in detachment (Belsky & Pascofearon, 2008; Slade, 2007; Sroufe, 2005; see **Figure 11.3**).

Multiple elements of the relationship can hinder or support this process of attachment formation between the infant and the parent. Some of these elements include: the infant temperament, the parent's attachment style and personality, marital relations and social support, past and current exposure to the adversity of parent and/or child (Belsky & Pascofearon, 2008; Slade, 2007; Sroufe, 2005), the parent's ability to function as a caregiver, and the parent's satisfaction with marital life, as well as family financial stability (George & Solomon, 2008).

These initial relationship patterns then influence one's relationships throughout life. How children and their parents manage the dance of proximity and protection, as well as how children continue to need their parents as a secure base for exploration, remains as important during later developmental periods (Marvin & Britner, 2008).

Developmental Phases of Attachment

The developmental phases of attachment begin at birth. During the first 3 months of a newborn's life, their response to caregiving is nondiscriminative; they respond to any adult caretaker who feeds them. Infants respond to familiar voices, favoring their mother's voice right from birth. They also respond to visual stimuli, preferring familiar faces to objects. An infant's behavior becomes more socially discriminative between 3 and 6 months of age. By 3 months, the infant is already familiar with attachment figures, forming a sequence of behaviors toward them. Between 6 and 36 months, the infant's growing locomotor skills, communications skills, and cognitive capacity allow them to control the need for proximity and to explore their surroundings. See **Figure 11.4**.

From 36 months onward, toddlers and preschoolers are more autonomous and possess the ability for self-control. They become more independent, self-reliant, and able to stay apart from primary attachment figures for longer periods. Children heavily rely on internalized working models when they are apart spending the majority of the day at a childcare facility or school. During that time, children form trusting relationships with other adult figures and peers.

Beyond their preschool years, there are no remarkable changes in attachment as it becomes

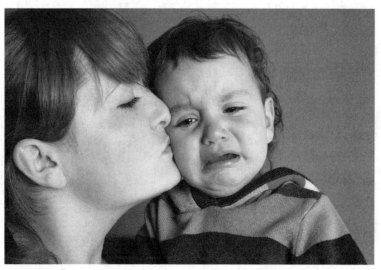

Figure 11.2 Secure attachment results in part from responsive and sensitive caregiving
© AlohaHawaii/Shutterstock.

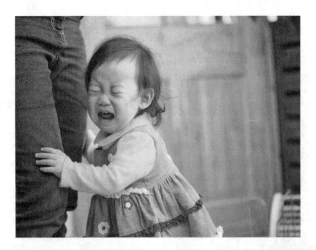

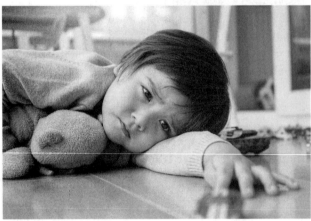

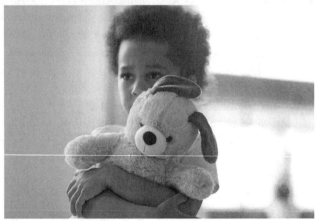

Figure 11.3 When a child's fear or uncertainty does not lead to consistent appropriate and comforting caregiver responses, the outcome can be clinginess, despair, or detachment

Top: Mcimage/Shutterstock; Left: © Ann in the uk/Shutterstock; Right: © fizkes/Shutterstock.

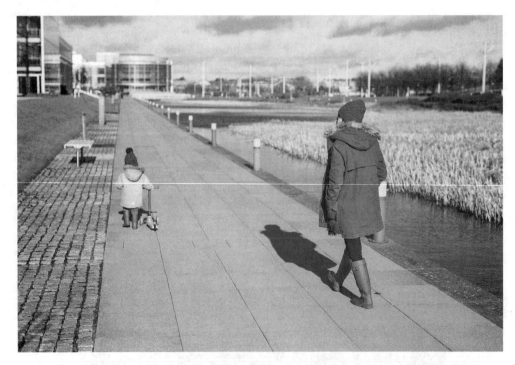

Figure 11.4 A child with secure attachment feels safe to explore, knowing that the caregiver functions as a "base" to return to

© Carlos G. Lopez/Shutterstock.

more sophisticated, abstract, and mentally operated. During middle childhood, around 6 to 11 years, children continue to return to their attachment figures as a secure base when facing danger or distress. At this phase, caregiving relationships are most important for their availability and emotional attunement rather than physical proximity. Adolescents' need for a secure base is mentally guided, supporting them in navigating stressful and challenging social interactions, yet immensely important for their sense of belonging (Marvin & Britner, 2008).

Attachment Styles

Through a specific assessment protocol called the strange situation, Ainsworth et al. (1978) developed classifications of attachment generally divided into secure or insecure attachment styles (see **Table 11.1**). The examiner evaluates the child's behavior toward the parent in response to him/her being separated and reunited with the parent several times. The secure style is a product of the parents' availability and sensitivity to the needs of the child and is characterized by the child's perception of confidence in situations of both nearness and separation from the parent (Kloth et al., 1998). In contrast, the insecure style is a product of a lack of parental availability and sensitivity and is expressed by the child as avoidance, resistance, or a combination of both, in response to stressful situations (Belsky, 1999b; Lowinger et al., 1995). Vast longitudinal experiments confirm the existence of attachment styles and subcategories (Chopik, Edelstein, & Grimm, 2019; Grossmann, Grossmann, & Waters, 2006; Sroufe, 2005).

Attachment Style and Impact on Parenting

The attachment style we develop as children continues to influence us as adults and as parents, thereby influencing our children's attachment development, a phenomenon that is referred to as intergenerational transmission of attachment relationships. Children's early experiences with their parents further internalize in adulthood as working models of caregiving, which guide their parenting (Banyard et al., 2003; Mikulincer et al., 2006). The internalized working models are implemented through psychological processes such as mentalizing and reflective functioning. Together, these processes, along with other psychological processes, create a coordinated caregiving system that either fosters or hinders the developing attachment bond with one's own child.

Mentalizing. Mentalizing is the capacity to understand we have separate minds and separate realities that guide our responses to others (Gergely & Watson, 1999; Oppenheim & Koren-Karie, 2002). Mentalization is the intergenerational vehicle of attachment transmission based on internalized working models of a parent formed throughout life (Humfrees et al., 2002). Parent reactions depend on the conscious and unconscious interpretation of an infant's signals, as well as their internalized working models (Belsky, 1999b). Explicit parental mentalizing is overt, conscious, verbal communications with an infant or child, while implicit mentalizing is unconscious, embodied behavior toward the infant (Shai & Belsky 2011a, 2011b).

Table 11.1 Attachment Styles Determined Through Observed Behaviors

Attachment Style	Behavioral Descriptions During the Strange Situation
Secure	Appears confident in situations of both nearness and separation from the parent; willing to explore and play.
Insecure avoidant	Shows little or no response to the attachment figure during separation or reunion situations; directs attention toward toys or objects.
Insecure resistant	Preoccupied with the attachment figure and presents both distress and resistance upon reunion; is hard to soothe.
Insecure disorganized	Presents inconsistent attachment responses at separation and reunion with expressions of fear, undirected movements and expressions (nonplay), and freezing of behavior and expression (emotional affect).

Data from Rutgers, A. H., Bakermans-Kranenburg, M. J., van Ijzendoorn, M. H., & van Berckelaer-Onnes, I. A. (2004). Autism and attachment: A meta-analytic review. *Journal of Child Psychology and Psychiatry, 45*, 1123–1134. https://doi.org/10.1111/j.1469-7610.2004.t01-1-00305.x.

A parent's mental capacity allows them to capture the infant's sensory signals (i.e., tactile, kinesthetic) and respond in an embodied manner. Indeed, parental implicit mentalizing promotes an infant's body ownership awareness and nonverbal interpersonal interaction. Securely attached mothers exhibited higher mentalizing capacity than mothers classified with an insecure attachment (Slade et al., 2005).

During parent–child play, the parent considers the child's inner world while holding an outside perspective based on reality. The example of a 3-year-old boy playing with his mother can assist us in understanding how play, attachment, and mentalization co-occur (see **Practice Example 11.1**).

The delicate balance between attachment and exploration allows infants and toddlers to explore their environment and play. If they feel threatened or afraid, young children will discontinue or not even begin to play. The parent role is to identify insecurities that activate the attachment system, and their ensuing response will depend on their mentalizing capacity and reflective functioning.

Reflective Functioning and Parental Sensitivity.
Reflective functioning assists a parent in responding to situations where a child grapples with a challenging task (Ordway et al., 2015; Slade, 2007). The parent reflects on a situation to respond in a supportive and attuned manner (Borelli et al., 2017). Parental reflective functioning has a crucial role in a child's ability to establish sustaining relationships (Fonagy &

Target, 1998; Slade, 2007). A parent's sensitive caregiving is considered an indicator of reflective functioning.

Parental reflective functioning likely plays a crucial role in the intergenerational transmission of attachment. Studies suggest that parental reflective functioning is related to child social competence, child reflective functioning, and child behavior (Benbassat & Priel 2012), as well as the parent's ability to parent with sensitivity (Oppenheim & Koren-Karie, 2002; Slade et al., 2005). Research suggests that parental sensitivity is related to later child behaviors (Zvara et al., 2018).

Maternal reflective functioning ability may be specifically protective for the child. For example, in a sample of mothers with trauma history, there was an intergenerational transmission of attachment disorganization, and this unresolved maternal trauma predicted infant disorganized attachment. However, those mothers with a history of abuse, but with high reflective functioning, had infants with organized attachment (Berthelot et al., 2015).

The Caregiving System.
The caregiving system was hypothesized by Bowlby to be the motivational heart of a parent's response to a child's distress or need for support (Shaver et al., 2010). The regulation of one's caregiving system originates developmentally in one's own primary attachment relationships. Under typical conditions, a parent gives priority to caregiving, especially when the child is vulnerable or threatened. The parent is expected to give priority to caregiving even when the threat extends to the self,

---

PRACTICE EXAMPLE 11.1 Toby, Molly, and Mentalizing

Toby is playing with a Playmobil set and trying to fit a person figure into a truck. The figure does not appear to fit into the driver's seat, and after several attempts, Toby throws both the truck and person figure in frustration.

Toby's mother, Molly, might respond in a variety of ways depending on their attachment and Molly's mentalizing. Consider what each might indicate. Imagine Molly looks at Toby and says, "I know you are upset honey, but please don't throw your toys, let's see what we can do about it," and she leans toward the toys to pick them up. Instead she could respond with "Don't throw your toys on the floor, let's see what we can do" as she picks up the truck and person figure and brings them to Toby. Or she could decide to respond, "Oh no, the little person got a boo-boo, let's pick it up ..." as she picks up the truck and the person.

In the first response, Molly reacts reflectively, acknowledging her child's feelings as she interpreted them, relying on her mentalizing capacity. This response is most likely to support her child in developing his mentalizing capacity. She differentiates herself from Toby by asking him not to throw toys, she offers to help him and follow up with an action (caregiving system). In the second example, Molly ignores Toby's mental state and responds in an attuned manner as she offers assistance accompanied by her actions. This response is supportive and helpful for the continuation of play at an explicit level. However, this response is not supportive at the implicit level and does not promote the development of Toby's mentalizing capacity. In the third response, Molly's concern is diverted from Toby to the person play figure. Her response is followed by an action, which might support the continuation of explicit play behavior, but does not explicitly or implicitly offer assistance. This response implies a lack of maternal mentalizing capacity and reflective functioning with an inability to identify and respond to Toby's emotional distress.

for instance, under conditions of domestic violence or environmental catastrophe.

Dysfunction in the caregiving system is manifested in either hyperactivation or deactivation, resulting, respectively, in anxious or avoidant caregiving dispositions.

Anxious caregiving is motivated, at least in part, by desires for acceptance, approval, and gratitude, which can impair sensitivity and lead to compulsive caregiving. Avoidant caregiving is characterized by efforts to detach oneself emotionally from the child's needs (Reizer & Mikulincer, 2007; Selcuk et al., 2010). Proper functioning of the caregiving system should foster quality caregiving, characterized by sensitivity and responsiveness to the child and commitment to meeting their needs (Bowlby, 1988). As seen in **Practice Examples 11.2**, **11.3**, and **11.4**, varied mother–infant dyads experience play differently because of their different attachment styles and caregiving capacity.

PRACTICE EXAMPLE 11.2 Jenifer, Barbara, and Avoidant Attachment

Observations: Jenifer crawls toward a toy rattle. Her mother, Barbara, sits across from her. Jenifer's hands grab the rattle. Then she brings it to her mouth. After a few moments, Jenifer crawls back to where Barbara sits, touching her knee as she approaches, then turning back to the toy rattle she left behind.

Analysis: Jenifer and Barbara's joint play is limited to physical contact (touching, cuddling, and eye contact) with no verbal exchanges. The physical contact is almost accidental or random. It is as if brief touch suffices as emotional support for Jenifer. Jenifer's behavior is not responsive or related to her mother's behavior. Barbara is present and is seated with proximity to Jenifer, but she provides no response to Jenifer's signals. This is an example of an avoidant infant attachment to a disconnected mother, who presents avoidant caregiving. Jenifer's avoidant attachment matches her mother's, which exemplifies the adaptive function of the infant's attachment response with that of the parent attachment style.

PRACTICE EXAMPLE 11.3 Samantha, Ann, and Dysfunction in the Caregiving System

Observations: Samantha sits in her mother Ann's lap, holding onto her. Samantha is looking around at the toys, her fists holding Ann's shirt tightly. Ann is reaching out to grasp a toy rattle to hand it to Samantha. Samantha shifts her gaze away from the rattle. Ann shakes the rattle and tries to move Samantha so she will sit next to her to allow her to hold the rattle in her hands. Samantha strengthens her grip and sharply turns her head away from the rattle.

Analysis: Samantha appears fearful as if exploration or play is a threat to the mother–child bond. Ann's invitation to play with the rattle is experienced as her attempt to distance herself from Samantha. In the presence of fear and anxiety, the attachment system is activated and the child's ability to explore and play diminished or immobilized. Ann's failure to respond to Samantha's increased separation anxiety and lack of verbalization and physical directionality suggest her caregiving system is activated. However, instead of eliciting a soothing caregiving response, it evokes a dismissing response to Samantha's fear.

PRACTICE EXAMPLE 11.4 Ally, Krista, Secure Attachment, and Joint Play

Observations: Ally sits on Krista's lap. She looks at the toys nearby. Krista looks at where Ally is looking and says softly while smiling, "Do you want to play with the rattle? So go and get it. I'm here." She then gently loosens her arms supporting Ally's pelvis as she shifts her weight from Krista's lap transitioning into a crawling position. Krista gently moves her feet with her hand softly touching Ally's hip as Ally is leaving "mom's secure base" and crawls toward the rattle. Krista says, "You are almost there" when Ally turns her head to look back at Krista, and they are both smiling at one another. Ally looks back at the rattle crawling at a faster pace now. She reaches the rattle, grasps it, and then sits holding the rattle, facing her mom. They both are smiling. Krista says, "You did it, you crawled right there! I am so proud of you!"

Analysis: Ally and Krista's play demonstrates a responsive and attuned chain of responses: verbal, behavioral, and sensory. Krista serves as a secure base for Ally to explore and play in the near environment. She responds to Ally's sensory signals of gaze and body movement and effortlessly picks up gestures and facial expressions. Ally is adapted to being understood and responds to her mom's bodily cues with an action. She is ready to explore and trust her mom to be there if she needs to fuel herself with a cuddle or a brief look back. Their emotional reactions are well synchronized and frame this brief moment of joint play.

How Does Attachment Support Exploration and Play?

Human relations are best understood in the family context. Bowlby believed in a fundamental and complementary relationship between an infant's attachment and exploratory behavior; that is, once a child's attachment system is organized, attachment-seeking behaviors are extinguished, and the child can then explore their environment (Bowlby, 1988). The relationship between the attachment system and the exploratory system is best understood in light of the separation-individuation theory conceptualization.

Separation is an infant's gradual extrication from their symbiotic fusion with the mother, while individuation is the child's perception of owning individual characteristics separate from their mother. Infants are essentially nonrelated or objectless at birth, then completely dependent on their mothers during the symbiosis phase. Infants' growing capacity to differentiate themselves from their mothers occurs in several subsequent developmental phases.

From birth through the first months of life, infants perceive themselves being part of their mothers, while mothers possess this perception as well, making it the symbiotic phase. As the infant is keenly interested in examining the mother's face and hair, differentiation begins then. With infant locomotor development, the ability to reach, crawl, and walk allows them to experience themselves physically apart from their mothers. While practicing locomotor capabilities in their proximate environment, the differentiation subphase is further established. Attachment theory scholars assert that at this phase, infants periodically seek the mother out as a "home base" for "emotional refueling" (Bowlby, 1988).

The next phase in the separation-individuation theory is rapprochement (15–24 months) initiated by the child's beginning awareness that the mother is, in fact, a separate person. Toddlers learn how to operate their environment using their communication skills with vocalization, gestures, and verbal bids. Here, they can communicate with their mothers negotiating for their desires. As soon as toddlers' cognitive capacity allows them to understand object constancy, the subphase of object constancy (24–36 months) has occurred, and toddlers possess internal images of both self and others (Brandell, 2010).

Mother–child interaction has a crucial role in a child's exploratory system development (Cooper, 2000; Winnicott, 1995, 1999). Play in infancy relies on parental capacity to attribute meaning to the infant's emotional states. It is therefore dependent on the engagement of the mother and her ability to give back in relation to what is being received from the infant (Desmarais,

2006; Winnicott, 1995, 1999). Through the separation from an attachment figure and the individuation process, children develop the capacity to be alone and explore their environment. Infants who are able to take on new challenges enthusiastically and are able to accept help without conflict achieve a balance between independence and dependence (Aoki et al., 2002).

As the child develops, play becomes more complex than exploratory play. According to Winnicott (1995, 1999), this play occurs when the infant or the child feels emotionally safe. This sense of safety is gradually developed along with maternal ability to allow the infant to be separated from her. This mutual separation process occurs in a space Winnicott refers to as "the secure space" (Winnicott, 1995, 1999). Realization of a secure space in childhood leads to the experience of mutual trust, play, and shared constructions (LaMothe, 2005). Social play between parent and child is a positive and significant indicator of that child's emotional, social, and cognitive development (Keren et al., 2005; Lindsey & Mize, 2000). Parent–child play is an enjoyable activity where the parent facilitates opportunities to choose, lead, and/or initiate play while responding accordingly (Keren et al., 2005; Weintraub & Waldman-Levi, 2009). Furthermore, during parent–child play, the child is being seen and heard, as well as understood, and in turn, the child's symbolic play provides the parent insight into the child's inner world (Desmarais, 2006).

Parent–Child Play

Parent–child play is a co-occupation, where both partners share physical space and objects, ideas, intentions, and emotions while interacting (Pickens & Pizur-Barnekow, 2009; Waldman-Levi & Bundy, 2016; Waldman-Levi, Grinion, et al., 2019a). The parent role during play is to support the child's engagement, exploration, and enjoyment in a playful manner (Waldman-Levi, Finzi-Dottan, et al., 2019; Waldman-Levi, Grinion, et al., 2019). See **Figure 11.5**. Parents' interaction styles during play with their children might differ based on their gender, attachment style, personality, level of education, role perception, and parenting beliefs, as well as their history and upbringing (Cabrera et al., 2017; Kwon et al., 2012; Waldman-Levi et al., 2015; Waldman-Levi, Grinion , et al., 2019; Weintraub & Waldman-Levi, 2009).

In parent–child play, the child's role is to practice their central occupation, play (Weintraub & Waldman-Levi, 2009), which is fundamental to their growth and development (Bundy & Du Toit, 2019). Through the act of playing with a responsive and supportive adult play partner, children learn social norms and rules. Children learn how to regulate their emotions

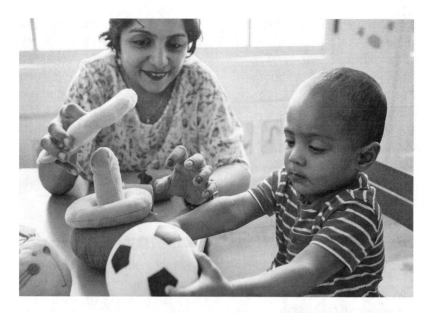

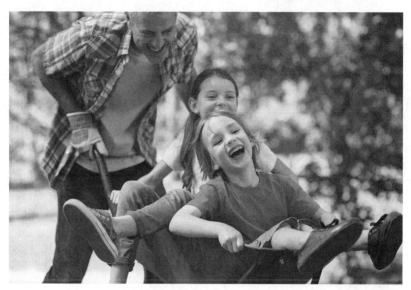

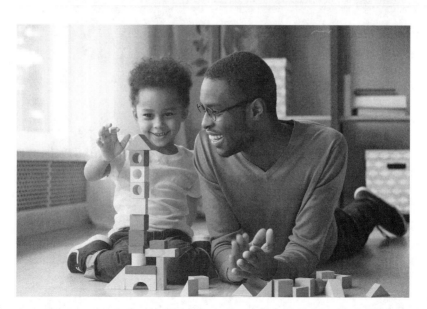

Figure 11.5 A caregiver's role during the co-occupation of play is to support the child's engagement, exploration, and enjoyment in a playful manner

and develop linguistic and cognitive skills (e.g.,;). A child's involvement in parent–child play consists of child-driven behaviors that affect the parent, such as the initiation of interactive bids, affect, vocalization, and alertness that make up a child's social involvement (Feldman & Eidelman, 2005).

Family Context

The family cultural context may influence parent–child joint play, as well as how often they play together (Kuhaneck et al., 2010; Weintraub & Waldman-Levi, 2009). Several studies have shown how mother–child play varies between families of different ethnicity or country of origin. For instance, mothers and children of American and European origin demonstrated child-led play, use of commercial games, toys, and probes, while encouraging symbolic and make-believe play. In contrast, mothers and children of Eastern origin exhibited parent-led play, imitation of real-life experiences during play, and values such as respect (Bazyk et al., 2003; Parham & Primeau, 2008).

Parental Roles

Life in the 21st century is financially demanding, and parents work for longer hours, leaving less time for mutual and spontaneous play (Swinth & Tanta, 2008). In recent years, societal and economic changes shifted family dynamics and resulted in some role reversal. The traditional roles of father as the sole or primary breadwinner and the mother as the primary caregiver are no longer the norm. Some fathers are now the primary caregivers, and in other families, parents share childrearing responsibilities (Bianchi et al., 2007; Cabrera, et al., 2011; Jones & Mosher, 2013). In a national survey of 10,403 fathers of children from infancy through 18 years old in the United States, researchers reported differences in fathers' involvement in their children's lives with fathers who were at home more reporting more time playing with their children. The difference in paternal involvement was linked to marital status, ethnicity, origin, age, and level of education (Jones & Mosher, 2013).

Parental Gender

Parental gender is an additional factor that may affect parent–child play. Mothers and fathers differ in the ways they play with their children. See **Figure 11.6**. Several studies reported that fathers tend to be more active and physical in the way they interact and play with their children, favoring rough-and-tumble play (John et al., 2013; St George & Freeman, 2017). Other researchers described fathers incorporating competitive play, challenges, and exhibiting age-mate behaviors during joint play (Cabrera & Roggman, 2017; Flanders et al., 2009) and toy play (St George et al., 2017). In a recent study, we found that the more frequently fathers displayed playful and supportive behaviors during joint play, the more playful and engaged their child was. Furthermore, when fathers displayed an increased quality of support for playful behaviors, the more skillful the child appeared during play (Waldman-Levi et al., 2020).

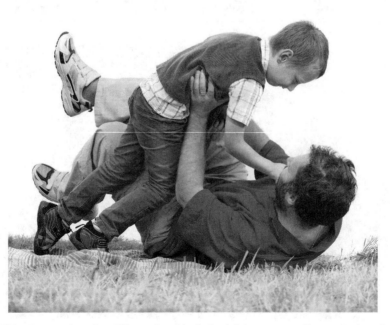

Figure 11.6 Parents of different gender play differently with their children, according to research. Fathers tend to engage in more active and physical play

© Kletr/Shutterstock.

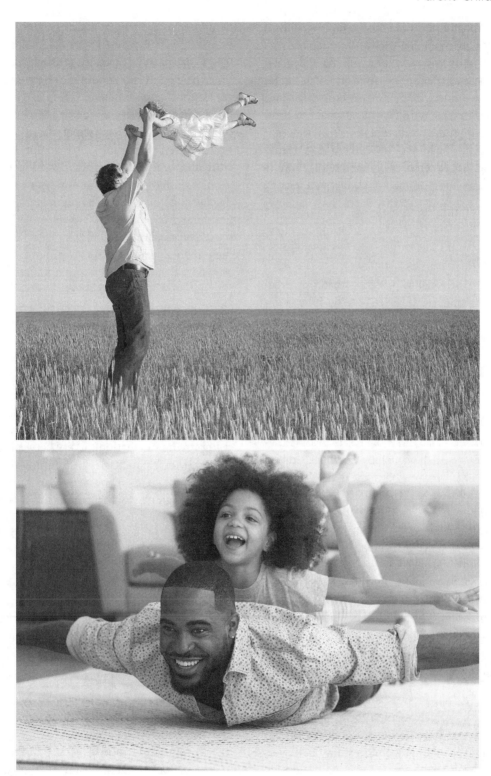

Figure 11.6 (Continued)
Top: © Gladskikh Tatiana/Shutterstock; Bottom: © fizkes/Shutterstock.

In contrast to fathers, mothers' play style is characterized as more structured. Both mothers and fathers are able to identify differences between their play style and that of their spouse (Waldman-Levi, Grinion, et al., 2019; Waldman-Levi et al., 2020). Fathers report their spouse to be more educational in their approach to joint play (Waldman-Levi et al., 2020). Mothers tend to demonstrate empathy as they guide, direct, and teach their children during joint play (John et al., 2013; Weintraub & Waldman-Levi, 2009), and they value play as an activity that allows them to connect with and educate their child (Waldman-Levi, Grinion et al., 2019). Mothers who support decision-making abilities over outcome-oriented behaviors and follow the child's lead during play have more playful children (Waldman-Levi, Grinion, et al., 2019).

Of interest, although parental play type differs by gender, overall parental playfulness may not (Menashe-Grinberg & Atzaba-Poria, 2017). However, mother and father playfulness may serve different purposes in child development and impact different areas of function (Cabrera et al., 2017; Menashe-Grinberg & Atzaba-Poria, 2017). Gender differences in parental playfulness may be particularly important for child outcomes in children with disabilities (Levavi, Menashe-Grinberg, Barak-Levy, & Atzaba-Poria, 2020).

Child Age

The child's age affects the nature of parent–child play experiences. During infancy, play is characterized by the exploration of the body, objects, and sensations (Schneider, 2009). At that time, the parent role is of a facilitator, as the child depends on the parent availability and response to validate interaction bids (Knox, 2008; Nakano et al., 2007; Weintraub & Waldman-Levi, 2009). Among infant–parent dyads, play consists of social (i.e., peek-a-boo and singing) and object-oriented play (Waldman-Levi et al., in preparation). In early toddlerhood and preschool years with growing cognitive and social-emotional capacities, differences in play emerge between boys and girls (Gmitrova et al., 2009; Holmes & Procaccino, 2009; Servin et al., 1999). Preschoolers playing with their parents engage in pretend play, book reading, or rough-and-tumble play (e.g., Cabrera & Roggman, 2017; Flanders et al., 2009; Waldman-Levi, Grinion, et al., 2019). During the middle-childhood period, parent–child dyads engaged mostly in board games and a few were observed using technology-based games (Waldman-Levi, Finzi-Dottan, et al., 2019).

Child Disability

When children exhibit developmental delays and/or disabilities, this influences the type and quality of their play (Childress, 2010; Lifter et al., 2011). Performance skill deficits challenge a child's ability to play as well as affect their interactions and parent–child play (Gale & Schick, 2009; Lifter et al., 2011). The child's disability may also alter the parent's perceptions of their abilities, perhaps leading to limitations in their autonomy for play and risk-taking (Beetham et al., 2019; Graham et al., 2015). For example, parents of children with a disability were less tolerant of risk-taking play compared to parents of typically developing children (Beetham et al., 2019).

One particularly important diagnosis to highlight is autism spectrum disorder (ASD), as children with ASD demonstrate a delay in social, symbolic, and pretend play skills. Their play appears disconnected and repetitive, with a lack of diversity, creativity, and playfulness. Their play often lacks spontaneity, joy, amusement, and continuous engagement (Baum, 2019; Godin et al., 2017). In turn, these deficits impose a great challenge on the parent–child play experience.

Children with ASD also demonstrate difficulties with attachment impacting parent–child play. Studies of children with ASD found they are less likely to display attachment security compared to their typically developing counterparts. However, variance in attachment security among children with ASD depends on their mental capacity, and symptom severity, as well as parental attachment representations and behavior (Rutgers et al., 2004; Seskin et al., 2010). For example, children whose parents demonstrated secure attachment and insightful behavior were better able to engage in parent–child play (Baker et al., 2015; Oppenheim et al., 2009; Seskin et al., 2010). Parental behaviors contributing to children's social engagement were positive affect, imitation, joint attention, initiation of social interaction, responsivity, and flexibility (Field et al., 2013; Nadel et al., 2008). Interventions aimed at improving interaction quality between children with ASD and their parents lead to improved social engagement (Baum, 2019; Dionne & Martini, 2011).

Although play with a parent elicits better play abilities than when children with disabilities play by themselves (e.g., Childress, 2010; De Falco et al., 2010), the benefits may vary based on which parent is playing with the child. For example, one study found when children played with their fathers, they demonstrated more symbolic play than when they engaged in play with their mothers (De Falco et al., 2010) The authors explained these differences with fathers' decreased tendency to overdemonstrate symbolic play, which may have promoted the progression of these skills.

Adversity

Exposure to childhood adversity in the form of maltreatment, poverty, and domestic violence negatively affects child development and predisposes children to posttraumatic stress disorder (PTSD) (Enlow et al., 2013). Adversity is most prevalent in low-income families with a host of effects on parenting capacity, child development, and academic performance (Bradbury et al., 2019; Cabrera et al., 2017; Demir & Küntay, 2014; Halfon et al., 2017; Narayan et al., 2017; Raffington et al., 2019). Among mothers and children exposed to domestic violence, children of mothers with PTSD were less playful than children whose mothers did not have PTSD. The quality of interaction observed during joint play of mothers with PTSD was of a lesser quality compared to mothers without PTSD (Waldman-Levi et al., 2015). Children exposed to adversity benefit from stable and nurturing relationships with adult caregivers and from safe, enriching, and play-conducive environments.

Mental Illness

Parental mental illness puts children at risk for developing a mental illness, behavioral disorders, and adjustment difficulties and predicts children's emotional and behavioral functioning (Gladstone et al., 2011; Risser et al., 2013). Parental mental illness impacts parental play behaviors and playfulness (Sethna, Murray, Edmondson, Iles, & Ramchandani, 2018) and thereby may influence parent–child play. A unique role for the occupational therapy practitioner may be working with a mother experiencing mental illness on parent–child play as a vehicle for the mother to connect with her child, enhance their relationship, and assist her to be a supportive play partner to her child (Olson, 2006a).

Parent–child play is also compromised when the child has a mental illness. Olson (2006b) describes the play challenges encountered at an in-patient psychiatric clinic with mentally ill children and their adult caregivers (i.e., a parent or legal guardian). The interactions between parent/caregiver and child lacked a playful attitude, attunement, and synchrony. It resulted in both play partners yearning for proximity, care, and a sense of belonging. "Little playful interaction occurring between parents and children … distant and superficial interaction … tense visits with outbursts and misconduct … need for positive interaction was not met" (p. 2). During occupational therapy activity groups, parents/caregivers and children were invited to either play or engage in an art or craft-type activity. Some parents/caregivers felt powerless facing their child's negative or disorganized emotions and disruptive behavior. Other parents/caregivers took control over the child's activity. Both parents/caregivers and children required concrete and constant assistance from the occupational therapy practitioner, which resulted in better play experiences.

Assessment of Parent–Child Play

To assess parent–child play, occupational therapists may consider evaluating child, parent, and dyadic aspects.

The child's play assessment is described in detail in Chapters 3-4 so this chapter will focus on the primary methods occupational therapists can use for assessing parental factors that are specific to parent–child play dyads.

Parental Behavior Assessment

Assessing parental behavior during play is complex, but there are two instruments that can be used by occupational therapists for this purpose. First, the Test of Environmental Supportiveness (TOES; Skard & Bundy, 2008) assesses the fit between the player/child and their physical and social environment. The TOES examines whether a child's physical and social environments support or hinder their playfulness behavior. Only a few items of the TOES can be used to evaluate parental support to their child during joint play, "the caregiver items" and "older playmate items." The way in which a therapist is able to assess caregiver and older playmate support of a child's play with the TOES is rather general; hence, it is most useful as a screening tool. If the occupational therapist discovers that parental support during joint play as measured by the TOES does not fit with the child's play needs, a second instrument is indicated to provide an in-depth look at the parent behavior.

The Parent/Caregiver's Support of Young Children's Playfulness Scale (Waldman-Levi & Bundy, 2016) is a 27-item criterion-referenced tool designed to assess how a parent or caregiver supports a child's playfulness based on observation of a 15-minute parent–child play session. The 27 items are scored on a scale of 1 (low) to 3 (high) on two scales. The first scale of 17 items measures the quality of the observed behaviors, and the second scale of 10 items measures their frequency. The scale has two factors. One is "Flow," consisting of nine items, which represent parent behaviors that frame the experience as well as the child's continued engagement in joint play. The second factor, "Creative," consists of 6 items, which represent parent behaviors that encourage creativity and use of humor. The scale has established psychometric properties (Waldman-Levi, Finzi-Dottan, et al., 2019; Waldman-Levi, Grinion, et al., 2019; Waldman-Levi et al., 2017).

Parental Perception Assessment

Another aspect worth considering when assessing joint play is parental perception regarding a child's play. Parental perception can be sought while incorporating a narrative approach to the evaluation process as well as to the entire intervention (Bryze, 2008; Mattingly & Fleming, 1994). A narrative approach involves meaningful conversations in which people's past and present experiences, attitudes, perceptions, thoughts, and feelings are explored and shared in a nonjudgmental manner. Therapists who practice a narrative approach use active listening skills, sensitivity, and self-reflection capacity to gather information and establish rapport with the parent to form a coherent and cohesive family play narrative. Freedman and Combs (1996) recommend using five different types of narrative questions: deconstruction questions, opening space questions, preference questions, story development questions, and meaning questions (see **Table 11.2**). **Table 11.3** presents a narrative-based interview of parents about play adapted for use in occupational therapy.

Promoting Parent–Child Play Within Families

Occupational therapy practitioners are equipped with knowledge and skills about human occupations and children's development to promote parenting skills and joint play as central occupations to support families. There is abundant research on the effectiveness of parent–child interventions in the psychology literature. For example, play is often used to improve other child behaviors such as aggression (Cosgrove & Norris-Shortle, 2015). Parent training approaches similarly have been used to improve child behaviors

Table 11.2 Categories and Descriptions of Narrative Questions

Question Categories	Description
Deconstruction	Assist individuals in unpacking their stories by distinguishing particular beliefs, practices, feelings, and attitudes. For example, does the situation you describe encourage particular feelings? What behaviors did you found yourself presenting in such situations as you described?
Opening space	Aim to discover something different from the problematic behavior in people's experiences. For example, are there situations in which your child behaves differently than you described?
Preference	Aim to let people choose between two possibilities to let them take charge of the direction of their story. For example, is this a good thing or a bad thing for you?
Story development	Invite people to relate the process and details, unfolded so far, and to connect it to a time frame, to a particular context, and other people. For example, how did you do it?
Meaning	Invite people into a reflective position from which they can regard different aspects of their stories, themselves, and various relationships. For example, what does this mean to you and your family?

Table 11.3 A Narrative-Based Play Interview

Narrative Interview Domain	Examples of Questions
The experience—story development	Can you tell me about a time when ...? Can you describe how your child plays at home and in school/daycare? Can you tell me about your family's daily routine? How would you describe the way your child plays? How do you react when she acts that way?
Thoughts—deconstruction	What do you think about play? (or playing with your child) How was it for you when you were a child? How do you perceive this behavior?
Feelings—deconstruction	How did you feel when ...? How do you think he/she feels when ...?
Values—deconstruction	How important play is to you as a parent? What types of activities do you promote for your family? Child?

and parenting ability (Gross et al., 2009; Kelly-Vance et al., 2013; Weisleder et al., 2016). Within occupational therapy, the Family Intervention for Improving Occupational Performance (FI-OP; Waldman-Levi, 2012; Waldman-Levi & Weintraub, 2015) stands alone as an intervention model to improve parent–child play; therefore, this will be the focus of the remainder of this chapter.

The FI-OP (Waldman-Levi, 2012) is an occupation-based, short-term intervention to address difficulties in the parent–child play experience of both the parent's supportive play behaviors and practices and the child's play functioning. The FI-OP originally was designed for mothers and their children who experienced severe domestic violence affecting maternal parenting capacity and child development. It is grounded in several theories: Attachment Theory (George & Solomon, 2008), Social-Cognitive Theory of Vygotsky and Feuerstein (Feuerstein, Klein, & Tannenbaum, 1991), Social-Learning Theory (Strand, 2002), Winnicott's concept of the secure base (1995, 1999), Reilly's (1974) Occupational Behavior Frame of Reference, and the occupational therapy literature on play (for example, Parham, 2008).

FI-OP Guidelines

The FI-OP is a two-armed intervention model. One arm focuses on improving parent–child interaction and support of the child during joint play. The second arm focuses on improving child play functions: play skills and playfulness behaviors. These two themes are the cornerstone for goal setting concerning the treated co-occupations, play and parenting/interaction. See **Table 11.4** for examples of goals and interventions related to these themes. The themes are tailored to each dyad's needs and adjusted across implementation. Each theme is addressed within spontaneous child-driven play interaction. As a result, it requires a high level of professional reasoning to adjust to these dynamics whether to support families of children with disabilities (see **Practice Example 11.5**) or families affected by trauma and adversity (Waldman-Levi & Weintraub, 2015; see **Practice Example 11.6**).

FI-OP Methods

The intervention methods are considered as "how to do," meaning, what clinical skills the intervening therapist uses to accomplish a certain goal. **Table 11.5** describes intervention methods used in the FI-OP model. As seen in **Figure 11.7**, it is anticipated that improving parent–child interaction during joint play will promote child's play functions and vice versa.

Session Structure

In the FI-OP model, each session has a constant organization (see **Figure 11.8**). The rationale for a well-defined session structure is grounded within the FI-OP theoretical background. According to attachment theory (George & Solomon, 2008) and

Table 11.4 Goals and Interventions to Address Different Themes in Parent–Child Play

Themes	Goal Areas to address	Intervention Examples	Professional Reasoning
Interaction: Parent/caregiver–child interaction during joint play	Developing, enabling and elaborating the parental sensitivity and responsiveness toward a child's needs, abilities, and preferences during joint play. Developing, enabling, and elaborating reciprocity between the parent and child.	The therapist verbalizes the child's behaviors to the parent (i.e., He is looking the other way; he is pointing to the dolls"). The therapist reinforces the parent when they demonstrate sensitive caregiving behaviors toward the child (i.e., "Yes, I think so too, he is not interested right now"). The therapist explains the importance of repetitions during play to facilitate joined play and synchrony as well as sense of security (i.e., he enjoys playing pick-a-boo again and again).	When children feel emotionally secure, they can play as well as learn new things. In the context of parent–child play, this sense of safety is achieved with parental sensitive and supportive play behaviors. Repetition provides emotional security and encourages additional experimentation, and, in turn, improves the child's ability to play. In and of itself, repetition creates a cycle of positive trials and a source of reward. Thus, the child can assimilate new information most efficiently.

(continues)

Table 11.4 Goals and Interventions to Address Different Themes in Parent–Child Play *(continued)*

Themes	Goal Areas to address	Intervention Examples	Professional Reasoning
Playfulness: Motivation, sense of control, freedom of constraints of reality, and framing	Developing, and encouraging a child's internal motivation, internal sense of control, freedom of constraints of reality, and ability to give and respond to social and communication cues.	*Internal motivation:* Encourage the child to investigate the environment and toys. Provide the child with verbal and nonverbal hints such as: "You can choose what you want to play with and what you do not wish to play with." The therapist should also reinforce a feeling of capability by saying things such as: "Wow, you are working so hard!" Providing reinforcements such as, "Well done, you made it all by yourself." "It is important to allow John to choose a toy for himself, if he has difficulty playing with it, we can help him." *Sense of Control:* "Here you go, I will hold the chair so you can climb and reach the shape container you wanted." *Freedom of Constraints of Reality:* The therapist expresses sense of humor, joking, mischievousness during play (i.e. silliness, embracing child's mistakes or own). Incorporate ideas or other ways to use play objects and materials in a creative way. Encourages role-playing *Framing/Social Communication:* Therapist's play initiative can be expressed through a variety of verbal or nonverbal hints (i.e., gestures, verbal statement or combination of the two).	When the parent validates child's selections and actions in play with verbal statement, or a positive gesture, it may motivate the child to continue playing Motivation and sense of control are interrelated playfulness behaviors. Positive reinforcement aimed to child abilities foster both these essential behaviors. *Sense of control* begins by building trusting relationships, while providing the child with a feeling of control and security in the environment. *Freedom of Constraints of Reality:* The process of play evokes internal feelings of fun, pleasure, and flow. To develop creativity, it is important to assist the parent and child to use ideas, people, space, and objects in varied ways that suit child's interest and capabilities. *Framing/Social Communication:* The therapist encourages child-led interaction and intervenes when invited to do so by the child. This rationale could be shared with the parent or reinforced when the parent exhibits it.
Play skills: Space and material management, symbolic and pretend play, and participation	Supporting the child in developing a variety of age-related play skills, such as practice play and symbolic or constructive play, as well as exploratory behavior and achievement behavior, parallel play and shared play.	Encourages development of play skills based on a child's preferences such as practice play (i.e., sorting shapes) or symbolic play (i.e., cooking dinner). Promote exploratory behavior (i.e., trial and error when playing something new the child is unfamiliar with), competency behavior (i.e., "Wow you figured it out, you tried and tried and did not give up, I am so proud of you"), solitary play, and parallel-cooperative play.	The therapist should first observe and identify the child's play skill level then intervene to develop it. It is important that the therapist keep in mind the frequency and duration of the child's quality of play skills so he/she can continue facilitating the play skills that need further development. In addition, the therapist should encourage transitioning to the next sequential level of play skill.

PRACTICE EXAMPLE 11.5 Assessment and Intervention for Dan and David's Joint Play

Observations of Joint Play: David, who is 61 years old, is playing with Dan, his 6-year-old son, who has a diagnosis of ASD. The play session starts with David forcefully holding Dan's hand and using it to push a button on a toy car. Dan. Moves away, lays down, and is not responding to his father's verbal prompts, but is playing independently with the cars. David tolerates silently watching Dan for a few moments, but eventually tries to move the car around and join in, which prompts Dan to leave/lose interest. David tries to interact with his son by taking one of two cars. Dan moves away from his father and up against a wall. When David follows, Dan leaves the toy cars and the area. Dan is not interested in interacting with his father and seems to be trying to create some space between them.

Dan is being pulled or directed, and choices are not often supported. However, David listens and adjusts when Dan makes it clear he wants to change play from cars and be Spiderman, but it takes David a minute to notice Dan is repeatedly stopping his father from putting the Spiderman mask over his eyes. David helps Dan self-advocate by having Dan repeat after him, "I want Spiderman." David allows for Dan's cape to be worn backwards and joins in with wearing it backwards. Dan appears to be interacting more with his own reflection than the father, but David tries to join in mirror play.

The occupational therapist (OT) rated the father's supportive behavior using the PCSYCP. David's scores indicates mild support for Dan's playfulness with better ability to support the flow of the joint play. He was better able to actively support Dan's engagement in free play, created a balance between the process of outcome-oriented play, and assisted Dan in overcoming barriers to continue playing as well as negotiate his needs during joint play. David also supported Dan in incorporating objects into play. However, other aspects were not as supportive, such as David's mild support in social play, transitions between play activities, modifying play, and incorporating fun, creativity, and mischief behavior. Also noted was a lack of praise and some overriding behavior (i.e., holding Dan's hand and physically directing him).

The OT rated Dan's playfulness behavior with the Test of Playfulness (ToP; Skard & Bundy, 2008). His scores indicated low playfulness. Dan appeared moderately motivated and engaged in the activities. He decided what he wanted to play with and when as well as maintained a level of safety (distanced himself when he did not want to comply). Dan seemed to play for sheer pleasure, mostly by himself, and at times indicated he wanted to play with his father (Spiderman). Dan's challenges lay in lack of skillful playfulness behavior, low level of creative use of objects or ideas, lack of pretend play, and ability to provide and respond to social cues as well as to maintain synchrony in joint play.

During the parent interview, David and his wife Caroline, shared their hopes of being able to play with their son as other parents they know do and how frustrating and challenging their joint play can be.

Intervention: The OT working with the family decided to incorporate the FI-OP model to support Dan's and David's joint play to improve Dan's play functioning. The OT set the following goals: (a) promote paternal sensitivity and responsiveness toward Dan's needs, abilities, and preferences during joint play; (b) encourage reciprocity between Dan and David as they engage in joint play; and (c) promote Dan's internal motivation, freedom of constraints of reality, and ability to give and respond to social and communication cues.

As the OT describes this plan, the parents agree it will be good that David will join the play sessions with Dan because he is mostly working and has less time to engage in play with Dan than Caroline has. Caroline had also mentioned that Dan seems to be looking more to interact with his father than with her in rough-and-tumble play. The OT and the family have decided they would meet one time a week for a triadic play session (Dan, David, and the OT) for 30 minutes, with the first 20 minutes for joint play and the last 10 minutes for debriefing. After the first 6 sessions, the OT will meet again with both parents to reassess the progress and decide together how to proceed.

During those six sessions, the OT directed David to support Dan in selecting and engaging in play activities that he likes by joining him and gradually incorporating new ideas or suggestions. She suggested they aim to find one activity in each session that both Dan and David could play on their own with some sort of exchange or turn-taking to create reciprocity in their joint play. Because Dan liked being Spiderman, they played that for as much as Dan wanted. David suggested one or two ideas at a session not to overwhelm Dan. The OT mainly framed the joint play experience and assisted in verbalizing each intention and gesture to promote reciprocity as well as social interaction in general. It appeared that the more they focused on small and enjoyable, fun moments of interaction, the more Dan and David felt at ease to simply play and be present for one another.

Winnicott's concept of the secure base (1995, 1999), young children benefit from a constant, secure, and safe environment where they maintain proximity with their attachment figure, yet are able to explore. Therefore, the session structure is designed to create this environment.

Each session begins with a greeting to both parent and child, creating a familiar ritual. Then the therapist invites the dyad to play for the next 20 minutes, where the child can also explore the environment in play. Once it is time to end the session, the therapist asks the parent and child to engage

PRACTICE EXAMPLE 11.6 Working with Families That Have Experienced Trauma and Adversity

Alice is a 28-year-old woman who is at a shelter where I run mother–child play sessions. When I first met Alice, the social worker had told me Alice had come from the hospital the night before and was reunited with her three children ages 6 years, 3 years, and 10 months. While Alice had been in the hospital receiving medical attention, her family members cared for her three children. The shelter staff informed me that Alice appeared disengaged for the past few hours, and her baby cried at night while she appeared to be in a deep sleep. A staff member had fed Alice's baby during the night, and the woman sharing a room with her took care of her 6-year-old daughter and 3-year-old son during the morning. The social worker had scheduled to meet with Alice after breakfast while her children attended the shelter daycare.

Alice's history was that her former boyfriend had raped and beaten her and she sustained severe physical injuries. As for her emotional injuries, details gradually unfolded as I got to know her. That first day, I met with Alice after she met with the social worker.

Parent Interview

Alice came in a few minutes late, and I greeted her and invited her to sit on the sofa across from me. I introduced myself and said that when a new woman with young children joins us, I meet with her alone, first, to learn about her needs and her children's needs. Alice listened; she was quiet and did not look at me. It seemed as if she was looking elsewhere. Her face had no expression. I continued with the family background questionnaire, and in the end, I asked about what had brought her to the shelter. She answered the questions while her face remained steel. She said her boyfriend attacked her in the presence of her baby, but she thinks she did not see or hear anything.

When I asked about the older children, she said they are fine with the move to the shelter, and there are no special developmental or emotional issues. I suggested we meet the following week so I could get to know her children and make time for play. I explained that we could take one child at a time for dyadic play. Alice said that was fine while her eyes looked at a spot in the wall behind me. Before I concluded our meeting, Alice suddenly said that she was experiencing a hard time with Andrew, her 3-year-old son. She stated that he didn't listen at all and could be aggressive and that he wasn't used to being with her. I asked her if she would rather we met first with Andrew or the girls. Alice wanted me to meet with her and all three of her children at the same time. She said that her 6-year-old, Megan, was helping her take care of Andrew and the baby, Shannon. I respected Alice's request regarding the meeting.

Initial Family Play Session

The following week I met with Alice and her three children. As they entered the room, I greeted them and invited them to sit on the carpet next to me. The playroom was set up with toys that suit children from infancy to 6 years. Alice held 10-month-old Shannon and sat on the carpet across from me; Megan sat next to her, which was also closer to me. Andrew was running around touching toys, and he seemed overwhelmed. Alice did not say anything. I asked Andrew if he wanted to meet my puppet and told him that the puppet wanted to say hi to him, his sisters, and his mom. Andrew kept running around, so I told him to "please join us when you are ready."

I started with a morning greeting, singing a song holding the puppet referring to Alice, Megan, and Shannon. The girls smiled back at me and held the puppet. Alice seemed distracted. I got up and greeted Andrew holding the puppet. Andrew grabbed the puppet and ran with it around the room. Megan said, "Andrew, that's not nice, come here." Andrew took a ball and kicked it. Alice said, "No Andrew." I suggested Megan choose a game she would like to play with and asked Alice, "What does Shannon like to play with?" pointing toward the basket with infant toys. She responded, "I don't know," pulled out a rattle, and gave it to Shannon, and then she put Shannon down on the carpet. Megan brought a puzzle and sat next to me. She took it out of the box and started to assemble the pieces. I suggested Alice join us. Megan did not look at Alice, and I said, "Alice come over here, there's a spot right here next to us." Alice moved and sat next to Megan and me. I handed a piece to Megan, asking if it would help her, Megan nodded and smiled. I continued, and it seemed she was waiting for me to hand her pieces. Baby Shannon was busy playing with the rattle, and Andrew was opening board games and taking the pieces out, moving from one game to the other. I suggested Alice switch roles with me and give puzzle pieces to Megan while I tried to see what Andrew would like to play with.

The only toy I had seen Andrew playing with for more than a few seconds was the ball. I approached Andrew and he moved quickly away. I stayed where I was and asked him if he wanted to play roll the ball with me. It seemed like a safe way to play ball with him having his baby sister on the carpet, his mom, and sister. Andrew took the ball and threw it across the other side of the room. I went to get the ball and he jumped over to grab it from me. I suggested we sit across from each other and roll the ball to see if we could catch it. I sat down and waited. Andrew threw the ball at me and I rolled it back to him saying: "Roll, roll, roll your ball." Andrew sat and I said, "Good job, Andrew, now roll, roll, roll the ball back to me." Andrew rolled the ball, then the next time he threw it. This parallel family play continued for a little longer until it was time to end the meeting.

I invited everyone to sit back in a circle and say good-bye to my puppet. Alice joined me, and Megan sat next to me. I suggested Alice bring Shannon, too, as I called Andrew to bring the ball and sit with us. Andrew came and sat next to Megan but outside the circle. I said that I enjoyed getting to know them all, and that next week I would like us to set time for joint play with each child separately. Alice said that was fine. Megan hugged me while Andrew rushed out yelling and kicking the ball.

Progression of Family Play

In the following weeks, I met with Alice and each of her children for short 15- to 20-minute joint play sessions. I observed her interactions with her children. I learned from the shelter staff that they as well as other women assisted Alice with parenting and everyday daily activities. As we developed a stronger therapeutic relationship. Alice shared with me bits and pieces of her story. From childhood, she had encountered sexual abuse and one traumatic event led to another. Her children were all exposed to her being assaulted by multiple partners, and Andrew's grandfather had physically abused him.

During the sessions, I was able to connect with Megan and Shannon. Alice gradually became a more active play partner and parented them. However, with Andrew, it was most challenging to find ways to connect. He was avoiding any gesture of human closeness or interaction. At one of our sessions, Alice, Andrew, and I were sitting on the carpet as we played with play dough. Suddenly, the alarm went off, and we jumped from its sharp sound. I looked for Andrew to check on him. Andrew was running around with a look of horror on his face. I knew he did not like to be touched, so I said, "It's okay, the alarm will stop soon. Come sit with us." Despite his fright and young age, Andrew did not seek an adult for protection. I then realized how profoundly he was affected by trauma. This incident as well as many other behaviors I witnessed taught me a lot about attachment, adversity, trauma, parenting, and play.

In the following sessions, I continued to respect each family member's emotional, social, and occupational needs. Alice needed someone who would care for her and her parenting needs without expecting anything relational in return. Megan needed a lot of reassurance, validation, and praise. Megan learned to get close when she needed and explored the play environment. She smiled back and responded and thrived during joint play. Andrew learned to sit next to us during play, to engage in play for longer periods, to ask for his needs to be met, and to respond to his mother and sisters.

Table 11.5 FI-OP Intervention Methods and Examples

Methods	Examples
Mediation: Several principles are used in mediating the interaction or child's play functioning (a) Intentionality and reciprocity—to encourage the child to perceive, understand, and experience an event on both cognitive and emotional levels. (b) Transcendence—the current interaction may be implemented in new situations beyond the current needs. (c) Meaning—the therapist provides meaning to different stimuli or to the interaction itself.	*Graded cues* ranging from general cue to more specific cue. To the child: "Where is the ball? Maybe it is hidden behind something or look over there (pointing) …" To the parent: When the child takes a bowl and puts it on a doll's head: "wait for him," "move closer," "follow her," "keep going." *Modeling*: The therapist serves as a "playful model" for the parent and/or the child, demonstrating certain playful behavior or supportive responses.
Environmental organization and adaptation: The play environment is designed to support and enhance interaction and playfulness.	The therapist designs and arranges a play space with a variety of toys and play materials that are safe to play with and adjusted to the child's play abilities and preferences. The play environment is well balanced in terms of the different stimulating factors in the room such as light and noise intensity, number of toys.
Consultation: Dissemination of knowledge while discussing ways to enhance positive interaction and to encourage or enable developing play skills and playfulness.	Discuss with the parent ways to modify the home play environment to match with the child and family needs. Encourage parental reflection on past play experiences and how it shaped how they play with their child. An additional topic that can stem from observing joint play: gender differences in play and how parental attributes affect joint play.

(continues)

Table 11.5 FI-OP Intervention Methods and Examples   (*continued*)

Methods	Examples
Reframing: Modifying the meaning of a situation by presenting new ways of viewing it. This method is applied in situations in which a parent perceives a child's behavior in a very negative light that interferes with their current joint play interaction.	The child throws a toy after having trouble manipulate it. The parent says "Well, he is aggressive," after which the therapist may say, "Maybe he is showing us that he has difficulty in manipulating the toy."
Reflection: Restating what the therapist observed or sensed of either the parent or child's behavior or feelings.	"Look, he is smiling at you. It seems like he is enjoying playing together."

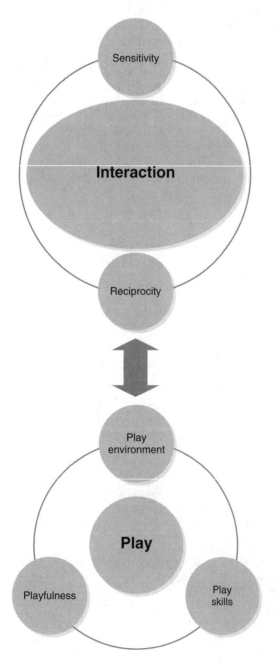

Figure 11.7 The FI-OP is a two-armed intervention model. One arm focuses on parent–child interaction, while the other focuses on improving child play

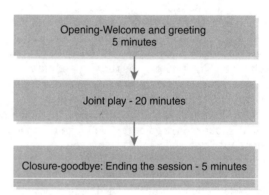

Figure 11.8 The FI-OP session structure

in the cleanup. Participating in cleanup allows the dyad to practice limit setting as well as gradually end the session. Right after cleanup time, the therapist invites both the parent and child to reconnect for "circle-closure time."

Research Support of FI-OP Intervention

In an effectiveness study, it was found that mother–child dyads who received 12 weekly FI-OP sessions compared to a control group, improved in several maternal, child, and dyadic aspects. Mothers demonstrated an improved interaction with their children during joint play and were more caring and affectionate toward their children. Children's play skills improved as well as their response to their mothers during joint play (Waldman-Levi & Weintraub, 2015).

Conclusion

Occupational therapists working with families and children recognize the centrality and importance of play to a child's growth and development. A child's engagement in play is relational and begins in the family context. Therefore, it is essential for occupational therapists to understand the essence of human relationships. Attachment theory provides an in-depth explanation for the parent–child bond and lays the foundation for understanding intimate relationships across the life span. Occupational therapists may assess parent–child play and use interventions such as the FI-OP model to promote play in families. Through parent–child play, occupational therapy practitioners jointly address both a parent's

interaction and support of the child in play together with the child's play skills and playfulness. Although early use has been primarily with families who had experienced domestic violence, professional reasoning may be used to determine application of the information provided in this chapter to support other families as well.

References

Ainsworth, M. D., Blehar, M., Waters, E., & Wall, S. (1978). *Patterns of attachment*. New York: Routledge.

Aoki, Y., Zeanah, C. H., Scott-Heller, S., & Bakshi, S. (2002). Parent–infant relationship global assessment scale: A study of its predictive validity. *Psychiatry and Clinical Neurosciences*, *56*, 493–497. https://doi.org/10.1046/j.1440-1819.2002.01044 .x011.03.004

Baker, J. K., Fenning, R. M., Howland, M. A., Baucom, B. R., Moffitt, J., & Erath, S. A. (2015). Brief report: A pilot study of parent–child biobehavioral synchrony in autism spectrum disorder. *Journal of Autism and Developmental Disorders*, *45*(12), 4140–4146. https://doi.org/10.1007/s10803-015-2528-0

Banyard, V. L., Williams, L. M., & Siegel, J. A. (2003). The impact of complex trauma and depression on parenting: An exploration of mediating risk and protective factors. *Child Maltreatment*, *8*(4), 334–349. https://doi.org/10.1177/1077559503257106

Baum, R. A. (2019). Learning to play and playing to learn: Enhancing interactions in young children with ASD. *Pediatrics*, *144*(3). https://doi.org/10.1542/peds.2019-1270e20191270

Bazyk, S., Stalnaker, D., Llerena, M., Ekelman, B., & Bazyk, J. (2003). Play in Mayan children. *American Journal of Occupational Therapy*, *57*, 273–283. https://doi.org/10.5014/ajot.57.3.273

Beetham, K. S., Sterman, J., Bundy, A. C., Wyver, S., Ragen, J., Engelen, L., … Naughton, G. (2019). Lower parent tolerance of risk in play for children with disability than typically developing children. *International Journal of Play*, *8*(2), 174–185. https://doi.org/10.1080/21594937.2019.1643980

Belsky, J. (1999a). Interactional and contextual determinants of attachment security. In J. Cassidy & P. R. Shaver (Eds.), *Handbook of attachment: Theory, research, and clinical applications* (pp. 249–264). New York: The Guilford Press.

Belsky, J. (1999b). Modern evolutionary theory and patterns of attachment. In J. Cassidy & P. R. Shaver (Eds.), *Handbook of attachment: Theory, research, and clinical applications* (pp. 141–161). New York: The Guilford Press.

Belsky, J., & Pascofearon, R. M. (2008). Precursors of attachment security. In J. Cassidy & P. R. Shaver (Eds.), *Handbook of attachment: Theory, research, and clinical application* (2nd ed., pp. 295–316). New York: The Guilford Press.

Benbassat, N., & Priel, B. (2012). Parenting and adolescent adjustment: The role of parental reflective functioning. *Journal of Adolescence*, *35*, 163–174. https://doi.org/10.1016/j .adolescence.2 011.03.004SRO

Berthelot, N., Ensink, K., Bernazzani, O., Normandin, L., Luyten, P., & Fonagy, P. (2015). Intergenerational transmission of attachment in abused and neglected mothers: The role of

trauma-specific reflective functioning. *Infant Mental Health Journal*, *36*, 200–212. https://doi.org/10.1002/imhj.21499

Bianchi, S. M., Robinson, J. P., & Milkie, M. A. (2007). *Changing rhythms of American family life*. New York: Russell Sage Foundation.

Borelli, J. L., Hong, K., Rasmussen, H. F., & Smiley, P. A. (2017). Reflective functioning, physiological reactivity, and overcontrol in mothers: Links with school-aged children's reflective functioning. *Developmental Psychology*, *53*, 1680–1693. https://doi.org/10.1037/dev0000371

Bowlby, J. (1969). *Attachment and loss*. (OKS Print.) New York: Basic Books.

Bowlby, J. (1988). *A secure base: Parent–child attachment and healthy human development*. New York: Basic Books.

Bradbury, B., Waldfogel, J., & Washbrook, E. (2019). Income-related gaps in early child cognitive development: Why are they larger in the United States than in the United Kingdom, Australia, and Canada? *Demography*, *56*(1), 367–390. https:// doi.org/10.1007/s13524-018- 0738-8

Brandell, J. R. (2010). Contemporary psychoanalytic perspectives on attachment. *Psychoanalytic Social Work*, *17*(2), 132–157.

Bryze, K. C. (2008). Narrative contributions to the play history. In L. D Parham & L. S Fazio (Eds.), *Play in occupational therapy for children* (2nd ed., 43–54). St. Louis, MO: Mosby.

Bundy, A., & Du Toit, S. H. J. (2019). Play and leisure. In B. A. B. Schell, G. Gillen, & M. E. Scaffa (Eds.), *Willard & Spackman's occupational therapy* (13th ed., pp. 805–823). Baltimore, MD: Lippincott Williams & Wilkins.

Cabrera, N. J., Hofferth, S. L., & Chae, S. (2011). Patterns and predictors of father–infant engagement across race/ethnic groups. *Early Childhood Research Quarterly*, *26*, 365–375. http://dx.doi.org/10.1016/j.ecresq.2011.01.001

Cabrera, N. J., Karberg, E., Malin, J. L., & Aldoney, D. (2017). The magic of play: Low-income mothers' and fathers' playfulness and children's emotional regulation and vocabulary skills. *Infant Mental Health Journal*, *38*(5), 1–14. https://doi.org/10.1002 /imhj.21682

Cabrera, N. J., & Roggman, L. (2017). Father play: Is it special? *Infant Mental Health Journal*, *38*(6), 706–708. https://doi .org/10.1002/imhj.21680

Caldwell, J. (2019). Let kids be kids. *FamilyFriend Poems*. https:// www.familyfriendpoems.com/poem/let-kids-be-kids

Childress, D. C. (2010). Play behaviors of parents and their young children with disabilities. *Topics in Early Childhood Special Education*, *29*(10), 1–9. https://doi.org/10.1177 %2F0271121410390526

Chopik, W. J., Edelstein, R. S., & Grimm, K. J. (2019). Longitudinal changes in attachment orientation over a 59-year period. *Journal of Personality and Social Psychology*, *116*(4), 598.

Cooper, R. J. (2000). The impact of child abuse on children's play: A conceptual model. *Occupational Therapy International*, *7*(4), 259–276. https://doi.org/10.1002/oti.127

Cosgrove, K., & Norris-Shortle, C. (2015). "Let's spend more time together like this": Fussy baby network infusion into a Baltimore homeless nursery program. *Zero to Three Journal*, *35*(3), 49–55.

De Falco, S., Esposito, G., Venuti, P., & Bornstein, M. H. (2010). Mothers and fathers at play with their children with Down syndrome: Influence on child exploratory and symbolic activity. *Journal of Applied Research in Intellectual Disabilities*, *23*(6), 579–605. https://doi.org/10.1111/j.1468-3148.2010.00558.x

Demir, Ö. E., & Küntay, A. C. (2014). Cognitive and neural mechanisms underlying socioeconomic gradients in language development: New answers to old questions. *Child Development Perspectives*, *8*(2), 113–118. https://doi.org/10.1111/cdep.12069

Desmarais, S. (2006). A space to float with someone: recovering play as a field of repair in work with parents of late-adopted children. *Journal of Child Psychotherapy*, *32*, 3, 349 –364. https://doi.org/10.1080/00754170600996879

Dionne, M., & Martini, R. (2011). Floor Time Play with a Child with Autism: A single-subject study. *Canadian Journal of Occupational Therapy*, *78*(3), 196–203. https://doi.org/10.2182/cjot.2011.78.3.8

Draper, P., & Beisky, J. (1990). Personality development in evolutionary perspective. *Journal of Personality*, *58*(1), 141–161.

Enlow, M.B., Blood, E., & Egeland, B. (2013). Sociodemographic risk, development competence, and PTSD symptoms in young children exposed to interpersonal trauma in early life. *Journal of Traumatic Stress*, *26*(6), 686-694. https://doi.org/10.1002/jts.21866

Feldman, R., & Eidelman, A. I. (2005). Does a triplet birth pose a special risk for infant development? Assessing cognitive development in relation to intrauterine growth and mother-infant interaction across the first 2 years. *Pediatrics*, *115*(2), 443-452. https://doi.org/10.1542/peds.2004-1137

Feuerstein, R., Klein, P. S., & Tannenbaum, A. J. (1991). *Mediated Learning Experience (MLE): Theoretical, psychosocial and learning implications*. London: Freund Publishing House, LTD.

Field, T. M., Ezell, S., Nadel, J., Grace, A., Allender, S., & Siddalingappa, V. (2013). Reciprocal imitation following adult imitation by children with Autism. *Infant and Child Development*, *22*(6), 642-648. https://doi.org/10.1002/icd.1812

Flanders, J.L., Leo, V., Paquette, D., Pihl, R.O., Séguin, J.R., & Séguin, J.R. (2009). Rough-and-tumble play and the regulation of aggression: an observational study of father–child play dyads. *Aggressive Behavior*, *35*(4), 285–295. https://doi.org/10.1002/ab.20309

Fonagy, P., & Target, M. (1998). Mentalization and the changing aims of child psychoanalysis. *Psychoanalytic Dialogues*, *8*, 87–114. https://doi.org/10.1080/10481889809539235

Freedman, J., & Combs, G. (1996). *Narrative therapy*. New York: W. W. Norton.

Gale, E., & Schick, B. (2009). Symbol-Infused joint attention and language use in mothers with deaf and hearing toddlers. *American Annals of the Deaf*, *153*(5), 484–503. http://www.jstor.org/stable/26234559

George, C., & Solomon, J. (2008). The caregiving system: A behavioral-system approach to parenting. In J. Cassidy & P. R. Shaver (Eds.), *Handbook of Attachment: Theory, Research, and Clinical Applications*, (2nd ed., pp. 833–856). New York: Guilford Press.

Gergely, G., & Watson, J.S. (1999). Early social-emotional development: Contingency perception and the social feedback model. In Rochat, P. (Ed.). *Early Social Cognition: Understanding Others in First Months of Life* (pp. 101–137). Hillsdale Erlbaum.

Gladstone, B.M., Boydell, K.M., Seeman, M.V., & McKeever, P.D. (2011). Children's experiences of parental mental illness: A literature review. *Early Intervention in Psychiatry*, *5*(4), 271–289. https://doi.org/10.1111/j.1751-7893.2011.00287.x

Gmitrova, V., Podhajecká, M., & Gmitrov, J. (2009). Children's play preferences: Implications for the preschool education. *Early Child Development and Care*, *179*(3), 339–351. https://doi.org/10.1080/03004430601101883

Godin, J., Freeman, A., & Rigby, P. (2017). Conceptual clarification of the playful engagement in social interaction of preschool-aged children with autism spectrum disorder (ASD). *Early Child Development and Care*, *189*(3), 430–440. https://doi.org/10.1080/03004430.2017.1324437

Graham, N. E., Truman, J., & Holgate, H. (2015). Parents' understanding of play for children with cerebral palsy. *American Journal of Occupational Therapy*, *69*, 6903220050. http://dx.doi.org/10.5014/ajot.2015.015263

Gross, D., Garvey, C., Julion, W., Louis, F., Sharon, T., & Hartmut, M. (2009). Efficacy of the Chicago Parent Program with low-income African American and Latino parents of young children. *Prevention Science*, *10*, 54–65. https://doi.org/10.1007/s11121-008-0116-7

Grossmann, K. E., Grossmann, K., & Waters, E. (Eds.). (2006). *Attachment from infancy to adulthood: The major longitudinal studies*. New York: Guilford Press.

Halfon, N., Larson, K., Son, J., Lu, M., & Bethell, C. (2017). Income inequality and the differential effect of adverse childhood experiences in US children. *Academic Paediatrics*, *17*, 70–78. https://doi.org/10.1016/j.acap.2016.11.007

Holmes, R. M., & Procaccino, J. K. (2009). Preschool children's outdoor play area preferences. *Early Child Development and Care*, *179*(8), 1103–1112. https://doi.org/10.1080/03004430701770694

Humfrees, H., O'Connor, T. G., Slaughter, J., Target, M., & Fongay, P. (2002). General and relationship-specific models of social cognition: Explaining the overlap and discrepancies. *Journal of Child Psychology and Psychiatry*, *43*(7), 873–883. https://doi.org/10.1111/1469-7610.0013_7

John, A., Halliburton, A., & Humphrey, J. (2013). Child–mother and child–father play interaction patterns with preschoolers. *Early Child Development and Care*, *183*(3–4), 483–497. https://doi.org/10.1080/03004430.2012.711595

Jones, J., & Mosher, W. D. (2013). Fathers' involvement with their children: United States, 2006–2010. *National Health Statistics Reports*, *71*, 1–21. Hyattsville, MD: National Center for Health Statistics.

Kelly-Vance, L., Dempsey, J., & Ryalls, B. (2013). The effect of a parent training program on children's play. *International Journal of Psychology*, *13*, 117–138. https://hdl.handle.net/20.500.12259/31798

Keren, M., Feldman, R., Namdari-Weinbaum, I., Spitzer, S., & Tyano, S. (2005). Relations between parents' interactive style in dyadic and triadic play and toddlers' symbolic capacity. *American Journal of Orthopsychiatry*, *75*(4), 599–607. https://doi.org/10.1037/0002-9432.75.4.599

Kloth, S., Janssen, P., Kraaimaat, F., & Brutten, G. J. (1998). Communicative styles of mothers interacting with their preschool-age children: A factor analytic study. *Journal of Child Language*, *25*, 149–168. https://doi.org/10.1017/S0305000997003334

Knox, S. (2008). Development and current use of the Revised Knox Preschool Play Scale. In L. D. Parham & L. S. Fazio (Eds.), *Play in occupational therapy for children* (2nd ed., pp. 71–93). St. Louis, MO: Mosby.

Kuhaneck, H. M., Spitzer, E., & Spitzer, S. L. (2010). *Activity analysis, creativity, and playfulness in pediatric occupational therapy: Making play just right*. Sudbury, MA: Jones and Bartlett Publishers.

Kwon, K. A., Jeon, H. J., Lewsader, J. T., & Elicker, J. (2012). Mothers' and fathers' parenting quality and toddlers' interactive behaviours in dyadic and triadic family contexts. *Infant and Child Development*, *21*(4), 356–373. https://doi.org/10.1002/icd.1746

LaMothe, R. (2005). Creating space: The fourfold dynamic of potential space. *Psychoanalytic Psychology*, *22*(2), 207–223. https://doi.org/10.1037/0736-9735.22.2.207

Levavi, K., Menashe-Grinberg, A., Barak-Levy, Y., & Atzaba-Poria, N. (2020). The role of parental playfulness as a moderator reducing child behavioural problems among children with intellectual disability in Israel. *Research in Developmental Disabilities*, *107*, 103793. https://doi.org/10.1016/j.ridd.2020.103793

Lifter, K., Foster-Sanda, S., Arzamarski, C., Briesch, J., & McClure, E. (2011). Overview of play: Its uses and importance in early intervention/early childhood special education. *Infants & Young Children*, *24*(3), 225–245. https://doi.org/10.1097/iyc.0b013e31821e995c

Lindsey, E. W., & Mize, J. (2000). Parent–child physical and pretense play: Links to children's social competence. *Merrill-Palmer Quarterly*, *46*(4), 565–588. https://www.jstor.org/stable/23092565

Lowinger, S., Dimitrovsky, L, Strauss, H., & Mogliner, C. (1995). Maternal social and physical contact: Links to early infant attachment behaviors. *The Journal of Genetic Psychology*, *156*(4), 461–476. https://doi.org/10.1080/00221325.1995.9914837

Marvin, R. S., & Britner, P. A. (2008). Normative development: The ontogeny of attachment. In J. Cassidy & P. R. Shaver (Eds.), *Handbook of attachment: Theory, research, and clinical application* (2nd ed., pp. 269–294). New York: The Guilford Press.

Mattingly, C., & Fleming, M. H. (1994). *Clinical reasoning: Forms of inquiry in a therapeutic practice*. Philadelphia, PA: F. A. Davis.

Menashe-Grinberg, A., & Atzaba-Poria, N. (2017). Mother–child and father–child play interaction: The importance of parental playfulness as a moderator of the links between parental behavior and child negativity. *Infant Mental Health Journal*, *38*(6), 772–784.

Mikulincer, M., Shaver, P. R., & Horesh, N. (2006). Attachment bases of emotion regulation and posttraumatic adjustment. In D. K. Snyder, J. A. Simpson, & J. N. Hughes (Eds.), *Emotion regulation in couples and families: Pathways to dysfunction and health* (pp. 77–99). Washington, DC: American Psychological Association.

Nadel, J., Martini, M., Field, T., Escalona, A., & Lundy, B. (2008). Children with autism approach more imitative and playful adults. *Early Child Development and Care*, *178*(5), 461–465. https://doi.org/10.1080/030044306008016

Nakano, S., Kondo-Ikemura, K., & Kusanagi, E. (2007). Perturbation of Japanese mother–infant habitual interactions in the double video paradigm and relationship to maternal playfulness. *Infant Behavior and Development*, *30*(2), 213–231. https://doi.org/10.1016/j.infbeh.2007.02.005

Narayan, A. J., Rivera, L. M., Bernstein, R. E., Harris, W. W., & Lieberman, A. F. (2017). Positive childhood experiences predict less psychopathology and stress in pregnant women with childhood adversity: A pilot study of the benevolent childhood experiences (BCEs) scale. *Child Abuse and Neglect*, *78*, 19–30. https://doi.org/10.1016/j.chiabu.2017.09.022

Olson, L. (2006a). When a mother is depressed: Supporting her capacity to participate in co-occupation with her baby—A case study. *Occupational Therapy in Mental Health*, *22*(3–4), 135–152. https://doi.org/10.1300/J004v22n03_09

Olson, L. (2006b). Introduction. *Occupational Therapy in Mental Health*, *22*(3–4), 1–10.

Oppenheim, D., Koren-Karie, N., Dolev, S., & Yirmiya, N. (2009). Maternal insightfulness and resolution of the diagnosis are associated with secure attachment in preschoolers with autism spectrum disorders. *Child Development*, *80*(2), 519–527. https://doi.org/10.1111/j.1467-8624.2009.01276.x

Oppenheim, D., & Koren-Karie, N. (2002). Mothers' insightfulness regarding their children's internal worlds: The capacity underlying secure child–mother relationship. *Infant Mental Health Journal*, *23*(6), 593–605. https://doi.org/10.1002/imhj.10035

Ordway, M. R., Webb, D., Sadler, L. S., & Slade, A. (2015). Parental reflective functioning: An approach to enhancing parent–child relationships in pediatric primary care. *Journal of Pediatric Health Care*, *29*, 325–334. https://doi.org/10.1016/j.pedhc.2014.12.002

Parham, D. L. (2008). Play and occupational therapy. In L. D. Parham & L. S. Fazio, *Play in occupational therapy for children* (2nd ed.), pp. 3–39. St. Louis, MO: Mosby.

Parham, L. D., & Primeau, L. A. (2008). Play and occupational therapy. In L. D. Parham & L. S. Fazio (Eds.), *Play in occupational therapy for children* (2nd ed., pp. 2–21). St. Louis, MO: Mosby, Inc.

Pickens, N. D., & Pizur-Barnekow, K. (2009). Co-occupational: Extending the dialogue. *Journal of Occupational Science*, *16*(3), 151–156. https://doi.org/10.1080/14427591.2009.9686656

Raffington, L., Czamarac, D., Mohnad, J. J., Falcka, J., Schmollc, V., … Shing, Y. L. (2019). Stable longitudinal associations of family income with children's hippocampal volume and memory persist after controlling for polygenic scores of educational attainment. *Developmental Cognitive Neuroscience*, *40*, 1–9. https://doi.org/10.1016/j.dcn.2019.100720

Reilly, M. (1974). *Play as exploratory learning*. Beverly Hills, CA: Sage Publications.

Reizer, A., & Mikulincer, M. (2007). Assessing individual differences in working models of caregiving: The construction and validation of the mental representation of caregiving scale. *Journal of Individual Difference*, 28, 227–239. https://doi.org/10.1027/1614-0001.28.4.227

Risser, H. J., Messinger, A. M., Fry, D. A., Davidson, L. L., & Schewe, P. A. (2013). Do maternal and paternal mental illness and substance abuse predict treatment outcomes for children exposed to violence? *Child Care in Practice*, 19(3), 221–236. https://doi.org/10.1080/13575279.2013.785932

Rutgers, A. H., Bakermans-Kranenburg, M. J., van Ijzendoorn, M. H., & van Berckelaer-Onnes, I. A. (2004). Autism and attachment: A meta-analytic review. *Journal of Child Psychology and Psychiatry*, 45, 1123–1134. https://doi.org/10.1111/j.1469-7610.2004.t01-1-00305.x

Schneider, E. (2009). Longitudinal observations of infants' object play behavior in the home context. *OTJR: Occupation, Participation and Health*, 29(2), 79–87. https://doi.org/10.3928/15394492-20090301-06

Selcuk, E., Günaydin, G., Sumer, N., Harma, M., Salman, S., Hazan, C., Dogruyol, B., & Ozturk, A. (2010). Self-reported romantic attachment style predicts everyday maternal caregiving behavior at home. *Journal of Research in Personality*, 44, 544–549. https://doi.org/10.1016/j.jrp.2010.05.007

Servin, A., Bohlin, G., & Berlin, L. (1999). Sex differences in 1-, 3-, and 5-year-olds' toy-choice in a structured play-session. *Scandinavian Journal of Psychology*, 40, 43–48. https://doi.org/10.1111/1467-9450.00096

Seskin, L., Feliciano, E., Tippy, G., Yedloutschnig, R., Sossin, K. M., & Yasik, A. (2010). Attachment and autism: Parental attachment representations and relational behaviors in the parent–child dyad. *Journal of Abnormal Child Psychology*, 38(7), 949–960. https://doi.org/10.1007/s10802-010-9417-y

Sethna, V., Murray, L., Edmondson, O., Iles, J., & Ramchandani, P. G. (2018). Depression and playfulness in fathers and young infants: A matched design comparison study. *Journal of Affective Disorders*, 229, 364–370.

Shai, D., & Belsky, J. (2011a). When words just won't do: Introducing parental embodied mentalizing. *Child Development Perspectives*, 5(3), 173–180. https://doi.org/10.1111/j.1750-8606.2011.00181.x

Shai, D., & Belsky, J. (2011b). Parental embodied mentalizing: Let's be explicit about what we mean by implicit. *Child Development Perspectives*, 5(3), 187–188. https://doi.org/10.1111/j.1750-8606.2011.00195.x

Shaver, P. R., Mikulincer, M., & Shemesh-Iron, M. (2010). A behavioral systems perspective on prosocial behavior. In M. Mikulincer & P. R. Shaver (Eds.), *Prosocial motives, emotions, and behavior: The better angles of our nature* (pp. 72–91). Washington, DC: American Psychological Association.

Skard, G., & Bundy, A. C. (2008). Test of playfulness. In L. D. Parham & L. S. Fazio (Eds.), *Play in occupational therapy for children* (2nd ed., pp. 71–93). St. Louis, MO: Mosby.

Slade, A., Grienenberger, J., Bernbach, E., Levy, D., & Locker, A. (2005). Maternal reflective functioning, attachment, and the transmission gap: A preliminary study. *Attachment & Human Development*, 7, 283–298. https://doi.org/10.1080/14616730500245880

Slade, A. (2007). Reflective parenting programs: Theory and development. *Psychoanalytic Inquiry*, 26, 640–657. https://doi.org/10.1080/07351690701310698

Sroufe, A. L. (2005). Attachment and development: A prospective, longitudinal study from birth to adulthood. *Attachment & Human Development*, 7(4), 349–367. https://doi.org/10.1080/14616730500365928

St George, J., Fletcher, R., & Palazzi, K. (2017). Comparing fathers' physical and toy play and links to child behaviour: An exploratory study. *Infant and Child Development*, 26(1). https://doi.org/10.1002/icd.1958

St George, J., & Freeman, E. (2017). Measurement of father–child rough-and-tumble play and its relations to child behavior. *Infant Mental Health Journal*, 38(6), 709–725. https://doi.org/10.1002/imhj.21676

Strand, P. S. (2002). Coordination of maternal directives with preschoolers' behavior: Influence of maternal coordination training on dyadic activity and child compliance. *Journal of Clinical Child and Adolescent Psychology*, 31(1), 6–15. https://doi.org/10.1207/153744202753441620

Swinth, Y., & Tanta, K. J. (2008). Play, leisure, and social participation in educational settings. In L. D. Parham & L. S. Fazio, *Play in occupational therapy for children* (2nd ed., pp. 301–317). St. Louis, MO: Mosby.

Waldman-Levi, A. (2012). *The efficacy of an intervention program for mothers and their children who reside in shelters for battered women, on mother's parental functioning, mother–child interaction and child's play functioning* (Unpublished doctoral dissertation). Hebrew University, Jerusalem, Israel.

Waldman-Levi, A., & Bundy, A. (2016). A glimpse into co-occupations: Parent's support of young children's playfulness scale. *Occupational Therapy in Mental Health*, 32(3). http://www.tandfonline.com/doi/full/10.1080/0164212X.2015.1116420

Waldman-Levi, A., Bundy, A., & Shai, D. (in preparation). *Playfulness development and cognitive ability among typically developing children: A longitudinal study* [Manuscript in preparation]. Occupational Therapy Department, Long Island University, Brooklyn.

Waldman-Levi, A., Finzi-Dottan, R., & Cope, A. (2019a). Balancing between synchrony and completion: A grounded theory approach to joint play at the latent period. *Journal of Child and Family Studies*, 1–22. https://doi.org/10.1007/s10826-019-01638-8

Waldman-Levi, A., Grinion, S., & Olson, L. (2019b). Effects of maternal views and support on childhood development through joint play. *The Open Journal of Occupational Therapy*, 7(4), 1–21. https://doi.org/10.15453/2168-6408.1613

Waldman-Levi, A., Katz, N., & Bundy, A. (2015). Playfulness and interaction: An exploratory study of past and current exposure to domestic violence. *Occupational Therapy Journal of Research*. https://doi.org/10.1177/1539449214561762

Waldman-Levi A., Olson, L., Apesa, S., Katz, H., Malks, T., Rychik, L., … Kohan, S. (2020). Father–child joint play experience and effects on child's playfulness. [poster abstract]. *The American Journal of Occupational Therapy*, 74(4_Supplement_1). https://doi.org/10.5014/ajot.2020.74S1-PO114

Waldman-Levi, A., Olson, L., Sheills, M., & Bundy. A. (2017). Co-occupations: Feasibility of a comprehensive in-depth assessment procedure. *The American Occupational Therapy Association Annual Conference*, Philadelphia, PA, US.

Waldman-Levi, A., & Weintraub, N. (2015). Efficacy of a crisis intervention for improving mother–child interaction and the children's play functions. *The American Journal of Occupational, Therapy, 69*, 1–11. https://doi.org/10.5014/ajot.2015.013375.

Weintraub, N., & Waldman Levi, A. (2009). Mother–child play. In R. Carlisle (Ed.), *Encyclopedia of play in today's society* (pp. 404–408). Thousand Oaks, CA: Sage. http://dx.doi .org/10.4135/9781412971935.n246

Weisleder, A., Brockmeyer-Cates, B., Dreyer, B. P., Berkule-Johnson, S., Huberman, H. S., Seery, A. M., … Mendelsohn, A. L. (2016). Promotion of positive parenting and prevention of socioemotional disparities. *Pediatrics, 137*(2). https://doi .org/10.1542/peds.2015-3239

Winnicott, D. W. (1995). *Playing and reality*. Tel-Aviv: Am-Oved.

Winnicott, D. W. (1999). *The child, the family and the outside world*. Tel-Aviv: Sifriat Poalim Publishing House Ltd.

Zvara, B. J., Sheppard, K. W., & Cox, M. (2018). Bidirectional effects between parenting sensitivity and child behavior: A cross-lagged analysis across middle childhood and adolescence. *Journal of Family Psychology, 32*, 484–495. https://doi.org/10.1037/fam0000372

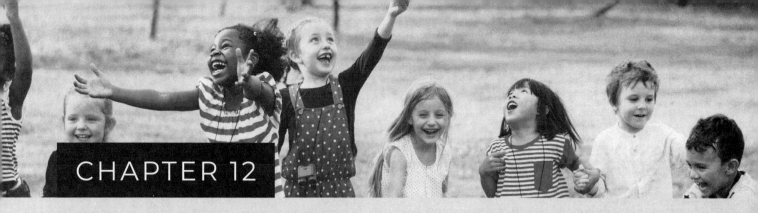

CHAPTER 12

Play to Promote Mental Health in Children and Youth

Lola Halperin, EdD, OTR/L

Sharon M. McCloskey, EdD, MBA, OTR/L, DipCOT

After reading this chapter, the reader will:

- Identify the benefits of play in relation to mental health.
- Describe the effects of adversity and mental health conditions on play.
- Make play "just right" for children with mental health concerns.
- Manage barriers to implementing play-based interventions for children with mental health concerns.

When we treat children's play as seriously as it deserves, we are helping them feel the joy that's to be found in the creative spirit. It's the things we play with and the people who help us play that make a great difference in our lives.

—Fred Rogers

Play contributes to the social emotional health of children (Ginsburg, 2007). Play is primarily a pleasurable experience that often results in positive emotions, which in turn, helps build a child's resilience and sense of well-being (Donaldson et al., 2011; Fredrickson, 2004; Seligman & Csikszentmihalyi, 2000). In contrast, mental illness can disrupt occupations (Krupa et al., 2009), including the essential occupation of play. Mental health conditions may become a barrier to play and have a negative effect on participation in other occupations (Keyes, 2007; Passmore, 2003; Singh & Anekar, 2018; Zawadzki et al., 2015). The benefit of play for mental health suggests that children and youth who have, or are at risk of, mental health conditions can benefit from a focus on play in occupational therapy. Occupational therapy practitioners therefore must understand the importance of play for children who experience trauma, adversity, and mental health conditions. This chapter presents play as a way to promote mental health and well-being as well as a desired outcome for children and youth with mental health conditions.

Mental Health

Mental health is the psychological foundation that supports all aspects of health and human development. Mental health is defined as a positive state of being and includes emotional, psychological, and social aspects of function (Galderisi et al., 2015). Mental health encompasses how one thinks and feels, how one manages social interactions, and how one regulates emotions and behaviors (American Occupational Therapy Association [AOTA], 2016a, 2016b).

Development of Mental Health in Children and Youth

The mental health of children and youth is a dynamic state of flourishing and functioning that includes elements of coping and resilience and changes over time depending on relationships, life situations, or stressors (Keyes, 2007). Recent research has broadened our understanding of the complex interplay of the impact on mental health from biological, family, community, and societal levels (National Academies of Sciences, Engineering, and Medicine, 2019; Ungar & Theron, 2020). Science informs us that fetal and early childhood experiences shape brain architecture and can strengthen or disrupt a child's emotional and mental health well-being (National Scientific Council on the Developing Child, 2012; Zhang et al., 2021). Positive relationships with responsive, caring adults are an important foundation for mental health as well as an ongoing protective factor (Mikulincer & Shaver, 2012; Rutten et al., 2013; please see Chapter 11 for more detail). Over time, advantages such as strong families, communities, and full societal inclusion continue to encourage the development of a healthy mind and body (National Academies of Sciences, Engineering, and Medicine 2019; Silva, Loureiro, & Cardoso, 2016).

Youth mental health development similarly includes positive and caring family and peer relationships, as well as learning about how to cope with mild or moderate levels of stress (Gunnar & Quevedo, 2007; Patalay & Fitzsimons, 2018; Spencer, Chun, Hartsock, & Woodruff, 2020; Triana, Keliat, & Sulistiowati, 2019; Ungar & Theron, 2020). Interrelated brain circuits and hormone systems that are specifically designed for youth to adapt to situations or environmental challenges allow for managing and coping with stress (Loman & Gunnar, 2010; Lupian, 2017; Van Der Kolk, 2014). In adolescence, science demonstrates the importance and complexity of the interaction between risk factors and resilience in relation to mental health (Gore & Colten, 2017).

Mental Health Conditions in Children and Youth

The development of a mental health condition is the result of a complex interplay of multiple internal and external factors and exposures, time/age, and exposure to unpredictable life events. Although they require a combination of biological, psychological, and environmental factors (Larson et al., 2017), in children and youth, mental health conditions are, however, quite common.

Prevalence of Pediatric Mental Health Conditions

In the United States, the prevalence of psychiatric conditions in youngsters has increased, now affecting 13–20% in a given year. Of children ages 2–17 years, 9.4 % have been diagnosed with ADHD, while 7.4% of children ages 3–17 years exhibit behavioral problems, 7.1% have been diagnosed with anxiety and 3.2% with depression. Anxiety, depression, and behavioral problems are even more common among children and adolescents living below the federal poverty level, affecting 22% of this population (Centers for Disease Control [CDC], 2019). These conditions often co-occur in the same child (CDC, 2020a). With this growing prevalence, researchers have become more interested in the factors leading to mental health conditions in children and youth.

Risk Factors

Structural brain abnormalities and/or chemical imbalances in the brain accompany most of the psychiatric conditions (American Psychiatric Association [APA], 2013; Bonder, 2015; CDC, 2021); however, biological vulnerabilities and genetic susceptibility interplay with other risk factors. Research suggests that many psychosocial vulnerabilities or stressors contribute to the development of psychopathology in children (Garfinkel et al., 1990; Meiser-Stedman et al., 2017). Maughan and Kim-Cohen (2015) describe epigenetic factors such as a child's stress response, individual vulnerabilities, and environmental or situational triggers. Some childhood psychiatric conditions are neurodevelopmental in nature, but other risk factors include parental and environmental stress and parental mental health conditions (Simmons et al., 2017; Yule, Houston, & Grych, 2019). Compromised early attachment patterns can negatively alter neural systems and neurodevelopment and contribute to neuropsychiatric problems, resulting in social and emotional difficulties later in life (Gaskill & Perry 2014). Intrinsic elements that influence the development of mental health conditions include temperament, insecure attachment, low self-esteem, shyness, and excessive worries or fears (Gartland, Riggs, Muyeen, et al., 2019). Extrinsic elements include poverty, deprivation, abuse, neglect, and exposure to other adverse childhood experiences (Basu & Banerjee, 2020).

Additional risk factors include adverse childhood experiences and trauma. The CDC (2020c) reports that one in seven children in the United States experience abuse, neglect, or adverse childhood experiences (ACEs). In the United States, approximately one million children are victims of maltreatment or trauma in any given year (National Child Traumatic Stress Network [NCTSN], 2020). Life events that cause adversity and traumatic stress in children and adolescents include physical, sexual, and emotional abuse and neglect; family dysfunction/mental illness or incarceration of a family member; institutional rearing; both community and domestic violence and/or substance abuse; human trafficking; natural disasters; mass shootings; terrorism and war/refugee experiences; life-changing accidents and illnesses; and losses of loved ones, such as sudden deaths or military deployment of family members, etc. (Cohen et al., 2010; NCTSN, 2020; Pizur-Barnekow, 2019).

Reactions to adverse events in children include negative emotional responses, attachment issues, developmental regression, behavioral changes/increased risk-taking and aggressiveness, disrupted sleeping and feeding patterns, and a variety of physical health problems (Felitti et al., 1998 as cited in Brown et al., 2019; NCTSN, 2020). Exposure to maltreatment, domestic violence, and other forms of adversity frequently results in developmental delays, trauma-and-stressor-related disorders, delinquency, or other mental health issues (APA, 2013; Cohen et al., 2010; Conradt et al., 2014; Enlow et al., 2013; Patterson et al., 2018; Sciaraffa et al., 2018). Psychiatric conditions in the trauma-and-stressor-related disorders category include reactive attachment and disinhibited social engagement disorders, adjustment disorder, acute stress disorder, posttraumatic stress disorder (PTSD), and persistent complex bereavement disorder, all of which are accompanied by disrupted play patterns in children and adolescents (APA, 2013; Bonder, 2015; Champagne, 2019).

Relationship to Age and Developmental Stage

Across the life span, there are frequent changes in both mental health and mental illness (Westerhof & Keyes, 2010). Certain mental health concerns can be experienced at any stage of childhood or adolescence; however, other emotional problems, such as anxiety or depression, and behavioral disorders, such as self-injury, noncompliance, and significant aggressions (verbal or physical), tend to occur in later childhood. Still other conditions, such as schizophrenia, are more often diagnosed in late adolescence or early adulthood (Kessler et al., 2007).

Threshold to Diagnosis

While most children and youth experience some level of stress and adversity, or mental health challenge at some point in their lives, not all emotional or behavioral responses are indicative of a psychiatric condition (Ogundele, 2018). Some behaviors can be a transient reaction to external circumstances. As children and youth grow, many experience occasional fears, worries, or behaviors such as impulsivity or tantrums. Early childhood behavior difficulties, such as being defiant or impulsive from time to time, becoming aggressive or losing one's temper, having a tantrum, and being deceitful or stealing occasionally, are considered an aspect of typical development in very young children and preschoolers (**Figure 12.1**). However, severe problem behaviors and prolonged emotional distress are generally indicative of a mental health condition (Galderisi et al., 2015). The challenge for practitioners is to distinguish a possible mental illness, which requires referral and intervention, from typical child

Figure 12.1 Not all behavioral difficulties indicate a mental health condition, as they are an occasional part of typical development

© Jill Tindall/Moment/Getty Images.

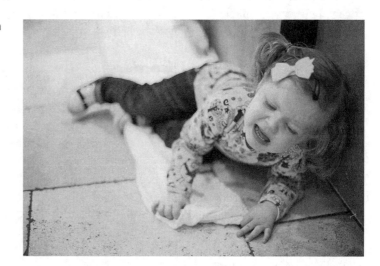

development or transient situational crisis, which can be managed without additional support.

Mental Health and Play
The Impact of Mental Health Conditions on Play

Mental health conditions and psychiatric conditions in childhood disrupt playfulness as well as the ability to participate and engage in the elements and patterns of play, both individually and with others (Pollack et al., 2016). Even though behavioral and emotional conditions in children are not always visible, how children with these conditions play and behave during play is observably different (Caprino & Stucci, 2017). For example, when a young child has a mental health condition, attunement play is disrupted (Whitcomb, 2012). The child may not have the capacity to effectively connect and engage with others. A child with a mental health condition may have difficulties deciding what to play, with whom, or how (Remsetter et al., 2010). As a result, object play, social play, and transformative-integrative and creative play patterns are altered. The form, function, and meaning of the play is different. Elements of playfulness, such as internal control, internal motivation, and the ability to suspend reality, may be disrupted (Bundy, 1997). If a child or adolescent is not feeling mentally well or in a "just right" emotional state, it can be difficult to be playful or to engage in play. Therefore, there will be observable altered play behaviors and patterns that result from mental ill-health such as refusal to participate in play, lack of spontaneity, persistent boredom, frequent temper tantrums/explosive behaviors, seeking to have his/her "own way" all the time, excessive need for reassurance, or difficulty taking turns or following the rules. Each mental health condition can negatively influence children's and adolescents' engagement, performance, and satisfaction across all areas of occupation, including play, in varied ways.

Neurodevelopmental Disorders and Play

There are a variety of neurodevelopmental disorders and each may impact play slightly differently. A child with an intellectual impairment might have a hard time participating in play activities due to cognitive and communication deficits, sensory processing issues, clumsiness, and social isolation. Children with intellectual impairments, although spontaneous and curious during play, may show less enjoyment of challenges presented in play activities (Messier, Ferland, & Majnemer, 2008). Multiple studies have documented

the way in which autism spectrum disorder (ASD) impacts play (Hobson, Lee, & Hobson, 2009; Jarrold, 2003). A child with ASD might exhibit restricted play preferences and repertoire due to difficulty with transitioning to novel situations (APA, 2013; Bonder, 2015; Tanner et al., 2015). In contrast, youngsters with a developmental coordination disorder (DCD) participate less in and are sometimes left out of team play and sport activities because of their clumsiness and inability to catch up with typically developing peers (APA, 2013; Bonder, 2015; Izadi-Najafabadia, 2019). Their play differs in other ways than merely motor skill (Rosenblum, Waissman, & Diamond, 2017), as they have fewer friends, less enjoyment in their play, and fewer play choices and opportunities. Preliminary evidence also shows that young children with DCD might be more prone than their typically developing peers to take part in aggressive play, both as victims and perpetrators (Kennedy-Behr et al., 2013). Children and adolescents affected by attention-deficit/hyperactivity disorder (ADHD) may struggle with sustaining attention and sequencing tasks, noticing details, following instructions, and controlling impulses. They often lose belongings, fidget during quiet tasks and seek movement excessively, present as more talkative than others, and intrude on conversations (APA, 2013; Bonder, 2015). Additionally, young people affected by ADHD demonstrate deficient social skills and less empathy for others when compared to their typically developing peers (Wilkes-Gillan et al., 2016). Studies of the play of those with ADHD suggest they are less likely to participate in cooperative play and may have more conflict, lack empathy, and be more likely to play indoors on the computer (Cordier, Bundy, Hocking, & Einfeld, 2010; Jasem & Delport, 2019; Normand et al., 2019).

Disruptive, Impulse-Control, and Conduct Disorders and Play

Issues with impulse control and lack of empathy are common among young individuals with oppositional defiant and conduct disorders, which are often characterized by poor social skills and hostility toward others. For example, a child with oppositional defiant behaviors might frequently bully peers, while an adolescent with conduct issues might violate rules, initiate physical altercations, show cruelty toward animals, and purposefully destroy property owned by others. Such behaviors can subsequently lead to social isolation and limited opportunities for age-appropriate play activities (APA, 2013; Bonder, 2015; Pollack et al., 2016). Compromised social skills are even more evident in children with complex symptomatology, such as ADHD combined with oppositional defiant disorder and higher levels of anxiety (Pollack et al., 2016). Moreover, behavioral problems in youngsters might eventually result in their placement in foster care or encounters with the juvenile forensic system (Engler, Sarpong, Van Horne, Greeley, & Keefe, 2020; Islam et al., 2020), which in turn might further decrease opportunities for developing healthy play/leisure habits.

Anxiety Disorders and Play

Anxiety can also impede play participation. For instance, a child diagnosed with separation anxiety might be able to play successfully in the presence of a trusted caregiver, yet refrain from any forms of play when feeling overwhelmed by the caregiver's absence, even if it is brief. An adolescent affected by social phobia might experience a similar discomfort when attempting to join play activities that involve peer interaction. Additionally, inflexible play patterns (e.g., unnecessarily repeating game steps or reordering toys or game parts) or compulsive cleaning up of toys may occur with obsessive-compulsive disorder (Brezinka, Mailänder, & Walitza, 2020). Research suggests that children with higher anxiety play less imaginatively, engage in more solitary play, express less positive affect in play, and demonstrate decreased organization in their play than those with less anxiety (Barnett, 1984; Christian, Russ, & Short, 2011).

Mood Disorders and Play

Play participation is often negatively influenced by affective symptoms, such as depression or mania. Unstable mood, anger, and irritability along with impulsive behaviors characterize young individuals diagnosed with disruptive mood dysregulation disorder and can be even more pronounced in those diagnosed with bipolar illness, often resulting in these youngsters being excluded from social play. Depression, on the other hand, often comes with diminished energy, impaired concentration, psychomotor retardation, poor self-esteem, and decreased ability to experience pleasure, all of which inevitably could limit a child's ability to enjoy playing (APA, 2013; Bonder, 2015). Children with depression play less and may engage in more nonplay than children without depression (Lous, de Wit, de Bruyn, Riksen-Walraven, & Rost, 2000).

Psychosis and Play

Psychosis is characterized by hallucinations (altered perceptions), delusions (fixed, unsubstantiated beliefs), distorted thought process, grossly disorganized speech and behavior, and negative symptoms, such as restricted emotional expression, diminished motivation, and diminished ability to enjoy daily activities. Psychosis can occur in children and adolescents as a result of different psychiatric conditions, such as schizophrenia spectrum disorders (SSD), bipolar illness, major depression and OCD, or due to exposure to trauma (APA, 2013; Green et al., 2015). Although less common than other mental health problems in pediatrics, when present, psychosis can challenge children's engagement in play by negatively affecting their cognition, language, imagination, and spontaneity during play (Green et al., 2015). Additionally, it is important to mention that children who are later diagnosed with SSD are also likely to demonstrate mild motor delays (APA, 2013; Hans et al., 2005), which further complicates their play participation.

Feeding and Eating Disorders and Play

Some of the childhood/adolescence psychiatric conditions impact play adversely because of the amount of time and energy the affected young individuals spend on the maladaptive routines that accompany their conditions. For example, an adolescent affected by anorexia nervosa or bulimia nervosa might be consumed by binging, purging, and exercising excessively, leaving little time for healthy leisure and socialization. In contrast, a child with pica may attempt to eat nonfood substances that are used in play (e.g., chalk, paint, strings, and pebbles) instead of playing with them (APA, 2013; Bonder, 2015; National Eating Disorders Association, 2020). Little research exists examining the relationships between these conditions and play or leisure specifically; however, one study identified restrictions in social leisure as the area of greatest perceived impairment reported by a group of individuals with anorexia (Tchanturia et al., 2013).

Substance-Related Disorders and Play

There is a relationship between leisure and substance use (Caldwell & Faulk, 2013; Sharp et al., 2011). Substance use can have a detrimental effect on play/leisure participation in young people. For instance, one of the symptoms of inhalant use disorder, which is more common in children ages 12–17 years than adults, is reducing or giving up social and recreational activities for the sake of using inhalant substances (APA, 2013; Bonder, 2015). Similarly, experimenting with other types of substances might have a negative impact on the developmental trajectory of children and adolescents, subsequently reducing their play/leisure opportunities and negatively affecting their quality. Engagement in healthy leisure, however, can be preventative (Caldwell & Faulk, 2013; Sharp et al., 2011). Occupational therapy practitioners may be able to assist youth in developing healthy leisure to prevent or reduce substance use.

Excessive substance use in adults can compromise children's play participation indirectly. For instance, children born to mothers who abuse alcohol might present with fetal alcohol spectrum disorders (FASD), which result in an array of sensory, motor, cognitive, social, and emotional deficits (CDC, 2020b), inevitably disrupting play skill acquisition in these children and their sense of mastery over play. Children with FASD have been shown to be less playful than those without the disorder (Pearton, Ramugondo, Cloete, & Cordier, 2014).

Gaming Addiction and Play

The era of technological advancements and social media has provided children and adolescents with augmented virtual opportunities, but has also created new mental health challenges for this population. Gaming addiction is now included in both the DSM-5 and the ICD-11 and is considered a significant public health concern that requires more research (APA, 2013; Kwak et al., 2020; Rumpf et al., 2018). While Internet gaming offers certain cognitive, motor, emotional, and even social benefits to young people and can be used therapeutically, when excessive, it is associated with disrupted daily routines, impulsivity, and poor behavioral control, especially in the absence of proper social supports (Kwak et al., 2020). Moreover, even though active video games might be less harmful than sedentary video games, when they replace active outdoor play, the effects on youths' mental health are still detrimental (Janssen, 2016; Montag & Elhai, 2020; Moore et al., 2020). On the other hand, decreased screen time (including video games) might be associated with lower rates of depressive symptoms in adolescents, while physical activity appears to improve attention in those affected by ADHD (Moore et al., 2020; Wagner, 2015). Occupational therapy practitioners are well positioned to help young clients plan their daily routines in a way that makes a balanced use of the virtual environments available to them (see Chapter 16 for details).

Gender Dysphoria and Play

Gender dysphoria refers to distress resulting from a discrepancy between one's gender identity and assigned gender. Gender-nonconforming choices may occur as early as preschool and may be associated with later gender dysphoria (Koehler et al., 2017; Roshan et al., 2019). Children may experience strong preferences for cross-dressing as well as for spending time with playmates of the opposite gender and choose play activities/objects and make-believe play roles that are typically assumed by the other gender. When the social environment does not accept an individual's gender identity, they can experience significant distress (Galupo, Pulice-Farrow, & Lindley, 2020; Syed, Afridi, & Dars, 2019). However, distress can be mitigated by the contexts that support children's desire to embrace the role of the other gender (Kimberly et al., 2018). It is, therefore, crucial for parents, caregivers, educators, health providers, and others to remain child-centered and to respect children's choices pertaining to play partners, roles, and objects. Occupational therapy practitioners may assist children and youth to engage in meaningful play and leisure occupations that fit their preferences, while educating others about the importance of such engagement for mental health (**Figure 12.2**).

Figure 12.2 Occupational therapy practitioners should assist children to play in ways that fit their preferences to support children's health

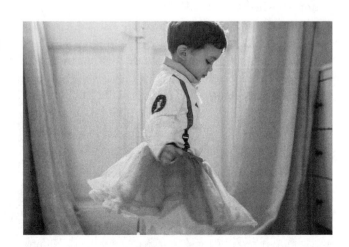

Additional Psychiatric Disorders and Play

Some psychiatric conditions in children impact their play participation indirectly. For example, elimination disorders, such as enuresis and encopresis (intentional or unintentional elimination of urine and feces into bed or clothing items) often contribute to a diminished self-esteem and social rejection and isolation of the affected child, perhaps eventually limiting their social play experiences (Lang et al., 2017). Similarly, sleep-wake disorders, which cause, among other symptoms, nightmares and sleepwalking in children, can create a significant distress for the child and their family (Gruber et al., 2014; Owens, 2007) eventually compromising their performance in all areas of occupation, including play.

Play in Twice-Exceptional Children and Adolescents

The term *twice-exceptional* refers to youngsters with disabilities who possess above-average intellectual ability. This phenomenon has been observed among young people with learning, communication, and autism spectrum disorders; ADHD; and emotional and behavioral issues. (National Association for Gifted Children [NAGC], 2020). These youngsters often demonstrate special talents and interests, as well as unusually high levels of curiosity, knowledge, creativity, imagination, and problem-solving and verbal abilities, while at the same time exhibiting motor, cognitive, emotional, and social deficits. As a result, they often display atypical play patterns, have difficulty forming friendships, and have a difficult time relating to and joining their peers during play, often seeking out older children or adults (**Figure 12.3**) (Bildiren, 2018; Chamberlin et al., 2007; Demina & Trubitsyna, 2016; NAGC, 2020; Sankar-DeLeeuw, 1999; Shechtman & Silektor, 2012.)

The Impact of Adversity on Play

Understanding play in children who have been exposed to traumatic events and other forms of adversity is of critical importance. The experience of significant adversity affects the developing brain and can have a negative impact on learning, social-emotional development, and emotional regulation (McKelvey et al., 2017; Nelson & Gabard-Durnam, 2020). Because younger children with a history of trauma cannot rely on the use of language to express their distress the way older children and adults do, they often exhibit posttraumatic play (PTP). PTP is characterized by inhibited or negative affect, rigid rituals that recreate traumatic events and utilize trauma-resembling objects, higher than usual presence of morbid themes, and increased levels of acting out/aggressivity (APA, 2013; Cohen & Gadassi, 2018; Cohen et al., 2010; Dripchak, 2007; NCTSN, 2020). While in certain contexts children may be asked to alter their play themes to those that are more acceptable, occupational therapy practitioners with additional play therapy training are well suited

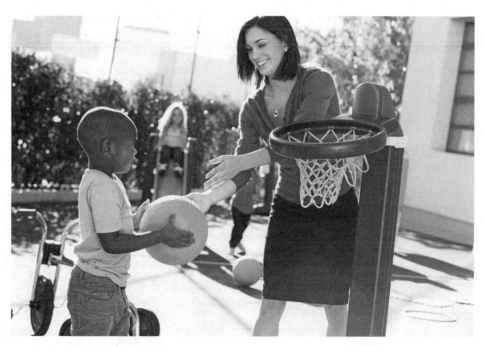

Figure 12.3 Some children with above-average intelligence may prefer to play with adults rather than other children
© Monkey Business Images/Shutterstock.

to support children and youth engaging in posttraumatic play to work through their distress with their play activities (Blunden, 2001; Cohen & Gadassi, 2018; Humble et al., 2019; Parker, Hergenrather, Smelser, & Kelly, 2021). By using trauma-informed approaches, practitioners help children build regulation through play (Fette, Lambdin-Pattavina, & Weaver, 2019).

The Reciprocal Relationship Between Mental Health and Play

As demonstrated earlier, mental health conditions impact one's play, but there is a reciprocal relationship between play and mental health. Play can also influence one's mental health. Research has demonstrated the importance of play in facilitating mental and social well-being. Engaged parenting and nurturing relationships, as they promote learning and adaptive behaviors, facilitate emotional regulation and provide an experience of joy (Bratton et al., 2005; Bratton et al., 2013). Understanding how mental well-being and play patterns interact in young individuals is crucially important for occupational therapy practitioners who work with the pediatric population.

Participation in play is fundamental to healthy cognitive, physical, social, and emotional development in childhood and adolescence (Ginsburg, 2007; Gray, 2011; Polatajko & Mandich, 2004). Play is also vital to the experience of positive mental health in children, which is essential to their overall well-being (Ginsberg, 2007; Zawadzki et al., 2015). The belief about play's influence on health and well-being is a basic tenet of occupational therapy practice (AOTA, 2020). Engagement in play contributes to flourishing, which refers to the experience of life going well, a combination of feeling good, participating, and functioning effectively in life (AOTA, 2011; Ginsburg, 2007; Huppert & So, 2013; Keyes, 2007; Nijhof et al., 2018). The amount of play and the type of play a child engages in may also signal the child's positive affect and general level of well-being (Ahloy-Dallaire, Espinosa, & Mason, 2018).

Spontaneous free play builds flexibility, coping skills, and resilience in emotional and social responses (Goldstein & Lerner, 2018; Slot, Mulder, Verhagen, & Leseman, 2017; Thibodeau, Gilpin, Brown, & Meyer, 2016). Through play, children can explore the social and emotional world and become comfortable with uncertainty and unpredictability. Play interactions with others afford the child opportunities to share, negotiate, cooperate, problem-solve, and self-manage emotions and behaviors. Pretend play fosters creativity and emotion regulation (**Figure 12.4**) (Goldstein & Lerner, 2018; Hofman & Russ, 2012). Free, unstructured play is also essential to acquiring social skills and empathy. Moreover, for younger boys in particular, rough play affords opportunities to learn how to manage one's anger and aggressivity (LaFreniere, 2011). As a child develops and grows through play, so too does their sense of relationship, identity, and feelings of belonging.

When young people are deprived of play, especially active outdoor play, they are essentially stripped of the opportunities to develop intrinsic interests and competencies; to learn how to regulate emotions, control behaviors, follow rules, and problem-solve; and restricted in their ability to make friends (Gray, 2011). All of these issues may contribute to the increase of psychiatric diagnoses, such as depression, anxiety, and ADHD, in this population (Belknap & Hazler, 2014; Chen et al., 2020; Gray, 2011; Montag & Elhai, 2020; Moore et al., 2020).

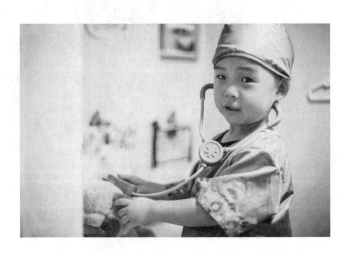

Figure 12.4 Pretend play fosters creativity and emotion regulation

© Nikola Stojadinovic/E+/Getty Images.

Addressing Mental Health with Play in Occupational Therapy

Given the impact of play on mental health and the impact of mental health conditions and adversity on play, it is clear why play is at the heart of occupational therapy practice in mental health settings. Occupational therapy practitioners serving youth with mental health conditions value and utilize play-based interventions in their practice (Halperin, 2020). An online survey of 31 therapist respondents who were working with youth with psychiatric diagnoses in 20 different states found that 77.42% rated the utilization of play-based interventions for pediatric populations with behavioral issues/psychiatric diagnoses as "extremely important." More than half (61.29%) of the therapists indicated that they incorporated play into their work daily, and they emphasized the role of play as an outlet for a young person's emotional distress. One of the therapists commented, "Play is a way to engage with traumatized or introverted kids."

Play, especially when child-driven, can significantly enhance the child's motor, cognitive, social and language development, self-esteem, coping skills, and ability to self-soothe. Productive play with parents or caregivers fosters a healthy attachment while at the same time promoting a sense of autonomy and self-control, and overall behavioral health (Cohen et al., 2010; Green et al., 2015; Haertl, 2019; Kjorstad et al., 2005; Patterson et al., 2018; Sigafoos et al., 1999; Waldman-Levi & Weintraub, 2015; Wilkes-Gillan et al., 2016). When channeled properly, play enables children to express their hidden thoughts and emotions and, by doing so, to accept their anxiety-provoking and even traumatizing experiences. Engaging in therapeutic play experiences can help children process the traumatic event, reduce stress, and facilitate coping (Cohen & Gadassi, 2018). Promoting playfulness in our clients may also be a way to facilitate better coping (Hess & Bundy, 2003; Magnuson & Barnett, 2013). Children can realize their strengths, hopes, and opportunities and problem-solve through play, all of which can have a healing effect (Dripchak, 2007). Moreover, play allows for interactions with typically developing peers and practice of social skills, while also fostering empathy for others (Rizk & Howells, 2019; Wilkes-Gillan et al., 2016).

Choosing Your Style as a Therapist

The importance of therapeutic use of self during play interventions is explained in Chapter 6 but

therapeutic style is an important consideration. Ideally, the way in which therapists facilitate therapeutic activities should match the client's needs, developmental level, and therapy goals, as well as the stage the client(s) and the therapist have reached together in terms of their therapeutic rapport and alliance. A facilitative style, defined as helping clients choose the activity and then guiding the process as needed, is frequently used (Halperin, 2020). The facilitative style is used especially with clients who are able to attend to a task and need less assistance, when working on making choices and fostering independence, and during pretend play. Another frequently used style is the directive style ("choosing the activity and providing ongoing instructions and guidance"), which is used more when working with clients on certain skills or novel activities, when addressing motor or cognitive delays, to help the client focus, to set limits, and "to help a child better understand their emotions." A third frequently chosen style is the advisory style, whereby clients choose/structure the play activity and engage in it independently, while the therapist stands by and intervenes only if necessary. An advisory style is used to assist young clients with developing social skills, such as collaboration and negotiation; with sequencing a task; and to ease the transition out of session. Although a facilitative style during play might be preferred by many therapists, both directive and advisory styles also offer benefits in certain situations.

Mental Health Settings

Occupational therapy practitioners work with children and youth with mental health conditions in many settings. Information on school-based practice and adolescent leisure intervention is provided in Chapters 10 and 13. In this chapter we focus more heavily on psychiatric hospitals, residential treatment centers, juvenile forensic centers, and group homes, which are the facilities where children and adolescents with more serious and complex mental health disorders receive care.

Assessment of and Through Play in Children with Mental Health Conditions

Assessment *of* play is described in Chapters 3 and 4 of this text, and the same general methods and tools can be used with children with mental health conditions. Here we discuss how we can use play to assess aspects of a child's or youth's social-emotional functioning, mental health, and well-being. So, this is a discussion of assessment *through* play.

Occupational therapists have unique knowledge, skills, and capacities to assess psychosocial and mental health issues in children and adolescents through play (Cahill & Bazyk, 2019; Champagne, 2019; Lane & Bundy 2011; Polatajko & Mandich, 2004). A mental health evaluation for a child emphasizes the barriers to a child's success, internal or external barriers, risk and protective factors and determines the challenges for the child that contribute to diminished emotional, social, cognitive, and behavioral engagement and participation. The occupational therapist often uses informal assessments such as activity analysis and observation (please see Chapter 4 for more guidance on informal assessment). The therapist may also evaluate the child through formal play assessment tools, such as the Parent Child Interaction Play Assessment Method (Smith, 2000) or the Test of Playfulness (Skard & Bundy, 2008).

Assessment through play can be more tolerable for the client, feel safer for the client, and allow the occupational therapist to see the client's strengths and weaknesses through the lens of a typical childhood activity. Play-based assessments are particularly valuable for children who are less verbal and expressive. Through play, the occupational therapist observes the child's ability to self-regulate with and without others. The therapist determines the child's preferences and motivations in play. The occupational therapist evaluates psychosocial behaviors and considers the child's sensorimotor performance. Somatosensory aspects of play afford the therapist an opportunity to evaluate a child's *window of tolerance* (Siegel, 1999) and consider the neurological foundations of social and emotional challenges. Through play assessment, the therapist might observe clumsiness and/or excessive fidgeting; overresponsiveness to touch or excessive seeking of a sensory input (e.g., an older child mouthing their toys); difficulty understanding/following directions; rigid play patterns (such as ordering toys excessively or resisting unfamiliar play objects/environments); limited ability to express thoughts and emotions about the play activity; hesitant or isolative play; restricted affect and limited engagement during play; difficulty taking turns; temper tantrums and explosive behavior toward peers or play objects; and play with "scary" themes. **Box 12.1** highlights some specific considerations in assessment through play for children and youth with mental health conditions.

Occupational therapy practitioners who address the needs of children and adolescents with mental

> **Box 12.1** Specific Play Assessment Considerations for Children and Youth with Mental Health Conditions
>
> - Careful examination of child preferences and how they exacerbate or mitigate mental health conditions.
> - Creation of boundaries and sense of safety, recognizing the child's prior trauma and potential fear(s).
> - Resist feeling offended by defiant or aggressive behaviors, but be prepared for them.
> - Examine and consider frustration tolerance and regulation during play activities.
> - Identify potential triggers for problematic behaviors in play.
> - Be prepared to provide comforting if needed.

health issues are likely to witness disruptive behaviors, aggression, inattention, dysregulation, unusual play behaviors, meltdowns, and a range of social-emotional behaviors among their clients. The occupational therapist needs to recognize that certain situations during the assessment can be traumatizing for a child. The therapist must be fully open to the child, in tune and calm with the child, and not be offended by defiant or aggressive behaviors.

Types of Interventions Using Play in Occupational Therapy

Occupational therapy practitioners select and design interventions to target mental health issues using play within occupation-based models of practice and frames of reference. Direct interventions with children and adolescents utilize play activities and promote capacities for occupational engagement. Examples of the types of play activities that may be used with children and youth with mental health conditions are provided in **Table 12.1**. Modifying play materials and environments, modeling for and imitating the child during play, creating "just right challenge," as well as therapeutic use of self/nurturing interactions with the child, and parent/caregiver education on play are all important strategies in this area of pediatric occupational therapy practice (Halperin, 2020). Interventions may be utilized in individual or group sessions. Therapists also adjust their style for clients and activities when delivering play-based intervention. See **Practice Example 12.1** for an example of the occupational therapy process in a mental health setting using play interventions.

Table 12.1 Common Play Activities Used in Occupational Therapy for Children and Adolescents with Psychiatric Diagnoses

Category of Play	Examples of Activities, Equipment, Supplies
Gross-motor/sensorimotor play	Obstacle courses, gym and sports-based play, outdoor and playground activities, challenge games, hide-and-seek, and yoga moves
Object play involving toys and sensory items	Small stretchy manipulatives, bubbles, kinetic sand, and cause-and-effect/exploratory toys
Social and team-based play	Peer interactions involving negotiation and collaboration
Pretend play	Pretend meal planning and preparation; playing "school" with focus on fine-motor tasks and relaxation strategies
Sensory integration-based/multisensory play	Suspended equipment; other vestibular and proprioceptive input
Play combined with storytelling/social stories	Storytelling using stuffed animals, dolls, toy houses, magnetic board/magnets
Expressive media-based play	Moving to music; drama play; drawings and arts and crafts
Board games	Both regular and therapeutic tabletop games
Play with symbolic themes	Puppets and popular movie/cartoon characters chosen by the child
Virtual reality-based play	Video and phone application-based games

Note: As reported by occupational therapy practitioners working in pediatric mental health (Halperin, 2020).

Data from Halperin, L. (2020). *Play-based occupational therapy in pediatric mental health: Therapists' perspective* (Unpublished manuscript). Graduate Program in Occupational Therapy, Sacred Heart University, Fairfield, CT.

Practice Example 12.1 Rohit and Play Within and Beyond a Psychiatric Facility

Rohit is an 8-year-old boy, who lives at home with his parents and three older siblings. Rohit's family immigrated to the United States from India a few months before he was born. When Rohit was 2.5 years old, he was diagnosed with an autism spectrum disorder (ASD). Rohit attends a special education school and receives outpatient treatment at a Child Guidance Center. Rohit frequently gets in trouble both at home and in school because of his out-of-control behaviors (screaming, hitting, biting, etc.). A week ago, during his visit to the Child Guidance Center, Rohit physically attacked his counselor and, as a result, was brought to the children's unit at the local inpatient psychiatric facility, where he is currently receiving medications, individual therapy with his social worker, and milieu and group occupational therapy.

On the unit, Rohit often giggles inappropriately and makes offensive comments toward his peers and some of the staff members. The charge nurse reports in the team meeting that Rohit comes across as "seeking negative attention and needing frequent redirection." Rohit's social worker at the hospital has been in touch with the Child Guidance Center. According to Rohit's counselor there, the father tends to use corporal punishment to discipline his children, despite her attempts to educate him about more appropriate parenting strategies. The social worker is considering referring Rohit to a residential program for children with behavioral problems.

You are an occupational therapist working at the hospital and running groups on the children's unit. You notice that during groups, Rohit presents with poor balance, bilateral coordination, and motor planning. For instance, he has difficulty throwing and catching balls and frequently bumps into people and objects around him. In addition, Rohit rarely establishes eye contact, often misses out on verbal directions provided to him, and frequently seeks tactile stimulation by touching peers, staff members, and various objects on the unit (such as the rug and the couch in the TV room).

You look through Rohit's chart and find a note indicating that Rohit had received an occupational therapy evaluation as a toddler (through the Birth-to-Three services), and that a home program was recommended to boost Rohit's sensorimotor development and to decrease his tantrums. The program consisted of vestibular and proprioceptive activities, including "rough play" with the father. There is no documentation in the chart indicating that Rohit has received any occupational therapy follow-up evaluation or treatment.

(continues)

PRACTICE EXAMPLE 12.1 Rohit and Play Within and Beyond a Psychiatric Facility   *(continued)*

How can you best help Rohit? As an occupational therapist situated in an acute setting, you can be instrumental with improving Rohit's quality of life during his short hospital stay; teaching him coping skills for dealing with his daily stressors; educating staff about the unique needs Rohit may have; and participating in monitoring his progress and planning his discharge in a way that will benefit him in the long run.

Play-based interventions, carried out either individually or in a group, are essential to Rohit's well-being during the hospitalization. Because Rohit presents with gross-motor deficits and exhibits behaviors suggesting that he might be seeking tactile and proprioceptive stimulation, it is important to provide him with safe movement opportunities and toys that are rich in texture. These play activities can incorporate supervised indoor or outdoor team/small-group games involving movement; construction with building blocks or large Lego pieces; pretend play/storytelling using stuffed animals or puppets; tabletop games, etc. While the hospital rules might not allow for toys or any types of play equipment to be left unattended on the unit, the occupational therapist can still advocate for Rohit to have access to a small durable stuffed animal or fidget toy/stress ball in between the activities he attends on the unit, so that he can experience the sensory input he appears to be seeking in socially acceptable ways.

It is also crucial to take into consideration the fact that Rohit has been subjected to corporal punishment at home and might be experiencing symptoms of trauma as a result, which may provide an additional explanation for his challenging behaviors and more insight about his current needs. The occupational therapist has to create a physically and emotionally secure play environment for Rohit and must refrain from unintentionally encouraging peer activities that might be perceived by Rohit as a potential threat (e.g., roughhousing).

Play activities can also be used to help Rohit begin to acquire the coping strategies and social skills he will need after his discharge to a residential program. While Rohit plays with his peers on the unit or at the hospital playground, the occupational therapist can praise his adaptive behaviors (such as following the game rules, sharing toys with other children, waiting for his turn, or addressing his playmates politely) and redirect his less-adaptive behaviors, such as touching others during play, ignoring his peers when they try to involve him in a game, or making hostile comments/pushing them when feeling upset. Moreover, conflicts that occur during play can serve as an opportunity for the therapist to teach Rohit simple grounding strategies, such as "Take a five," "Reach for the sky as you breath in, lower your arms and breathe out slowly," "Count to five," "Squeeze your stress ball," and "Use your words to tell us how you feel."

One of the most challenging tasks you may encounter in your role as Rohit's occupational therapist might have to do with his discharge planning. For instance, because other disciplines might not be fully aware of the sensory processing differences that often accompany ASD and the effects these differences have on one's behavior, daily functioning and play patterns, occupational therapists have the duty of educating their coworkers on these important topics and advocating for discharge referrals that take into consideration clients' sensory differences. In Rohit's case, it might be crucial for us to convey to the rest of the treatment team that Rohit would benefit from sensory modifications in his residential program and direct occupational therapy, particularly play- and sensory integration-based interventions.

Top-Down and Bottom-Up Interventions

Occupational therapy practitioners use professional reasoning to determine whether to use a top-down approach, a bottom-up approach, or a combination of both. (Please see **Table 12.2** for examples of both approaches.) Both top-down and bottom-up approaches refer to the order of areas of the brain being addressed based on neurodevelopmental principles. The therapist determines which approach is a better match for the child's development and abilities.

When we design play-based interventions from a *top-down* approach, we are engaging the neocortex, the rational brain, which controls thinking, language, personality, and decision making (Van Der Kolk, 2014). An example of a top-down approach is the use of cognitive behavioral therapy (CBT). This approach teaches the child to examine thoughts, emotions, and behaviors. Once the child has a shift in thinking to gain insights into their emotions and behaviors and develops the capacity to modify dysfunctional beliefs, changes occur in their emotional responses and behaviors. Because of the focus on thinking and language, top-down interventions require that the client has adequate cognitive and language processing to support their use or that caregivers are available to assist (Lillas, TenPas, Crowley & Spitzer, 2018; Martini, Cramm, Egan, & Sikora, 2016).

Table 12.2 Top-Down and Bottom-Up Play-Based Interventions for Children and Youth with Mental Health Conditions

Intervention	Description/Examples
Top-Down	
Cognitive behavioral	Cognitive restructuring/reframing before, during, and after play experiences such as: ■ Positive self-talk strategies ■ Play scenarios that afford opportunities for expression and interpersonal relating ■ Meaning making with use of symbols and metaphors during play
Executive function	■ Cognitive and self-management strategies during play ■ Play activities that require focus and attention ■ Problem-solving and goal-directed strategies during play ■ Understanding possible outcomes during structured play scenarios ■ Play for development of decision making
Positive Behavioral Interventions and Supports (PBIS)	■ School-based context initiative of three-tiered approach to creating a positive environment for children ■ Child taught social skills and appropriate social behaviors during play and recess time, with and without others
Cognitive-based emotional regulation	■ Cognitive awareness of emotional responses, identification of triggers, and selection of emotional regulation strategies during play. ■ Use of social-emotional checklists or measures during play. ■ Identification and use of self-regulation and calming strategies. ■ Instruction in specific sensory/emotional regulation programs during play (for example, Kuypers & Winner, 2011; Oetter, Richter, & Frick, 2019; Williams & Shellenberger, 1995)
Behavioral interventions	■ Training of child in appropriate play behaviors ■ Use of positive reinforcement and external motivators during play ■ Use of behavioral charts during play
Social skills training	■ Unstructured and structured play activities with others ■ Emphasis on connection with others through play ■ Development of Social Stories™ (Gray, 2015) in preparation for and implementation during play
Bottom-Up	
Sensory supports and techniques	■ Creation of play/sensory environment that is comfortable and safe for the child ■ Before, during, and after play, emphasis on use of the body and the sensory play space; calming and organizing strategies (breathing; rhythm; deep pressure; movement; sound and vibration) ■ Use of attachment principles—coregulation and joint attention during play ■ Use of arousal principles—seeking window of tolerance during play; seeking "just-right" state of being; emotions, arousal, and behavioral changes affected through vestibular activation during play ■ Sensory diet strategies (use of weight, chewy toys, swings, rough-and-tumble play)
Specific sensory/emotional regulation programs during play	The following programs first require top-down instruction; however, once learned, the strategies can be used with a child for a bottom-up approach to self-regulation during play: ■ Zones of Regulation: A curriculum designed to foster self-regulation and emotional control (Kuypers & Winner, 2011) ■ The Alert Program (Williams & Shellenberger, 1995) ■ The MORE Program: Integrating the mouth with sensory and postural functions (Oetter et al., 2019)

(continues)

Table 12.2 Top-Down and Bottom-Up Play-Based Interventions for Children and Youth with Mental Health Conditions

(continued)

Intervention	Description/Examples
Mind–body awareness strategies	■ Mindfulness ■ Progressive muscular relaxation ■ Guided imagery ■ Therapeutic yoga ■ Dance
Nature and outdoors	Sensory awareness through play: breath, smells, sound, touch, movement, etc.
Physical activity and sport	■ Exercise—walking, running, climbing, swimming ■ Ball games—throwing, bouncing ■ Team games—basketball, soccer, volleyball, baseball
Contextual interventions	■ Modify play materials ■ Modify physical environment ■ Modify social environment ■ Parent/caregiver education

When an occupational therapist designs play interventions from a *bottom-up* approach, the focus is on engaging the brain stem functions (e.g., arousal, breathing, somatic awareness, etc.) and the limbic system, the parts of the brain that process emotions and memory, regulate autonomic or endocrine function in response to emotional stimuli and are also involved in regulating emotional and behavioral responses (Van Der Kolk, 2011). The bottom-up approach emphasizes somatosensory and sensorimotor interventions (e.g., practicing mindfulness as a strategy for emotional regulation in preparation for play or during play participation).

Use of Consequences and Behavioral Strategies

Employing natural and logical consequences can promote adaptive behaviors in young people. While natural consequences represent the inevitable ramifications of one's actions at some point in the future, logical consequences are reasonable immediate disciplinary measures that make the most sense, considering the nature of the undesirable behavior, and can be explained to a young person clearly and without power struggles (Dreikurs & Soltz, 1992). For example, a child who constantly refuses to share play objects with peers might eventually discover that other children avoid playing with them, which is a natural consequence of their behavior. However, if a child uses outdoor playground equipment unsafely despite the supervising adult's redirections, the adult may replace playground time with indoor activities for the day, which represents a logical consequence for the child's actions. Natural and logical consequences are often more powerful than either punishments or material rewards because they are more conducive to a young person's learning and better foster their sense of responsibility, "contribution, participation and satisfaction" (Dreikurs & Soltz, 1992, p. 75).

When relying on behavioral strategies in a therapeutic environment, it is important that therapists use them wisely. Often it is best to ignore the child's undesirable, but not dangerous behaviors and instead compliment their desirable behaviors; apply natural and logical consequences rather than punishments if simply ignoring the negative behavior does not work; and refrain from using a child's basic needs, such as food, affection, or play, as rewards for a positive behavior and instead offer praise or special privileges (e.g., watching a movie or going on trips). The importance of not withholding play from young clients to punish undesirable behaviors cannot be overemphasized. As one of our study participants noted, many of these youngsters "... have been through trauma and may have lost their childhood or never really experienced one to begin with. Incorporating play into their group and individual therapy is vital for their overall mental health" (Halperin, 2020).

Child-Centered Play Therapy and Adlerian Play Therapy

Child-Centered Play Therapy (CCPT) has been recognized as one of the most effective evidence-based modalities that help children overcome aggressivity, poor impulse control, disruptive behaviors, and other emotional and behavioral issues (Axline, 1974, as cited in Landreth, 2012; Bratton et al., 2013; Meany-Walen & Teeling, 2016; Ray, 2011, as cited in Wilson & Ray, 2018). CCPT is based on Carl Rogers's person-centered theory that children show a natural desire to do well when exposed to nurturing relationships and that their undesirable behaviors mirror their inner conflicts that need to be understood before these behaviors can be changed. CCPT also assumes that children rely on play as a form of self-expression (Axline, 1974, as cited in Landreth, 2012; Meany-Walen & Teeling, 2016; Ray, 2011, as cited in Wilson & Ray, 2018). Helping children reflect on their emotions and thoughts, while providing encouragement, returning responsibility, and setting limits during play, assists them with developing empathy, self-regulating better, and assuming responsibility for their actions (Wilson & Ray, 2018).

CCPT prioritizes creating a safe space, allowing the child to choose and lead the play activity, paraphrasing their statements (to reflect feelings and content), inviting her/him to label their experiences, and establishing boundaries (Landreth, 2002, as cited in Patterson et al., 2018). Dripchak (2007) also recommends the use of storytelling during play, with gentle redirection from the therapist, to guide "scary" play toward more acceptable resolutions. For example, if a child uses dolls to reenact an abusive scene, the therapist can intervene and model for the child how the dolls instead can "talk to each other" in order to resolve the imaginary conflict between them. Such redirection, however, is most effective after therapeutic rapport has been established, and the child has had enough opportunities to express self through play, with the therapist observing rather than directing it (Dripchak, 2007).

Adlerian play therapy (AdPT) is a powerful, evidence-based treatment modality grounded in Alfred Adler's individual psychology theory (Dillman Taylor & Bratton, 2014; Meany-Walen & Teeling, 2016). AdPT consists of building a trusting, collaborative rapport with the young client; gathering information about their interests and beliefs (including misperceptions); and enhancing their insight as well as teaching them coping and social skills through creative play, storytelling, and similar activities (Dillman Taylor & Bratton, 2014; Meany-Walen & Teeling, 2016).

While both CCPT and AdPT were developed outside of the occupational therapy realm and are predominantly used by play therapists, psychologists, counselors, social workers, and so forth, many of their guiding principles are widely accepted and might be instrumental to other disciplines serving pediatric populations, including occupational therapy. Moreover, these principles are in agreement with the therapeutic modes already used in occupational therapy practice, such as empathizing, collaborating, and problem solving with a client and encouraging and instructing them (Taylor, 2008). For instance, an occupational therapist witnessing angry nonverbal behaviors during play (e.g., throwing or kicking stuffed animals) in a verbal child might say to the child in a calm voice, "You seem to be upset. Can you try to use your words to tell me what is upsetting you right now?" If the child is able to identify what has triggered their behavior, the therapist can then say, "You did a really good job telling me what makes you angry. I can see why you are upset. But it makes me sad when you throw or kick things. Let's see if we can play again and this time try to be gentler." If the child is not able to verbalize how they feel, the therapist should still set limits by saying, "I am sorry to see you so upset. I would really like to keep playing with you, but please try to be more careful with the toys." In both cases, the therapist can also offer options to the child, such as, "We can keep playing with the same toys or try something different, if you would like, but we have to play nicely. What do you think we should play with next?" Every time the child shows more caution when handling toys, the therapist should reward them with a positive comment, until aggression toward play objects becomes a nonissue.

Group Interventions

Group interventions provide opportunities for social learning in the presence of a therapist, who can guide the group process appropriately. Group play can be particularly beneficial, and occupational therapy practitioners working in pediatric psychiatric institutions often design group play activities that foster cognition, emotion regulation, and motor and social skills all at once. Please see **Practice Example 12.2** for a description of the use of a modified board game with a group.

PRACTICE EXAMPLE 12.2 **A Modified Board Game for a Social Group**

An occupational therapist modified an older version of the commercially available SAFETY FIRST™ board game for a social group she facilitated with elementary school-age children in an acute psychiatric setting. This game came with cards describing real-life scenarios pertaining to community mobility, school/playground/fire safety, and so on for the children to discuss and problem-solve. In the modified version, each child received the same number of cards and two plastic cups of different colors, an empty one and one with a fixed number of poker chips in it.

Players took turns solving the situations described on their cards. After each child presented their solution to a specific safety-related scenario on their card, other group members used poker chips from their "Give away" cup to evaluate their peer's answer on a 1–3 scale and explained their decision, while the therapist assisted them with providing constructive and respectful feedback to each other. Children used empty cups to collect the chips they received from peers. The child who collected the largest amount of chips by the end of the group won the game. Modifications made to this game provided opportunities for the players to exercise impulse control, make judgements about potentially dangerous situations, communicate with peers effectively, and experience a sense of mastery.

Consultation

Parents of children with mental health conditions may use the recommendations of occupational therapy practitioners to improve their ability to encourage family play. Practitioners working in community settings for mental health or in the schools may find the consultant role quite important for facilitating participation. Please see **Practice Example 12.3**, Lucy and Alex, for an example of how an occupational therapist might consult with a family to recommend appropriate play activities for children with mental health conditions.

PRACTICE EXAMPLE 12.3 Lucy and Alex

Lucy and her brother, Alex, are 9-year-old twins born in Belarus, where they were institutionalized at an orphanage. At the age of 2.5 years, they moved to the United States, where they since have lived with their adopted parents. Lucy has fetal alcohol syndrome and an IQ of 55. She attends a private school for persons with intellectual disabilities. She usually plays with a couple of children at her school, but often misperceives social cues, has a low frustration tolerance, and cries easily. Lucy occasionally becomes explosive and physically aggressive and sometimes engages in name-calling when she feels intimidated.

Her brother, Alex, attends the local public school. Alex has a history of being violent toward his classmates. At home, he has recently been aggressive with his family members and intentionally destroyed the family's laptop. He cropped the family dog's ears with a pair of scissors, which resulted in the dog's placement in a shelter and the initiation of mental health services.

The occupational therapist met with their mother, who is especially concerned about the after-school hours, when both twins are at home. They fight constantly. Alex teases Lucy and can be physically aggressive with her. Lucy is nervous around him and often becomes verbally assaultive toward him, which then further escalates his aggressive behaviors at home.

The parents have attempted to engage Lucy and Alex in family play/leisure activities, such as playing board games, shooting basketball, and playing tug-of-war, but they did not seem to relieve the tension between the children. Lucy's mother would like the therapist to recommend leisure activities for all of them to participate in as a family.

The occupational therapist completes an informal play observation of the two children together and finds:

- High levels of competition between the children
- Alex has better cognition
- Alex's activity choices are too hard for Lucy so she gets frustrated

Given these observations, the occupational therapist recommends noncompetitive activities for the family that are easily completed by individuals with various levels of ability such as nature walks in different locations, kicking or throwing a ball to each other, playing with bubbles, dancing/moving to music, looking for bugs, mud play, simple meal preparation tasks, movie night, and acting out stories from movies.

For Lucy, the occupational therapist also recommends activities she is able to complete independently so she can experience mastery. Specifically, these activities include chalk play, arts and crafts, specific toys, and books.

Addressing Barriers and Challenges to Play-Based Occupational Therapy with Children and Youth with Mental Health Conditions

Many practitioners in the mental health field report having faced challenges that result from both complex clients' presentation and contextual obstacles within the settings they have practiced (Halperin, 2020; Preyde et al., 2009). Challenges pertaining to clients' status/symptoms include inattentiveness, difficulty with following instructions, emotional dysregulation, poor impulse control, and lack of interest. Institutional challenges include limited access to age-appropriate play materials due to lack of funding and restrictions pertaining to supplies/equipment; lack of a safe play space; stringent policies regarding play privileges; restricted use of touch when interacting with clients; insufficient time; limited training among staff; and therapist's lack of confidence. For example, pretend play could lead to reenactment of experienced trauma beyond a therapist's comfort level or felt scope of practice. Because the primary aim of inpatient psychiatric facilities in the United States is to ensure immediate safety, the length of stay in these institutions is usually limited to a number of days, with treatment focusing on stabilization and discharge planning, which leaves little time for more rehabilitative approaches and often results in occupational therapy being delivered in groups rather than individually (Mahaffey et al., 2019). Diverse needs and high levels of symptom severity among patients in acute psychiatric settings often jeopardize their daily structure and create an environment of constant safety monitoring and restricted physical space. Additionally, varying training levels of staff members and frequent misconceptions about the need for overly controlling and forceful patient management practices also contribute to a challenging atmosphere in these facilities (Delaney & Hardy, 2008). Moreover, budget cuts significantly compromise the quality of care across psychiatric institutions (Baker & Gutheil, 2011), inevitably limiting access to nonmedical equipment and supplies. The aforementioned issues also might be encountered in outpatient, residential, community-, and school-based settings serving children and adolescents with psychiatric diagnoses, even if to a lesser degree. Expectations from caregivers, teachers, and other team members that reflect limited understanding of the occupational therapy role and lack of parental involvement are also reported (Halperin, 2020). However, many of these challenges can be mitigated by addressing maladaptive play and environmental and activity modifications.

Managing Maladaptive Play in Children with Mental Health Conditions

Managing the behaviors of children with mental health conditions requires special considerations on the part of the occupational therapy practitioner. Creating a "just right" and nurturing play environment; catering to young client's intrinsic motivation, while simultaneously setting limits and enforcing social rules; modeling play behaviors for the child; and involving typically developing peers and caregivers in the play process can all be helpful when addressing maladaptive play behaviors/patterns in children and adolescents (Rizk & Howells, 2019; Wilkes-Gillan et al., 2016). However, managing aggressive or "scary" play might require continued effort and additional competencies.

As discussed earlier, some children may experience posttraumatic play (PTP). When guided by a skillful adult and coupled with storytelling (and retelling of it in a more adaptive way), PTP can help traumatized children relive their trauma in a therapeutic manner and experience a sense of mastery and control over their lives, eventually leading to a resolution of the traumatic experience. Children may be able to relive the event through play but in a less passive role, thus through fantasy becoming the hero or at least demonstrating one's capabilities as opposed to being a victim (Chazan & Cohen, 2010). However, when the PTP is not handled properly (e.g., the therapist either dismisses the distress signaled by the child or becomes overly directive while trying to resolve it too early in the therapeutic process), children might become retraumatized, "stuck" in their trauma, and exhibit symptom worsening and even developmental regression with continued negative play patterns (Dripchak, 2007).

Many adults become concerned when witnessing aggressivity in children. However, themes of potential danger and fear are commonly present in children's play. Moreover, some levels of impulsivity and aggression are evident in most young children and represent an age-appropriate developmental milestone (Wilson & Ray, 2018). Playful aggression may, in fact, serve beneficial purposes and has been suggested as an important aspect of young play that should be allowed (Hart & Nagel, 2017). Playful aggression can be defined as "verbally and physically cooperative play behaviour involving at least two children, where all participants enjoyably and voluntarily engage in reciprocal role playing that includes aggressive make-believe themes, actions, and words; yet lacks intent to harm either emotionally or physically" (Hart & Tannock, 2013, p. 108). Therapists need to determine the level of aggression they are witnessing in play and whether it is typical.

In typical development, children's verbal abilities, emotion regulation, and sense of mastery over the outer environment increase, leading to a reduction in aggressive behaviors, usually between ages 6 and 10. However, when signs of persistent aggression continue to manifest in a child, they might be predictive of future misconduct, school-related difficulties, social deficits, and diminished mental health (Wilson & Ray, 2018). Additionally, externalizing behaviors (such as aggression, rule breaking, and other forms of disruptive conduct) often signal emotional distress in children, and increased awareness regarding this phenomenon among caregivers may result in more support and better outcomes for affected children (Meany-Walen & Teeling, 2016).

Safety Concerns in Play

In some instances, explosive behaviors during play become unsafe to a point where play might need to be modified or terminated. For example, one of this chapter's authors has witnessed young clients attempt to push, bite, spit, and swing chairs at their peers and staff out of frustration during group play in an inpatient psychiatric facility. Because of the severity of these behaviors, a behavioral approach was necessary. This particular facility used the "three warnings rule" to encourage the acting out-of-control child or adolescent to use words instead. After three warnings and opportunities to change behavior, the client was required to leave the activity and was escorted to their room to take a break and talk to staff about what had happened and how a similar incident could be avoided in the future. To be able to participate in the next activity, the youngster had to demonstrate that they were able to regain control by interacting with others without physical outbursts. If aggressive behaviors reoccurred in the next group activity, the young client was removed from groups for the rest of the day and offered to engage in one-to-one activities (including play) with staff members instead, while practicing coping strategies, to earn group privileges for the following day. While this approach departed somewhat from the child-centered principles, it helped ensure

safety on the unit and taught children and adolescents that their behaviors had consequences.

Recognizing New Trauma and Stress

Another important consideration pertaining to maladaptive play patterns in youth has to do with reporting newly observed signs of distress during play. For instance, children and adolescents who have experienced sexual trauma may reenact it by using drawings, dolls, puppets, or stuffed animals; choose play themes with an unhappy ending; make threats toward play objects imitating the person who abused them; present as detached and stare into space while playing; and exhibit regressive behaviors (e.g., an older child sucking on a pacifier during play). While some of these behaviors can also result from more commonly encountered stressful events, such as familial conflicts or a birth of a sibling, it is essential that therapists note them, inquire about the reasons behind these behaviors (e.g., by gently pointing them out to the youngster and waiting for her/his response), and report the signs of suspected abuse to child protection services (Brown et al., 2008). Occupational therapy practitioners who witness such play behaviors in their young clients should document them and follow their treatment facility's reporting procedures.

Overcoming Environmental Barriers to Play in Mental Health Settings

Occupational therapy practitioners working with this population across various facilities often resort to following the "Do what you can with what you have where you are" principle, to promote play opportunities and other meaningful activities for their young clients. With careful planning, creativity, and positive attitude, our profession can make a difference, even when situated in challenging contexts and environments.

Overcoming Material Barriers

Both individual and group play activities can be facilitated while operating on a limited budget. For instance, stuffed animals, dolls and puppets, building blocks, play dough, kinetic sand, and basic arts and crafts supplies are examples of affordable materials that can be used for expressive play. Play with simple sensory objects, such as stress balls, bean bags, and soap bubbles helps young people self-soothe and can be introduced to them as a coping strategy to use outside of the treatment session. Many inexpensive board games promote cognition and social interaction skills.

Yet one of the biggest challenges with all of the listed materials is that potentially they can be used by young clients who are in distress to harm self or others (e.g., glue can be sniffed, soap bubbles and kinetic sand can be ingested, building blocks and stress balls can be thrown at a peer, intentional or unintentional misuse of jump ropes can cause strangulation, etc.), which indicates that close supervision is needed when utilizing these objects in play-based interventions. Moreover, it may also be necessary to have policies requiring that all materials, including toys, be screened for safety; stored outside of the hospital units; counted before being used in therapeutic activities; and then collected, recounted, and returned to the storage room right after the activity is over.

Overcoming Physical Environment Barriers

Outdoor play can be more complicated for many psychiatric facilities, due to stringent safety policies and, in some instances, a dominant culture of token economy use. For example, a psychiatric hospital may have access to a playground, but rarely make use of it if the staff members believe that children must earn the "privilege" of playing outdoors by behaving appropriately indoors. In such instances, the occupational therapist might need to educate her/his colleagues about play being a basic need and an important energy outlet for children and to suggest that other activities, such as watching TV, be used as a reward for positive behaviors instead. However, if the treatment team disagrees with this recommendation, the therapist will have to compromise and find creative ways to engage children in gross-motor activities indoors.

In some situations, children may not be able to participate in outdoor play safely due to acute symptoms and challenging behaviors (e.g., suicidality, aggression toward peers, risk of elopement), and playground visits might need to be temporarily replaced with indoor activities for them. When outdoor play is not available, the therapist may use indoor gross-motor activities such as parachute games, indoor obstacle courses built with reasonably safe materials (e.g., large balls, hula-hoops, cones), or yoga games, while also ensuring that a sufficient number of staff members are available to help supervise these activities. A valuable alternative to an outdoor playground is a sensory space, which uses colorful paths/activity maps incorporating curved lines, mazes, Lego walls,

and more, and can be installed in hallways, classrooms, offices, or homes to promote play, physical activity, fine-motor skills, core academic competencies, and social/emotional development (including self-regulation and decision making) among children (Action for Healthy Kids, 2020). Because sensory spaces are usually designed utilizing affordable materials, occupational therapy practitioners working with young people in psychiatric settings should consider advocating for installing these spaces in their facilities. Sensory kits, carts (trolleys), or boxes represent another effective, easy-to-implement and affordable intervention (Adams-Leask et al., 2018; Martin & Suane, 2012; OT-Innovations, 2020; Scanlan & Novak, 2015). They allow for carefully selected sensory items that are tailored to clients' needs to be delivered to the unit, used individually or in groups under staff supervision, and stored outside of the unit in between therapy sessions.

Should an institution serving youngsters with mental health concerns gain access to additional funds (e.g., private donations, grants), it may be beneficial for the occupational therapy practitioner(s) employed by it to introduce the idea of designing a sensory room at the facility to their peers and administration. Sensory rooms (otherwise called sensory modulation rooms) are sensory-friendly therapeutic spaces designed to help prevent and manage emotional crisis by achieving "just right" levels of arousal. Sensory rooms offer a promising intervention for pediatric facilities (Bobier et al., 2015). While some companies design sensory rooms with pricey and sophisticated multimedia equipment, therapeutic spaces can also be created relying on inexpensive items and play materials, such as bean bags, yoga mats, therapy balls, small trampolines, rock waterfalls, weighted objects, stuffed animals, stress balls/fidgets, arts and crafts supplies, playing cards, and tabletop games (Bobier et al., 2015; OT-Innovations, 2020). Due to clients' symptom acuity, the use of sensory spaces in inpatient facilities might need to adhere to a certain schedule and require consistent staff supervision. Staff members might need to limit access to a sensory room for a child/adolescent in the midst of a behavioral crisis, when she/he is acting out-of-control, if it would be perceived by them as a reward for an undesirable behavior. Instead, it can be provided to a youngster who is reporting distress, but is still able to contain it, or, after the out-of-control behavior has de-escalated and the young client has had the opportunity to reflect on her/his actions. This approach will allow them the opportunity to internalize the strategies they learned in the sensory room as coping skills for the future.

Conclusion

Play is essential to children's development and mental health. Play fosters therapeutic rapport making play-based occupational therapy interventions both legitimate and valuable. Psychiatric conditions, exposure to adversity, and other mental health concerns jeopardize young people's participation in play. However, when proper supports are provided, engagement in play significantly improves outcomes for this client population. Occupational therapy practitioners can utilize play-based interventions and impact mental health and well-being through "making play just right." Sensorimotor activities, object play, and social/team-based play are commonly used by occupational therapy practitioners serving pediatric clients with mental health issues. Pretend play, storytelling and expressive/symbolic play, as well as board games and virtual-reality-based activities, can also serve as successful treatment modalities for this population. Therapeutic style as well as top-down and bottom-up interventions are matched to the present needs of the child and the activity demands. A child-centered approach should be considered whenever possible. Creative problem-solving can overcome contextual barriers. More robust training on specific play-based interventions including play therapy for occupational therapy practitioners serving pediatric populations with developmental and behavioral issues, as well as further research in this field are warranted.

References

Action for healthy kids. (2020). *Sensory hallways.* https://www.actionforhealthykids.org/activity/sensory-hallways/

Adams-Leask, K., Varona, L., Dua, C., Baldock, M., Gerace, A., & Muir-Cochrane, E. (2018).The benefits of sensory modulation on levels of distress for consumers in a mental health emergency setting. *Australias Psychiatry, 26*(5), 514–519. http://dx.doi.org/DOI:10.1177/1039856217751988

Ahloy-Dallaire, J., Espinosa, J., & Mason, G. (2018). Play and optimal welfare: Does play indicate the presence of positive affective states?. *Behavioural Processes, 156,* 3–15.

American Occupational Therapy Association (AOTA). (2011). *Building play skills for healthy children & families.* https://www.aota.org/-/media/Corporate/Files/Practice/Children/Browse/Play/Building%20Play%20Skills%20Tip%20Sheet%20Final.pdf

American Occupational Therapy Association (AOTA). (2016a). *Mental health promotion, prevention, and intervention: Across the lifespan* [Fact Sheet]. https://www.aota.org/~/media/Corporate/Files/Practice/MentalHealth/Distinct-Value-Mental-Health.pdf

American Occupational Therapy Association (AOTA). (2016b). *Occupational therapy's role in mental health with children and youth* (Fact Sheet). https://www.aota.org/-/media/Corporate/Files/AboutOT/Professionals/WhatIsOT/MH/Facts/MH%20in%20Children%20and%20Youth%20fact%20sheet.pdf

American Occupational Therapy Association (AOTA). (2020). Occupational therapy practice framework: Domain and process (4th ed.). *American Journal of Occupational Therapy, 74* (Supplement 2). Advance online publication.

American Psychiatric Association (APA). (2013). *Diagnostic and statistical manual of mental disorders* (5th ed.). Washington, DC: American Psychiatric Publishing.

Baker, J. O., & Gutheil, T. G. (2011). "Are you kidding?"; Effects of funding cutbacks in the mental health field on patient care and potential liability issues. *Journal of Psychiatry and Law, 39*(3), 425–440.

Barnett, L. A. (1984). Research note: Young children's resolution of distress through play. *Journal of Child Psychology and Psychiatry, 25*(3), 477–483.

Basu, S., & Banerjee, B. (2020). Impact of environmental factors on mental health of children and adolescents: A systematic review. *Children and Youth Service Review, 119.* https://doi.org/10.1016/j.childyouth.2020.105515

Belknap, E., & Hazler, R. (2014). Empty playgrounds and anxious children. *Journal of Creativity in Mental Health, 9*(2), 210–231.

Bildiren, A. (2018). Developmental characteristics of gifted children aged 0–6 years: Parental observations. *Early Child Development and Care, 188*(8), 997–1011.

Blunden, P. (2001). The therapeutic use of play. In L. Lougher (Ed.), *Occupational therapy for child and adolescent mental health* (pp. 67–86). Edinburgh, Scotland: Churchill Livingstone.

Bobier, C. M., Boon, T., Downward, M., Loomes, B., Mountford, H., & Swadi, H. (2015). Pilot investigation of the use and usefulness of a sensory modulation room in a child and adolescent psychiatric inpatient unit. *Occupational Therapy in Mental Health, 31*(4), 385–401.

Bonder, B. R. (2015). *Psychopathology and function* (5th ed.). West Deptford, NJ: SLACK Inc.

Bratton, S. C., Ceballos, P. L., Sheely-Moore, A. I., Meany-Walen, K., Pronchenko, Y., & Jones, L. D. (2013). Head start early mental health intervention: Effects of child-centered play therapy on disruptive behaviors. *International Journal of Play Therapy, 22*(1), 28.

Bratton, S. C., Ray, D., Rhine, T., & Jones, L., (2005). The efficacy of play therapy with children: A meta-analytic review of treatment outcomes. *Professional Psychology: Research and Practice, 36*(4), 376–390.

Brezinka, V., Mailänder, V., & Walitza, S. (2020). Obsessive compulsive disorder in very young children—a case series from a specialized outpatient clinic. *BMC Psychiatry, 20*(1), 1–8.

Brown, C., Stoffel, V. C., & Munoz, J. P. (2019). *Occupational therapy in mental health; A vision for participation* (2nd ed.). Philadelphia, PA: F. A. Davis.

Brown, S., Brack, G., & Mullis, F. (2008). Traumatic symptoms in sexually abused children: Implications for school counselors. Professional School *Counselling, 11*(6), 368–379. https://www.jstor.org/stable/42732850

Bundy, A. C. (1997). Play and playfulness. In L. D. Parham & L. S. Fazio (Eds.), *Play in occupational therapy for children* (pp. 52–66). St. Louis, MO: Mosby.

Cahill, S., & Bazyk, S. (2019). School-based occupational therapy. In J. O'Brien & H. Kuhaneck (Eds.), *Case-Smith's occupational therapy for children and adolescents* (8th ed., pp. 627–658). St. Louis, MO: Elsevier.

Caldwell, L. L., & Faulk, M. (2013). Adolescent leisure from a developmental and prevention perspective. In *Positive leisure science* (pp. 41–60). Dordrecht: Springer.

Caprino, F., & Stucci, V. (2017). Play in children with multiple disabilities. In S. Best, V. Stancheva-Popkostadinova, & D. Bulgarelli (Eds.), *Play development in children with disabilities* (pp. 147–153). Berlin: DeGruyter.

Centers for Disease Control and Prevention (CDC). (2019). *Data and statistics on children's mental health.* https://www.cdc.gov/childrensmentalhealth/data.html.

Centers for Disease Control and Prevention (CDC). (2020a). *Children's mental health. Data and statistics.* https://www.cdc.gov/childrensmentalhealth/data.html

Centers for Disease Control and Prevention (CDC). (2020b). *Fetal alcohol spectrum disorders.* https://www.cdc.gov/ncbddd/fasd/facts.html

Centers for Disease Control and Prevention (CDC). (2020c). *Preventing child abuse and neglect.* https://www.cdc.gov/violenceprevention/childabuseandneglect/fastfact.html

Centers for Disease Control and Prevention (CDC). (2021). *About mental health.* https://www.cdc.gov/mentalhealth/learn/index.htm

Chamberlin, S. A., Buchanan, M., & Vercimak, D. (2007). Serving twice-exceptional preschoolers: Blending gifted education and early childhood special education practices in assessment and program planning. *Journal for the Education of the Gifted, 30*(3), 372–394.

Champagne, T. (2019). Trauma and stressor-related disorders. In C. Brown, V. C. Stoffel, & J. P. Munoz (Eds.), *Occupational therapy in mental health: A vision for participation* (2nd ed., pp. 211–224). Philadelphia, PA: F. A. Davis.

Chazan, S., & Cohen, E. (2010). Adaptive and defensive strategies in posttraumatic play of young children exposed to violent attacks. *Journal of Child Psychotherapy, 36*(2), 133–51.

Chen, S., Cheng, Z., & Wu, J. (2020). Risk factors for adolescents' mental health during the COVID-19 pandemic: A comparison between Wuhan and other urban areas in China. *Global Health, 16*(1). https://doi.org/10.1186/s12992-020-00627-7.

Christian, K. M., Russ, S., & Short, E. J. (2011). Pretend play processes and anxiety: Considerations for the play therapist. *International Journal of Play Therapy, 20*(4), 179–192. https://doi.org/10.1037/a0025324

Cohen, E., Chazan, S., Lerner, M., & Maimon, F. (2010). Posttraumatic play in young children exposed to terrorism. *Infant Mental Health Journal, 31*(2), 159–181.

Cohen, E., & Gadassi, R. (2018). The function of play for coping and therapy with children exposed to disasters and political violence. *Current Psychiatry Reports, 20*(5), 1–7.

Conradt, E., Abar, B., Lester, B. M., LaGasse, L. L., Shankaran, S., Bada, H., & Hammond, J. A. (2014). Cortisol reactivity to social stress as a mediator of early adversity on risk and adaptive outcomes. *Child Development, 85*(6), 2279–2298. http://dx.doi.org/org.10.1111/cdev.12316

Cordier, R., Bundy, A., Hocking, C., & Einfeld, S. (2010). Empathy in the play of children with attention deficit hyperactivity disorder. *OTJR: Occupation, Participation and Health, 30*(3), 122–132.

Delaney, K. R., & Hardy, L. (2008). Challenges faced by inpatient child/adolescent psychiatric nurses. *Journal of Psychosocial Nursing, 46*(2), 21–24.

Demina, E. V., & Trubitsyna, A. N. (2016). A case-study of inclusion of an intellectually gifted adolescent with autism spectrum disorder in a general education school: Risk factors and developmental resources. *Psychological Science and Education, 21*(3). http://dx.doi.org/10.17759/pse.2016210313

Dillman Taylor, D., & Bratton, S. C. (2014). Developmentally appropriate practice: Adlerian play therapy with preschool children. *Journal of Individual Psychology, 70*(3), 205–219.

Donaldson, J. M., Vollmer, T. R., Krous, T., Downs, S., & Berard, K. P. (2011). An evaluation of the good behavior game in kindergarten classrooms. *Journal of Applied Behavior Analysis, 44*(3), 605–609.

Dreikurs, R., & Soltz, V. (1992). *Children: The challenge.* New York: Penguin Group.

Dripchak, V. L. (2007). Posttraumatic play: Towards acceptance and resolution. *Clinical Social Work Journal, 35*, 125–134. http://dx.doi.org/10.1007/s10615-006-0068-y

Engler, A. D., Sarpong, K. O., Van Horne, B. S., Greeley, C. S., & Keefe, R. J. (2020). A systematic review of mental health disorders of children in foster care. *Trauma, Violence, & Abuse*, 1524838020941197.

Enlow, M. B., Blood, E., & Egeland, B. (2013). Sociodemographic risk, development competence, and PTSD symptoms in young children exposed to interpersonal trauma in early life. *Journal of Traumatic Stress, 26*(6), 686–694. http://dx.doi.org/DOI:org/10.1002/jts.21866

Felitti, V. J., Anda, R. F., Nordenberg, D., Williamson, D. F., Spitz, A. M., Edwards, V., . . . Marks, J. S. (1998). Relationship of childhood abuse and household dysfunction to many of the leading causes of death in adults: The Adverse Childhood Experiences (ACE) Study. *American Journal of Preventive Medicine, 14*(4), 245–258. http://dx.doi.org/https://doi.org/10.1016/s0749-3797(98)00017-8

Fette, C., Lambdin-Pattavina, C., & Weaver, L.L. (2019). Understanding and applying trauma-informed approaches across occupational therapy settings. *OT Practice.* https://www.aota.org/-/media/Corporate/Files/Publications/CE-Articles/CE-Article-May-2019-Trauma.pdf

Fredrickson, B. L. (2004). The broaden-and-build theory of positive emotions. *Philosophical Transactions of the Royal Society of London. Series B: Biological Sciences, 359*(1449), 1367–1377.

Galderisi, S., Heinz, A., Kastrup, M., Beezhold, J., & Sartorius, N. (2015). Toward a new definition of mental health. *World Psychiatry, 14*(2), 231–233. https://doi.org/10.1002/wps.20231

Galupo, M. P., Pulice-Farrow, L., & Lindley, L. (2020). "Every time I get gendered male, I feel a pain in my chest": Understanding the social context for gender dysphoria. *Stigma and Health, 5*(2), 199.

Garfinkel, B., Carlson, G., & Weller, E. (1990). *Psychiatric disorders in children and adolescents*. Philadelphia, PA: W. B. Saunders.

Gartland, D., Riggs, E., Muyeen, S., Giallo, R., Afifi, T. O., MacMillan, H., . . . Brown, S. J. (2019). What factors are associated with resilient outcomes in children exposed to social adversity? A systematic review. *British Medical Journal Open*, 9, 1–14. http://dx.doi.org/10.1136/bmjopen-2018-024870

Gaskill, R. L., & Perry, B. D. (2014). The neurobiological power of play: Using the neurosequential model of therapeutics to guide play in the healing process. In C. A. Malchiodi & D. A. Crenshaw (Eds.), *Creative arts and play therapy. Creative arts and play therapy for attachment problems* (pp. 178–194). New York: Guilford Press.

Ginsburg, K. R. (2007). *The importance of play in promoting healthy child development and maintaining strong parent-child bonds*. https://pediatrics.aappublications.org/content/pediatrics/119/1/182.full.pdf

Goldstein, T. R., & Lerner, M. D. (2018). Dramatic pretend play games uniquely improve emotional control in young children. *Developmental Science*, 21(4), e12603.

Gore, S., & Colten, M. E. (2017). Introduction: Adolescent stress, social relationships, and mental health. In *Adolescent stress* (pp. 1–14). New York: Routledge.

Gray, C. (2015). *The new social story™ book* (15th anniversary ed.). Arlington, TX: Future Horizons.

Gray, P. (2011). The decline of play and the rise of psychopathology in children and adolescents. *American Journal of Play*, 3(4), 443–463.

Green, E. J., Fazio-Griffith, L., & Parson, J. (2015). Treating children with psychosis: An integrative play therapy approach. *International Journal of Play Therapy*, 24(3), 162–176.

Gruber, R., Carrey, N., Weiss, S. K., Frappier, J. Y., Rourke, L., Brouillette, R. T., & Wise, M. S. (2014). Position statement on pediatric sleep for psychiatrists. *Journal of the Canadian Academy of Child and Adolescent Psychiatry*, 23(3), 174.

Gunnar, M., & Quevedo, K. (2007). The neurobiology of stress and development. *Annual Review of Psychology*, 58, 145–173.

Haertl, K. (2019). Coping and resilience. In C. Brown & V. Stoffel (Eds.), *Occupational therapy in mental health: A vision for participation*. Philadelphia, PA: F. A. Davis.

Halperin, L. (2020). Play-based occupational therapy in pediatric mental health: Therapists' perspective. Unpublished manuscript, *Graduate Program in Occupational Therapy*, Sacred Heart University, Fairfield, CT.

Hans, S. L., Auerbach, J. G., Auerbach, A. G., & Marcus, J. (2005). Development from birth to adolescence of children at-risk for schizophrenia. *Journal of Child and Adolescent Psychopharmacology*, 15(3), 384–394.

Hart, J. L., & Nagel, M. C. (2017). Including playful aggression in early childhood curriculum and pedagogy. *Australasian Journal of Early Childhood*, 42(1), 41–48.

Hart, J. L., & Tannock, M. T. (2013). Playful aggression in early childhood settings. *Children Australia*, 38(3), 106–114. https://doi.org/10.1017/ cha.2013.14

Hess, L. M., & Bundy, A. C. (2003). The association between playfulness and coping in adolescents. *Physical & Occupational Therapy in Pediatrics*, 23(2), 5–17.

Hobson, R. P., Lee, A., & Hobson, J. A. (2009). Qualities of symbolic play among children with autism: A social-developmental perspective. *Journal of Autism and Developmental Disorders*, 39(1), 12–22.

Hoffmann, J., & Russ, S. (2012). Pretend play, creativity, and emotion regulation in children. *Psychology of Aesthetics, Creativity, and the Arts*, 6(2), 175.

Humble, J. J., Summers, N. L., Villarreal, V., Styck, K. M., Sullivan, J. R., Hechler, J. M., & Warren, B. S. (2019). Child-centered play therapy for youths who have experienced trauma: A systematic literature review. *Journal of Child & Adolescent Trauma*, 12(3), 365–375. https://doi.org/10.1007/s40653-018-0235-7

Huppert, F. A., & So, T. T. (2013). Flourishing across Europe: Application of a new conceptual framework for defining well-being. *Social Indicators Research*, 110, 837–861.

Islam, H., Mosa, A. S., Srivastava, H. K., Mandhadi, V., Rajendran, D., & Young-Walker, L. M. (2020). Discovery of comorbid psychiatric conditions among youth detainees in juvenile justice system using clinical data. *ACI Open*, 4(02), e136–e148.

Izadi-Najafabadia, S., Ryan, N., Ghafooripoor, G., Gill, K., & Zwicker, J. G. (2019). Participation of children with developmental coordination disorder. *Research in Developmental Disabilities*, 84, 75–84. http://dx.doi.org/10.1016/j.ridd.2018.05.011

Janssen, I. (2016). Estimating whether replacing time in active outdoor play and sedentary video games with active video games influences youth's mental health. *Journal of Adolescent Health*, 59(5), 517–522.

Jarrold, C. (2003). A review of research into pretend play in autism. *Autism*, 7(4), 379–390.

Jasem, Z. A., & Delport, S. M. (2019). Mothers' perspectives on the play of their children with attention deficit hyperactivity disorder. *Occupational Therapy International*, https://doi.org/10.1155/2019/6950605

Kennedy-Behr, A., Rodger, S., & Mickan, S. (2013). Aggressive interactions during free-play at preschool of children with and without developmental coordination disorder. *Research in Developmental Disabilities*, 34(9), 2831–2837. http://dx.doi.org/10.1016/j.ridd.2013.05.033

Kessler, R. C., Amminger, G. P., Aguilar-Gaxiola, S., Alonso, J., Lee, S., & Ustun, T. B. (2007). Age of onset of mental disorders: A review of recent literature. *Current Opinion in Psychiatry*, 20(4), 359.

Keyes, C. L. (2007). Promoting and protecting mental health as flourishing: A complimentary strategy for improving national mental health. *American Psychologist*, 62, 95–108.

Kimberly, L. L., Folkers, K. M., Friesen, P., Sultan, D., Quinn, G. P., Bateman-House, A., . . . Salas-Humara, C. (2018). Ethical issues in gender-affirming care for youth. *Pediatrics*, 142(6).

Kjorstad, M., O'Hare, S., Soseman, K., Spellman, C., & Thomas, P. (2005). The effects of post-traumatic stress disorder on children's social skills and occupational play. *Occupational Therapy in Mental Health*, 39–57.

Koehler, A., Richter-Appelt, H., Cerwenka, S., Kreukels, B. P., Watzlawik, M., Cohen-Kettenis, P. T., . . . Nieder, T. O. (2017). Recalled gender-related play behavior and peer-group preferences in childhood and adolescence among adults applying for gender-affirming treatment. *Sexual and Relationship Therapy*, 32(2), 210–226.

Krupa, T., Fossey, E., Anthony, W. A., Brown, C., & Pitts, D. B. (2009). Doing daily life: How occupational therapy can inform psychiatric rehabilitation practice. *Psychiatric Rehabilitation Journal, 32*, 155–166.

Kupyers, L. M., & Winner, M. G. (2011). *The zones of regulation: A curriculum designed to foster self-regulation and emotional control.* Santa Clara, CA: Think Social Publishing.

Kwak, K. H., Hwang, H. C., Kim, S. M., & Han, D. H. (2020). Comparison of behavioral changes and brain activity between adolescents with internet gaming disorder and student pro-gamers. *International Journal of Environmental Research and Public Health, 17*(2), 441.

LaFreniere, P. (2011). Evolutionary functions of social play: Life histories, sex differences, and emotion regulation. *American Journal of Play, 3*(4), 464–488.

Landreth, G. L. (2012). *Play therapy: The art of the relationship.* New York: Routledge.

Lane, S. J., & Bundy, A. C. (2011). *Kids can be kids: A childhood occupations approach.* Philadelphia, PA: F. A. Davis.

Lang, R., McLay, L., Carnett, A., Ledbetter-Cho, K., Sun, X., & Lancioni, G. (2017).Complications and side effects associated with a lack of toileting skills. In *Clinical guide to toilet training children* (pp. 19–31). Cham: Springer.

Larson, S., Chapman, S., Spetz, J., & Brindis, C. D. (2017). Chronic childhood trauma, mental health, academic achievement, and school-based health center mental health services. *Journal of School Health, 87*(9), 675–686.

Lillas, C., TenPas, H., Crowley, C., & Spitzer, S.L. (2018). Improving regulation skills for increased participation for individuals with ASD. In R. Watling & S.L. Spitzer (Eds.), *Autism across the lifespan: A comprehensive occupational therapy approach* (4th ed., pp. 319-338). Bethesda, MD: AOTA press.

Loman, M., & Gunnar, M. R. (2010). Early experience and the development of stress reactivity and regulation in children. *Neuroscience and Biobehavioral Reviews, 34*(6), 867–876.

Lous, A. M., de Wit, C. A., de Bruyn, E. E., Riksen-Walraven, J. M., & Rost, H. (2000). Depression and play in early childhood: Play behavior of depressed and nondepressed 3-to 6-year-olds in various play situations. *Journal of Emotional and Behavioral Disorders, 8*(4), 249–260.

Lupian, S. (2017). Helping teenagers develop resilience in the face of stress. In R. Dahl, A. Suleiman, B. Luna, S. Choudhury, K. Noble, S. J. Lupien, … M. R. Uncapher (Eds.), *The adolescent brain: A second window to opportunity.* New York: UNICEF. https://repositorio.minedu.gob.pe/bitstream/handle/20.500.12799/5746/The%20Adolescent%20Brain%20A%20second%20window%20to%20opportunity.pdf?sequence=1

Magnuson, C. D., & Barnett, L. A. (2013). The playful advantage: How playfulness enhances coping with stress. *Leisure Sciences, 35*(2), 129–144.

Mahaffey, L., Dallas, J., & Munoz, J. P. (2019). Supporting individuals through crisis to community living: Meeting a continuum of service needs. In C. Brown, J. C. Stoffel, & J. P. Munoz (Eds.), *Occupational therapy in mental health: A vision for participation* (2nd ed., pp. 655–671). Philadelphia, PA: F. A. Davis.

Martin, B. A., & Suane, S. N. (2012). Effect of training on sensory room and cart usage. *Occupational Therapy in Mental Health, 28*(2), 118–128. http://dx.doi.org/10.1080/016421 2X.2012.679526

Martini, R., Cramm, H., Egan, M., & Sikora, L. (2016). Scoping review of self-regulation: What are occupational therapists talking about? *American Journal of Occupational Therapy, 70*, 7006290010. https://doi.org/10.5014/ajot.2016.020362

Maughan, B., & Kim-Cohen, J. (2015). Continuities between childhood and adult life. *British Journal of Psychiatry, 187*, 301–303.

McKelvey, L. M., Selig, J. P., & Whiteside-Mansell, L. (2017). Foundations for screening adverse childhood experiences: Exploring patterns of exposure through infancy and toddlerhood. *Child Abuse and Neglect, 70*, 112–121.

Meany-Walen, K. K., & Teeling, S. (2016). Adlerian play therapy with students with externalizing behaviors and poor social skills. *International Journal of Play Therapy, 25*(2), 64–77.

Meiser-Stedman, R., Smith, P., Yule, W., Glucksman, E., & Dangleish, T. (2017). Posttraumatic stress disorder in young children three years post-trauma: Prevalence and longitudinal predictors. *Journal of Clinical Psychiatry, 78*(3), 334–339.

Messier, J., Ferland, F., & Majnemer, A. (2008). Play behavior of school age children with intellectual disability: Their capacities, interests and attitude. *Journal of Developmental and Physical Disabilities, 20*(2), 193–207.

Mikulincer, M., & Shaver, P. R. (2012). An attachment perspective on psychopathology. *World Psychiatry: Official Journal of the World Psychiatric Association (WPA), 11*(1), 11–15.

Montag, C., & Elhai, J. D. (2020). Discussing digital technology overuse in children and adolescents during the COVID-19 pandemic and beyond: On the importance of considering Affective Neuroscience Theory. *Addictive Behaviors Reports* (12). doi:10.1016/j.abrep.2020.100313

Moore, S. A., Faulkner, G., Rhodes, R. E., Brussoni, M., Chulak-Bozzer, T., Ferguson, L. J., . . . Tremblay, M. S. (2020). Impact of the COVID-19 virus outbreak on movement and play behaviours of Canadian children and youth: A national survey. *International Journal of Behavioral Nutrition and Physical Activity, 17*(85). https://doi.org/10.1186/s12966-020-00987-8.

National Academies of Sciences, Engineering, and Medicine. (2019). *Fostering healthy mental, emotional, and behavioral development in children and youth: A national agenda.* Washington, DC: The National Academies Press. doi: https://doi.org/10.17226/25201. https://www.ncbi.nlm.nih.gov/books/NBK551842/pdf/Bookshelf_NBK551842.pdf

National Association for Gifted Children (NAGC). (2020). *Ensuring gifted children with disabilities receive appropriate services: Call for comprehensive assessment.* https://www.nagc.org/sites/default/files/Position%20Statement/Ensuring%20Gifted%20children%20with%20Disabilities%20Receive%20Appropriate%20Services.pdf

National Child Traumatic Stress Network (NCTSN). (2020). *About child trauma.* https://www.nctsn.org/what-is-child-trauma/about-child-trauma

National Eating Disorders Association. (2020). *PICA.* https://www.nationaleatingdisorders.org/learn/by-eating-disorder/other/pica

National Scientific Council on the Developing Child. (2012). *Establishing a level foundation for life: Mental health begins in early childhood: Working paper 6.* Updated Edition. http://www.developingchild.harvard.edu

Nelson III, C. A., & Gabard-Durnam, L. J. (2020). Early adversity and critical periods: Neurodevelopmental consequences of violating the expectable environment. *Trends in Neurosciences*, 43(3), 133–143.

Nijhof, S. L., Vinkers, C. H., van Geelen, S. M., Duijff, S. N., Achterberg, E. J. M., van der Net, J., . . . Lesscher, H. M. B. (2018). Healthy play, better coping: The importance of play for the development of children in health and disease. *Neuroscience and Behavioral Reviews*, 95, 421–429.

Normand, S., Soucisse, M. M., Melançon, M. P. V., Schneider, B. H., Lee, M. D., & Maisonneuve, M. F. (2019). Observed free-play patterns of children with ADHD and their real-life friends. *Journal of Abnormal Child Psychology*, 47(2), 259–271.

Oetter, P., Richter, E. W., & Frick, S. M. (2019). *M. O. R. E.: Integrating the Mouth with Sensory and Postural Functions.* Framingham, MA: Therapro.

Ogundele M. O. (2018). Behavioral and emotional disorders in childhood: A brief overview for pediatricians. *World Journal of Clinical Pediatrics*, 7, 9–26.

OT-Innovations. (2020). *Sensory rooms in mental health.* https://www.ot-innovations.com/clinical-practice/sensory-modulation/sensory-rooms-in-mental-health-3/

Owens, J. (2007). Classification and epidemiology of childhood sleep disorders. *Sleep Medicine Clinics*, 2(3), 353–361.

Parker, M. M., Hergenrather, K., Smelser, Q., & Kelly, C. T. (2021). Exploring child-centered play therapy and trauma: A systematic review of literature. *International Journal of Play Therapy*, 30(1), 2–13. https://doi.org/10.1037/pla0000136

Passmore, A. (2003). The occupation of leisure: Three typologies and their influence on mental health in adolescence. *OTJR: Occupation, Participation, and Health*, 23(2), 76–83.

Patalay, P., & Fitzsimons, E. (2018). Development and predictors of mental ill-health and wellbeing from childhood to adolescence. *Social Psychiatry and Psychiatric Epidemiology*, 53(12), 1311–1323.

Patterson, L., Stutey, D. M., & Dorsey, B. (2018). Play therapy with African American children exposed to adverse childhood experiences. *International Journal of Play Therapy*, 24(7), 215–226. http://dx.doi.org/10.1037/pla0000080

Pearton, J. L., Ramugondo, E., Cloete, L., & Cordier, R. (2014). Playfulness and prenatal alcohol exposure: A comparative study. *Australian Occupational Therapy Journal*, 61(4), 259–267.

Pizur-Barnekow, K. (2019). Early intervention: A practice setting for infant and toddler mental health. In C. Brown, V. C. Stoffel, & J. P. Munoz (Eds.), *Occupational Therapy in Mental Health: A Vision for Participation* (2nd ed., pp. 573–584). Philadelphia, PA: F. A. Davis.

Polatajko, H., & Mandich, A. (2004). *Enabling occupation in children: The cognitive orientation to daily occupational performance approach.* Ottawa, Canada: CAOT.

Pollack, B., Hojnoski, R., DuPaul, G., & Kern, L. (2016). Play behavior differences among preschoolers with ADHD: Impact of comorbidity ODD and anxiety. *Journal of Psychopathology and Behavior Assessment*, 38, 66–75.

Preyde, M., Adams, G., Cameron, G., & French, K. (2009). Outcomes of children participating in mental health residential and intensive family services: Preliminary findings. *Residential Treatment for Children & Youth*, 26(1), 1–29.

Remstetter, C. L., Murray, R., & Garner, A. S. (2010). The crucial role of recess in schools. *Journal of School Health*, 80(11), 517–526.

Rizk, S., & Howells, V. (2019). Leisure and play. In C. Brown, V. C. Stoffel & J. P. Munoz (Eds.), *Occupational therapy in mental health: A vision for participation* (2nd ed., pp. 896–908). Philadelphia, PA: F. A. Davis.

Rosenblum, S., Waissman, P., & Diamond, G. W. (2017). Identifying play characteristics of pre-school children with developmental coordination disorder via parental questionnaires. *Human Movement Science*, 53, 5–15.

Roshan, G. M., Talaei, A., Sadr, M., Arezoomandan, S., Kazemi, S., & Khorashad, B. S. (2019). Recalled pre-school activities among adults with gender dysphoria who seek gender confirming treatment—An Iranian study. *Asian Journal of Psychiatry*, 42, 57–61.

Rumpf, H. J., Achab, S., Billieux, J., Bowden-Jones, H., Carragher, N., Demetrovics, Z., . . . Poznyak, V. (2018). Including gaming disorder in the ICD-11: The need to do so from a clinical and public health perspective: Commentary on: A weak scientific basis for gaming disorder: Let us err on the side of caution (van Rooij et al., 2018). *Journal of Behavioral Addictions*, 7(3), 556–561.

Rutten, B. P., Hammels, C., Geschwind, N., Menne-Lothmann, C., Pishva, E., Schruers, K., . . . Wichers, M. (2013). Resilience in mental health: Linking psychological and neurobiological perspectives. *Acta Psychiatrica Scandinavica*, 128(1), 3–20.

Sankar-DeLeeuw, N. (1999). Gifted preschoolers: Parent and teacher views on identification, early admission and programming. *Roeper Review*, 21(3), 174–179.

Scanlan, J. N., & Novak, T. (2015). Sensory approaches in mental health: A scoping review. *Australian Occupational Therapy Journal*, 62(5), 277–285. http://dx.doi.org/10.1111/1440-1630.12224

Sciaraffa, M. A., Zeanah, P. D., & Zeanah, C. H. (2018). Understanding and promoting resilience in the context of adverse childhood experiences. *Early Childhood Education Journal*, 46, 343–353. http://dx.doi.org/10.1007/s10643-017-0869-3

Seligman, M. E. P., & Csikszentmihalyi, M. (2000). Positive psychology: An introduction. *American Psychologist*, 55(1), 5–14.

Sharp, E. H., Coffman, D. L., Caldwell, L. L., Smith, E. A., Wegner, L., Vergnani, T., & Mathews, C. (2011). Predicting substance use behavior among South African adolescents: The role of leisure experiences across time. *International Journal of Behavioral Development*, 35(4), 343–351.

Shechtman, Z., & Silektor, A. (2012). Social competencies and difficulties of gifted children compared to nongifted peers. *Roeper Review*, 34(1), 63–72.

Siegel, D. J. (1999). *The developing mind: How relationships and brain interact to shape who we are.* New York: Guilford Press.

Sigafoos, J., Roberts-Pennell, D., & Graves, D. (1999). Longitudinal assessment of play and adaptive behavior in young children with developmental disabilities. *Research in Developmental Disabilities*, 20(2), 147–162.

Silva, M., Loureiro, A., & Cardoso, G. (2016). Social determinants of mental health: A review of the evidence. *The European Journal of Psychiatry*, 30(4), 259–292.

Simmons, J. G., Schwartz, O. S., Bray, K., Deane, C., Pozzi, E., Richmond, S., . . . Yap, M. B. H. (2017). Study protocol: Families and childhood transitions study (FACTS)—a longitudinal investigation of the role of the family environment in brain development and risk for mental health disorders in community based children. *BMC Pediatrics, 17*(1), 153.

Singh, P., & Anekar, U. (2018). The importance of early identification and intervention for children with developmental delays. *Indian Journal of Positive Psychology, 9*, 233–237.

Skard, G., & Bundy, A. C. (2008). Test of playfulness. In L. D. Parham & L. S. Fazio (Eds.), *Play in occupational therapy for children* (2), 71–93. St. Louis, MO: Mosby.

Slot, P. L., Mulder, H., Verhagen, J., & Leseman, P. P. (2017). Preschoolers' cognitive and emotional self-regulation in pretend play: Relations with executive functions and quality of play. *Infant and Child Development, 26*(6), e2038.

Smith, D. T. (2000). Parent–child interaction play assessment. In K. Gitlin-Weiner, A. Sandgrund, & C. Schafer (Eds.), *Play diagnosis and assessment* (2nd ed., pp. 340–370). New York: Wiley.

Spencer, R. L., Chun, L. E., Hartsock, M. J., & Woodruff, E. R. (2020). Neurobiology of stress–health relationships. In *The Wiley encyclopedia of health psychology* (pp. 21–35). Hoboken, NJ: Wiley

Syed, I. A., Afridi, M. I., & Dars, J. A. (2019). An artistic inquiry into gender identity disorder/gender dysphoria: A silent distress. *Asian Journal of Psychiatry, 44*, 86–89.

Tanner, K., Hand, B. N., O'Toole, G., & Lane, A. E. (2015). Effectiveness of interventions to improve social participation, play, leisure, and restricted and repetitive behaviors in people with autism spectrum disorder: A systematic review. *American Journal of Occupational Therapy, 69*(5), 1–12.

Taylor, R. R. (2008). *The intentional relationship: Occupational therapy and use of self.* Philadelphia, PA: F. A. Davis.

Tchanturia, K., Hambrook, D., Curtis, H., Jones, T., Lounes, N., Fenn, K., . . . Davies, H. (2013). Work and social adjustment in patients with anorexia nervosa. *Comprehensive Psychiatry, 54*(1), 41–45.

Thibodeau, R. B., Gilpin, A. T., Brown, M. M., & Meyer, B. A. (2016). The effects of fantastical pretend-play on the development of executive functions: An intervention study. *Journal of Experimental Child Psychology, 145*, 120–138.

Triana, R., Keliat, B. A., & Sulistiowati, N. M. D. (2019). The relationship between self-esteem, family relationships and social support as the protective factors and adolescent mental health. *Humanities & Social Sciences Reviews, 7*(1), 41–47.

Ungar, M., & Theron, L. (2020). Resilience and mental health: How multisystemic processes contribute to positive outcomes. *The Lancet Psychiatry, 7*(5), 441–448.

Van Der Kolk, B. (2014). *The body keeps the score: Brain, mind, and body in the healing of trauma.* New York: Penguin Books.

Wagner, K. D. (2015). Mental health benefits of exercise in children. *Psychiatric Times, 32*(1), 37–37.

Waldman-Levi, A., & Weintraub, N. (2015). Efficacy of a crisis intervention for improving mother–child interaction and the children's play functions. *American Journal of Occupational Therapy, 69*, 1–11. http://dx.doi.org/10.5014/ajot.2015.013375

Westerhof, G. J., & Keyes, C. L. (2010). Mental illness and mental health: The two continua model across the lifespan. *Journal of Adult Development, 17*(2), 110–119.

Whitcomb, D. A. (2012). Attachment, occupation, and identity: Considerations in infancy. *Journal of Occupational Science, 19*, 271–282.

Wilkes-Gillan, S., Buncy, A., Cordier, R., & Lincoln, M. (2016). Child outcomes of a pilot parent-delivered intervention for improving the social play skills of children with ADHD and their playmates. *Developmental Neurorehabilitation, 19*(4), 238–245. http://dx.doi.org/10.3109/17518423.2014.948639

Williams, M. S., & Shellenberger, S. (1995). *The alert program.* Albuquerque, NM. TherapyWorks, Inc.

Wilson, B. J., & Ray, D. (2018). Child-centered play therapy: Aggression, empathy, and self-regulation. *Journal of Counseling & Development, 96*, 399–409.

Yule, K., Houston, J., & Grych, J. (2019). Resilience in children exposed to violence: A meta-analysis of protective factors across ecological contexts. *Clinical Child and Family Psychology Review, 22*(3), 406–431.

Zawadzki, M. J., Smyth, H. M., & Costigan, H. J. (2015). Real-time associations between engaging in leisure and daily health and well-being. *Annals of Behavioral Health, 49*, 605–615.

Zhang, Z., Li, N., Chen, R., Lee, T., Gao, Y., Yuan, Z., . . . Sun, T. (2021). Prenatal stress leads to deficits in brain development, mood related behaviors and gut microbiota in offspring. *Neurobiology of Stress, 15*, 100333.

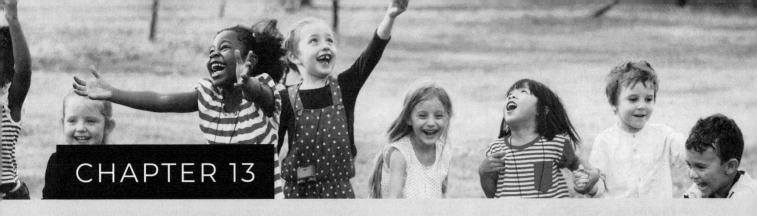

CHAPTER 13

Creative Play and Leisure for Adolescents

Susan Bazyk, PhD, OTR/L, FAOTA

After reading this chapter, the reader will:

- Describe the impact of leisure participation on important developmental changes.
- Discuss how playfulness applies to leisure participation.
- Describe both the benefits and risks associated with leisure participation.
- Explain how the context, breadth, and density of leisure participation influence positive outcomes.
- Identify significant barriers to leisure participation.
- Apply environment-focused, coaching, and strength-based methods for promoting leisure participation in occupational therapy.
- Promote leisure participation within a multitiered public health framework at the universal, targeted, and intensive levels.
- Develop individual, group, and whole school occupational therapy strategies for promoting leisure participation in adolescents with and without disabilities and/or mental health challenges.

It is widely claimed that positive leisure pursuits contribute to the development of self-fulfilled and mentally healthy young people.

—Passmore and French (2001)

A major aim of occupational therapy is to help people participate in and enjoy a range of occupations, including leisure, to promote health and quality of life across the life span (American Occupational Therapy Association [AOTA], 2020a; Wilcock & Hocking, 2015). Through occupations we define who we are, where we have been, and where we are going. When people learn to enjoy complex occupations that provide challenges corresponding to their skills, they are more likely to develop innate abilities, experience a positive self-esteem, and be happier overall

(Csikszentmihalyi, 1993). The focus of this chapter is on occupational therapy practitioners' role in promoting play and leisure in adolescents. Consistent with research and society's use, I will focus on leisure as the primary form of play in adolescence. Nonetheless, this is meaningful leisure rooted in and informed by a thorough knowledge of play.

Leisure is presented from a multitiered, public health perspective (Bazyk, 2011a; Wilcock & Hocking, 2015). The emphasis is on addressing the leisure participation needs of all youth with and without disabilities and/or mental health challenges at the level of a whole population, at-risk individuals, and those with identified leisure challenges. Application of the occupational therapy process in addressing adolescents' leisure participation in diverse school, clinic, and community contexts is described. Clinical examples highlight the occupational therapist's role in embracing occupational justice—that all youth have a right to explore and engage in a range of meaningful and health-promoting leisure occupations (Townsend, 1999).

Adolescence, Play, and Leisure

Adolescence can be broadly defined as the second decade of life and developmental period straddling the transition from childhood to adulthood (Bell, 2016). Development during middle childhood (6–12 years) provides a critical foundation for later success and adjustment in adolescence and adulthood (Newman & Newman, 2018). During this stage, children develop skills in friendship formation, skill learning, team play, and self-evaluation. Adolescence brings about further changes in thinking, emotions, and social relationships (Pavlova & Silbereisen, 2015). Adolescents can think in more abstract and complex ways that allow them to reflect on relevant life issues such as future goals, personal interests, cultural differences, and sexual relationships (Newman & Newman, 2018).

Youth gradually shift allegiance to a peer group, where they spend the majority of their time and learn how to function within a group, deal with hostility and dominance, make close friends, and develop communication and interaction skills (Denworth, 2020; Florey & Greene, 2008). Friendships help teens develop social perspective-taking and cognitive flexibility, helping them become less self-centered. They have the ability to analyze social problems, empathize with another's feelings, and eventually accept individual differences in personality or abilities (Newman & Newman, 2018). Friendships often develop between youth who enjoy the same leisure activities and share common interests.

Exposure to a range of opportunities beyond merely family and school reflects the expanded social world of adolescents and fosters psychosocial autonomy from parents (Passmore & French, 2001). Leisure, freely chosen activities during free time, is important for developing this autonomy (Pavlova & Silbereisen, 2015). The context of leisure also offers opportunities for personal and social identity exploration and development because it allows for more freedom of choice as compared to academics or work. Adolescents take an active role in shaping their interests by selecting and repeating activities based on the quality of the experience (Delle Fave & Bassi, 2000).

Having access to diverse leisure opportunities that are both socially desirable and enjoyable is critical to identity development in adolescence.

Play and Playfulness in Adolescence

Historically, occupational therapy literature on play reflects the premise that play mirrors development and thus increases in complexity over time (Bryze, 2008). For example, according to The Play History (Takata, 1974), play during adolescence focuses on recreation and organized activities during leisure time. Publications over the past 20 years concentrate heavily on leisure participation during adolescence (Henry, 2008; Mahoney et al., 2005; Wilson et al., 2010). As such, content in this chapter focuses on the occupational therapy practitioner's role in fostering leisure participation. Bundy (1993), however, has challenged therapists to expand our view of play to consider the importance of playfulness. Because playfulness is defined by its characteristics rather than the activity, it can occur in the context of any activity, including leisure, academics, or work.

Considered a personality trait associated with health outcomes and quality of life, playfulness has been studied across the life span (Proyer, 2017; Proyer et al., 2018). Playfulness can be described as a style of interaction characterized by flexibility, manifest joy, and spontaneity (Bundy, 1993). Proyer (2017) defines playfulness as a personality trait that "allows people to frame or reframe everyday situations in a way such that they experience them as entertaining, and/or intellectually stimulating, and/or personally interesting" (p. 114). Playful people seek out opportunities to interact playfully with others (e.g., playful teasing) and may use their playfulness under difficult situations to diffuse tension.

Research has linked a number of positive outcomes to playfulness, such as coping, creativity, performance at work, and innovation (Proyer et al., 2018). In a study of playfulness in adolescent males (ages 13 to 17), Hess and Bundy (2003) found that those rating high in playfulness displayed higher degrees of internal control, intrinsic motivation, the freedom to suspend reality, and coping skills. Results suggest that adolescent playfulness may help predict appropriate social interactions and the ability to deal with teasing and bullying (Hess & Bundy, 2003). When exploring the relationship between playfulness in adolescents (ages 12 to 19 years) with perceived daily stress, Staempfli (2007) found that while playful adolescents did not experience fewer daily stressors, they did report higher levels of self-confidence, positive affect, and satisfaction about health. It is important to note that the association of playfulness with emotional well-being was mediated during youth's leisure participation (Staempfli, 2007). This suggests the importance of embedding playfulness during leisure activities in order to foster emotional well-being. In a recent correlational study of adolescents (Proyer & Tandler, 2020), while playfulness was unrelated to self-reported grades and goal achievement orientation, it did correlate positively with life satisfaction (social life, self, friends) and intrinsic goals.

These research findings suggest the importance of tuning in to playfulness in adolescence and recognizing how playfulness could be used to help youth manage difficult social situations and deal with challenges at school or during leisure (Proyer & Tandler, 2020). Additionally, it is important for occupational therapy practitioners to acknowledge the potential benefits of using playfulness when interacting with adolescents as a way to build relationships, increase motivation, and foster group cohesion.

Leisure in Adolescence

Leisure participation is strongly associated with the customs of adolescence particularly in Western societies (Passmore & French, 2001). In studies of time use during adolescence, leisure accounts for 40–57% of a young person's time on average (Csiszentmihalyi & Larson, 1984; Farnworth, 1999; Larson & Kleiber, 1993). Demographic differences in leisure participation have been noted based on gender (e.g., females report spending less time in sports and playing video games), ethnicity (e.g., Latino and African American adolescents in the United States participate less in extracurricular activities and spend more time with family than White counterparts), and socioeconomic status (Pavlova & Silbereisen, 2015). A young person's developmental status, motivation, and abilities may also constrain leisure participation (Mahoney et al., 2005). Although discretionary time outside of school provides an important context for promoting adolescent development, the potential for growth depends in part on how the time is used (Sharp et al., 2015). Structure, active involvement, breadth, and amount of leisure, as well as the role of context are critical factors that occupational therapy practitioners address.

Defining and Categorizing Leisure

Leisure is defined as freely chosen, intrinsically motivated, and enjoyable activities pursued during discretionary time that provide a sense of personal meaning (Henry, 2008; Passmore, 2003; Zhang et al., 2014). In contrast to academics, self-care, and work, leisure provides opportunities for activities that are freely chosen based on individual preferences. Given opportunities to explore a variety of leisure activities, adolescents gradually develop personal preferences for different kinds of activities (Passmore & French, 2001). One's leisure interests reveal what makes a person unique (Zhang et al., 2014). A variety of terms are used in the literature outside of occupational therapy to describe leisure participation for youth such as structured leisure activities, organized out-of-school activities, and extracurricular activities, to name a few (Bazyk, 2011a). For the purposes of this chapter, leisure activities refer to all these variations.

Leisure activities have been categorized in a number of ways primarily based on the amount of structure, personal involvement, investment of skills, and nature of activity as detailed in **Table 13.1**. In addition, others have categorized leisure based on the type of activity such as mass media, social, outdoor, sports, cultural, and hobbies (Lloyd & Auld, 2002).

Benefits of Structured Leisure Participation

The contribution of adolescent leisure to physical and mental health, quality of life, and better life outcomes is well documented (Brajsa-Zganec et al., 2011; Mahoney et al., 2004; Passmore & French, 2003; Trainor et al., 2010). Research has consistently demonstrated a positive relationship between participation in structured leisure and positive youth development, which emphasizes building and improving assets that enable youth to grow and flourish throughout life (Fredricks & Eccles, 2006; Larson, 2000; Leversen et al., 2012). Larson (2000) emphasizes the development of initiative as a core quality of positive youth development and makes a case for participation in structured leisure activities as an important context for such development. The quality of the leisure experience is also an important consideration. Csikzentmihalyi & Larson (1984) found that the most intrinsically rewarding leisure occupations were highly structured and organized, had rules, and required the development and use of skills. In addition, these types of activities were found to promote flow—a state of consciousness characterized by deep concentration and absorption associated with identity formation and optimal experience (Csikszentmihalyi, 1993; Csikszentmihalyi & Larson, 1984). Research using youth inventories of participation and focus groups yield similar findings—that participation in structured leisure is associated with both personal and interpersonal development (Dworkin et al., 2003; Hansen et al., 2003; Mahoney et al., 2005; Trainor et al., 2010).

Table 13.1 Categorizations of Leisure by Specific Characteristics

Characteristic	Categories	Examples
Amount of structure (Eccles et al., 2003; Mahoney & Stattin, 2000)	**Structured leisure** ■ Associated with regular participation schedules ■ Directed by one or more adult ■ Rule-guided interaction ■ Emphasize skill ■ Performance requires sustained active attention and the provision of feedback ■ Higher social complexity involving peer cooperation, support from family members, and guidance from adult role models	School and community-sponsored athletics, music organizations, after-school clubs (e.g., Scouts), theatre, dance
	Unstructured leisure ■ Spontaneous ■ Occur without formal rules and adult direction ■ Include few opportunities for skill development	Watching television, playing video games, hanging out with friends, listening to music
Nature of activity (Passmore & French, 2001)	**Achievement leisure** ■ Demanding and often competitive ■ Provide a sense of personal challenge	Sports, dance, playing a musical instrument, hobbies, creative arts
	Social leisure ■ Engaged in for the primary purpose of being with others	Hanging out with friends, talking on the phone, use of social media
	Time-out leisure ■ Low demand ■ Relaxation ■ Way to pass time	Watching TV, using social media, playing video games
Investment of skills (Stebbins, 2007)	**Casual leisure** ■ Pleasant activities ■ Do not require much training for enjoyment ■ May contribute to social relationships when done in a group	Going out to eat, hiking in a park, swimming at a pool
	Serious leisure ■ Skill-based activities requiring effort and persistence ■ Provides the benefits of self-expression, self-actualization, and self-enrichment with like-minded peers	Playing chess, photography, pottery, playing a musical instrument in a band
	Project-based leisure ■ Time-limited ■ Moderately complicated ■ Creative undertakings that require planning, effort, and skills	Making a mosaic frame, knitting a scarf, woodworking projects
Amount of effort (Nishino & Larson, 2003)	**Active leisure** ■ Involves some challenge ■ Combines effort and enjoyment with opportunities for learning a skill (for example, musical, social, physical)	Rock climbing, playing in a band, backpacking
	Passive leisure ■ Activities for the purpose of pleasure, relaxation, coping with stress, or filling free time	Pleasure reading, watching TV, using social media, hanging out with friends

Personal Development. Several areas of personal development have been identified as benefitting from participation in structured leisure (Hansen et al., 2003; Trainor et al., 2010). First, participation provides opportunities to facilitate identity work. Exposure to and participation in a variety of leisure activities allows a young person to explore, express, and refine one's identity and passion (Zhang et al., 2014). During these activities, youth assess their talents, interests, values, and place in the social structure. Choices communicate to self and others that "This is who I am" or "What I am meant to do" and are based on the person's expectations for successful performance and enjoyment of the activity (Barber et al., 2005, p. 188).

Second, organized activities have been viewed as providing a context for the development of initiative and autonomy (Larson, 2000). Initiative reflects the self-motivation needed to devote effort over time to achieve a challenging goal, a core quality that individuals need in order to transition to the complexities of adult life and future work (Wilson et al., 2010). Three elements of initiative include intrinsic motivation (wanting to do the activity), concerted engagement, and commitment over time (Larson, 2000). Additionally, because leisure is self-initiated and based on personal choice, it serves an important context for the development of autonomy, which is critical for the transition to adulthood (Leversen et al., 2012).

Third, structured activities are associated with greater skill development (Hansen et al., 2003; Wilson et al., 2010). Participation in structured leisure is associated with higher academic achievement (Passmore, 2003), the development of positive habits contributing to physical health especially with sports (Mahoney et al., 2005), skill development (e.g., athletic, artistic, homemaking), and beginning work skills (Dworkin et al., 2003; Mahoney & Stattin, 2000). In addition to these benefits, Gilman (2001) found that structured leisure participation promoted greater satisfaction at school, stronger identification with the school culture, and a more positive academic self-concept than time spent in low-structured leisure activities.

Finally, participation in structured leisure is associated with greater subjective well-being and positive mental health (Leversen et al., 2012). In a recent study exploring leisure physical activity, increased positive affect and less negative affect was found in adolescents reporting greater amounts of physically active leisure (White et al., 2018). Additionally, a number of emotional competencies have been associated with participation in structured leisure, including managing feelings, controlling impulses, increasing self-esteem, and reducing stress (Mahoney et al., 2005; Trainor et al., 2010). In terms of positive mental health, Csikszentmihalyi (1993) found that when people learn to enjoy complex occupations that provide challenges corresponding to their skills, they are more likely to develop innate abilities, experience positive self-esteem, and be happier overall.

Interpersonal Development. A second outcome from structured leisure is interpersonal development, which focuses on the development of social connections. Structured leisure activities expand the social world of adolescents and involve greater social complexity requiring higher-level interpersonal skills. First, participation in shared structured leisure provides an important context for the development of new peer friendships with youth who have similar interests. Many structured leisure pursuits involve interaction with peers who are typically outside the youth's immediate network, providing opportunities to interact with peers of different ages, racial and ethnic backgrounds, and socioeconomic status (Dworkin et al., 2003; Trainor et al., 2010). Second, youth activities provide opportunities to develop a variety of social skills, including working effectively with others, giving and receiving feedback, and learning how to interact appropriately across settings (Hansen et al., 2003; Mahoney et al., 2005). The third attribute of interpersonal development is the growth of close connections to adults with social capital, such as coaches, artists, dancers, musicians, and other valued community members. These adults offer special skills and knowledge to youth and provide a sense of belonging to a network of people valued in the community. Close relationships with adults with social capital may provide long-term sources of emotional support and social networking such as access to information about future jobs or colleges.

Preparation for Future Work. According to Passmore (1998), participation in leisure appears to provide positive training ground for many of the requirements for work. Many structured leisure pursuits require intelligence, concentration, task commitment, persistence, and teamwork—all critical for success at work. These abilities are typically encouraged and modeled by adult supervisors. The actual structure of leisure pursuits imposes organization on youth time, helping in the development of time management and health-promoting daily habits for independent living such as maintaining a balance of work, rest and leisure. Involvement in positive structured extracurricular activities has important implications regarding a young person's perceptions of and investment in their future (Bazyk, 2005).

Outcomes from Unstructured and Passive Leisure

Outcomes associated with participation in unstructured and passive forms of leisure are mixed. Some leisure scientists contend that certain forms of unstructured leisure (e.g., attending concerts, hiking, and going out to dinner) contribute to positive adolescent development (Caldwell & Faulk, 2013). Such activities are chosen for enjoyment, or personal interests and may occur in isolation or in a group without adult supervision. However, other studies consistently link engagement in unstructured or passive leisure (e.g., hanging out with peers, watching TV, and playing video games) with poor academic performance, antisocial behaviors, and becoming young offenders (Farnworth, 1999; Mahoney & Stattin, 2000).

The social context of unstructured leisure is different in that adult supervision is typically lacking, allowing for greater opportunities to engage in at-risk behaviors such as drinking, unsupervised sex, and drugs (Mahoney & Stattin, 2000). Furthermore, less time spent in structured activities is associated with less time with positive adult role models and, subsequently, an increased risk of developing maladaptive attitudes about school and the future in general (Sharp et al., 2015). Trainor et al. (2010) found that youth who are psychologically healthy tend to participate in structured activities, while those with low self-esteem and poor psychological functioning tend to engage in unstructured activities that lack challenge.

Passive forms of leisure generally lack complexity and can be characterized as providing little or no mental or physical challenge or requiring no skills, which may result in boredom. Boredom is a subjective experience that there is nothing meaningful to do and that time is passing slowly (Csikszentmihalyi & Csikszentmihalyi, 1988; Spaeth et al., 2015). Feelings of dissatisfaction, stress, and annoyance may accompany boredom. During these times, the person may actually experience a sense of bodily tension and restlessness (fidgeting, sighing, yawning) from an underaroused nervous system. As a result, boredom may lead a person to seek stimulation from any activity (even illegal) that is interesting or challenging in order to reach an optimal level of arousal (Farnworth, 1999). Adolescent boredom may occur when families, schools, and communities do not offer a range of developmentally appropriate leisure opportunities and contexts.

Leisure Context, Breadth, and Density

Both exposure to a range of potential leisure occupations and the availability of resources to support engagement are critical factors linked with the likelihood that youth will develop and maintain healthy leisure interests. Furthermore, simply participating in structured leisure may not always result in positive outcomes—the context, breadth, and density are also important considerations.

Context. Occupational therapy practitioners must consider the physical, social, and emotional aspects of where leisure is occurring. Eight key features of the leisure context are associated with positive youth development and include: physical and psychological safety, appropriate structure, supportive relationships, opportunities for belonging, positive social norms, support for efficacy and mattering, opportunities for skill building, and integration of family, school, and community efforts (Mahoney et al., 2005). Although many organized leisure activities incorporate several, if not all, of these features, therapists can screen and advocate for such features in youth programming.

Breadth. Although benefits are consistently associated with participation in structured versus unstructured leisure activities, involvement in a greater breadth of activities has also been advocated. In a study of rural adolescents, it was found that those who participated in the most structured and unstructured activities did better in terms of grades, school attachment, and future educational expectations (Sharp et al., 2015). Adolescents with low breadth of involvement in both structured and unstructured leisure showed poorer outcomes. These findings are important to consider because youth in rural and lower SES settings report limited options for organized activities compared to suburban youth. It is important for occupational therapists to encourage participation in a variety of activities (both structured and unstructured) in order to help teens explore interests, skills, and personal characteristics across settings (Sharp et al., 2015).

Density. In terms of leisure, density means frequency of participation. In a study of leisure participation in Norwegian adolescents, Leverson et al. (2012) found a strong relationship between participation in leisure and life satisfaction. Results suggested that density of participation was important in addition to the variation of activities. The more often adolescents participated in various leisure activities, the higher their feelings of competence and relatedness. Leisure activities engaged in frequently and over time provide opportunities for skill development, allowing adolescents to feel that they are good at something (Leverson et al., 2012; Mahoney et al., 2005). Developing new skills, forming new behaviors, and building relationships take time.

Influences on Leisure Participation

In order to experience the benefits of leisure, youth must participate. The home, school, and community environments may either support or undermine youth's engagement in complex activities that they can learn to enjoy. Both exposure to a range of potential leisure occupations and the availability of resources to support engagement are critical factors influencing the likelihood that adolescents will develop and maintain healthy leisure interests (Mahoney et al., 2005). Resources such as parks, organized sports, other community programs, and competent adults to oversee the activities are essential. If only mindless or aggressive opportunities for action are available, youth will miss the opportunity to seek out and experience health-promoting challenges (Bazyk & Bazyk, 2009; Farnworth, 1999). Occupational therapy practitioners need to be aware of the multiple factors that may limit the availability of and access to healthy leisure activities, such as systemic racism, cultural bias, or gender-related issues (AOTA, 2020b). It is important to recognize how such factors might limit an adolescent's leisure participation and advocate to minimize disparities affecting marginalized groups. For example, therapists need to become aware of and support community-driven initiatives aimed at providing healthy recreation, sports, and after-school activities in low-income environments.

Finances and Transportation. Adolescents living in low-income environments may have less access to leisure participation due to issues related to availability and affordability. An important predictor of structured leisure participation is financial capital. Youth from families with higher socioeconomic status (SES) have greater financial capacity to pursue a larger range of leisure activities (Bazyk, 2011b; Farnworth, 1999). Most structured leisure activities (organized sports, dance lessons, and Scouts) require some sort of transportation and fee for participation. Many also require expensive equipment or specialized clothing. Low-income urban and rural youth generally have less opportunity to engage in structured leisure because of limited finances and/or transportation (Bazyk, 2011b).

Disability. Despite the importance of leisure and its positive impact on health outcomes, participation in community-based leisure occupations is significantly restricted among youth with various types of disabilities in comparison to their peers without disabilities (Batya Engel-Yeger et al., 2009; Bedell et al., 2013; Law et al., 2015). Those with more significant functional impairment tend to report lower levels of participation in leisure activities (Schreuer et al., 2014). A North American study found that 37% of youth with disabilities never took part in organized physical activities compared to only 10% among nondisabled peers (Bedell et al., 2013). Research has also found that youth with physical disabilities tend to participate more in informal, unstructured activities alone at home and less in structured community-based leisure (Law et al., 2006). Youth experiencing depression and peer rejection are at higher risk of boredom and leisure deprivation and may benefit from services aimed at fostering meaningful leisure participation and peer-related social skills (Spaeth et al., 2015).

Promoting Leisure Participation Within a Public Health Framework in Occupational Therapy

Given the developmental, mental, and physical health benefits of participation in a range of leisure occupations, it is important for occupational therapy practitioners to address the leisure needs of *all* adolescents—those with and without disabilities and/or mental health challenges. A multitiered, public health framework has been described (Bazyk, 2011c) and applied by therapists to address mental health in youth. This framework has been effective in helping practitioners to articulate and advocate our distinct value in mental health promotion, prevention, and intervention with children and youth (Bazyk et al., 2015). As a part of this work, this framework has also been applied in addressing leisure (Bazyk, 2011c).

A public health framework is compatible with occupational therapy's commitment to promoting health and participation of clients including persons, groups, and populations through engagement in occupation (AOTA, 2020a). It is timely for occupational therapy practitioners to reframe how we address leisure to include promotion and prevention in addition to occupational therapy's traditional focus on intervention for those with limitations due to disability, illness, injury, or poverty. Such a shift in thinking requires practitioners to reflect on who we should serve and where, followed by a strategic conceptualization of what services might entail (Bazyk, 2011c). In order to address the leisure needs of all adolescents, the following sections will provide descriptions of occupational therapy services at the universal, targeted, and individualized levels with practice examples representing diverse settings (school, clinic, and community). Although occupational therapy's emphasis will vary depending on context, all efforts share a common belief in the positive relationship between participation in meaningful and health-promoting leisure and health (Bazyk, 2011a).

Key Intervention Approaches Applied to Promote Leisure Participation

Based on current literature on adolescent leisure participation and intervention, it is important for occupational therapy practitioners to foster leisure exploration and participation in a variety of structured activities within natural contexts. The following intervention approaches guide efforts to promote successful and enjoyable leisure participation. It is important that they be applied at the universal, targeted, and individualized levels of service provision.

Use of an Ecological Model

An ecological model, focusing on the relationship between person–occupation–environment (P–E–O), has been widely supported in occupational therapy (Law et al., 1996). Just as factors within the person may support or impede occupational performance, so too can the environment have a positive or negative influence. A core skill for all occupational therapy practitioners is activity analysis, which is the ability to analyze the relationship between the person, environment, and occupation and determine factors needed for successful participation (as detailed in Chapter 4). When the activity-environment demands are greater than the person's abilities, then adaptation of the environment or the activity may be provided to foster successful participation (Bazyk, 2011c).

Environment-Focused Interventions

Environmental barriers and restricted social supports have been linked to decreased leisure participation in youth with disabilities (Anaby et al., 2014). In particular, community access to leisure facilities and programs may be limited, which discourages participation. Although environmental factors are

critical to participation, therapy has primarily focused on improving performance component functioning (Anaby et al., 2016; Law et al., 2015). However, with environment-focused interventions, the therapist, youth, and family collaborate to remove environmental barriers, provide the necessary supports (e.g., physical, social, activity-based), and build on strengths to enhance successful participation (Anaby et al., 2016; Law & Darrah, 2014).

Context Therapy. Research supports context therapy (Darrah et al., 2011), an intervention focusing on modifying environmental conditions and activity demands to foster leisure participation rather than focusing primarily on improving the young person's component skills. For example, in order to decrease the activity demands of independent performance during a dance class, a peer buddy (e.g., a child with higher skills and positive social interaction) may dance alongside a child with autism to provide the needed environmental supports (e.g., verbal and physical prompts) for successful participation.

Leisure Coaching. Environment-focused intervention has involved a coaching element (Graham, Rodger, & Ziviani, 2009) where the therapist coaches the adolescent and parent on identifying and implementing effective strategies to improve leisure participation (Anaby et al., 2016). Evidence of effectiveness in implementing this type of environment-focused context therapy among youth with physical disabilities has been demonstrated (Law et al., 2015). For example, in a 12-week occupational therapy intervention involving environmental modifications and coaching with six adolescents with disabilities, Anaby et al. (2016) found clinically significant improvements in occupational performance. Contemporary approaches emphasize the importance of targeting modifiable factors within real-life environments rather than focusing solely on "fixing a deficit" within the adolescent to foster leisure participation.

Focus on Strengths

"All young people possess a unique combination of strengths, struggles, interests, personality traits, and passions" (Carter et al., 2015, p. 116). However, "disability has long been defined and described in the language of deficits" (Carter et al., 2015, p. 101). An overemphasis on the remediation of deficits for youth with disabilities may have important limitations, particularly related to transition to adulthood. Participating in the community and developing relationships are heavily dependent on personal strengths. In a mixed-method study of youth and young adults with intellectual disability and/or autism, it was found that youth who participated in a higher number of community-based after-school activities, were reported to have a higher number of personal and interpersonal strengths. Assisting adolescents to develop leisure interests and activities that enhance and showcase their strengths may provide a relevant context within which youth develop and deepen strengths over time (Carter et al., 2015).

Embed Playfulness

When promoting leisure, it is important for occupational therapy practitioners to embed playful interactions to communicate "having fun" together. Playfulness can be used to diffuse tension and to move beyond resistance to participate. For example, one teenage female refused to participate in a mock TV production during an after-school leisure group by stating, "That's stupid." The skilled therapist quickly quipped in a joking manner, "I'll tell you what, why don't you do the activity and afterwards, you can tell me how much you hated it." This made the teen laugh. She participated in the activity and told the therapist afterwards how much she loved it and that she wanted to do it again. Playfulness can be powerful in building relationships between therapists and adolescents, increasing motivation and the possibility of having fun together. It is also important to recognize and encourage a young person's playfulness by explicitly pointing it out as an important character strength to both the young person and parents. For example, "Max has a great sense of humor. He makes us all laugh, which adds to our fun and wanting to spend time together!"

Approaches Within the Multitiered Public Health Framework

A multitiered public health framework supports a change in thinking from an individually focused deficit-driven model of occupational therapy intervention, to a whole-population strength-based approach. The three major tiers of service can be depicted in a pyramid (see **Figure 13.1**) and include: Tier 1—universal leisure promotion (for all), Tier 2—targeted prevention (for those at risk of limited leisure), and Tier 3—individualized (for those with leisure deficits). Universal leisure promotion emphasizes competence enhancement as well as environmental modifications to support leisure participation for all

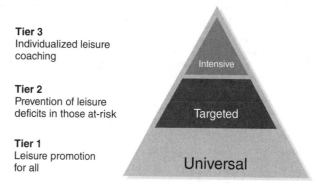

Figure 13.1 Multitiered public health framework for addressing leisure in occupational therapy

adolescents with and without limitations. Targeted prevention efforts focus on reducing the occurrence of leisure deficits in youth at risk (e.g., those with disabilities, social challenges, limited finances) by providing targeted services. Individualized intervention focuses on leisure coaching with the adolescent and family in order to foster successful leisure participation for those with leisure deficits (Bazyk, 2011a).

The occupational therapy process in addressing leisure in adolescence within a multitiered framework follows a traditional process of evaluation, intervention, and targeting outcomes (AOTA, 2020a). It is important to remember that "client" is defined broadly and includes the adolescent, parents and family, peer groups, school community, clinic setting, and community (Bazyk, 2011d).

In the following sections, information specific to the occupational therapy process focusing on leisure participation is presented for each of the three levels of service provision within a public health framework along with occupational therapy examples of implementation and outcomes. Although these are presented separately, there is often overlap in actual practice. Examples of occupational therapy services representing each tier are provided in **Table 13.2**. Occupational therapy examples of addressing the leisure needs of adolescents are derived from Every Moment Counts' Making Leisure Matter initiative. Background information and a summary of this initiative can be found in **Box 13.1**.

Tier 3: Individualized Evaluation and Intervention

Occupational therapy services at this level focus on helping youth with disabilities and/or mental health challenges who have little or no leisure participation to explore and participate in meaningful and healthy leisure interests. The occupational therapy process therefore begins with an evaluation of the

Table 13.2 Examples for Promoting Adolescent Leisure Participation in a Multitiered Public Health Framework

Tier	Intervention Type	Population Served	Strategies
3	Individualized Occupational Therapy Leisure Coaching	Youth with identified limitations in leisure participation	■ Include leisure participation as a part of every occupational therapy evaluation. ■ Begin with open-ended questions such as "What do you do for fun after school and on weekends?" ■ Identify leisure strengths, limitations, and barriers to participation. ■ Interview parents to learn about their child's leisure experiences, opportunities, and interests. ■ Educate youth, parents, and school personnel about occupational therapy's role in promoting leisure participation. ■ Use individual occupational therapy (OT) leisure coaching strategies over time to strategically foster structured leisure participation in one or more activities.
2	Targeted Occupational Therapy Leisure Groups	Youth at risk of leisure deprivation	■ Tune in to youth who might be at risk of limited leisure participation, such as those with challenges related to disabilities, mental health issues, sensory processing disorders, and/or obesity. ■ Screen for leisure deficits. ■ In addition to providing Tier 1 strategies, provide small-group interventions targeting those at risk during recess or after school focusing on exposure and participation in a variety of leisure activities. Unless exposed to leisure activities, youth will not discover interests and talents. Consider including peers with established leisure skills to lead various group activities. Youth often learn best from peer role models.

Tier	Intervention Type	Population Served	Strategies
1	Schoolwide Leisure Promotion	All students in the school (with and without disabilities and mental health challenges)	■ Explore local, state, and national resources focusing on inclusive community-based leisure. ■ Educate youth, families, and school providers about the mental and physical health benefits of structured leisure participation, and advocate for participation in a variety of activities (arts, music, theater, sports, clubs). ■ Implement Every Moment Counts' Refreshing Recess program to promote participation in healthy play and leisure for all students (https://everymomentcounts.org/refreshing-recess/). ■ Help develop schoolwide inclusive leisure activities such as The Sparkle Effect inclusive cheerleading (www.generationspirit.org) or inclusive drama clubs. ■ Develop and share a handout highlighting the benefits of structured leisure participation and a list of school- and community-sponsored options.

young person's leisure participation. An occupational profile may be used initially to explore the young person's leisure interests and participation as well as to identify opportunities and barriers. This information can easily be obtained with informal conversations using open-ended questions such as, "What do you do for fun after school and on weekends?" "Tell me about a typical weekend," "What are your favorite hobbies and interests?" and "What new leisure activity would you like to learn and do?" Such informal interviews with the young person are critical for gaining their perspectives. Although there are a number of leisure inventories and assessment tools (see **Table 13.3**), we have found that taking the time to complete them is not necessary for the evaluation when an adolescent indicates little or no leisure participation.

Evaluation also involves gathering information from other important "clients" including parents/caregivers and the school and community context. Conversations with parents/caregivers provide an opportunity to explore their priorities and concerns related to their adolescent's leisure participation and perceptions of strengths and challenges.

Although parents may have a sense of their adolescent's interests, it is important to talk individually with the young person to gain their views. For example, when an occupational therapist used an interest inventory with pictures, a young girl with Down syndrome and intellectual impairment pointed to pictures of softball and camping. Her parents exclaimed, "We never knew she was interested in these activities!" Based on this evaluation, the occupational therapist worked with the parents and young girl to find a local softball team and provided informal coaching to foster successful participation. The parents were excited to have their daughter be a part of a team and experience joy and success in participating. This example demonstrates how parents may make assumptions about their young person's interests or lack thereof. Communicating directly with the adolescent fosters exploration and independent decision making which contributes to the development of autonomy.

Evaluation of the context is critical for gathering important information used during the intervention process. Whether the occupational therapy practitioner works in a school, clinic, or community, being aware of available leisure activities is essential

Box 13.1 Every Moment Counts' Making Leisure Matter Initiative

The practice examples included throughout this chapter are derived from work completed as a part of Every Moment Counts (EMC). Originally funded by the Ohio Department of Education (2012–15), EMC is a multipronged mental health promotion initiative developed to help all children and youth become mentally healthy in order to succeed in school, at home, and in the community (Bazyk, 2019; Bazyk et al., 2015). This initiative emphasizes mental health promotion, inclusion of children with disabilities and/or mental health challenges in school and community settings, integrating occupational therapy services in natural settings throughout the day (classroom, recess, cafeteria, and after school), and collaborating with all relevant stakeholders to enhance their ability to be mental health promoters (refer to www .everymomentcounts.org).

Making Leisure Matter is one of EMC's initiatives that originally developed as an exploratory research study (2014–16). A convenience sample of 20 occupational therapists and occupational therapy assistants committed to working together over a period of 2 years in order to strategically foster leisure participation in youth with disabilities and/or mental health challenges who were identified as engaging in few or no leisure occupations. Practitioners worked in a variety of schools, private practice outpatient, and community-based settings.

Occupational therapy practitioners involved in this initiative, selected youth (ages 8–20 years) on their caseloads that they knew had little or no leisure participation. Youth with a variety of diagnoses were represented. After learning about the benefits and barriers associated with structured leisure participation (Anaby et al., 2016; Graham et al., 2009) during an orientation session, the therapists used a number of strategies (coaching, strength-based, environmental modifications) over time that would result in participation in one or more community- or school-based leisure occupations.

Participation in one or more structured leisure activities on a routine basis (minimum of once per week) over an extended period of time (minimum of 2 months) was the targeted outcome. Nineteen of the 20 youth involved in Phase 1 successfully identified and participated in one or more leisure activities within 3 to 9 months of OT leisure coaching. A range of leisure activities were chosen based on the young person's interests, family resources, and community availability (e.g., pottery, crocheting, bird watching, adapted football, running, softball, theater, horticulture, cooking). It is important to note that a variety of interest inventories were used as a part of the OT leisure coaching process in order to educate and expose the young person to possible leisure pursuits. Therapists noted that both adolescents and parents

were often unaware of the wide variety of possibilities. Once an interest was sparked, the therapist and young person explored community options using online resources with parent input.

The one participant who was not successful had parents who decided not to support their son's pursuit of joining a softball team. This was a young teen who struggled with obesity, self-esteem issues, and depression. His parents reported that he was happy playing video games at home. In situations such as this one, it is important not to "give up," but to explore other strategies for working with the young person and family. The occupational therapist was able to involve the young male in softball and other active play during school recess.

In some cases, the occupational therapy practitioner noted that "success bred further success." Parents were excited to observe their son's or daughter's successful participation in the community and the associated benefits of expressed joy, new friends, expanded skills, and independence. Occupational spin-off was noted, which represents the notion that success and enjoyment experienced during a new leisure occupation may lead to further leisure exploration (Rebiero & Cook, 1999). Parents were observed as feeling more confident in their ability to find leisure activities in the community and in the belief that their daughter or son could be successful in a community-sponsored activity. OT leisure coaching not only helps youth in expanding leisure interests, but also helps parents develop the skill and confidence needed to search for options and complete the registration process.

During Phase 2 of the Making Leisure Matter initiative, therapists began to brainstorm, develop, and implement Tier 1 and 2 strategies for promoting leisure participation at the universal and targeted levels in school and community settings. With increased attention to youth at risk of leisure deprivation, therapists realized that they were not effectively promoting leisure participation. Given occupational therapists' ability to facilitate occupation-based groups, several therapists developed and implemented groups to foster both social emotional learning and leisure participation. Other therapists identified leisure needs at the universal, whole-school, and community level. Creative ways to promote leisure at school such as the development of Special Olympics and walking and running clubs occurred. Other therapists brought community leisure organizations into the school or offered leisure groups at local recreation centers. The longer therapists were involved in the Making Leisure Matters initiative, the more their services expanded to the universal and targeted levels.

Table 13.3 Assessments Related to Leisure Participation

Assessment and Author	Availability	Population	Characteristics	Clinical Use
Children's Assessment of Participation and Enjoyment (CAPE) and Preferences for Activities of Children (PAC) King et al. (2004)	Pearson Assessments at http://www .pearsonclinical.com	Ages 6 to 21 years	■ Standardized self-report ■ Assesses five types of activities (recreational, social, active physical, skill-based, self-improvement) ■ Takes about 30–45 minutes	Measures children's participation in and enjoyment of out-of-school recreation and leisure Identifies youth's exposure to and preferences in social and leisure activities to plan leisure participation
Devereux Student Strengths Assessment (DESSA) LeBuffe, Shapiro, & Robitaille (2018)	https://apertureed.com/?s=DESSA	Kindergarten through eighth grade Can be used individually or with a whole class	■ Standardized norm-referenced, strength-based rating scale of social-emotional competencies ■ Completed by parents/ guardians, teachers, or school staff ■ Assesses competencies in eight dimensions: self-awareness, social awareness, self-management, goal-directed behavior, relationship skills, personal responsibility, decision making, and optimistic thinking	Identifies social-emotional skills in order to enhance competencies in weaker areas
Measure of Environmental Qualities of Activity Settings (MEQAS) King et al. (2014) King, Rigby, & Avery (2016)	https://hollandbloorview.ca/research -education/bloorview-research -institute/outcome-measures /measure-environmental-qualities-2	Children & adolescents	■ Observer-completed measure of environmental qualities of leisure activity settings for young people ■ Good to excellent psychometric properties ■ Assesses the environment in: social activities, physical activities, quality of the physical environment, opportunities for choice, opportunities for personal growth, and opportunities to interact with adults	Assesses overall quality of a leisure activity for clinical use and to improve environments for participation

(continues)

(continued)

Table 13.3 Assessments Related to Leisure Participation

Assessment and Author	Availability	Population	Characteristics	Clinical Use
Pediatric Interest Profile: Surveys of Play for Children & Adolescents Henry (2000)	Publisher: UIC http://www.cade.uic.edu/moho/	6–21 years (different versions for three different age ranges) Can be used with children and adolescents with and without disabilities	■ Nonstandardized interview checklists ■ Child self-reports interest and participation in activities	Assists in identifying a student's play and leisure participation and also identifies potential areas of interest
Refreshing Recess Environmental Analysis Bazyk (2021)	Download from http://s3.us-east-2.amazonaws.com/s3.everymomentcounts.com/wp-content/uploads/2021/03/01192600/RR_EnvironmentalAnalysis_FINAL_fillable_3-1-21.pdf	Kindergarten through 12th grade	■ Nonstandardized structured observation of recess ■ Part of the Refreshing Recess program ■ Considers areas of: playground toys/equipment, recess supervisors, behavior expectations, students' social interaction, students' physical activity, students' play activities & games, opportunities for structured and unstructured play, inclusion of students with disabilities and/or emotional challenges, and transition to and from recess	Identifies positive and negative aspects of recess to implement strategies for promoting a positive recess experience
School Setting Interview (SSI) Hemmingsson, Egilson, , & Kielhofner (2005)	Publisher: UIC https://www.moho.uic.edu/productDetails.aspx?aid=10	Elementary & high school	■ Nonstandardized ■ Client-centered semistructured interview ■ Assesses student–environment fit and identifies need for accommodations in physical or social contexts such as classroom, playground, gym, and field trips	Identifies student's perceptions of his or her social and leisure participation and enjoyment of school
Social Profile—Child Version Donohue (2013)	AOTA Press https://myaota.aota.org/shop_aota/product/1244	Kindergarten through 12th grade	■ Assesses activity participation, social interaction, and group membership/roles ■ Focus is on interaction within a group	Evaluates a student's cooperation and participation in group activities

in helping young people and families make informed choices. For example, therapists can complete a leisure environmental scan in the young person's community. This involves searching for potential community-based options for participation in a wide array of areas, including sports, outdoor nature activities, theater, arts and crafts, music, and cooking, to name a few. Although this task may be time consuming initially, a growing awareness of community resources will evolve over time as therapists make leisure a part of their everyday work with youth. Whenever possible, sharing resources with other occupational therapists is important for fostering a greater awareness of community-based options for participation. Additionally, a formal assessment of the environment, such as the *Measure of Environmental Qualities of Activity Settings* (MEQAS), can be completed to evaluate social and physical aspects of community-based leisure activities (King et al., 2014). Refer to Table 13.3 for details about the MEQAS. As a standardized measure, this can also be used for research purposes as well.

Tier 3 individualized intervention involves a variety of approaches, as described earlier, including an ecological P–E–O analysis, environment-focused services, embedding playfulness, strength-based strategies, and leisure coaching. Specific to youth with physical disabilities, the Pathways and Resources for Engagement and Participation (PREP) intervention has been shown to be effective in improving performance in meaningful community-based activities (Anaby et al., 2018; Anaby et al., 2016; Law et al., 2015). This 12-week client-centered intervention focuses on enhancing participation by focusing on strengths, removing environmental barriers, and coaching adolescents and parents. The five steps guiding intervention include (1) making goals, (2) mapping out a plan, (3) making it happen, (4) measuring process and outcomes, and (5) moving forward (Law et al., 2016). In an interrupted time series design study involving 28 adolescents with physical disabilities, the PREP intervention resulted in statistically significant improvements in leisure participation (Anaby et al., 2018). A similar intervention approach focusing on coaching youth with developmental disabilities and/or mental health challenges was developed as OT leisure coaching in the Every Moment Counts initiative.

Individualized OT Leisure Coaching. The vision guiding OT leisure coaching is that all children and youth have a right to participate in and enjoy healthy hobbies and interest in inclusive school and community settings. The overall objective of leisure coaching is participation in one or more structured leisure activities on a routine basis (minimum of once per week) over an extended period of time (e.g., 3 or more months). The focus is to help all children and youth explore, select, and participate in extracurricular leisure activities in order to develop enjoyable hobbies and interests. The occupational therapy practitioner serves as an:

- *Educator*, sharing information about the health benefits of participation in enjoyable hobbies and interests with youth, families and school personnel;
- *Facilitator* of the change process, by working collaboratively with youth to help them explore and participate in enjoyable leisure activities; and
- *Advocate* of inclusive leisure participation, by promoting involvement in integrated school- and community-sponsored extracurricular activities (Every Moment Counts, 2021).

The coaching process combines the use of emotional support and encouragement, information exchange, and a structured process of planning for and participating in chosen activities. Emotional support and encouragement is provided to build trust and help the youth and family explore and pursue leisure participation. The occupational therapist uses listening, empathy, reframing abilities, guiding, and encouraging. Information is exchanged between the occupational therapist, youth, and family. The therapist shares information about the health benefits of leisure participation. The youth shares information about potential leisure interests. The family shares information about available resources (financial, transportation, time, etc.) and values related to leisure participation. A structured process is used to identify interests, explore options, plan, and engage in the leisure activity. This process often involves activity analysis, problem solving, and scaffolding the experience; advocating for the child/youth/family; and therapeutic use of self to enable successful participation. Refer to **Practice Example 13.1** for a description of Tier 3 OT leisure coaching.

Six key steps to OT leisure coaching help foster successful participation outcomes. Each is described with an example of their application by an occupational therapist (Kelly) providing outpatient services after school to a young 10-year-old male with autism (Alex).

Step One: Start the Conversation Start the conversation about the importance of leisure with the youth and the parents, and educate them about the health benefits of participation in meaningful hobbies and interests during out-of- school time. Obtain parental buy-in and support, and begin to develop a trusting relationship.

PRACTICE EXAMPLE 13.1 Individual Occupational Therapy Leisure Coaching with Dori

Dori, a 13-year-old with mitochondrial disease, has been receiving outpatient OT and PT at The Cleveland Clinic since she was an infant. Some of her challenges include limitations in physical strength and coordination, gross-motor development, and social participation. Strengths include perseverance and her love of swimming.

Dori has participated in individual adapted aquatics lessons since she was 5 years old with her OT instructor, Mary Lou Kennedy, OTR/L. Because Dori struggled with self-esteem in groups and difficulty making friends, Mary Lou felt that she would benefit from being a part of a swim team, both socially and emotionally. Although Mary Lou found a local Paralympics swim team and had parental support, Dori was reluctant to join.

Because Dori had a close and trusting relationship with Mary Lou, she agreed to meet at a swim practice session to observe. Having Mary Lou there as a support and advocate helped Dori decide to go. Dori was so excited seeing the swimmers that she borrowed an extra swimsuit from another swimmer and joined the practice. This example demonstrates the benefits of Mary Lou's OT leisure coaching. She found the Paralympics swim program (i.e., the right match), made contact with the coach and arrangements to observe, and accompanied Dori and her mother to the practice. These seemingly small strategies were huge in helping Dori overcome her reluctance to try something new.

Dori joined the swim team and swims three times a week (see **Figure 13.2**). She competes in meets and expanded her circle of friends both in and out of school. Dori gained strength and coordination as a result of the increased amount of swimming per week, which, in turn, decreased her need for OT and PT services to monthly consultation.

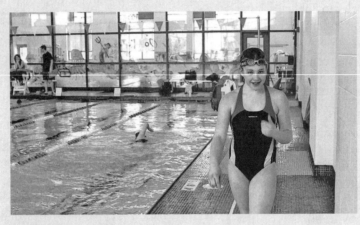

Figure 13.2 Dori at the pool
Courtesy of Susan Bazyk.

Application: Kelly met with Alex's mother, who indicated that he is on a soccer team but "hates" going to the point of tears. She would like for him to be involved in an out-of-school activity, but is not sure what he might like. Alex struggles with social interaction in groups and making friends. Kelly shared information about the importance of helping Alex be exposed to and find leisure activities that are enjoyable and align with his strengths and interests. Alex and his mother were excited about working together to explore options outside of soccer that he might want to try.

Step Two: Spark an Interest Complete an interest inventory with the youth and provide education about a variety of creative arts, sports, and nature-based activities. Help the youth prioritize the list of interests. Share this with caregivers.

Application: Kelly used an interest inventory with Alex to discuss a range of leisure activities. One of the creative arts activities was pottery, about which Alex was curious. They went online to read information and look at pictures and videos about pottery. Alex was excited about learning how to make pottery, and his mother was supportive.

Step Three: Explore School- or Community-Sponsored Options Explore available options for participation such as through using the Internet and with consideration of family resources. Engage the youth and the family in this process as much as possible. It is important to know your community and venues for inclusive participation!

Application: Using the Internet, Kelly explored community-based pottery classes with Alex and his mother.

Step Four: Make a Match and a Plan Discuss the school- and/or community-sponsored options for participation with the youth and caregivers. Plan for registration and entry into the activity, and contact the program instructor/coach (if necessary) to discuss relevant information regarding the youth's strengths and needs related to accommodations and successful participation.

Application: Based on his mother's availability and financial resources, Alex agreed to attend an introductory pottery class for 8- to 12-year-old children at a nearby recreation center. Kelly talked privately with Alex's mother about what information, if any, should be shared with the pottery teacher ahead of time related to Alex's diagnosis and strategies to support social participation. With the mother's approval, Kelly talked with the pottery teacher about Alex's strengths and needs related to social interaction. The teacher, having taught pottery to children for over 10 years, exclaimed, "I think I've got this!"

Step Five: Just Do It! The youth participates in the activity with OT leisure coaching provided to foster success. Importantly, coaching occurs only as much as needed such as when adapting entry into the activity, modifying the environment, or supporting the instructor/coach).

Application: Kelly checked in with Alex and his mother after the first couple of pottery classes in order to problem-solve any challenges or needs. Neither reported any concerns, noting that Alex looked forward to going and came home excited about what was done.

Step Six: Occupational Reflection and Future Plans Following participation, be sure to talk with the youth and caregivers separately about the experience. Explore what the teen liked or disliked about the activity. Foster ongoing exploration and participation in a variety of healthy hobbies and interests.

Application: At the end of the class, Kelly asked Alex what he thought, and he exclaimed, "Pottery is perfect." He wanted to take private pottery lessons because the group class was not offered again for 3 months. His mother was in full support and happy that Alex developed a strong interest in a leisure activity. She also gained confidence in Alex's ability to succeed in an out-of-school activity independently and in her own ability to search for community-sponsored classes. Alex and his mother continued to explore other activities available for children through their local recreation center.

Tier 2: Targeted Leisure Groups

Tier 2 services are developed and implemented with youth at risk of developing limited leisure participation. Those at risk include adolescents with disabilities and/or mental health challenges who may struggle with social interaction and friendship, anxiety and/or depression, and being bullied (Bazyk, 2011b). Adolescents experiencing obesity may struggle with self-esteem issues as well as physical challenges (Bazyk & Winne, 2013). Additionally, specific efforts to promote leisure participation with youth at risk due to restricted access and availability (e.g., low-income urban contexts or rural areas) may be provided (Bazyk & Bazyk, 2009). Targeted services emphasize both the prevention of limitations related to leisure (e.g., boredom, lack of structured leisure, participation in risky unstructured activities) as well as the promotion of a variety of healthy and meaningful leisure interests (Bazyk, 2011b).

Evaluation at this level involves strategically tuning in to youth at risk and exploring what they do for fun during free time. Similar to Tier 3 services, evaluation also includes having an awareness of school and community leisure options and identifying those that might be a good fit for youth with developmental, physical, and/or mental health challenges. Visiting settings and meeting youth directors or coaches can serve a dual purpose of advocating for inclusion as well as assessing whether a setting values having youth with challenges participate and making accommodations to ensure enjoyment and success.

Occupational Therapy Leisure Groups.
Occupation-based groups focusing on leisure exploration can be an important strategy for fostering leisure interests in youth at risk of limited participation. There is strong evidence to support activity-based social skills groups targeting leisure for enhancing children and youth's social participation and mental health (Arbesman et al., 2013). All occupational therapy practitioners obtain entry-level skills and experience in developing and facilitating occupation-based groups with children and youth (Olson, 2011). By "doing" together, occupation-based groups help participants work together in a cooperative manner, experience group cohesion, and build friendships (Bazyk & Bazyk, 2009). Groups may be more effective in helping at-risk youth develop important social skills and friendships. At the same time, youth are exposed to novel activities, giving them opportunities to try out something new, identify hidden strengths, and develop new leisure interests. Furthermore, occupation-based groups have the ability to reach more youth in a given

---

PRACTICE EXAMPLE 13.2 Opening Doors for Leisure Groups in School

One occupational therapist, Teri LaGuardia, MOT, OTR/L, identified that it is important to "look for the open doors" for providing needed services. At two separate IEP meetings, concerns about students' struggles with anxiety, making friends, and being bullied were discussed. Based on this awareness and the principal's support, Teri developed a group called "Friendship and Activity Detectives," which was offered 1 day per week for 8 weeks during recess targeting students who struggled as well as nondisabled peer mentors. The groups focused on playing games, leisure exploration, friendship promotion, and social and emotional learning. Because the groups were so successful in helping the students have fun and make friends, the principal supported continued implementation.

Another occupational therapist, Chrystal Boyd, MS, OTR/L, developed an after-school gaming club, initially targeting youth with disabilities at Hudson City Schools in Ohio. She was aware that several high school students on her caseload had few friends and nothing to do after school. With principal support, space was provided for the teens to meet and play video games, hang out, and enjoy a snack under the supervision of the occupational therapist. Soon, the club attracted teens without disabilities and has grown to be an inclusive club for students with and without disabilities to play games, have fun, and make friends.

---

session. While the primary goal of these groups is to expose youth to a variety of leisure occupations in order to foster the development of leisure interests, occupational therapy practitioners need to make the case that such groups can address a number of occupational performance goals in order to implement these groups in school, clinic, and community settings.

Making the Case for Occupational Therapy Leisure Groups in Schools. For practitioners in school settings, it is critical to be aware of and to educate others on how the Individuals With Disabilities Education Act (IDEA) (Pub. L. 108–446) (2004) supports services that promote play and leisure in natural contexts throughout the day. First, IDEA mandates that schools must provide nonacademic and extracurricular services and activities in the manner necessary to afford students with disabilities an equal opportunity for participation in those services and activities (see Section 300, Nonacademic Services). These services and activities may include athletics, recreational activities, special-interest clubs, and recess activities. Second, schools must ensure that each student with a disability participates with nondisabled peers in the extracurricular services and activities to the maximum extent possible (least restrictive environment). Further, supplementary aids and services deemed necessary by the IEP team need to be provided to help students participate in nonacademic settings.

Armed with this knowledge, occupational therapy practitioners need to talk about the importance of leisure participation with students, families, and school personnel and, based on the law, actively advocate for services that promote leisure participation during recess and after school. For example, small groups that integrate students both with and without disabilities can be offered during recess to enhance play,

leisure, and social participation. Such recess groups, despite occurring over a short amount of time, can be effective in exposing youth to games (e.g., card games, board games, four square) or simple crafts (e.g., making friendship bracelets), building friendships, and reducing bullying. See **Practice Example 13.2** for descriptions of occupational therapists successfully implementing leisure groups in schools.

Making the Case for Occupational Therapy Leisure Groups in After-School Clinic and Community Settings. Youth with disabilities and/or mental health challenges receiving outpatient services are often seen during the after-school hours. Providing individual services focusing on performance component functioning (e.g., fine-motor skills, sensory processing, social skills) may limit opportunities to explore leisure activities within a social context. Given that youth with disabilities are at greater risk of leisure deprivation and being bullied (Bazyk, 2011b), developing and providing occupation-based groups is an important service delivery option for outpatient clinic settings. Participation in groups provides opportunities to develop friendships. Having high-quality friendships, or at least one best friend, can help prevent youth from being a victim of bullying (Bazyk, 2011b). Offering a range of leisure groups as a way to expose youth to a variety of structured leisure (games, art, horticulture) can also provide opportunities to address performance goals such as fine-motor skills, self-regulation, and sensory processing. Refer to **Practice Example 13.3** for a description of leisure groups in a clinic setting.

Making the Case for Occupational Therapy Leisure Groups in the Community. Community-based groups offered in natural settings such as recreation centers can foster

PRACTICE EXAMPLE 13.3 Clinic-Based Occupational Therapy Leisure Groups

At Cleveland Clinic's outpatient services, Jenny Negrey, MOT, OTR/L, noted that most of the youth on her caseload reported having few friends, limited leisure pursuits (with most being unstructured video gaming), and anxiety. With the realization that individual therapy sessions were limited in the ability to foster social interaction and friendship skills, Jenny and colleagues developed and implemented several theme-based leisure groups targeting at-risk youth and exposing them to a variety of activities. The first group, coled with Julie Jesinski, MOT, OTR/L, focused on playing games and targeting youth on their caseloads with limited leisure participation, friendship challenges, and families with limited financial resources. Each week, a small group of seven youth learned and played one game (e.g., Uno, dominoes, Pictionary, Trivial Pursuit). Families received an information sheet about the game so that they could follow up at home if they desired. During the group, pro-social skills such as turn-taking, how to be a good friend, and how to win or lose gracefully were reinforced. Not only did the youth benefit from participation, but parents also recognized the value of participating in leisure activities and making friends. A short video of this "Game Break" group can be viewed on the Every Moment Counts website (https://everymomentcounts. org/view.php?nav_id=193). As a result of this group's success, the therapists developed other leisure groups focusing on art (Young Artists), horticulture (Green Thumbs Up), yoga (Mindful Movements), and hobby exploration (Positive Pursuits).

PRACTICE EXAMPLE 13.4 Occupational Therapy Leisure Groups at a Recreation Center

Maria Llerena, OTR/L, and two colleagues, a speech therapist and an ABA therapist, developed a business with the purpose of offering cooking groups at a local recreation center for children and youth with ASD (see www. thekidnectionsgroup.com). Parents enjoyed being able to drop their son or daughter off at a recreation center to engage in group activities under the skilled facilitation of therapists. Based on demand and parent feedback, the groups expanded to include other leisure activities (e.g., crafts, Legos®, games) and peers without disabilities. Other benefits of this type of program are that the therapists do not have the added expenses of paying for clinic space, and parents may prefer to have their youth participate at a recreation center instead of an outpatient clinic.

participation in leisure. Recreation centers often offer a variety of classes for children and youth that require registration and class fee for participation. Refer to **Practice Example 13.4** for an example of occupational therapy leisure groups offered in a recreation center.

Occupation-based groups can also be embedded in after-school youth programs. Payment for services are possible if parents are able to obtain insurance coverage or pay out of pocket. This is not always feasible, especially in low-income urban contexts. Community-based after-school programs almost always lack the finances needed to provide occupational therapy services. Low-income urban youth are at risk of occupational deprivation in the area of leisure due to lack of family and financial resources. One way to meet the structured leisure and social and emotional needs of this population is through university-led occupational therapy service learning programs (see **Practice Example 13.5** for details about a preventive leisure group for low-income youth).

Tier 1: Universal School and Community-Based Leisure Promotion

It is critical that parents and school personnel be made aware of the multiple benefits of structured leisure for their children—that participation in self-selected structured leisure provides positive opportunities for fostering health, identity work, and life skill development. Given occupational therapy practitioners' scope of practice in the areas of play, leisure, and social participation combined with skills in analyzing P–E–O, it is important that we provide services at the universal level.

This is feasible in school settings given that IDEA mandates that students with disabilities receive services in the least restrictive environment (LRE) to the maximum extent possible (34 C.F.R. § 300.114(A)(2) (i)). This means that whenever possible, occupational therapy practitioners need to be integrating services in natural contexts throughout the day (both academic and nonacademic) as opposed to providing exclusively individual therapy in isolated settings (Cahill & Bazyk, 2019). For example, a therapist implementing a universal, schoolwide program might embed accommodations and supports for students with disabilities in order to ensure successful and enjoyable participation (Mohler, Kerns, & Bazyk, 2014).

Another reason for providing integrated services is that theories of motor learning indicate that the practice of activities in a natural context is most effective for achieving new skills (O'Brien & Lewin, 2008). When

PRACTICE EXAMPLE 13.5 Preventive OT Leisure Groups with Low-Income Youth

The Occupational Therapy Groups for HOPE (Healthy Occupations for Positive Emotions) were developed to address the occupation-based, social-emotional, and interaction needs of low-income urban youth. They have been offered by Cleveland State University occupational therapy students since 2004 (Bazyk, 2006).

Under the supervision of the project director (S. Bazyk), two graduate occupational therapy students coplan and facilitate the weekly groups with 6 to 10 youth ages 6–14 years. Each group is 8 weeks in length. The groups promote:

- **Participation in Meaningful Leisure Occupation:** The HOPE groups expose youth to a variety of structured leisure occupations such as games, drumming, horticulture, and arts and crafts (**see Figure 13.3**). Activities are selected by the occupational therapy students based on input from the youth with the goal of exposing them to new activities and the development of new hobbies and interests.
- **Social and Emotional Learning (SEL) Activities:** SEL activities are embedded and focus on the development of social competencies (e.g., understanding the relationship among feelings, thoughts, and behaviors; empathy), friendship skills, conflict-resolution skills, and anger management skills. The social-emotional aspects help youth recognize their emotions, think about their feelings and how one should act, and regulate their behavior based on thoughtful decision making. The strategies for teaching appropriate ways to express anger are adapted from *Volcano in My Tummy: Helping Children to Handle Anger* (Whitehouse & Pudney, 1996).
- **Group Process:** The small groups provide a supportive environment and an opportunity to develop positive relationships with caring adults. Through "doing together" the HOPE groups foster peer interaction and teamwork leading to a sense of group cohesion.
- **Positive Behavioral Interventions and Supports (PBIS):** PBIS promotes the use of proactive strategies to prevent problem behavior by altering a situation before problems escalate and to concurrently teach appropriate alternatives. Examples of strategies embedded during the HOPE groups include clearly communicating group rules and creating a warm and positive group environment.
- **Mental Health Literacy:** Youth learn about positive mental health (feeling good, doing well, coping with challenges) and strategies for managing stress. By participating in various leisure activities, they learn firsthand the relationship between enjoyable occupations and feeling good emotionally.

Organization of the Group Sessions

Group sessions are structured into the following three segments:

- Conversation time focuses on introducing the SEL theme for the session, setting the emotional tone, and promoting group cohesion.
- The occupation-based project activity is considered the "heart" of the group because it exposes the children to activities that may develop into long-term interests and allows them to practice the social-emotional skill introduced during conversation time. Examples of projects and activities include making greeting cards using rubber stamping, crocheting scarves, creating papier mâché masks, and doing yoga. The project activities focus on exposing children to a variety of structured leisure occupations to broaden their repertoire of interests and promote the development of hobbies.
- Closure involves revisiting the SEL theme and occupational reflection—an opportunity to think about the influence of activity on emotional and physical health.

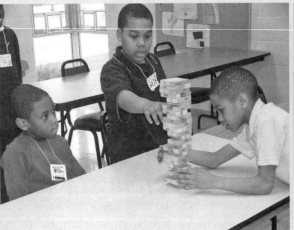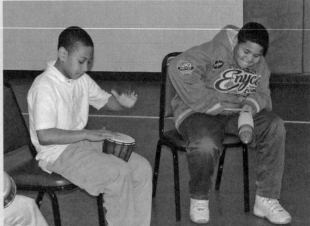

Figure 13.3 Youth are exposed to a variety of structured leisure occupations such as games and drumming

Courtesy of Susan Bazyk.

Research Outcomes

- **Meaning for Youth: Becoming Hooked on Doing.** Results from a phenomenology study revealed that the youth perceive the groups to be *fun* (occupational meaning) because of engagement in novel and challenging projects and talking about feelings within a supportive group context (occupational form). Participation in creative leisure occupations that allow for choice transforms mood so that youth experience happiness and forget their problems (occupational function). The children enjoy the projects and activities and express wanting to do more. Children are often heard saying, "What are we going to do today?" or "I wish you could come every day." They become hooked on doing and experience firsthand the power of occupation, that participating in creative occupations fosters positive feelings. In addition, as the weeks pass, the youth begin to interact as a cohesive group—sharing materials and praising each other's accomplishments. Youth also indicated that they enjoy being able to talk about their feelings.
- **Meaning for OT students: Becoming an Occupational Therapist.** By planning and facilitating the HOPE groups, OT students experienced professional growth over the 8 weeks. Professional reasoning progressed from mechanical procedural reasoning to flexible forms of conditional reasoning. "By providing preventive occupation-based groups, students observed the power of the just-right occupation on fostering active participation and enjoyment in children. No longer just a concept, occupation-based practice was experienced first-hand and became real" (Bazyk et al., 2010, p. 185).

integrating services, practitioners have opportunities to observe how students on their caseload participate in play and leisure during recess and also tune in to students who demonstrate limited participation or who are at risk but not on one's caseload. As such, integrated services maximize the impact of occupational therapy, giving practitioners the opportunity to address the leisure needs of more students and educate teachers and other school providers about occupational therapy's full scope of practice (Cahill & Bazyk, 2019).

In terms of evaluation and intervention at the universal level, occupational therapy practitioners focus on opportunities for quality play and leisure during recess and extracurricular after-school activities. During the school day, recess is a critical time of the day to promote active play, friendship, teamwork, and inclusion of students with disabilities and/or mental health challenges. Due to the unstructured nature of recess combined with supervisors who are often unprepared to foster positive play and social interaction among large groups of students, there are often higher incidents of bullying and behavior challenges. Embedding occupational therapy services during recess can contribute to the promotion of enjoyable participation in healthy play and leisure activities for all students (refer to **Practice Example 13.6** for a universal occupational therapy recess program).

PRACTICE EXAMPLE 13.6 A Universal Recess Program

As a part of Every Moment Counts, Refreshing Recess focuses on creating a positive recess experience for students. Detailed information on how to implement this program with downloadable materials such as posters, newsletters, and lesson plans are available online (https://everymomentcounts.org/view.php?nav_id=62).

Evaluation consists of observing recess and completing a Recess Environmental Scan (Mohler, Kerns, & Bazyk, 2014).The occupational therapy practitioner analyzes the occupations of play and leisure as well as the physical, social, and emotional contexts to determine

- Do children and youth engage in enjoyable and healthy forms of play and leisure?
- Are there students who struggle to fit in?
- Do recess supervisors interact with students in positive ways and encourage a variety of play activities?

Strengths and challenges specific to the recess experience are identified to help shape implementation of the Refreshing Recess program.

What does the program involve? This is a 6-week, 1 day/week, program embedded into recess, which includes the following interventions:

- **Educating** recess supervisors, school administrators, teachers, and students about how to create a positive recess experience for all students by offering a variety of activity ideas and embedding strategies for promoting positive behaviors and social interactions during recess. Occupational therapy practitioners use a variety of educational methods such as an orientation session, newsletters, talking points, posters, and bookmarks (several are available to download from the website).
- **Embedding weekly activities** by an occupational therapist in order to encourage children to engage in active play, develop new interests, form friendships, interact positively with peers, include others, and decrease bullying. Any structured activities that are provided are strictly optional, so students may choose whether or not they would like to participate.

(continues)

PRACTICE EXAMPLE 13.6 A Universal Recess Program *(continued)*

- **Occupational therapy coaching** with recess supervisors to model positive social interaction with students, resolve conflicts, help problem-solve behavior challenges, suggest a variety of enjoyable recess activities, and create opportunities for inclusion of all students with and without disabilities.

Each week has a theme along with a suggested activity.

- **Week 1: Kickoff: Let's get started!** Students receive the Refreshing Recess bookmark. The occupational therapist provides an orientation to recess supervisors and explores challenges and needs.
- **Week 2: Let's make friends and have fun together.** Students participate in a friendship scavenger hunt or game that fosters teamwork. Recess supervisors learn about fostering friendships.
- **Week 3: Let's play and work together.** Students create something together with a variety of art materials. Recess supervisors learn about teamwork and conflict resolution.
- **Week 4: Let's get fit and get along.** Students engage in a "Fitness Trail" with stations of different physical activities. Recess supervisors learn about Positive Behavioral Interventions & Supports (PBIS).
- **Week 5: Let's respect differences and include everybody.** Students engage in a game of tag that allows children to work together to bring back into the game those who had been tagged. Recess supervisors learn how to promote inclusion.
- **Week 6: Let's make sure everyone has fun.** Students engage in a game of untying knots together. Recess supervisors learn about bullying prevention.

Outcomes

Preliminary findings from survey data indicate that the Refreshing Recess program resulted in statistically significant changes in students perceiving outdoor recess to be fun, students being engaged in active play, the number of games that adults promote, and students looking forward to recess. Recess supervisors reported positive changes in the following areas: feeling adequately trained to supervise recess, having the necessary supports to promote play, knowing how to interact socially with students, and knowing how to successfully resolve conflict. (Mohler, Kerns, & Bazyk, 2014).

Developing an awareness of the school and communities' extracurricular activities is also important so that the occupational therapy practitioner can foster exploration and participation for students receiving IEP services as well as those at risk. Being knowledgeable about community-based options for leisure participation is useful for actively advocating for inclusive participation—another important aspect of the therapist's role within a school. For example, the occupational therapy practitioner can complete a leisure environmental scan of school and community-based activities and compile them in a handout to share with students and parents. When families have limited financial and transportation means, the practitioner can target and share low-cost activities that can be accessed by bus or on foot. An occupational therapy practitioner can promote whole-school strategies targeting leisure participation as exemplified in **Practice Examples 13.7** and **13.8.**

PRACTICE EXAMPLE 13.7 Universal Whole-School Leisure Promotion

David Weiss, OTR/L, has been an occupational therapist at Positive Education Program's Prentiss Autism Center for 16 years. This is an alternative school for children and youth with ASD and significant developmental and emotional disabilities. A majority of the students have one or more comorbid mental health challenges (e.g., anxiety, depression, severe behavioral disorders).

David is an original participant in the Every Moment Counts' Making Leisure Matter initiative. He began by providing individual OT Leisure Coaching, helping students to participate in adapted football and soccer. This success motivated him to do more. Because the school did not offer any extracurricular sports or leisure activities, with the support of the school's principal, David developed a number of whole-school leisure-promotion initiatives over the past 6 years. In order to ensure school personnel "buy-in" and participation, David initially involved colleagues in brainstorming ways to embed leisure activities and programs as a part of the school culture. He believes that it is critical to bring events to the table with enthusiasm and convey how leisure activities benefit students' development of skills (gross motor, communication, self-regulation, math), mental and physical health, relationships, and participation in the community. David ensures success by utilizing best practices to help students participate such as visual schedules, social stories, and predictable routines.

Special Olympics

In 2015, David developed an official schoolwide Special Olympics program. He collaborated with the adaptive physical education teacher to embed sports training into the curriculum including basketball, football, soccer, cheerleading, and running. All students participate either in a sporting event or in making signs and materials for the parade. All families have opportunities to participate and attend the annual games and parade. This program has been so successful and enjoyable that it has become a part of annual activities and the school culture.

Walking Club and Running Marathon Program

Autistic adolescents are less likely to be physically active, leading to greater risk for other health problems such as overweight and obesity, diabetes, and poor physical endurance. In 2016, the walking/running club was initiated as a simple strategy to foster more movement throughout the day. Why promote walking and running at school? Walking and running has little associated cost, can be done individually or as a group, and uses the strengths of people with autism (e.g., thrive on structure, routine, and repetition). Many physical and emotional benefits are associated with walking and/or running such as decreasing anxiety and depression, elevating mood, and increasing physical fitness. The walking club is built into the school's schedule after lunch for 30 minutes.

The Walking/Running Marathon Program became an extension of the walking club. It was also developed by David and implemented with two others (Robert Zachary, teacher, and Doug Bletcher, autism personal coach). Students participate in two to three training sessions per week for 2–3 months as a part of their school day. Training involves stretching, race etiquette, socializing with peers, and tracking miles. Students have a goal of completing 25 miles and participating in a practice race before completing a community race (from 1.2 miles to 26.2-mile marathon distance). The race is attended by family and friends. Students that complete the community race earn a medal, shirt, free pair of running shoes, and celebration banquet. The Marathon Program participation has grown from 3 students in 2016 to 15 students in 2019.

Zachary's Success

Zachary is an adolescent with autism who struggles with prolonged engagement, sensory defensiveness, and verbal communication. He has participated in the Marathon Program for 3 years as well as Special Olympics and the school's football, soccer, and basketball competitions. Participation has resulted in improvements in affect, communication, and staying engaged in activities. He has completed six 5k races, two 10k races, and a half marathon. In 2019, he received a Gold and Silver Medal in the Special Olympics Ohio Summer Games. Zachary's parents are thrilled about his success. Zachary is passionate about running, and his parents, extended family, and friends enjoy going to see him race. Participation in running is an established and enjoyable leisure occupation for Zachary and his parents. It has resulted in improved mental and physical health and quality of life (see **Figure 13.4**).

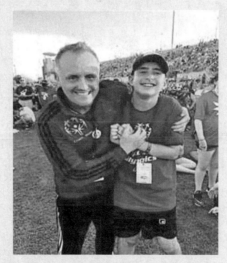

Figure 13.4 Zachary, an adolescent with autism, participates in activities like running, which has improved his mental and physical health

Courtesy of Susan Bazyk.

PRACTICE EXAMPLE 13.8 Bringing Community Leisure Programs to School

Maria Llerena, OTR/L, brought community-based leisure programs to be guest presenters at The Achievement Centers for Children Autism School in Westlake, Ohio. She found that an overwhelming number of community programs (e.g., martial arts, ballet, theater) wanted to include youth with disabilities and/or mental health challenges. Leaders from various community programs talked about their program, performed demonstrations, and involved students in sample activities. These minisessions provided students with an opportunity to try out a variety of leisure activities in order to spark an interest and pursue community-based participation. The programs also provided written materials to parents about their specific program schedule and registration information.

Conclusion

Adolescent leisure participation promotes skill development, health, and positive life outcomes. With a commitment to occupational justice, occupational therapy practitioners are guided by the belief that all youth have a right to participate in and enjoy meaningful and health-promoting leisure, despite barriers such as disabilities or poverty. Occupational therapy practitioners realize this commitment by promoting leisure participation within a multitiered public health framework. Occupational therapy leisure scenarios provided examples of individual leisure coaching, leisure groups for those at risk, and whole-school initiatives that advocate for and result in inclusive leisure participation for all youth.

References

American Occupational Therapy Association (AOTA). (2020a). Occupational therapy practice framework: Domain and process (4th ed.). *American Journal of Occupational Therapy, 74* (Supplement 2).

American Occupational Therapy Association (AOTA). (2020b). *AOTA's guide to acknowledging the impact of discrimination, stigma, and implicit bias on provision of services.* https://www.aota.org/~/media/Corporate/Files/Practice/Guide-Acknowledging-Impact-Discrimination-Stigma-Implicit-Bias.pdf

Anaby, D., Law, M., Coster, W., Bedell, G., Khetani, M., Avery, L., & Teplicky, R. (2014). The mediating role of the environment in explaining participation of children and youth with and without disabilities across home, school, and community. *Archives of Physical Medicine and Rehabilitation, 95*(5), 908–917.

Anaby, D. R., Law, M., Feldman, D., Majnemer, A., & Avery, L. (2018). The effectiveness of the Pathways and Resources for Engagement and Participation (PREP) intervention: Improving participation of adolescents with physical disabilities. *Developmental Medicine & Child Neurology, 60*(5), 513–519. https://doi.org/10.1111/DMCN.13682

Anaby, D. R., Law, M. C., Majnemer, A., & Feldman, D. (2016). Opening doors to participation of youth with physical disabilities: An intervention study. *Canadian Journal of Occupational Therapy, 83*(2), 83–90. http://doi.org/10.1177/0008417415608653

Arbesman, M., Bazyk, S., & Nochajski, S. M. (2013). Systematic review of occupational therapy and mental health promotion, prevention, and intervention for children and youth. *American Journal of Occupational Therapy, 67,* e120–e130. https://doi.org/10.5014/ajot.2013.008359

Barber, B. L., Stone, M. R., Hunt, J. E., & Eccles, J. S. (2005). Benefits of activity participation: The roles of identify affirmation and peer group norm sharing. In J. L. Mahoney, R. W. Larson, & J. S. Eccles (Eds.), *Organized activities as contexts of development: extracurricular activities, after-school and community programs* (pp. 185–210). Mahwah, NJ: Erlbaum.

Batya Engel-Yeger, B., Jarus, T., Anaby, D., & Law, M. (2009). Differences in patterns of participation between youths with cerebral palsy and typically developing peers. *American Journal of Occupational Therapy, 63,* 96–104. https://doi.org/10.5014/ajot.63.1.96

Bazyk, S. (2005). Exploring the development of meaningful work for children and youth in Western contexts. WORK: A Journal of Prevention, *Assessment, & Rehabilitation, 24,* 11–20.

Bazyk, S. (2006). Creating occupation-based social skills groups in after-school care. *Occupational Therapy Practice, 11,* 13–18.

Bazyk, S. (2011a). *Mental health promotion, prevention, and intervention with children and youth: A guiding framework for occupational therapy.* Bethesda, MD: AOTA Press.

Bazyk, S. (2011b). Enduring challenges and situational stressors during the school years: Risk reduction and competence enhancement. In S. Bazyk (Ed.), *Mental health promotion, prevention, and intervention with children and youth: A guiding framework for occupational therapy* (pp. 119–139). Bethesda, MD: AOTA Press.

Bazyk, S. (2011c). Promotion of positive mental health in children and youth: A guiding framework for occupational therapy. In S. Bazyk (Ed.), *Mental health promotion, prevention, and intervention with children and youth: A guiding framework for occupational therapy* (pp. 3–20). Bethesda, MD: AOTA Press.

Bazyk, S. (2011d). Occupational therapy process: A public health approach to promoting mental health in children and youth. In S. Bazyk (Ed.), *Mental health promotion, prevention, and intervention with children and youth: A guiding framework for occupational therapy* (pp. 21–44). Bethesda, MD: AOTA Press.

Bazyk, S. (2019). Occupational therapy's role in school mental health. In C. Brown, V. Stoffel, & J. Munoz (Eds.), *Occupational therapy in mental health: A vision for participation.* (2nd ed., pp. 809–837). Philadelphia, PA: F. A. Davis Company.

Bazyk, S., & Bazyk, J. (2009). The meaning of occupational therapy groups for low-income youth: A phenomenological study. *The American Journal of Occupational Therapy, 6,* 69–80. https://doi.org/10.5014/ajot.63.1.69

Bazyk, S., Demirjian, L., LaGuardia, T., Thompson-Repas, K., Conway, C., & Michaud, P. (2015). Building capacity of occupational therapy practitioners to address the mental health needs of children and youth: Mixed methods study of knowledge translation. *American Journal of Occupational Therapy, 69,* 6906180060p1–6906180060p10. https://doi.org/10.5014/ajot.2015.019182

Bazyk, S., Gordon, R., Haines, J., Percociante, M., & Glorioso, M. (2010). Service learning: The process of doing and becoming an occupational therapist. *Occupational Therapy in Health Care, 24*(2), 171–187. http://doi.org/10.3109/07380571003681194

Bazyk, S., & Winne, R. (2013). A multi-tiered approach to addressing the mental health issues surrounding obesity in children and youth. *Occupational Therapy in Health Care, 27*(2), 84–98. http://doi.org/10.3109/07380577.2013.785643

Bedell, G., Coster, W., Law, M., Liljenquist, K., Kao, Y. C., Teplicky, R.,... Khetani, M. A. (2013). Community participation, supports, and barriers of school-age children with and without disabilities. *Archives of Physical Medicine and Rehabilitation*, 94(2), 315–323. http://doi:10.1016/j.apmr.2012.09.024

Bell, B. T. (2016). Understanding adolescents. In L. Little, D. Fitton, B. Bell, & N. Toth (Eds.), *Perspectives on HCI research with teenagers* (pp. 11–27). Cham: Human-Computer Interaction Series, Springer.

Brajsa-Zganec, A., Merkas, M., & Sverko, I. (2011). Quality of life and leisure activities: How do leisure activities contribute to subjective well-being? *Social Indicators Research*, 102(1), 81–91. http://dx.doi.org/10.1007/s11205-010-9724-2

Bryze, K. (2008). Narrative contributions to The Play History. In L. D. Parham & L. S. Fazio (Eds.), *Play in occupational therapy for children* (2nd ed., pp. 43–54). St. Louis, MO: Mosby, Inc.

Bundy, A. (1993). Assessment of play and leisure: Delineation of the problem. *American Journal of Occupational Therapy*, 47(3), 217–222. https://doi.org/10.5014/ajot.47.3.217

Cahill, S., & Bazyk, S. (2019). School based occupational therapy. In J. Case-Smith & J. O'Brien (Eds.), *Occupational therapy for children* (8th ed., pp. 627–658). St. Louis, MO: Mosby.

Caldwell, L., & Faulk, M. (2013). Adolescent leisure from a developmental and prevention perspective. In T. Freire (Ed.), *Positive leisure science* (pp. 41–60). New York: Springer. http://doi.org/10.1007/978-94-007-5058-6_3

Carter, E. W., Boehm, T. L., Biggs, E. E., Annandale, N. H., Taylor, C. E., Loock, A. K., & Liu, R. Y. (2015). Known for my strengths: Positive traits of transition-age youth with intellectual disability and/or autism. *Research and Practice for Persons with Severe Disabilities*, 40(2), 101–119. https://doi.org/10.1177/1540796915592158

Csikszentmihalyi, M. (1993). Activity and happiness: Towards a science of occupation. *Occupational Science: Australia*, 1(1), 38–42. https://doi.org/10.1080/14427591.1993.9686377

Csikszentmihalyi, M., & Csikszentmihalyi, I. S. (Eds.). (1988). *Optimal experience: Psychological studies of flow in consciousness*. New York: Cambridge University Press.

Csikszentmihalyi, M., & Larson, R. (1984). *Being adolescent: Conflict and growth in the teenage years*. New York: Basic Books.

Darrah, J., Law, M. C., Pollock, N., Wilson, B., Russell, D. J., Walter, S. D.,... Galuppi, B. (2011). Context therapy: A new intervention approach for children with cerebral palsy. *Developmental Medicine and Child Neurology*, 53, 615–620. http://doi:10.1111/j.1469-8749.2011.03959.x

Delle Fave, A., & Bassi, M. (2000). The quality of experience in adolescents' daily lives: Developmental perspectives. *Genetic Social and General Psychology Monographs*, 126(3), 347–367.

Denworth, L. (2020). The outside influence of your middle-school friends. *The Atlantic*. https://www.theatlantic.com/family/archive/2020/01/friendship-crucial-adolescent-brain/605638/

Donohue, M. V. (2013). *Social profile: Assessment of social participation in children, adolescents, and adults*. Bethesda, MD: AOTA Press.

Dworkin, J. B., Larson, R., & Hansen, D. (2003). Adolescents' accounts of growth experiences in youth activities. *Journal of Youth and Adolescence*, 32, 17–26. https://doi.org/10.1023/A:1021076222321

Eccles, J. S., Barber, B. L., Stone, M., & Hunt, J. (2003). Extracurricular activities and adolescent development. *Journal of Social Issues*, 59, 865–889. https://doi.org/10.1046/j.0022-4537.2003.00095.x

Every Moment Counts. (2021). *Occupational therapy leisure coaching: Helping children and youth develop healthy and enjoyable hobbies & interests*. http://s3.us-east-2.amazonaws.com/s3.everymomentcounts.com/wp-content/uploads/2021/03/10141231/Leisure_Coaching_Info_Brief_2021.pdf

Farnworth, L. (1999). Time use and leisure occupations of young offenders. *The American Journal of Occupational Therapy*, 54(3), 315–325. https://doi.org/10.5014/ajot.54.3.315

Florey, L. L., & Greene, S. (2008). Play in middle childhood. In L. D. Parham & L. S. Fazio (Eds.), *Play in occupational therapy for children* (2nd ed., pp. 279–300). St. Louis, MO: Mosby, Inc.

Fredricks, J. A., & Eccles, J. S. (2006). Is extracurricular participation associated with beneficial outcomes? *Concurrent and longitudinal relations. Developmental Psychology*, 42(4), 698–713. https://psycnet.apa.org/doi/10.1037/0012-1649.42.4.698

Gilman, R. (2001). The relationship between life satisfaction, social interest, and frequency of extracurricular activities among adolescent students. *Journal of Youth and Adolescence* 30, 749–767. https://doi.org/10.1023/A:1012285729701

Graham, F., Rodger, S., & Ziviani, J. (2009). Coaching parents to enable children's participation: An approach for working with parents and their children. *Australian Occupational Therapy Journal*, 56(1), 16–23. https://doi.org/10.1111/j.1440-1630.2008.00736.x

Hansen, D., Larson, R., & Dworkin, J. B. (2003). What adolescents learn in organized youth activities: A survey of self-reported developmental experiences. *Journal of Research on Adolescence*, 13(1), 25–55. https://doi.org/10.1111/1532-7795.1301006

Hemmingsson, H., Egilson, S., Oshrat, H., & Kielhofner, G. (2005). *The school setting interview: SSI version 3.0*. Stockholm: Swedish Association of Occupational Therapists.

Henry, A. D. (2000). *Pediatric interest profiles: Surveys of play for children and adolescents, kid play profile, preteen play profile, adolescent leisure interest profile*. San Antonio, TX: Therapy Skill Builders.

Henry, A. (2008). Assessment of play and leisure in children and adolescents. In L. D. Parham & L. S. Fazio (Eds.), *Play in occupational therapy for children* (2nd ed., pp. 95–193). St. Louis, MO: Mosby.

Hess, L. M., & Bundy, A. C. (2003). The association between playfulness and coping in adolescents. *Physical & Occupational Therapy in Pediatrics*, 23(2), 5–17. https://doi.org/10.1080/J006v23n02_02

Individuals With Disabilities Education Improvement Act of 2004, Pub. L. 108–446, 20 U. S. C. §§ 1400–1482.

King, G., Law, M., King, S., Hurley, P., Hanna, S., Kertoy, M., Rosenbaum, P., & Young, N. (2004). *Children's assessment of participation and enjoyment (CAPE) and preferences for activities of children (PAC)*. San Antonio, TX: Harcourt Assessment, Inc.

King, G., Rigby, P., & Avery, L. (2016). Revised measure of environmental qualities of activity settings (MEQAS) for youth leisure and life skills activity settings. *Disability and Rehabilitation*, 38(15), 1509–1520.

King, G., Rigby, P., Batorowicz, B., McMain-Klein, M., Petrenchik, T., Thompson, L., & Gibson, M. (2014). Development of a direct observation measure of environmental qualities of activity settings. *Developmental Medicine & Child Neurology*, 56(8), 763–769. https://doi:10.1111/dmcn.12400

Larson, R. W. (2000). Toward a psychology of positive youth development. *American Psychologist, 55,* 170–183. https://psycnet.apa.org/doi/10.1037/0003-066X.55.1.170

Larson, R. W., & Kleiber, D. A. (1993). Daily experiences of adolescents. In P. Tolan & B. Cohler (Eds.), *Handbook of clinical research and practice with adolescents* (pp. 125–145). Wiley: New York

Law, M., Anaby, D., Imms, C., Teplicky, R., & Turner, L. (2015). Improving the participation of youth with physical disabilities in community activities: An interrupted time series design. *Australian Occupational Therapy Journal, 62*(2), 105–115. https://doi.org/10.1111/1440-1630.12177

Law M,. Anaby D., Teplicky R., & Turner L. (2016). *Pathways and resources for engagement and participation (PREP): A practice model for occupational therapists* [Internet]. https://www.canchild.ca/en/shop/25-prep

Law, M., Cooper, B., Strong, S., Stewart, D., Rigby, P., & Letts, L. (1996). The person-environment-occupation model: A transactive approach to occupational performance. *Canadian Journal of Occupational Therapy, 63*(1), 9–23. https://doi.org/10.1177/000841749606300103

Law, M., & Darrah, J. (2014). Emerging therapy approaches: An emphasis on function. *Journal of Child Neurology, 29,* 1101–1107. http://doi.org/10.1177/0883073814533151

Law, M., King, G., King, S., Kertoy, M., Hurley, P., Rosenbaum, P., et al. (2006). Patterns of participation in recreational and leisure activities among children with complex physical disabilities. *Developmental Medicine & Child Neurology, 48*(5), 337–342. https://doi.org/10.1017/S0012162206000740

LeBuffe, P. A., Shapiro, V. B., & Robitaille, J. L. (2018). The Devereux student strengths assessment (DESSA) comprehensive system: Screening, assessing, planning, and monitoring. *Journal of Applied Developmental Psychology, 55,* 62–70.

Leversen, I., Danielsen, A. G., Birkeland, M. S., & Oddrun, S. (2012). Basic psychological need satisfaction in leisure activities and adolescents' life satisfaction. *Journal of Youth and Adolescence, 41,* 1588–1599. http://doe:10.1007/s1094-012-9776-5

Lloyd, K. M., & Auld, C. J. (2002). The role of leisure in determining quality of life: Issues of content and measurement. *Social Indicators Research, 57,* 43–71. https://doi.org/10.1023/A:1013879518210

Mahoney, J. L., Larson, R. W., & Eccles, J. S. (2005). Organized activities as developmental contexts for children and adolescents. In J. L. Mahoney, R. W. Larson, & J. S. Eccles (Eds.), *Organized activities as contexts of development: extracurricular activities, after-school and community programs* (pp. 3–22). Mahwah, NJ: Erlbaum.

Mahoney, J. L., & Stattin, H. (2000). Leisure activities and adolescent antisocial behavior: The role of structure and social context. *Journal of Adolescence, 23*(2), 113–127. https://doi.org/10.1006/jado.2000.0302

Mahoney, J. L., Stattin, H., & Lord, H. (2004). Unstructured youth recreation centre participation and antisocial behaviour development: Selection influences and the moderating role of antisocial peers. *International Journal of Behavioral Development, 28*(6), 553–560.

Mohler, R., Kerns, S., & Bazyk, S. (2014). *Refreshing recess.* http://www.everymomentcounts.org/view.php?nav_id=62

Newman, B. M., & Newman, P. R. (2018). *Development through life: A psychosocial approach.* Belmont, CA: Wadsworth/Thomson Learning.

Nishino, H. J., & Larson, R. (2003). Japanese adolescents' free time: Juku, Bukatsu, and government efforts to create more meaningful leisure. *New Directions for Child and Adolescent Development, 99,* 23–35.

O'Brien, J., & Lewin, J. E. (2008). Part 1: Translating motor control and motor learning theory into occupational therapy practice for children and youth. *OT Practice, 13*(21), E 1–8C.

Olson, L. (2011). Development and implementation of groups to foster social participation and mental health. In S. Bazyk (Ed.), *Mental health promotion, prevention, and intervention with children and youth: A guiding framework for occupational therapy* (pp. 95–115). Bethesda, MD: AOTA Press.

Passmore, A. (1998). Does leisure support and underpin adolescents' developing worker role? *Journal of Occupational Science, 5*(3), 161–165.

Passmore, A. (2003). The occupation of leisure: Three typologies and their influence on mental health in adolescents. *OTJR: Occupation, Participation, and Health, 23,* 76–83. https://doi.org/10.1177%2F153944920302300205

Passmore, A., & French, D. (2001). Development and administration of a measure to assess adolescents' participation in leisure activities. *Adolescence, 36,* 67–75.

Passmore, A., & French, D. (2003). The nature of leisure in adolescence: A focus group study. *British Journal of Occupational Therapy, 66*(9), 419–426.

Pavlova, M. K., & Silbereisen, R. K. (2015). Leisure activities choices among adolescents. in J. D. Wright (Ed.), *International encyclopedia of the social & behavioral sciences* (2nd ed., pp. 830–837). Amsterdam: Elsevier. https://doi.org/10.1016/B978-0-08-097086-8.26003-0.

Proyer, R. T. (2017). A new structural model for the study of adult playfulness: Assessment and exploration of an understudied individual differences variable. *Personality and Individual Differences, 108,* 113–122. https://doi.org/10.1016/j.paid.2016.12.011

Proyer, R. T., Gander, F., Bertenshaw, E. J., & Brauer, K. (2018). The positive relationships of playfulness with indicators of health, activity, and physical fitness. *Frontiers in Psychology, 9,* 1–16. https://doi.org/10.3389/fpsyg.2018.01440

Proyer, R. T., & Tandler, N. (2020). An update on the study of playfulness in adolescents: Its relationship with academic performance, well-being, anxiety, and roles in bulling-type-situations. *Social Psychology of Education, 23,* 73–99. https://doi.org/10.1007/s11218-019-09526-1

Rebeiro, K., & Cook, J. (1999). Opportunity, not prescription: An exploratory study of the experience of occupational engagement. *Canadian Journal of Occupational Therapy, 66*(4), 176–187. https://doi.org/10.1177%2F000841749906600405

Schreuer, N., Sachs, D., and Rosenblum, S. (2014). Participation in leisure activities: Differences between children with and without physical disabilities. *Research in Developmental Disabilities 35*(1), 223–233. https://doi.org/10.1016/j.ridd.2013.10.001

Sharp, E. H., Tucker, C. J., Baril, M. E., Van Gundy, K. T., & Rebellon, C. J. (2015). Breadth of participation in organized and unstructured leisure activities over time and rural adolescents' functioning, *Journal of Youth & Adolescents*, *44*. 62–76. http://doi.org/10.1007/s10964-014-0153-4

Spaeth, M., Weichold, K., & Silbereisen, R. K. (2015). The development of leisure boredom in early adolescence: Predictors and longitudinal associations with delinquency and depression. *Developmental Psychology*, *51*(10), 1380–1394. https://psycnet.apa.org/doi/10.1037/a0039480

Staempfli, M. B. (2007). Adolescent playfulness, stress perception, coping and well-being. *Journal of Leisure Research*, *39*(3), 393–412. https://psycnet.apa.org/doi/10.1080/00222216.2007.11950114

Stebbins, R. A. (2007). *Serious leisure: A perspective for our time*. New Brunswick, NJ: Transaction Publishers.

Takata, N. (1974). Play as prescription. In M. Reilly (Ed.), *Play as exploratory learning* (pp. 209–246). Thousand Oaks, CA: Sage Publications.

Townsend, E. (1999). Enabling occupation in the 21st century: Making good intentions a reality. *Australian Occupational Therapy Journal*, *46*, 147–159.

Trainor, S., Delfabbro, P., Anderson, S., & Winefield, A. (2010). Leisure activities and adolescent well-being. *Journal of Adolescence*, *33*(1), 173–186. https://psycnet.apa.org/doi/10.1016/j.adolescence.2009.03.013

White, R. L., Parker, P. D., Lubans, D. R., MacMillan, F., Olson, R., Astell-Burt, T., & Lonsdale, C. (2018). Domain-specific physical activity and affective wellbeing among adolescents: An observational study of the moderating roles of autonomous and controlled motivation. *International Journal of Behavioral Nutrition and Physical Activity*, *15*(1), 1–13.

Whitehouse, E., & Pudney, W. (1996). *A volcano in my tummy: Helping children to handle anger*. Gabriola Island, BC, Canada: New Society Publishers.

Wilcock, A. A., & Hocking, C. (2015). *An occupational perspective of health*. Thorofare, NJ: Slack.

Wilson, D. M., Gottfredson, D. C., Cross, A. B., Rorie, M., & Connell, N. (2010). Youth development in after-school leisure activities. *Journal of Early Adolescence*, *30*(5), 668–690. https://doi.org/10.1177%2F0272431609341048

Zhang, S., Shi, R., Liu, X., & Miao, D. (2014). Passion for leisure activity, presence of meaning, and search for meaning: The mediating role of emotion. *Social Indicators Research*, *115*(3), 1123–1135. https://psycnet.apa.org/doi/10.1007/s11205-013-0260-8

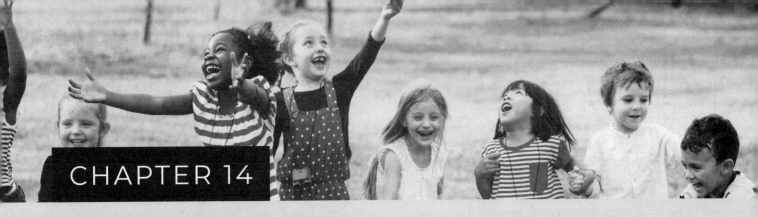

CHAPTER 14

Improving Social Play and Friendships Through Play in Groups

Sarah E. Fabrizi, PhD, OTR/L

After reading this chapter, the reader will:

- Explain the importance and benefits of social play and friendships throughout childhood.
- Discuss the development of play in groups.
- Describe theories guiding play with groups.
- Identify types of playgroups and potential outcomes for participation.
- Design occupational therapy playgroups based on desired outcomes.

Playing with friends is a victory.

—**Fuzzy Zoeller**

Throughout this text, authors have described the significance of play in the lives of children and its importance for health and well-being. Play does not only occur alone, but also with others. Many hours of childhood are spent playing with friends. When going well, play happens with parental figures[1] and siblings and then expands to include a larger group of caregivers, extended family, and small social groups in the community where the family lives. Interacting in groups with family and friends provides the opportunity to develop nurturing relationships and socialization, as well as promote mental health and resilience (Szekely et al., 2016; Yogman et al., 2018).

Children with general developmental delays, autism spectrum disorder (ASD), and other disabilities may be at risk for difficulties interacting with peers despite a desire for social play and friendships (Bradley & Male, 2017; Guralnick, 2010; Potter, 2015; Wolfberg et al., 2015).

Occupational therapy practitioners use play in groups to support creativity, play performance, and social participation. Creating child-focused environments fosters positive relationships between the parent and child and the child and peers (Yu et al., 2011). Innovation and creativity are required to meet practice demands with the limits of current available information (Golinkoff & Hirsh-Pasek, 2016). Occupational therapy practitioners promote innovation and creative capacity with children by incorporating peers

---

[1] Because families come in diverse forms, the use of the word *parent* throughout this chapter is intended to encompass all those in parental roles including guardians, foster-parents, caregivers, and so on.

in group play to work on projects of passion with a playful spirit. Interacting in groups with family and friends provides the opportunity to develop nurturing relationships and socialization, as well as to promote mental health and resilience (Szekely et al., 2016; Yogman et al., 2018). Play in groups and creative learning appear to develop in tandem. Through playgroups, occupational therapy practitioners deliver tailored play-based therapy while facilitating parent support and community connections (Armstrong et al., 2020). This chapter provides an overview of playgroups, with a focus on the role of occupational therapy to improve social play and friendships in children using groups.

Social Play

Social play happens when children play with other adults or children (see **Figure 14.1**). The foundations for social play develop from infant interactions with caregivers and expand to include other family members and siblings and then other children and adults. The demands of the social environment provide considerable challenges for all children, and for many, social play can be hard work.

Social play can take on many forms. The play can be unstructured or structured. The play can center around the use of objects and can also include use of pretending and imagination. Social play can look like peek-a-boo, playing with musical instruments or pots and pans, building a fort, or playing tag. Contextual factors, including international and national policies, community resources, and cultural norms, shape social play.

Social play has changed over time, most recently in two major ways (Shonkoff & Phillips, 2000). First, families are having fewer children. Fewer siblings means less opportunity to play with built-in playmates at home. Next, with parents working, children may enter childcare at a younger age. Parents that keep children at home may need to put an increased emphasis on social play. It is possible that some young children have fewer opportunities for social play, while others may have more exposure to other children with less adult scaffolding and support during play interactions. Context can therefore influence development.

The Development of Social Play

Play becomes more complex and social throughout early childhood. Babies show interest in each other as early as 2 months, and giant leaps in sustained interaction occur between 1 and 2 years. Social play parallels emotional development as described in **Table 14.1**. Social play often begins at home with parents and siblings, and skills can later translate to play with extended family, family friends, peers at school and in sports and leisure activities, and later peer groups.

The social play of toddlers can be demanding. Adult structuring of play during this age is paramount for success, and playing with a familiar playmate is shown to expand social play (Shonkoff & Phillips, 2000). The intensity and conflict of toddler social play does appear to decrease during the preschool years, and peer rejection in groups is often of children who are either overly aggressive or shy and withdrawn.

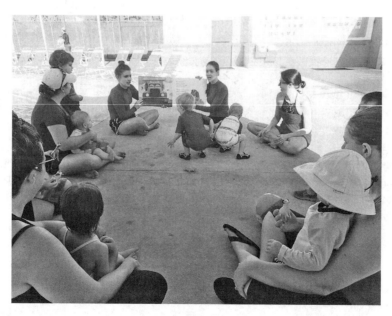

Figure 14.1 Young children and their caregivers play and learn together in parent–child playgroups
Courtesy of Sarah Fabrizi.

Table 14.1 The Relationship of Social Play and Emotional Development

Age	Social Play Stage	Emotional Development	Description
Birth–3 months	Unoccupied play	Noticing emotions; showing interest; responsiveness	Babies discover how the body moves. Play with caregivers and siblings on floor during tummy time. Babies are born with the need and desire to connect with others around them. They show and share emotions.
Birth–2 years	Solitary play	Social referencing (6 months); self–other differentiation; emotion regulation	Focus is mostly on exploring alone and sharing interest with others. Babies look to parents or loved ones to gauge their reaction.
2 years	Spectator/onlooker play	Theory of mind developing gradually (18–24 months); empathetic responsiveness	Toddlers discover that they have their own thoughts and so might others (different from their own). Children observe other children playing, but may not join in. Children share in another's distress or joy.
2+ years	Parallel play	Expressing emotions; helping behaviors; verbal and facial concern over others' distress	Children play alongside others, with the same play activity or a different one. Children experiment with expressing emotions in new ways.
3–4 years	Associate play	Managing emotions	Children begin to interact with others in a play activity. Children must develop new coping skills to navigate new social environments.
4+ years	Cooperative play	Ability to understand another's perspective	Children play together with others with interest in both the play activity and the other children.

Data from Parten, M. B. (1932). Social participation among preschool children. *Journal of Abnormal and Social Psychology*, 27(3), 243–269. https://pathways.org/kids-l earn-play-6-stages-play-development/; McDonald, N. M. & Messinger, D. S. (2011). The development of empathy: How, when, and why. In A. Acerbi, J. A. Lombo, & J. J. Sanguineti (Eds.), *Free will, emotions, and moral actions: Philosophy and neuroscience in dialogue*. Vatican City: IF-Press..

The Benefits of Social Play

There are myriad benefits from social play throughout childhood. These include a sense of belonging, identity development, social skills, positive relationships, and empathy.

Social play is essential for the feeling of belonging to occur as children get older (Kang, 2020). When children feel a sense of belonging, they develop a strong sense of self-identity. This connection with others builds confidence and mutual respect, important skills in navigating conflicts and challenges.

Social play shapes the way that a person thinks about themselves and others. During social play, children share their personal ideas and interests and express their feelings. This expression of self occurs while bargaining with others and reaching compromises for play to continue.

As children play with others, they learn to navigate their social environment using their imagination to construct new realities. Competence in social play allows a child to participate in a wide range of social environments.

In social play, children learn the skills to figure out interactions with others, while building and expanding their social networks. These social skills can include communication skills, emotional regulation, cognitive skills, and social problem solving (Grover et al., 2020). Social skills developed during play support a child's ability to listen to directions, pay attention, solve disputes with words, and focus on a task without constant supervision (Diamond, Barnett, Thomas, & Munro, 2007). Good social skills mean higher social self-efficacy, the individual belief that they have control over their own motivation and behavior and can impact the social environment.

Playing in groups with family and friends provides the opportunity to develop nurturing relationships. Peer relationships are an important factor for a child's mental health (Szekely et al., 2016). Positive relationships buffer against toxic stress and build social-emotional resilience (Yogman et al., 2018). Resilience and social self-efficacy can protect against depression and loneliness, giving the child a dynamic capacity to achieve career success and, ultimately, health and well-being throughout their lifetime.

Playing with others successfully means listening, responding to social cues, and taking on a playmate's perspective—key in the development of empathy. Empathy is the ability to understand and share the feelings of others. Playing with others can moderate, or have an interacting and strengthening effect, on the development of empathy. Empathy has also been found to be related to high-quality friendship (Van den Bedem, Willems, Dockrell, Van Alphen, & Rieffe, 2018).

Social Play in Children with Special Needs

Children with developmental disabilities and those at risk may need additional support in developing the skills needed for social play. Without adult facilitation, children with disabilities may play alone, isolating themselves from peers and social activities (Wong & Kasari 2012). Cognitive and intellectual disabilities put children at an increased risk for less time in play with peers (Tonkin et al., 2014). Playing alone decreases the number of contextually relevant opportunities that children with disabilities have to develop social skills when compared to their peers of the same age (Barton, 2015; Movahedazarhouligh, 2018). There is a relationship between poor social skills and poor outcomes for mental and physical health later in life (Segrin, 2019), making this an important area for intervention.

The social play participation of children with special needs demonstrates varied patterns. Although all children appear to have similar interests, children with special needs participate more in social activities with family and at locations closer to home (Kreider et al., 2015; Tonkin et al., 2014). Occupational therapy practitioners can support the development of social play by identifying risk, promoting opportunities, creating social play scripts to initiate interactions with others who have shared interests, and helping individuals develop an awareness of their unique social skills.

Friendship

A friendship is a relationship of shared affection between two or more people. Children have a natural tendency to seek out friendships. Friendships are influenced by the physical and social environment and can include a shared play activity or interest. Friendships are all about having fun and playing together. Making friends usually involves talking or having things in common, and shared experiences maintain friendships over time. Having a friend, or friends, is important. Early friendships play an important role in the development of social play and learning how to maintain and deepen social relationships.

The Development of Friendship

Friendships based on interest, affection, and social play can be established as early as the end of the first year. Infants and toddlers pay attention to each other and influence one another's behavior through the use of imitation. Imitation becomes the basic way that young children communicate and socially interact. Toddlers have been observed to imitate each other's behaviors, almost exactly, creating a similarity that distinguishes the interaction as friendship (Over & Carpenter, 2013; Whaley & Rubenstein, 1994). The mirrored exchanges create a reciprocity and shared activity between young children, which demonstrate the desire to belong to a group even very early on. See **Table 14.2** for the developmental stages of friendship in children.

Relationships with friends may be most important from middle childhood into adolescence. In adolescence, friendships allow for sharing of experiences and reflection on self. Adolescents appear to be particularly impressionable, where negative experiences in friendships may have a stronger impact on individuals than positive ones (Schwartz-Mette et al., 2020). The function of friendship during this time in development is identity exploration. When friendship is reciprocated, children feel better about who they are, and they are able to identify with their peers (Maunder & Monks, 2019). The effects of socialization with a friend group are intense in adolescence then decrease from young adulthood on (Wrzus & Neyer, 2016).

Social skills and personality are two factors that influence both the development and maintenance of friendship groups. Social skills can influence the child's role as friend, how they perceive themselves as a friend to others, and who they identify as being their

Table 14.2 The Developmental Stages of Children's Friendships

Stage of Friendship	Age	Description
Interest	2–6 months	As early as 2 months, infants get excited and stare at one another.
Social bids	6–9 months	Infants smile and babble at one another and sometimes initiate and return the social bid.
Imitation	9–12 months	Infant play begins as two infants exchange actions.
Reciprocity	1–2 years	Longer and more complex interactions and reciprocal interaction consistent with emerging theory of mind.
Momentary playmates	3–7 years	Friendships are about having fun together. Children view their friends as momentary playmates.
One-way assistance	4–9 years	Friendships go beyond any one activity. Children care about having friends. Friends are thought of as children who do nice things.
Two-way fair weather cooperation	6–12 years	Friends are able to share perspectives and are concerned about fairness and reciprocity. Friendships are formed around similar interests.
Intimate, mutually shared relationships	11–15 years	Friends help each other to solve problems and share thoughts and feelings.
Mature friendship	12–adulthood	Friendships emphasize trust and support.

Data from Selman, R. L. (1981). The child as friendship philosopher. In S. R. Asher, and J. M. Gottman (Eds.), *The development of children's friendships* (pp. 242–272). Cambridge: Cambridge University Press; Shonkoff, J. P., Phillips, D. A., & National Research Council. (2000). Rethinking nature and nurture. In *From neurons to neighborhoods: The science of early childhood development.* National Academies Press (US).

friends throughout middle childhood. For example, children use social communication to seek things in common with peers and show interest in others' experiences. Personality traits shape the selection of friends and how these friendships develop over time.

Requirements for Friendship

Friendship requires social competence in self-regulation, positive self-identity, cultural competence, effective communication, cooperation, understanding another's perspective, and problem solving (Barnett, 2018; Han & Kemple, 2006). A friend must learn to identify different feelings, respond appropriately, and manage their own emotional response to keep a friendship going over time.

The Impact of Friendship

Friends can have a profound impact on the development of identity, and friendship also shapes personality. Through friendships, children learn more about themselves. Early-childhood friendships are frequently overlooked as a positive developmental influence. Research shows the importance of friendship and its impact on mental and physical health (Almquist, 2012). In early childhood, friends provide an important opportunity for social play. The social context a friendship provides can be a safe place for children to practice managing social relationships.

Friendships can support the development of social skills. Friendships during the childhood years allow for social communication as children learn the rules of conversation. Children also observe, imitate, and learn age-appropriate behavior. Friends learn to take on another's perspective and manage and match emotions (Cleary et al., 2018).

Friendships create a sense of belonging and contribute to the child's quality of life. In reciprocal friendships, children can make each other feel special as well as provide emotional support and validation. It should be noted that even unilateral friendship, or the perception of having a friend that may not be reciprocated, can be protective in depression and loneliness (Schwartz-Mette et al., 2020). Challenges with friendships early in life are associated with anxiety, depression, and loneliness and may impact adult well-being (Sakyi et al., 2015; Schwartz-Mette et al., 2020).

Friendships in Children with Special Needs

Children with special needs can have unique patterns in both making and keeping friends. Children with special needs may have difficulty entering into social play groups as well as keeping play going. Children who have difficulty joining in play with others or who are rejected by peers are at risk to miss out on social play opportunities and the lifelong benefits of friendship.

Students with special education needs report fewer friendships than peers without special needs (Schwab, 2019). The likelihood of friendship for children with special needs may be more dependent on the individual than the setting (Webster & Carter, 2007). Individual challenges impact friendship development as the patterns for social interaction over time are so dynamic.

Specific groups of children are more at risk for challenges with friendship. For example, children with attention-deficit/hyperactivity disorder (ADHD) may have negative social behaviors, such as impulsivity or aggression, and are twice as likely to report having no friends (Fox et al., 2020). Social isolation and negativity from fewer friendships can have additional risks in adolescence from conduct disorders to depression. Young children with ASD and other developmental disabilities often are the least-preferred play partners (Barnett, 2018; Guralnick, 1999). The difficulties that some children with special needs demonstrate in interacting with peers does not mean that they do not have the desire or the capacity to participate in play (Wolfberg et al., 2015). A key theme that emerges from the perspective of young children with ASD is the importance of the opportunity to make friends and the friendships that are formed from these opportunities (Bradley & Male, 2017; Potter, 2015).

Children with special needs face many obstacles in the development of friendships, and intervention early in development, beginning with the family, is essential. Children at risk for difficulties in friendship development may benefit from group play to focus on sharing interests, interpreting the social play, and interacting positively with others. Successful inclusive friendships share these features as well as being developed outside of school and having active support from both sets of parents (Webster & Carter, 2007).

Theories Guiding Play in Groups

There are a variety of theories to describe why individuals seek out play opportunities with others, and why occupational therapy practitioners might use play in groups to improve social play and friendships. While this is not a comprehensive list, this section describes a selection of theories that have contributed to how social play is understood and explores how these theories influence occupational therapy's use of play groups.

Social Development Theory

Developmental theorists suggest that play provides the context for learning to occur. Parents and other caregivers are the initial source for social development and continue to influence a child's social awareness through modeling. Parental figures also promote opportunities for playing with other children. Children enlist the help of another to engage and therefore become socialized (Vandervert, 2017). Another person of greater skill, through scaffolding, can assist children to complete activities they are unable to do alone if those activities are within the range of ability or zone of proximal development (Vygotsky, 1980). Occupational therapy practitioners apply social development theory when modeling skills through play, selecting and coaching peer models, and grading social skill development within the child's range of ability.

A prominent occupational therapist, Lela Llorens (1970), provided an interpretation of developmental theories, which described how development facilitates growth in both a horizontal and longitudinal process. Whereas individuals develop longitudinally advancing through life stages, horizontal growth of self (such as in social-cultural aspects) occurs during each cycle of development. Occupational therapists might select facilitating activities and relationships during each cycle of development that include play in small groups, teams, and clubs as interpersonal relationships grow over time.

Social Cognitive Theory

According to social cognitive theory, people learn by observing and supporting others. The focus is on self-determination and social participation (Cole & Tufano, 2020). Self-determination can be described as the control individuals have over their own life. Social participation is described not as a separate category, but a constant and interdependent factor in the life of an individual. The role of a child as a friend cannot be separated from the occupation of social play. A child thrives when they are given some agency to play a role in their learning (Hirsh-Pasek et al., 2015). Occupational therapy practitioners can use social learning as a strategy for change in playgroups by integrating self-determination, social participation, and opportunities for friendship.

Social Cultural Theory

Social cultural theories suggest that development and learning are consequences of a child's meaningful social interactions. A resurgence in play research at the end of the 20th century examined play and learning in the family home cross-culturally (McLean et al., 2016). Rogoff (2016) describes that, from infancy and into early childhood, children engage with others in shared endeavors. Child development is a process that involves active, interrelated roles of children and their social, cultural worlds known as guided participation. Rogoff (2016) describes a specific form of guided participation, called Learning by Observing and Pitching In (LOPI, n.d.), where children are included in a wide range of activities by the family and community. In LOPI, the goal of learning is to transform children's social participation, increase their level of responsibility, and help them to contribute to the community.

Playgroups

Playgroups provide the opportunity to improve social skills and for children to develop friendships and sense of belonging. Play in groups can provide opportunities for a small group of children to play with toys, make choices about activities and playmates, and learn to get along with others.

Playgroups in Occupational Therapy

Group intervention in occupational therapy provides an alternative to individual intervention, allowing the therapist to meet both individual needs for social play and the needs of multiple children in a group at one time. Survey research indicates that approximately 40% to 60% of pediatric physical and occupational therapists use group intervention at least occasionally in practice (LaForme Fiss, 2012). Group intervention is the use of distinct knowledge of the dynamics of group and social interaction and leadership techniques to facilitate learning and skill acquisition across the life span. Whereas systematic inclusion of children with special needs in all aspects of participation is paramount to a healthy society, targeted intervention in smaller groups will have more of an effect on building social skills that are important for developing friendship and participating in group play (Barnett, 2018; Guralnick, 2010).

Because of a core belief in the positive relationship between occupation and health (American Occupational Therapy Association [AOTA], 2020), occupational therapy practitioners are interested in the relationship of the occupations of play and social participation, including friendships, to health and well-being. Occupational therapy practitioners use their training and skills to provide targeted intervention using play in groups. Occupational therapy playgroups focus on social play and friendships through implementing a range of approaches, developing shared interests, addressing occupational roles, and building social interaction skills.

Occupational therapy practitioners implement playgroups with different approaches tailored for various children. For example, a developmental parent and child playgroup may promote parent–child interaction and parent responsiveness for the general population. A social skills group for preschoolers with ASD alongside typically developing peers may establish social skills and build friendships, preventing rejection and isolation. An after-school activity group for middle schoolers in at-risk communities can help to establish social-emotional skills necessary for cooperation and building friendships, preventing occupational deprivation.

Cultivating shared interests provides a foundation for building social play and friendship . Children with limited play interests may have fewer opportunities for friendships to develop. An occupational therapy practitioner may work with a child to incorporate a wider range of play interests, especially those compatible with peers' interests or modify or negotiate interests within the group (see Chapter 16 for detailed suggestions on this topic).

Occupational therapy practitioners also may focus on the habits, routines, roles, and rituals of the child and how each contributes to patterns of social participation. A therapist may work with a family to set aside a routine for free play with siblings and caregivers each day. The family can work with play objects they already have in a safe, familiar place.

Occupational therapy practitioners use roles as a way of organizing a client's occupations including play. A role is a set of behaviors expected by society and shaped by culture and context (AOTA, 2020). The role of friend carries with it social activities such as greeting, joining in play, and keeping things going. Therapists may assist the child in building role competence so that the tasks associated with being a friend are performed according to the expectations of the peer group. Social roles (friend) and occupations (social play participation) are inseparable and should both be considered with play in groups.

The occupational therapist evaluates and monitors the child's capacity for social play with a focus on social interaction skills. This includes initiating, terminating, producing, physically supporting, shaping content, maintaining flow, verbally supporting, and adapting social interactions (AOTA, 2020). Ineffective performance skills of an individual group member can impact the collective group outcome (AOTA, 2020). For example, a child may repeatedly walk around the circle during a shared reading activity during playtime, demonstrating difficulty regulating their behavior during the social interaction. In this case, the occupational therapy practitioner might offer a familiar play object to help the child transition to circle time and engage with the other play objects and peers.

Types of Playgroups

Playgroups have been used both in the United States and internationally across many countries and both within and outside occupational therapy. The types of playgroups vary in terms of their focus, purpose, and location. In early childhood, partnering with the family as a recipient of services and providing education and social support is essential. While the role of the family is still significant in middle childhood, the playgroup focus shifts to building social skills and social play during participation with a peer group. Playgroups that focus on building specific skills and self-efficacy around a shared area of interest have promise in achieving social play and friendships that extend beyond intervention.

Parent–Child Playgroups in Early Intervention (Birth to 3)

Playgroups are embedded in the early intervention framework in countries around the globe. The playgroup prevention model has been used in Australia, the United Kingdom, Ireland, the Netherlands, and New Zealand (Williams et al., 2018). Over 60% of Australian children have attended a playgroup (Hancock et al., 2012). In these playgroups, caregivers and their children gather to engage in play-based learning. The desired outcomes of these playgroups are threefold: to promote child learning and development, support parenting skills, and increase families' social and community connections (Armstrong et al., 2020). There is an added emphasis on the facilitation of play in these playgroups. The focus on both parental involvement and facilitation of play highlights the potential to support young children's learning and parental engagement in communities (McLean et al., 2014).

There are three main types of parent–child playgroups: community, supported, and therapeutic playgroups (Armstrong et al., 2020; Armstrong et al., 2018; Commerford & Robinson, 2017; Wright et al., 2019). Community playgroups are parent-led, unfunded, and do not always have a strategic focus on improving outcomes. Supported or facilitated playgroups are usually set up to provide a service to families who may not have access to community playgroups. These playgroups are led by a hired playgroup facilitator and funded by not-for-profit organizations. Supported playgroups engage at-risk families and children (Jackson, 2013). Therapeutic playgroups, also referred to as intensive supported playgroups, are designed for children with a developmental delay or disability. Therapeutic playgroups often utilize a skilled and qualified facilitator along with a social worker, working in partnership with parents and providing information and strategies (Armstrong et al., 2020). Please see **Table 14.3** for a list of the active ingredients supporting benefits in parent–child therapeutic playgroups from the perspective of early intervention professionals.

Table 14.3 Active Ingredients of Parent–Child Therapeutic Playgroups

Active Ingredient	Description
Facilitator characteristics	Facilitating skills, relational skills, technical skills (qualification and training), partnership, teamwork
Family characteristics	Clarifying and meeting parental expectations, shared experiences, parent led
Structural components	Consistent routine, natural learning opportunities, indoor/outdoor resources, peer modeling, inclusive, interagency collaboration
Information provision	Content/format of information delivery
Playgroup logistics and information	Accessible, parking

Data from Armstrong, J., Elliott, C., Wray, J., Davidson, E., Mizen, J., & Girdler, S. (2020). Defining therapeutic playgroups: Key principles of therapeutic playgroups from the perspective of professionals. *Journal of Child and Family Studies*, 29, 1029–1043. https://doi.org/10.1007/s10826-019-01622-2.

Parent Interaction and Playfulness in Groups.

In parent–child playgroups, the provider interacts and engages primarily with the caregiver instead of the child, resulting in outcomes of parent competence and confidence (McCollum, Santos, & Weglarz-Ward, 2018). For example, the Parents Interacting with Infants (PIWI) interdisciplinary intervention uses playgroups to strengthen and enhance parent–child relationships, child social-emotional development, and child communication skills (McCollum & Yates, 1994; McCollum et al., 2001). The PIWI developmental topic plans were developed for children with delays in social-emotional development and are located on the Center on the Social Emotional Foundations for Early Learning website (http://csefel.vanderbilt.edu). The playgroup facilitator establishes the context for parent–child interaction, recognizes parenting competence, focuses the parents' attention, provides developmental information, models, and suggests using these strategies in a least to most approach (where setting up the context is the least amount of support, and suggesting what the parent might try would be the most). See **Practice Example 14.1** for an example of the PIWI playgroup.

Another early intervention playgroup focused on parent-to-child and child-to-child play activities once weekly for 8 consecutive weeks. The semistructured group included children ages 15 months to 36 months who were enrolled in early intervention and recruited by their primary service providers based on relevant family goals such as playing with friends, playing in a group, and getting ready for preschool. This playgroup took place at a community park with an indoor and outdoor area accessible to all playgroup members both during and after playgroup. The hour-long playgroup included a period of sensorimotor exploration; constructive play with objects with high sharing, social, and imaginative potential (blocks, large Legos, music instruments); social play with caregivers and peers; and emerging cooperative and pretend play (kitchen items, play food, trucks/cars, baby play, dress up, birthday party, animals, puppets, outdoor objects). Social play was promoted by opportunities for positive caregiving and child playfulness, as well as modifications to the physical and social environment to practice play skills and achieve success (see **Figure 14.2**).

Sensory Processing and Ayres Sensory Integration in Groups.

Sensory-based therapy groups implemented by occupational therapy practitioners in early intervention use play and other activities to address challenging behaviors in children and create a support network for

---

PRACTICE EXAMPLE 14.1 Aiden in a Parent–Child Playgroup

Aiden was a 2-and-a-half-year-old boy diagnosed with ASD. His father noted that Aiden was beginning to initiate play at home, but he didn't seem very interested in the other children at family birthday parties or on the playground. He was worried for Aiden to start preschool. He was working with an occupational therapist, Joanne, in early intervention, who, because of this, suggested he attend a regional weekly playgroup with other parents and similar-aged children in their area. Joanne thought that a playgroup would be a great way for Aiden to practice some of the social skills he was initiating at home with his parents. She also thought it was a good idea for Aiden's parents to connect with other parents and children and expand some of the activities in which they typically participate in the community. Finally, Joanne felt that a playgroup was a great place to solve any potential challenges that arise during group play with an adult facilitator to build his parents' confidence before he began preschool.

Joanne facilitated the playgroup once a month, and Aiden's father agreed that it might be a good time to give it a try. At first during playgroup, Aiden stayed away from the group activities. However, he was very interested in trains and joined the group to pick up a train during a play activity. His father joined in conversation with another child's mother, who shared how it took her son a few weeks to get used to the group. Aiden and his family decided to continue attending the weekly playgroup, facilitated by a different member of the early intervention team each week. Joanne let Aiden's family know that she would come to the first few sessions and then as much as needed.

During the playgroup sessions, the group facilitator would always have children greet each other, introduce different developmental topics for the parents and children to discuss, and set up various play activities. Aiden's parents enjoyed the playgroup discussion about managing behavior, where they read about monkeys jumping on the bed, played with monkey puppets, tried to imitate expressions from monkey faces, and practiced going and stopping while jumping on bubble wrap. Over the course of several months attending playgroup, Aiden learned to wave hello to friends during circle time. He would join in during the play activities, mostly playing alongside his peers but occasionally watching what others were doing. His parents felt more confident that they were able to provide the support he needed to transition to preschool, and they were able to replicate some of the activities that Aiden enjoyed in playgroup at home.

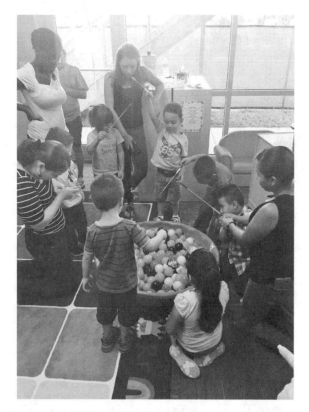

Figure 14.2 Children fish for rubber ducks at a center-based early childhood playgroup

Courtesy of Sarah Fabrizi.

caregivers. For example, in a rural center based early intervention program, 10 mothers and their 2- to 3-year-olds participated in The Wiggly Worm Sensory Processing Playgroup (Gee & Nwora, 2011). The eight sessions included parent education while children engaged in sensory activities. Each group included sensory/gross-motor play, tactile/fine-motor activities, a sensory-based snack activity, and music activities (see **Figure 14.3**). Although sensory group therapy may be less optimal for addressing

sensory processing than individualized, structured sensory therapy, a sensory playgroup offers a socially rich environment for addressing social play and including parents more so that they can carry over sensory play activities at home and generate other activities of their own.

Interdisciplinary Sensory-Enriched Early Intervention (ISEEI) is a group early intervention program based on the use of sensory strategies, including an enriched environment, and is guided by sensory integration theory (Blanche et al., 2016). Potential outcomes include communication, self-regulation, and social emotional abilities. An occupational therapist, a physical therapist, and a speech-language-pathologist designed ISEEI to be used by teachers and aides in direct consultation with therapists. Teachers and aides follow a prescribed protocol, with monthly themes covering developmental areas (social interaction, gross and fine motor, language and communication, and cognition) (Blanche et al., 2016). The adult-to-child ratio is 1:3, where participating children also spend 30–45 minutes daily in a sensory-enriched gym that meets the fidelity requirements for Ayres Sensory Integration.

Early Peer Playgroups

Peer playgroups for preschoolers and others with similar developmental abilities generally focus on the development of skills necessary for social play and provide the social environment that supports practice of these skills.

Cognitive–Functional (Cog–Fun) Groups.

The Cognitive–Functional (Cog–Fun) intervention is an occupational therapy approach to improving underlying executive function deficits and self-efficacy

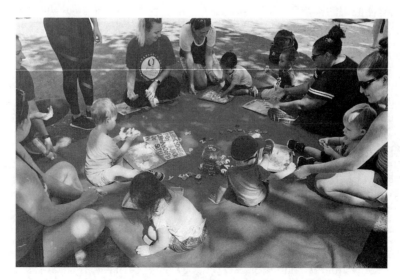

Figure 14.3 Children engage in sensory play during an early intervention playgroup

Courtesy of Sarah Fabrizi.

and was adapted for group intervention (Rosenberg et al., 2015). The Cog–Fun playgroup was implemented to address, among other challenges, social skill deficits in preschoolers diagnosed with ADHD. This group intervention is provided over 11 weekly 45-minute group treatment sessions and is conducted by two occupational therapist group leaders. Parents alternate weekly between participating in the group with their children or participating in a group session with the center's social worker and joining the children for the last 5 minutes. The group intervention teaches six specific executive function strategies (I listened, I waited for my turn, I asked for help, I have an idea, I made an effort, and I helped a friend) during play, self-care, and social participation. Games and activities were used during the sessions to practice the strategies, and parents were encouraged to use the games to carry the strategies over to home.

Playgroups for Young Children with ASD.
The integrated play groups (IPG) model (Wolfberg et al., 2015) focuses on the development of meaningful peer relationships and social play participation for children with ASD. The National Clearinghouse on Autism Evidence and Practice (Steinbrenner et al., 2020) recognizes playgroups as evidence-based practice for individuals with ASD under the category of Peer-Based Instruction and Intervention (PBII). The group facilitator guides child participation through strategies such as: supporting play initiations, guiding social communication, and scaffolding play within the zone of proximal development. IPG includes active engagement in play with peers that vary in skill. Some players develop play skills, while other peers learn to adapt their social play. The typical number of children in an IPG is three to five total playmates, with a higher ratio of expert to novice players. The playgroup site remains consistent, and the play session is structured to include an opening and closing ritual and 40 minutes of guided participation in play. Playmates meet twice a week for 12 weeks.

Three strategies that have been identified to promote social and play skills for young children with ASD that should be considered for use in inclusive playgroups include the use of visual scripts, video modeling, and embedding choice (Barnett, 2018). Scripts are explicit scenarios or prompts that can be written and practiced to focus a child's engagement in a specific activity that impacts participation such as initiating play, requesting and sharing toys, and inviting friends to join. Video modeling involves watching a short video of the performance of an activity. Video modeling can support the correct use of play objects

with peers during playgroup. Providing children choices in a playgroup supports self-determination and has a positive impact on motivation.

Playgroups for School-Age Children
The following examples of playgroups have been described for use with school-age children. In most of these groups, the role of the parent and/or adult is less prominent than in early childhood. Some playgroups, such as the IPG, described earlier, have evidence to support utilization with both preschool and school-age children. In order for social skills, social play, and friendship to generalize from the therapeutic playgroup to other settings, it is important to consider when and where the opportunity for peer interaction can happen again. For example, a group that meets outside of school in a clinic or community setting may need additional parent support and/or regularly scheduled activities (park, club, sports). Skills addressed in school-based playgroups may be able to influence skills and friendships that happen at school. Ideally, the child would have social play opportunities for both.

Activities-Based ENGAGE.
ENGAGE intervention includes a greater number of typically developing peers in a school playgroup along with about two to three classmates with ASD. Sessions are scheduled during recess for 30 minutes twice a week for 8 weeks. Typical peers are chosen based on friendships and peer relationships in the classroom as well as teacher suggestions. The playgroup is based on shared interest and collectively decides on activities to include during conversation, structured games, free play, storytelling, and music. The group leader facilitates play as needed, but fades out as children are able to play independently.

Cognitive Orientation to Daily Occupational Performance (CO-OP).
CO-OP is an occupation-based cognitive approach designed to help individuals master skills (Dawson, McEwen, & Polatajko, 2017). CO-OP uses child-chosen goals to foster children's motivation and engagement in the learning process. When implemented as a playgroup, the children in the group develop both individual goals and shared goals. Groups are formed by occupational therapists based on shared areas of interest and need. A child's verbal ability is important to consider in the formation of CO-OP groups (Anderson et al., 2017). Groups typically include weekly sessions, as well as parent involvement and education. When implemented as a playgroup for

children with developmental coordination disorder, children reported feelings of competence and a sense of belonging (Anderson et al., 2017). Feeling accepted by peers, feeling like a part of the group, and knowing that they are not alone are important outcomes related to social play and friendship. Working in a group increases opportunities for social play and builds the child's confidence for social play away from the CO-OP group.

Facilitated Peer Play Dyads. A clinic-based peer play program can address the social play and friendship challenges of children with ADHD (Wilkes-Gillan et al., 2016). One program pairs children with ADHD with a typically developing playmate. The playmate can be known to the child or a sibling to promote friendship development. Each pair has 1-hour weekly sessions for 10 weeks. In sessions 1–3, 5, 7, and 10, the occupational therapist shows the children and parents a 3-minute video of themselves at play. In the video, green slides indicate desired social skills, and red slides show social skills needing improvement. Verbal cues identify actions to make play more fun. The child identifies three key things to remember (with support as needed) before entering into a playroom. In the playroom, the therapist uses social skill modeling and verbal cues to link back to the video session during 25 minutes of mutually enjoyable cooperative play. The therapist also facilitates identification of the peer's emotional states during play. Parent education takes place in session 7, and home sessions take place during weeks 8 and 9.

Social Play and Friendship Groups for Older and At-Risk Children

Children who enter middle and high school with social skill and friendship challenges will likely continue to need support, direct instruction, and practice. Often, there is less time during the school day to address social play and friendship as the child gets older. Occupational therapy practitioners working in the school may consider small-group projects and weekly social skills groups similar to those utilized with younger children. Providing training and practice opportunities over a wide range of settings (including after-school project groups, clubs, and sports) will support generalizing social skills into real life. See **Figure 14.4** for an example of a group activity creating a community garden. Social playgroups with older children may also include self-awareness, emotional regulation, and fostering prosocial interactions with peers.

Project Groups. Low-income urban youth may be at risk for occupational deprivation, not having a safe place to engage in social play and build friendships. After-school and summer groups often take place in neighborhood community centers. While limited evidence and funding for programs exist, occupational therapy practitioners have an opportunity to promote social play and friendship through occupation-based project groups. In one example, groups of occupational therapy student facilitators supervised by an occupational therapist implemented

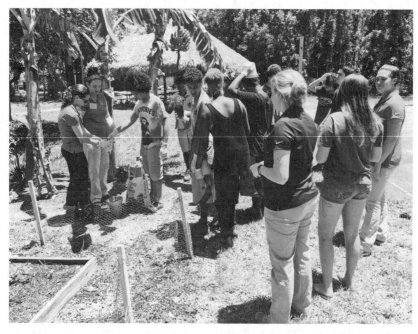

Figure 14.4 Teens participate in creating a community garden during a group activity
Courtesy of Sarah Fabrizi.

a yearly 9-week group program once a week for 1 hour for 8–10 youth (Bazyk & Bazyk, 2009). The group consisted of an introductory discussion, participation in an activity, and a short closing discussion. Social-emotional themes were introduced in the discussion. Projects included making bracelets, clothespin art, yarn projects, rubber stamping cards, papier mâché masks, knitting, and yoga. Potential benefits include self-awareness, emotional regulation, and cooperation. Occupational therapists may work with local children's advocacy groups or community centers to explore opportunities in this area. Partnerships with local universities and graduate students seeking fieldwork opportunities are also options for developing project groups.

Group Sports. Another important consideration for social play and friendship is involvement in group sports. Specific studies examined the impact of a 14-week karate intervention for boys with ASD and found significant reductions in social skill deficits and communication deficits (Bahrami et al., 2016). Another study (Kang et al., 2011) found significant improvements in cooperativeness after a 6-week sports intervention group for children with ADHD. Occupational therapy practitioners can create groups based on sports interest areas, support families as they join youth and recreational sports programs, or a combination of both.

Evidence for the Benefit of Playgroups and Future Research Needs

Multiple studies of playgroups across many countries, settings, ages, and diagnoses have noted a variety of benefits including, but not limited to, academic performance, behavior, cognition, communication, joint attention, mental health, play and playfulness, school readiness, and social participation. (Please see **Table 14.4** for an overview of some of the research evidence regarding playgroups.) However, many unanswered questions remain. Future research is needed on social play and friendship in middle and high school children and young adults and to determine the use of different types of playgroups with diverse populations.

Table 14.4 Evidence Supporting the Use of Playgroups

Type of Playgroup	Benefit	Citation
Community parent–child playgroups	Promote young children's developmental outcomes; encourage positive interactions between parent and child in play.	McLean et al., 2016
	Build community capacity.	Keam et al., 2018
	Provide social and economic benefits.	McShane, et al., 2016; Strange, Bremner, Fisher, Howat, & Wood, 2016
	Promote health and well-being.	Lakhani & Macfarlane, 2015
	Influence communities to broaden social support and other community involvements.	Keam et al., 2018
Community parent–child playgroups—OT led	Significant increases in child playfulness; improved parent confidence and child playfulness.	Fabrizi, Ito, & Winston, 2016; Fabrizi & Hubbell, 2017; Fabrizi, 2015
Supported parent–child playgroups	Connect with parents and foster parental knowledge about play; enrich child learning and enhance positive parenting behaviors; improve parents' social supports; may improve children's sociability and transition to school.	Commerford & Robinson, 2017; McLean et al., 2018; Williams, Berthelsen, Viviani, & Nicholson, 2018
Therapeutic parent–child playgroups	Improve parenting distress, goal achievement, family support, children's social and emotional development; build parent's confidence and social support networks; provide opportunities for social interaction and a source of motivation for children as they learn from peers.	Armstrong et al., 2020; Hung & Pang, 2010

(continues)

Table 14.4 Evidence Supporting the Use of Playgroups *(continued)*

Type of Playgroup	Benefit	Citation
PIWI	Increase child communication and parent facilitation and interaction.	Green et al., 2018
Mother's groups	Build relationships with others in the local community, enhance feelings of connectedness.	Strange et al., 2014
The Wiggly Worm Sensory Processing Playgroup	Improve caregiver understanding of sensory activities, their children's responses to sensory stimuli, and sensory processing concepts following the program.	Gee & Nwora, 2011
ISEEI	Significant improvement in all areas of development except fine-motor skills; children without sensory processing difficulties showed significant improvement in language and cognition.	Blanche et al., 2016
Cog–Fun group	Significantly improved daily functioning, executive function, and social functioning for the children who demonstrated clinical impairment.	Rosenburg et al., 2015
IPG	Strong evidence to support children with ASD participating with typically developing peers in playgroups. Children that participate in the IPG model have demonstrated significant gains in symbolic and social play that generalizes to unsupported play with unfamiliar peers.	Wolfberg et al., 2015
ENGAGE	Affect both peer engagement during recess as well as peer acceptability.	Kasari et al., 2011, 2016
CO-OP group	Improve self-esteem, a sense of belonging, self-awareness, and self-determination, as well as motor skills.	Anderson et al., 2017
Facilitated peer play (for children with ADHD)	Significant improvement in social play skills, pragmatic language, and problem solving postintervention. Good maintenance of social skills.	Fox et al., 2020; Wilkes-Gillan et al., 2016
After-school playgroups	At-risk participants described their experience as fun. The children enjoyed creative projects and working together.	Bazyk et al., 2009

Note: Type of playgroup is listed in the same order of presentation in the text.

While the body of research on playgroups is promising, occupational therapy practitioners should carefully consider the many contributing factors to group intervention. One of the challenges to building a body of evidence on playgroups has been the lack of a consistent model that would include a shared definition along with specific principles for practice. In order to advance playgroup efficacy, there is still a need for more research to determine the active ingredients of the therapeutic playgroup, given the complexity of the many variables that need to be considered (Armstrong et al. 2018; Williams et al., 2018).

Further research is required to develop the evidence base regarding parental education about play in playgroups and the most appropriate form of parental education across playgroup types (McLean, Edwards, Evangelou, et al., 2017). A systematic review of evidence to improve mental health and positive behavior (social skills) in children birth through age 5 indicated that group-based parent training should be implemented with caution due to methodological flaws in the current evidence (Kingsley et al., 2020). Occupational therapists implementing playgroups should think about how they are providing education to parents and monitor whether parents are able to use this information effectively in their everyday lives.

How to Create and Design Playgroups

Information from theory and evidence about play in groups can guide occupational therapy practitioners to create and design playgroups that translate to the specific practice settings and their clients that would benefit. Occupational therapy practitioners utilize this information to systematically proceed with planning, implementing, and measuring the outcomes of play in groups (AOTA, 2020). See **Practice Example 14.2** for an example of an occupational therapist creating and designing a playgroup for children on her caseload.

Evaluations for Using Playgroups

Creating a playgroup begins with identifying the needs of the population or client group. This can be done both formally and informally, by asking questions, giving a short survey, or even doing a formal needs assessment. A needs assessment looks at what is missing between currently available services and the services that families or children want. As many pediatric playgroups are provided by a team of providers, it is also important to consult with the interprofessional team of providers in your practice setting that share an interest in playgroups. Through this process, you can target who might benefit from improving social play and building friendships in group intervention. You can also start to think about what types of groups the evidence describes for the identified population.

Each of the individual children and families will need to be interviewed prior to beginning group. Find out what the parent/child expectations of group participation are and what they are hoping to get out of the playgroup. Each individual member of the group should

---

PRACTICE EXAMPLE 14.2 Lorin's Design of a New Playgroup

Lorin is an occupational therapist working at a private outpatient clinic. She currently has three children on her caseload of similar age and developmental abilities whose families have reported challenges with play with others and making friends at school. To address these needs, Lorin wants to offer a playgroup for these children. Lorin first discusses her thoughts with the facility management and mentors where she works and where the playgroup will be held. Her clinic thinks playgroups are a great idea and can even think of other children who may benefit once things get going. She checks and determines that the children's insurance covers group services. The clinic also agrees to offer the playgroup at a flat rate private pay option. Then she shares the idea with the families of the children, who feel that the playgroup will support some of the goals they have for their children with regard to social play and friendship.

The children Lorin has in mind for the playgroup are Enzo, age 11; Brooke, age 10; and Marc, age 12. Two of the children have a diagnosis of developmental coordination disorder, and the third has signs of sensory processing disorder. Lorin has used the CO-OP model in individual treatment and is interested in the application of CO-OP in a group format. Lorin knows that all three children are very interested in comics and superheroes, and she is thinking this will be a great way to create mutually enjoyable activities.

During individual treatment sessions, Lorin has each child come up with individual goals for participating in the group. Marc mentions he wants to be able to go all the way across the monkey bars. Brooke wants to make new friends. Enzo wants to be able to play soccer during school recess.

At the first group session, the three children decide on the group goal, which will be to play with new friends during recess at school. Lorin observes the children interacting together and uses a dynamic performance analysis to determine where any breakdowns in social skills and social play are. Lorin introduces goal-plan-do-check with a jumping jack example, as all kids were able to successfully complete the activity and learn the process. Lorin encourages the parents to observe as many sessions as they are able to help the children practice skills they are learning at home and in other community settings. The children are asked to keep a notebook and write down what they do on a daily basis to meet their goals. During each session, Lorin has the children complete a superhero mission that involves playground games and activities. At the end of each session, the children are asked to reflect on how well they initiated the play activity, how they were able to keep it going, and what challenges came up interacting with others and how they handled them.

The children report they enjoy working together in a group, and they are now friends. They are making progress in meeting both their individual goals and the group goal. Their parents believe they are more confident and have better reports back from school about making friends and playing on the playground.

be assessed for occupational performance, performance skills and patterns, and client factors. An increased focus on the demands of social play and friendship such as communication, emotional regulation, cognitive skills, social problem solving, positive self-identity, cultural competence, cooperation, and empathy is indicated. The impact of each individual's attitude and performance on the group should be considered. Group composition can be an important factor in the success of a playgroup.

Next, conduct an activity analysis of the playgroup based on the session plan and structure you design (see **Table 14.5**). The context for the playgroup must also be assessed, including the physical environment, equipment and technology, the social environment, and any policies and/or systems affecting playgroup participation. If an interprofessional team will be providing the group play, this can be a topic for a planning meeting to determine team roles and collaboration.

Playgroup Physical Environment

Aspects of the physical environment can support or act as a barrier to play in groups. Indoor and outdoor play opportunities should be explored. Natural play spaces foster self-determination in early childhood (Kochanowski & Carr, 2014). Some studies (Larrea et al., 2019) have reported greater social participation and more complex forms of play among peers in the outdoor environment.

Objects in the environment can impact social play as well. A systematic review of loose-parts play in school-age children (Gibson et al., 2017) reported mixed results on the impact on social development. Null results were found for peer acceptance, social competence, and social skills, but observed increases were seen in cooperative play. Shared reading experiences with books and reading props were found to be connected to social, cognitive, and emotional developmental outcomes as well as social play (Kohm

Table 14.5 Sample Activity Analysis of a Caregiver–Child Playgroup Session

Playgroup Activities	Time Required	Space Required	Activity Description	Safety Precautions	Objects Needed	OT Facilitator Role
Greeting/hello song	5 minutes	Small-group space; circle or outdoor blanket	Group faces and greets each other	None	None	Greet all parents and children, sing hello song with each child's name
Topic introduction/ shared book reading	5 minutes	Small-group space; circle or outdoor blanket	Introduce developmental topic; read book; children play with props and share reading	Watch that small props are not mouthed	Large book, small books, props related to topics in books	Educate on topic, encourage parents to engage children in the book, suggest and model animation, props, visual and tactile cues, modify as needed
Parent–child sensorimotor play	10 minutes	Indoor or outdoor playground if available; space to explore	Parents follow child's lead to explore various sensory and motor activities	Watch that smaller objects are not mouthed; watch outdoor exploration especially for fall risks	Tactile exploration bin, play tunnel, bubbles	Set up the environment, acknowledge parent attempts, model following child's lead, draw parent's attention to child's cues

Playgroup Activities	Time Required	Space Required	Activity Description	Safety Precautions	Objects Needed	OT Facilitator Role
Parent–child and child–child constructive play	10 minutes	Small-group space; outdoor blanket	Parent–child and child–child play with objects, longer play interactions and cooperation and sharing	Watch that smaller objects are not mouthed	Large blocks/ Legos, boxes, arts and crafts	Bring out objects, support and extend parent–child and child–child play such as offering and sharing items
Parent–child pretend play	10 minutes	Indoor or outdoor playground if available; space to explore	Parents and child use objects in both functional and creative ways	Watch outdoor exploration especially for fall risks, unsafe object use	Scarves, laundry basket, recycled objects/loose parts	Provide objects; support parents in observing child, following their lead, and responding; model pretend play ideas
Snack and conversation	5 minutes	Small table or outdoor blanket so group can sit together	Children are seated together supported by parents; parents talk about topics of interest	Any food allergies, dietary restrictions, choking hazards	Snack, small cups, water	Support parents to help children develop skills, facilitate shared conversation
Come together song/game	10 minutes	Small-group space; circle or outdoor blanket	Group sings song, uses hand motions, props as needed	None	Musical instrument/ parachute	Initiate song, support parents and children to participate, modify pace and use repetition as needed
Topic review, goodbye song	5 minutes	Small-group space; circle or outdoor blanket	Brief discussion about the developmental topic and some of the noteworthy events of the playgroup	None	None	Review developmental topic and describe examples of related parent–child and child–child interactions

et al., 2016). Electronic toys may act as a barrier to social play as they can be more solitary, whereas more traditional toys (such as books, blocks, balls, bubbles) may support opportunities for initiating and maintaining social play.

Playgroup Social Environment

Peers support a playful environment and play skills. Children can acquire knowledge by sharing in pretend play with more knowledgeable play partners (Sutherland

& Friedman, 2013). Peer-mediated learning strategies (PMLS) involve teaching typically developing peers to interact with children with disabilities. This buddy training can increase the frequency and duration of children's cooperative play (Hu et al., 2018; Hughett et al., 2013). Collaboration can be particularly beneficial for lower-ability children. However, high-ability children either regressed or did not benefit when paired with lower-ability participants (Sills et al., 2016). Interventions involving typically developing peers in friendship groups united by shared interests seem to result in improved generalization (Chapin et al., 2018; Fox et al., 2020).

Family members can create a playful experience. Encouraging siblings and extended family to attend playgroups supports inclusion and makes it easier for parents to attend. This can also provide additional opportunities to educate the child's extended family (Armstrong et al., 2020). Parents can also learn from each other in playgroups. Sharing between parents is enhanced with group diversity in ability and experience, inclusion of siblings, and facilitator skill (Armstrong et al., 2020). Parents have reported they value the following activities in group play: free play with a large range of toys and good-quality equipment, sing-alongs, live animals, and guest professionals who give information or teach about a topic (Commerford & Robinson, 2017).

Playgroup Intervention

The intervention plan will include the information from the evaluation and incorporate best available evidence on play in groups. The plan should include setting up the physical and social environment, parent participation and/or education, facilitation of social skills through coaching and modeling, and providing varied opportunities for practice using structured and unstructured social play activities and games. The occupational therapy practitioner may choose to utilize an existing evidence-based program, modify a playgroup plan, or develop a program of their own. Playgroup implementation involves carrying out the group play intervention and monitoring both individual child and group progress. Formal notes should include how each child is responding to play in groups, their progress toward agreed-upon goals, and how individual performance impacts the group process. For example, you would note whether or not a child initiated play with another group member. Another noteworthy event would be a conflict, such as not wanting to share a play object. You may want to describe how each child handles the conflict, how much adult support is needed, and how long it takes

them to return to play. Keeping track of attention, imitation, and how long play interactions last between children can also be valuable. The playgroup plan can be modified to meet the dynamic needs of the participating children and families.

Playgroup Structure

The structure of the playgroup session itself deserves special attention. The purpose and the outcome of each playgroup structure and session should center around improving the social play and friendship of each playmate. Matching the structure of the group to the needs of the children, parents, and group will achieve the best results. At times, the specific type of group play will dictate the structure of the session. For example, instruction in social skills and early practice may require more of a structured approach whereas exploration, creativity, and imagination would be achieved with free play in a carefully constructed play environment.

There is value in including both structured play and free play. The child-directed nature of free play allows for playfulness, the "secret sauce" for play. Structured play provides opportunities for supporting play and building play skills, while still allowing the child self-determination through play choices. It may be beneficial to begin a playgroup session with more structure and planning, and then allow for more unfolding of spontaneous social play interactions over time.

Developmental topics and play themes allow for parent education on topics of interest, shared interests among children, collaborative play projects, and creativity of both facilitators and participants. Children with more involved social play challenges may initially need more adult support and guidance, and a smaller carefully thought-out group composition.

Playgroup Facilitator

Occupational therapy practitioners that facilitate play in groups to improve social play and build friendships must meet the needs of the children and families while embedding goals into play opportunities. Play in groups requires providing parents with developmental information on play and selecting specific strategies for engagement. Information may be in the form of structured talks and handouts, or through informal conversations during the playgroup session (Armstrong et al., 2020). The degree of job satisfaction and level of training of facilitators may be an important factor in supporting families' rates of attendance, which, in turn, influences the benefit families receive from the playgroup (Berthelsen et al., 2012). Effective facilitators are organized, are adaptable, focus on strengths, manage group dynamics, and resolve conflicts (Armstrong, 2020). Facilitating playgroups with children also requires a playful nature, while still instructing in skills. Coaching can also be effective in supporting friendship in children (King & Keenan, 2021). With older children, facilitators must balance playfulness with managing behavior and keeping the group therapeutic.

An important skill of the playgroup facilitator is knowing when to add supports and when to fade out support and guidance. This is determined through careful observations of play interactions. After a new play ability has been supported, the therapist provides opportunities to play with this skill in the group. If the play is going smoothly, the therapist does not intervene but intently observes, ready to support and guide if needed. Signs of fatigue, frustration, dysregulation, or disengagement are indicators that supports or modifications are needed. The therapist must be authentically present to notice small signs quickly before they escalate and become too disruptive to the group, and the therapist must utilize rapid professional reasoning to be ready to intervene appropriately to support individuals and the group.

Measurement of Playgroup Outcomes

In order to show change as a result of play in groups it is essential to assess progress toward outcomes using the same measures agreed upon during intervention planning and in relation to achievement of goals. Change can be described in both the individual and the group. The interprofessional team may provide input on outcome measures to demonstrate individual and group response to playgroup intervention.

Collective playgroup goals should be established. Three primary goals are relevant to peer competence and can be measured at the time of assessment, during intervention, and after the group concludes (Guralnick, 2010). These include peer-group entry, conflict resolution, and maintaining play.

Outcomes of play in groups should be related to the child's ability to engage in social play and build friendships. See **Box 14.1** for suggested child and parent outcomes. Specific goal measures should be reliable and valid and sensitive to show change as a result of participation.

Box 14.1 Outcomes and Goal Areas for Playgroups

Child Outcomes	Play
	Playfulness
	Social play
	Social communication
	Emotional regulation
	Social problem solving
	Cultural competence
	Cooperation
	Self-efficacy
	Self-determination
	Friendship
	Empathy
	Play participation
	Social participation
	Quality of life
	Belonging and acceptance
Parent Outcomes	Parenting self-efficacy
	Parent–child interaction
	Parent responsiveness
	Social support
	Reduced parenting stress
	Parental well-being
	Belonging and acceptance

Conclusion

Social play and friendships are incredibly important for meaningful relationships and social competence in all environments throughout a lifetime. Social play and friendships contribute to communication, emotional regulation, and social problem solving. Play in groups can support self-efficacy, resilience, empathy, a sense of belonging, and a positive trajectory for mental health. For many of the children we see in occupational therapy, social play and friendship do not come easily or develop typically. However, children can learn appropriate social behaviors from modeling others and peer practice in play, essential components of playgroup interventions. There are many types of playgroups available for occupational therapy practitioners to choose from, most with some research evidence supporting their use. For the therapist interested in creating or designing a playgroup, there are important considerations such as the physical and social play environments available, the structure of the playgroup, who will facilitate sessions, and the specific needs of the families and children looking to promote or improve social play and friendships.

References

Almquist, Y. M. (2012). Childhood friendships and adult health: Findings from the Aberdeen Children of the 1950s Cohort Study. *European Journal of Public Health, 22*(3), 378–383. https://doi.org/10.1093/eurpub/ckr045

American Occupational Therapy Association (AOTA). (2020). Occupational therapy practice framework: Domain & process(4th ed.). *American Journal of Occupational Therapy, 74*(Supplement 2), 7412410010. https://doi.org/10.5014/ajot.2020.74S2001

Anderson, L., Wilson, J., & Williams, G. (2017). Cognitive Orientation to daily Occupational Performance (CO-OP) as group therapy for children living with motor coordination difficulties: An integrated literature review. *Australian Occupational Therapy Journal, 64*, 170–184. https://doi.org/10.1111/1440-1630.12333

Armstrong, J., Elliott, C., Wray, J., Davidson, E., Mizen, J., & Girdler, S. (2020). Defining therapeutic playgroups: Key principles of therapeutic playgroups from the perspective of professionals. *Journal of Child and Family Studies, 29*, 1029–1043. https://doi.org/10.1007/s10826-019-01622-2

Armstrong, J., Paskal, K., Elliott, C., Wray, J., Davidson, E., Mizen, J., & Girdler, S. (2018). What makes playgroups therapeutic? A scoping review to identify the active ingredients of therapeutic and supported playgroups. *Scandinavian Journal of Occupational Therapy, 26*(2), 1–22. https://doi.org/10.1080/11038128.2018.1498919

Bahrami, F., Movahedi, A., Marandi, S. M., & Sorensen, C. (2016). The effect of karate techniques training on communication deficit of children with autism spectrum disorders. *Journal of Autism and Developmental Disorders, 46*(3), 978–986.

Barnett, J. H. (2018). Three evidence-based strategies that support social skills and play among young children with autism spectrum disorders. *Early Childhood Education Journal, 46*, 665–672. https://doi.org/10.1007/s10643-018-0911-0

Barton, E. (2015). Teaching generalized pretend play and related behaviors to young children with disabilities. *Exceptional Children, 81*(4), 489–506. https://doi.org/10.1177/0014402914563694

Bazyk, S., & Bazyk, J. (2009). Meaning of occupation-based groups for low-income urban youths attending after-school care. *American Journal of Occupational Therapy, 63*(1), 69–80.

Bazyk, S., Michaud, P., Goodman, G., Papp, P., Hawkins, E., & Welch, M. A. (2009). Integrating occupational therapy services in a kindergarten curriculum: A look at the outcomes. *American Journal of Occupational Therapy, 63*(2), 160–171.

Berthelsen, D., Williams, K., Abad, V., Vogel, L., & Nicholson, J. (2012). *The parents at playgroup research report: Engaging families in supported playgroups.* Brisbane: Queensland University of Technology; Playgroup Association of Queensland.

Blanche, E. I., Chang, M. C., Gutierrez, J., & Gunter, J. S. (2016). Effectiveness of a sensory-enriched early intervention group program for children with developmental disabilities. *American Journal of Occupational Therapy, 70*, 7005220010. http://dx.doi.org/10.5014/ajot.2016.018481

Bradley, K., & Male, D. (2017). "Forest School is muddy and I like it": Perspectives of young children with autism spectrum disorders, their parents and educational professionals. *Educational and Child Psychology, 34*(2), 80–96.

Chapin, S., McNaughton, D., Boyle, S., & Babb, S. (2018). Effects of peer support interventions on the communication of preschoolers with autism spectrum disorder: A systematic review. *Seminars in Speech and Language, 39*(5), 443–457. https://doi.org/10.1055/s-0038-1670670

Cleary, M., Lees, D., & Sayers, J. (2018). Friendship and mental health. *Issues in Mental Health Nursing, 39*(3), 279–281. https://doi.org/10.1080/01612840.2018.1431444

Cole, M., & Tufano, R. (2020). *Applied theories in occupational therapy: A practical approach.* Thorofare, NJ: SLACK.

Commerford, J., & Robinson, E. (2017). Supported playgroups for parents and children: The evidence for their benefits. *Family Matters, 99*, 42–51. https://www.aifs.gov.au/cfca/

Dawson, D., McEwen, S., & Polatajko, H. (Eds.). (2017). *Cognitive orientation to daily occupational performance in occupational therapy: Using the CO-OP approach to enable participation across the lifespan.* Bethesda, MD: AOTA Press.

Diamond, A., Barnett, W. S., Thomas, J., & Munro, S. (2007). Preschool program improves cognitive control. *Science, 318*(5855), 1387–1388.

Fabrizi, S. E. (2015). Splashing our way to playfulness! An aquatic playgroup for young children with autism: A repeated measures design. *Journal of Occupational Therapy, Schools, and Early Intervention, 8*(4), 292–306. https://doi.org/10.1080/19411243.2015.1116963

Fabrizi, S., & Hubbell, K. (2017). The role of occupational therapy in promoting playfulness, parent competence, and social participation in early childhood playgroups: A pretest posttest design. *Journal of Occupational Therapy, Schools, & Early Intervention, 10*(4), 346–365. http://dx.doi.org/10.1080/19411243.2017.1359133

Fabrizi, S. E., Ito, M. A., & Winston, K. (2016). Effect of occupational therapy–led playgroups in early intervention on child playfulness and caregiver responsiveness: A repeated-measures design. *American Journal of Occupational Therapy, 70*, 7002220020. http://dx.doi.org/10.5014/ajot.2016.017012

Fox, A., Dishman, S., Valicek, M., Ratcliff, K., & Hilton, C. (2020). Effectiveness of social skills interventions incorporating peer interactions for children with attention deficit hyperactivity disorder: A systematic review. *American Journal of Occupational Therapy, 74*, 7402180070. https://doi.org/10.5014/ajot.2020.040212

Gee, B. M., & Nwora, A. J. (2011). Enhancing caregiver perceptions using center-based sensory processing playgroups: Understanding and efficacy. *Journal of Occupational Therapy, Schools, & Early Intervention, 4*(3–4), 276–290. https://doi.org/10.1080/00220671.2012.635588

Gibson, J. L., Cornell, M., & Gill, T. (2017). A systematic review of research into the impact of loose parts play on children's cognitive, social and emotional development. *School Mental Health, 9*, 295–309. https://doi.org/10.1007/s12310-017-9220-9

Golinkoff, R., & Hirsh-Pasek, K. (2016). *Becoming brilliant: What science tells us about raising successful children.* Washington, DC: APA Press.

Green, K. B., Towson, J. A., Head, C., Janowski, B., & Smith, L. (2018). Facilitated playgroups to promote speech and language skills of young children with communication delays: A pilot study. *Child Language Teaching and Therapy*, 34(1), 37–52.

Grover, R. L., Nangle, D. W., Buffie, M., & Andrews, L. A. (2020). Defining social skills. In Nangle, D. W., Erdley, C. A., & Schwartz-Mette, R. A. (Eds.), *Social Skills Across the Life Span* (pp. 3–24). San Diego, CA: Academic Press.

Guralnick, M. J. (1999). The nature and meaning of social integration for young children with mild developmental delays in inclusive settings. *Journal of Early Intervention*, 22(1), 70–86.

Guralnick, M. J. (2010). Early intervention approaches to enhance the peer-related social competence of young children with developmental delays: A historical perspective. *Infants and Young Children*, 23(2), 73–83. https://doi.org/10.1097/IYC.0b013e3181d22e14

Han, H. S., & Kemple, K. M. (2006). Components of social competence and strategies of support: Considering what to teach and how. *Early Childhood Education Journal*, 34, 241–246. https://doi.org/10.1007/s10643-006-0139-2

Hancock, K., Lawrence, D., Mitrou, F., Zarb, D., Berthelsen, D., Nicholson, J., & Zubrick, S. (2012). The association between playgroup participation, learning competence and social-emotional wellbeing for children aged four–five years in Australia. *Australian Journal of Early Childhood*, 37(2), 72–81.

Hirsh-Pasek, K., Zosh, J. M., Golinkoff, R. M., Gray, J. H., Robb, M. B., & Kaufman, J. (2015). Putting education in "educational" apps: Lessons from the science of learning. *Psychological Science in the Public Interest*, 16(1), 3–34.

Hu, X., Zheng, Q., & Lee, G. T. (2018). Using peer-mediated LEGO play intervention to improve social interactions for Chinese children with autism in an inclusive setting. *Journal of Autism and Developmental Disorders*, 48, 2444–2457. https://doi.org/10.1007/s10803-018-3502-4

Hughett, K., Kohler, F. W., & Raschke, D. (2013). The effects of a buddy skills package on preschool children's social interactions and play. *Topics in Early Childhood Special Education*, 32(4), 246–254. https://doi.org/10.1177/0271121411424927

Hung, W. W., & Pang, M. Y. (2010). Effects of group-based versus individual-based exercise training on motor performance in children with developmental coordination disorder: A randomized controlled study. *Journal of Rehabilitation Medicine*, 42, 122–128.

Jackson, D. (2013). Creating a place to "be": Unpacking the facilitation role in three supported playgroups in Australia. *European Early Childhood Education Research Journal*, 21(1), 77–93.

Kang, K. D., Choi, J. W., Kang, S. G., & Han, D. H. (2011). Sports therapy for attention, cognitions and sociality. *International Journal of Sports Medicine*, 32(12), 953–959. https://doi.org/10.1055/s-0031-1283175

Kang, S. (2020). The power of play. *American Journal of Health Promotion*, 34(5), 573–575. https://doi.org/10.1177/0890117120920488e

Kasari, C., Dean, M., Kretzmann, M., Shih, W., Orlich, F., Whitney, R.,... King, B. (2016). Children with autism spectrum disorder and social skills groups at school: A randomized trial comparing intervention approach and peer composition. *The Journal of Child Psychology and Psychiatry*, 57(2), 171–179.

Kasari, C., Locke, J., Gulsrud, A., & Rotheram-Fuller, E. (2011). Social networks and friendships at school: Comparing children with and without ASD. *Journal of Autism and Developmental Disorders*, 41(5), 533–544.

Keam, G., Cook, K., Sinclair, S., & McShane, I. (2018). A qualitative study of the role of playgroups in building community capacity. *Health Promotion Journal of Australia*, 29(1), 65–71. https://doi.org/10.1002/hpja.4

King, G., & Keenan, S. (2021). Solution-focused coaching for friendship in pediatric rehabilitation: A case study of goal attainment, client engagement, and coach stances. *Physical & Occupational Therapy in Pediatrics*, 1–18. https://doi.org/10.1080/01942638.2021.1947435

Kingsley, K., Sagester, G., & Weaver, L. L. (2020). Interventions supporting mental health and positive behavior in children ages birth–5 yr: A systematic review. *American Journal of Occupational Therapy*, 74, 7402180050. https://doi.org/10.5014/ajot.2020.039768

Kochanowski, L., & Carr, V. (2014). Nature playscapes as contexts for fostering self-determination. *Children, Youth and Environments*, 24(2), 146–167. https://doi.org/10.7721/chilyoutenvi.24.2.0146

Kohm, K. E., Holmes, R. M., Romeo, L., & Koolidge, L. (2016). The connection between shared storybook readings, children's imagination, social interactions, affect, prosocial behavior, and social play. *International Journal of Play*, 5(2), 128–140. https://doi.org/10.1080/21594937.2016.1203895

Kreider, C. M., Bendixen, R. M., Young, M. E., Prudencio, S. M., McCarty, C., & Mann, W. C. (2015). Réseaux sociaux et participation avec les autres, chez des adolescents ayant des troubles d'apprentissage, de l'attention et du spectre de l'autisme[Social networks and participation with others for youth with learning, attention, and autism spectrum disorders]. *Canadian Journal of Occupational Therapy*, 83(1), 14–26. https://doi.org/10.1177/0008417415583107

LaForme Fiss, A. (2012). Group intervention in pediatric rehabilitation. *Physical & Occupational Therapy in Pediatrics*, 32(2), 136–138. https://doi.org/10.3109/01942638.2012.668389

Lakhani, A., & Macfarlane, K. (2015). Playgroups offering health and well-being support for families a systematic review. *Family & Community Health*, 38, 180–194. https://doi.org/10.1097/FCH.0000000000000070.

Larrea, I., Muela, A., Miranda, N., & Barandiaran, A. (2019). Children's social play and affordance availability in preschool outdoor environments. *European Early Childhood Education Research Journal*, 27(2), 185–194. https://doi.org/10.1080/1350293X.2019.1579546

Llorens, L. A. (1970). Facilitating growth and development: The promise of occupational therapy. *American Journal of Occupational Therapy*, 24, 93–101.

LOPI. (n.d.). Overview of learning by observing and pitching in (LOPI). https://learningbyobservingandpitchingin.sites.ucsc.edu/overview/

Maunder, R., & Monks, C. P. (2019),Friendships in middle childhood: Links to peer and school identification, and general self-worth. *British Journal of Developmental Psychology*, 37, 211–229. https://doi.org/10.1111/bjdp.12268

McCollum, J. A., Gooler, F., Appl, D. J., & Yates, T. J. (2001). PIWI: Enhancing parent–child interaction as a foundation for early intervention. *Infants & Young Children*, 14(1), 34–45.

McCollum, J. A., Santos, R. M., & Weglarz-Ward, J. M. (2018). *Interaction: Enhancing children's access to responsive interactions*

(*DEC Recommended Practices Monograph Series No. 5*). Washington, DC: Division for Early Childhood.

McCollum, J. A., & Yates, T. J. (1994). Dyad as focus, triad as means: A family-centered approach to supporting parent–child interactions. *Infants and Young Children*, 6(4), 54–63. https://doi.org/10.1097/00001163-199404000-00008

McDonald, N. M., & Messinger, D. S. (2011). The development of empathy: How, when, and why. In A. Acerbi, J. A. Lombo, & J. J. Sanguineti (Eds.), *Free will, emotions, and moral actions: Philosophy and neuroscience in dialogue*. Vatican City: IF-Press.

McLean, K., Edwards, S., & Colliver, Y. (2014). Supported playgroups in schools: What matters for caregivers and their children? *Australian Journal of Early Childhood*, 39(4), 73–80.

McLean, K., Edwards, S., Evangelou, M., & Lambert, P. (2018). Supported playgroups in schools: Bonding and bridging family knowledge about transition to formal schooling. *Cambridge Journal of Education*, 48(2), 157–175. https://doi.org/10.1080/0305764X.2016.1268569

McLean, K., Edwards, S., Evangelou, M., Skouteris, H., Harrison, L. J., Hemphill, S. A.,... Lambert, P. (2017). Playgroups as sites for parental education. *Journal of Early Childhood Research*, 15(3), 227–237. https://doi.org/10.1177/1476718X15595753

McLean, K., Edwards, S., Morris, H., Hallowell, L., & Swinkels, K. (2016). *Community playgroups—Connecting rural families locally pilot. A Research Report Prepared for Playgroup* Victoria. Melbourne: Australian Catholic University.

McShane, I., Cook, K., Sinclair, S., Keam, G., & Fry, J. (2016). *Relationships Matter: The Social and Economic Benefits of Community Playgroups*. Melbourne, Australia: RMIT University. http://dx.doi.org/10.2139/ssrn.2814527

Movahedazarhouligh, S. (2018). Teaching play skills to children with disabilities: Research-based interventions and practices. *Early Childhood Education Journal*, 46, 587–599. https://doi.org/10.1007/s10643-018-0917-7

Over, H., & Carpenter, M. (2013). The social side of imitation. *Child Development Perspectives*, 7(1), 6–11.

Parten, M. B. (1932). Social participation among preschool children. *Journal of Abnormal and Social Psychology*, 27(3), 243–269. Retrieved from https://pathways.org/kids-learn-play-6-stages-play-development/

Potter, C. (2015). "I didn't used to have much friends": Exploring the friendship concepts and capabilities of a boy with autism and severe learning disabilities. *British Journal of Learning Disabilities*, 43(3), 208–218. https://doi-org/10.1111/bld.12098

Rogoff, B. (2016). Culture and participation: A paradigm shift. *Current Opinion in Psychology*, 8, 182–189. https://doi.org/10.1016/j.copsyc.2015.12.002

Rosenberg, L., Maeir, A., Yochman, A., Dahan, I., & Hirsch, I. (2015). Effectiveness of a cognitive–functional group intervention among preschoolers with attention deficit hyperactivity disorder: A pilot study. *American Journal of Occupational Therapy*, 69, 6903220040. http://dx.doi.org/10.5014/ajot.2015.014795

Sakyi, K. S., Surkan, P. J., Fombonne, E., Chollet, A., & Melchior, M. (2015). Childhood friendships and psychological difficulties in young adulthood: An 18-year follow-up study. *European Child & Adolescent Psychiatry*, 24(7), 815–826. https://doi.org/10.1007/s00787-014-0626-8

Schwab, S. (2019). Friendship stability among students with and without special educational needs. *Educational Studies*, 45(3), 390–401. https://doi.org/10.1080/03055698.2018.1509774

Schwartz-Mette, R. A., Shankman, J., Dueweke, A. R., Borowski, S., & Rose, A. J. (2020). Relations of friendship experiences with depressive symptoms and loneliness in childhood and adolescence: A meta-analytic review. *Psychological Bulletin*, 146(8), 664–700. https://doi.org/10.1037/bul0000239

Segrin, C. (2019). Indirect effects of social skills on health through stress and loneliness. *Health Communication*, 34(1), 118–124.

Selman, R. L. (1981). The child as friendship philosopher. In S. R. Asher & J. M. Gottman (Eds.), *The development of children's friendships* (pp. 242–272). Cambridge: Cambridge University Press.

Shonkoff, J. P., Phillips, D. A., & National Research Council. (2000). Rethinking nature and nurture. In J. P. Shonkoff & D. A. Phillips (Eds.), *From neurons to neighborhoods: The science of early childhood development*. Washington, DC: National Academies Press (US).

Sills, J., Rowse, G., & Emerson, L. M. (2016). The role of collaboration in the cognitive development of young children: A systematic review. *Child: Care, Health & Development*, 42(3), 313–324. https://doi-org.ezproxy.fgcu.edu/10.1111/cch.12330

Steinbrenner, J. R., Hume, K., Odom, S. L., Morin, K. L., Nowell, S. W., Tomaszewski, B.,... Savage, M. N. (2020). *Evidence-based practices for children, youth, and young adults with autism*. Chapel Hill: The University of North Carolina at Chapel Hill, Frank Porter Graham Child Development Institute, National Clearinghouse on Autism Evidence and Practice Review Team.

Strange, C., Bremner, A., Fisher, C., Howat, P., & Wood, L. (2016). Mothers' group participation: Associations with social capital, social support and mental well-being. *Journal of Advanced Nursing*, 72(1), 85–98. https://doi.org/10.1111/jan.12809

Strange, C., Fisher, C., Howat, P., & Wood, L. (2014). Fostering supportive community connections through mothers' groups and playgroups. *Journal of Advanced Nursing*, 70(12), 2835–2846. https://doi-org.ezproxy.fgcu.edu/10.1111/jan.12435

Sutherland, S. L., & Friedman, O. (2013). Just pretending can be really learning: Children use pretend play as a source for acquiring generic knowledge. *Developmental Psychology*, 49(9), 1660–1668. https://doi.org/10.1037/a0030788

Szekely, E., Pappa, I., Wilson, J. D., Bhamidi, S., Jaddoe, V. W., Verhulst, F. C.,... Shaw, P. (2016). Childhood peer network characteristics: Genetic influences and links with early mental health trajectories. *Journal of Child Psychology & Psychiatry*, 57(6), 687–694. https://doi-org./10.1111/jcpp.12493

Tonkin, B. L., Ogilvie, B. D., Greenwood, S. A., Law, M. C., & Anaby, D. R. (2014). Étude de délimitation de l'étendue de la participation des enfants et des jeunes handicapés à des activités en dehors du contexte scolaire [The participation of children and youth with disabilities in activities outside of school: A scoping review]. *Canadian Journal of Occupational Therapy*, 81(4), 226–236. https://doi.org/10.1177/0008417414550998

Van den Bedem, N. P., Willems, D., Dockrell, J. E., Van Alphen, P. M., & Rieffe, C. (2018). Interrelation between empathy and friendship development during (pre)adolescence and the moderating effect of developmental language disorder: A longitudinal study. *Social Development*, 28, 599–619. https://doi.org/10.1111/sode.12353

Vandervert, L. (2017). Vygotsky meets neuroscience: The cerebellum and the rise of culture through play. *American Journal of Play, 9*(2), 202–227.

Vygotsky, L. S. (1980). *Mind in society: The development of higher psychological processes* (M. Cole, V. John-Steiner, S. Scribner, & E. Souberman, Eds.). Cambridge, MA: Harvard University Press.

Webster, A., & Carter, M. (2007). Social relationships and friendships of children with developmental disabilities: Implications for inclusive settings. A systematic review. *Journal of Intellectual & Developmental Disability, 32*, 200–213. https://doi.org/10.1080/13668250701549443.

Whaley, K. L., & Rubenstein, T. S. (1994). How toddlers "do" friendship: A descriptive analysis of naturally occurring friendships in a group child care setting. *Journal of Social and Personal Relationships, 11*(3), 383–400. https://doi.org/10.1177/0265407594113005

Wilkes-Gillan, S., Bundy, A., Cordier, R., Lincoln, M., & Chen, Y. W. (2016). A randomised controlled trial of a play-based intervention to improve the social play skills of children with attention deficit hyperactivity disorder (ADHD). *PLoS One, 11*, e0160558. https://doi.org/10.1371/journal.pone.0160558

Williams, K. E., Berthelsen, D., Viviani, M., & Nicholson, J. M. (2018). Facilitated parent–child groups as family support: A systematic literature review of supported playgroup studies. *Journal of Child and Family Studies, 27*(8), 2367–2383. https://doi.org/10.1007/s10826-018-1084-6

Wolfberg, P., DeWitt, M., Young, G. S., & Nguyen, T. (2015). Integrated play groups: Promoting symbolic play and social engagement with typical peers in children with ASD across settings. *Journal of Autism and Developmental Disorders, 45*, 830–845. https://doi.org/10.1007/s10803-014-2245-0

Wong, C., & Kasari, C. (2012). Play and joint attention of children with autism in the preschool special education classroom. *Journal of Autism and Developmental Disorders, 42*(10), 2152–2161.

Wright, A. C., Warren, J., Burriel, K., & Sinnott, L. (2019). Three variations on the Australian supported playgroup model. *International Journal of Social Welfare, 28*(3), 333–344.

Wrzus, C., & Neyer, F. J. (2016). Co-development of personality and friendship across the lifespan. *European Psychologist, 21*, 233–236. https://doi.org/10.1027/1016-9040/a000277

Yogman, M., Garner, A., Hutchinson, J., Hirsh-Pasek, K., Golinkoff, R. M., & Committee on Psychosocial Aspects of Child and Family Health. (2018). The power of play: A pediatric role in enhancing development in young children. *Pediatrics, 142*(3).

Yu, S., Ostrosky, M., & Fowler, S. (2011). Children's friendship development: A comparative study. *Early Childhood Research & Practice, 13*(1). https://files.eric.ed.gov/fulltext/EJ931228.pdf

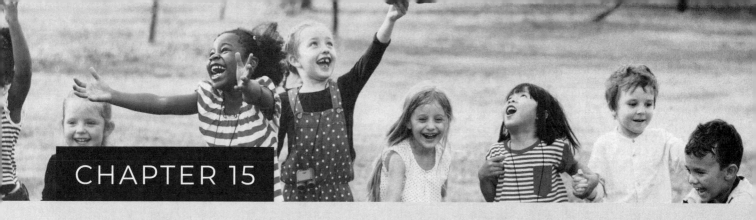

CHAPTER 15

Perspectives on the Meaning of Play: International, Cultural, and Individual Contexts

Helen Lynch, PhD, MSc, Dip COT, Dip Montessori

After reading this chapter, the reader will:

- Describe play occupation from contrasting sociocultural contexts and from child and adult perspectives.
- Compare and contrast play as a universal concept versus play as a cultural concept.
- Identify reasons for protecting a child's right to play.
- Describe the core international documents that address a child's right to play.
- Explain challenges in occupational therapy for enabling play in international contexts.
- Apply play-centered occupational therapy that reflects local sociocultural and policy contexts.
- Formulate ways to enable play, informed by international examples of good practice.

A fundamental problem with universal claims about play is that they basically ignore the contrasting realities of childhood experiences and the cultural forces that may help shape caregiver's ideas about play and early learning, and children's role in their own play.

—The Oxford Handbook of the Development of Play.

Play is a phenomenon evident in cultural communities across all continents of the world (Lancy, 2007; Roopnarine, 2011). Although play is a universal behavior recognized in humans (Burghardt, 2014), play develops as a synthesis of nature *and* nurture. Indeed, the United Nations Committee on the Rights of the Child (CRC) General Comment 17, has contextualized play as a cultural expression whereby "children reproduce, transform, create and transmit culture through, for example, their imaginative play, songs, dance, animation, stories, painting, games, street theatre, puppetry, festivals, etc." (CRC, 2013, p. 5). Consequently, we need to ask: Does this mean that play is not universal after all? And how does play differ across cultures?

Occupational therapy practitioners who are committed to enhancing play for the children they serve, must understand how the form, function, and meaning of play can differ in different cultures. Occupational therapists need to understand play as a cultural phenomenon and not just a developmental one in order to build capacity to design interventions that have a goodness of fit for the child and family (Pierce, 2003). To strengthen their therapeutic power, therapists need

© Rawpixel.com/Shutterstock.

399

to endeavor to practice with cultural sensitivity and ask questions about play from a cultural perspective, when working with children and families: What does play mean to this child? Is play important to this family? How does this child express play when free to do so? What does play "look like" in this community?

This chapter aims to explore play from an international cultural perspective, building on earlier content in this text. By taking an ecological approach, the chapter will examine play in relation to diverse sociocultural contexts from the child to the family and community, including policy. The meaning of play internationally across cultures will be explored and contextualized to understand cultural barriers and enablers of play that frame play-in-practice. Central to this analysis will be a focus on what play means to children themselves, as experts in their own lives. Current research evidence from occupational science and therapy will be used to inform the content, with examples from international play initiatives utilized to examine potential ways of expanding practice in the future, in an evidence-informed way. Before delving into the discussion of play internationally, however, some clarification of terminology is important, particularly in relation to culture.

Occupational Therapy Perspectives on Culture and Play

Culture can be defined as the passing on of specific attributes across generations based on beliefs and values, which are evident in *the habits, rituals, and practices of daily life* (Shonkoff & Phillips, 2000). Within the *Occupational Therapy Practice Framework*, 4th edition (OTPF4), habits and routines are known as *performance patterns*, whereby individuals and their occupational lives are influenced by their family and community contexts and cultural norms *over time* (American Occupational Therapy Association [AOTA], 2020). Hence, culture is not static, but rather it is a collective, dynamic phenomenon (Dickie, 2004; Hasselkus, 2002). It is constantly emergent, with evidence "that it is learned, shared, patterned, evaluative, and persistent but changeable" (Bonder et al., 2004, p. 159). Culture is inherently historical, located in tradition and folklore, and has a strong evolutionary character that requires an understanding of past as well as present influences. Therefore, the study of play in humans fundamentally requires a study of sociocultural and historical contexts. See **Box 15.1** for a reflection on the history of play and cultural values.

The profession of occupational therapy has long understood the need to be concerned with cultural competence and, more recently, cultural safety and humility (Hammell, 2013). Underpinning these concepts is the realization that occupational therapy practice is heavily influenced by Western, minority world values and traditions (Lindsay et al., 2014). In fact, little to date has been written about diverse sociocultural contexts and their influence on play as occupation, to inform the design of interventions that are tailored to the child. Perhaps due to the strong commitment to the psychological perspective of childhood in occupational therapy, with its associated normative approach, there is an acceptance that play is universal and does not need to be personalized. We have learned about the developmental sequences of social, cognitive, and object play (e.g., Parten, 1932;

Box 15.1 The Necessity of Understanding History in Relation to Studies of Play and Play Values

Research on play has been documented as part of the general exploration of ancient cultures and artifacts over centuries, such as those from the Indus valley civilization in Northern India from 2000 years BC, where it was found that play was a recognized part of childhood and provided for among that society, which is different to how it is valued there today (Oke et al., 1999). Similar variances over time were found from a review of multiple ethnographic studies of play, where Lancy cites a quote from the U.S. Department of Labor Children's Bureau in 1914 that spoke out against play, as being dangerous for babies, as it ruins their nerves (Wolfenstein, 1955, as cited in Lancy, 2007). However, Wolfenstein notes that whereas once play was considered wicked, then viewed as harmless, it has now become accepted as a duty for parents in some cultures.

Therefore, as an important point of reflection, any sociocultural study of play serves to illuminate only a given point in time and can be assumed to be evolving and changing even as the research paper is being published: The pace of change across societies has accelerated with the influence of globalization, new technologies, changing economies, and migrant communities, resulting in the need for ongoing and persistent study to capture and document the concurrent changing nature of play across culture and time.

See Toy Industry Europe for a timeline of the history of play (search the word "timeline" on the TIE website to access the pdf): https://www.toyindustries.eu/wp-content/uploads/2016/11/tie_toy_timeline_brochure_-_final_17_12_2013-1.pdf.

Piaget, 1962; Smilansky, 1968). Yet we also know from developmental studies of motor development that developmental sequences can differ across cultures (Adolph et al., 2010). Adolf et al.'s review of cross-cultural motor development research found that childrearing practices and contextual factors have a significant influence on motor development and consequently result in differing trajectories of development in different communities. Hence this evidence confirms and reaffirms basic principles of occupational science and therapy, that we need to consider specificity[1] as well as universality. We need to examine individuals in their contexts and explore the fit between the environment, the child, and the behavior, i.e., the person–environment–occupation transaction.

Considering the Occupation of Play from Contrasting Sociocultural Contexts

In occupational therapy, the concept of the developmental niche is often adopted to ensure that practice is culturally and contextually relevant. The developmental niche was coined by Super and Harkness (1986) to capture the embedded characteristics of family-centered, sociocultural practice and involves three main subsystems: "the physical and social setting in which the child lives, culturally regulated customs of childcare and childrearing, and the psychology of the caretakers" (Super & Harkness, 1986, p. 552). Examples of cultural attributes that may relate to play include parenting goals and expectations for their children, values related to routines and discipline, and gender roles and beliefs about play. Hence, central in any exploration of sociocultural perspectives on play is the examination of families and family occupations: doing, being, becoming, and belonging from the past into the present.

Play Materials Across Cultures and Family Occupations

Cultural studies of play have been conducted over recent decades by anthropologists, ethnographers, and folklorists such as Schwartzman (1979), Opie and Opie (1969), Whiting and Edwards (1992), and Gaskins, Haight, and Lancy (2007). Although multiple play forms (such as social play or object play)

have been studied with children across cultures, imaginative or pretend play is one play form that most clearly links with culture, due to the artifacts and materials associated with it. This is most apparent in studies where children commonly model adult activities within their culture, which is most observable in cultures that are less globalized with less exposure to products from the industrial world (Lancy, 2007). For example, in north Botswana cultures, in East Africa, and in Zanzibar, children were noted to play out adult rituals and routines such as debating, playing adult board games, cooking, or herding animals (Berinstein & Magalhaes, 2009; Chick, 2015). Similarly, in a New Guinea culture, Heider found that it was common for boys to play with spears and herd flowers representing animals, while Gosso identified that girls liked to play at pounding flour in north Brazil in a similar manner to the adults (Gosso, 2010; Heider, 1997). Hence, Chick noted that many of the objects for play were miniatures of the adult world and included toy bows and arrows, guns, vehicles, and kitchen utensils. See **Practice Opportunity 15.1** for an example of play reproducing cultural context.

Examples of objects used for play have been noted in many other studies also, where any object can become a plaything depending on what is available to the child (see **Figure 15.1**). For example, in Edwards' research across six cultures, children from the more subsistence agricultural cultures within Kenya, Mexico, Philippines, Japan, and India used predominantly natural materials for play compared to the more industrialized culture in the United States, where children had more commercial toys and play materials (Edwards, 2000). Similarly, in a study in India, children were observed to adapt their play and improvise with shells, bottle tops, tins, and household utensils, according to the affordances and availability of objects and spaces (Oke et al., 1999). From these findings across cultures, children's play consistently reflected the social culture within which the children played. Outcomes for children are that they can gain knowledge of cultural routines through play and therefore gain mastery of cultural processes: "Play serves as a mechanism through which children acquire the cultural values with which they construct and reconstruct their daily interactions" (Holmes, 2013, p. 8).

Aside from play with everyday objects and miniatures of adult tools, toys to support fantasy play were noted in Edwards' (2000) research. These commercial

[1] *Specificity* is the term used by many researchers of culture, including Adolph and Wachs, who sought to identify the influence of sociocultural contexts on child development (Wachs, 1987).

Practice Opportunity 15.1 Exploring Play in Cultural Contexts

When you read reports from children about their play, you can see inside their play worlds and begin to notice their cultural contexts. Here is an example from a group of children, ages 4 to 5 years, in San Juan, Puerto Rico, playing together in school:

> J. knocks on the door to a playhouse on the playground in which L., R., N., M., J., A1., & E. are hiding. A2. stands next to him at the door. "We're visiting," J. says. "Open up the door for visitors." Children inside the house scream and hold the door closed. "No, they're witches!" one child inside the house cries. "Witches!" several other children shout, laughing and screaming. "Open the door. We won't eat you," A2. says. "We aren't even hungry." He laughs. The children inside the house scream and laugh and hold the door closed. "It is witches!" one unidentified child shouts. "Hold the door!" (Trawick-Smith, 2010, p. 552).

Their play is focused on a common play event where children try to frighten each other, and in this case, it involves witches. Witches are a feature of many diverse cultures, have a historical and sometimes religious relevance, and, in children's fairy tales, often represent evil. In some cultures, witches are primarily regarded as being part of festivals such as Halloween. These children are reproducing their cultural contexts through their play and using a shared notion of what is scary to enhance the risk and excitement in their play.

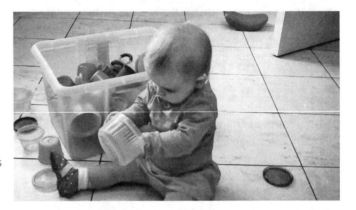

Figure 15.1 An Irish infant plays with kitchen containers. In this family context, the infant's mother keeps a box of small items for her child to play with, while she is working in the kitchen. Such orchestration of playspaces has been noted in many studies of family play, where play is enabled through strategies for inclusion or segregation. Segregation is the keeping of play activity separate from daily routines or housework while inclusion is the embedding of play in daily routines (Primeau, 1998)

Courtesy of Helen Lynch.

toys for play were more prevalent within cultures where children are given more novelty and stimulation and involved toys relating to heroes and magic carpets (Sutton-Smith, 1986). Other studies identified that toys were valued differently across cultures. For example, while digital toys were commonly valued in Japanese cultures, Ruckenstein noted in 2010 that in Nordic countries, they were seen as unnatural. So, toys have cultural characteristics that may not translate globally (Ruckenstein, 2010).

Adult–Child Play Across Cultures

Play is a universal phenomenon; however, adult–child play demonstrates both similarities and differences within and between cultures.

Similarities and Differences

While some of the ethnographic and anthropological research involved a significant focus on how and where children played, common across such studies is the cultural context of the family home, with a focus on adult–infant play in order to examine cultural scripts and developmental niches. Culture flows through communities primarily from parent to child; therefore, the study of the relationship between culture and play has focused extensively on the study of adult–child play, where play is shaped by the value or belief systems passed down or restructured across generations (Roopnarine, 2011). Hence while play in childhood is a focus of importance, it is evident that play is enacted within cultural contexts and can therefore be shaped and, as some researchers note, dominated by the adults within those worlds (Ramugondo, 2012).

Mother–infant play has been the most researched area of adult–child play to date. This form of play is common across cultures, especially in infancy but rare in many cultures beyond early childhood (Lancy, 2007) and differs across the world in terms of frequency. For example, in a study of mother–toddler play in Guatemala, Turkey, India, and the United States, researchers found that mothers in Guatemala were less likely to play with their toddlers compared to those from the United States and India (Göncü et al., 2000). In another study conducted by Lancy (2007), who reviewed evidence of mother–child play across 186 ethnographies, comparative differences were found across cultures of the game of peek-a-boo. Although there is no evidence to confirm peek-a-boo is a universal game, it is found across Europe, Japan, Brazil, India, Malaysia, South Africa, and America, among others (Fernald & O'Neill, 1993). In Lancy's review, it was common for mothers to play peek-a-boo-type games with their infants in Western societies; however, it was rare elsewhere. Yet, even among Western societies, there were differences where British mothers played fewer social games like peek-a-boo with their infants compared to American mothers (Lancy, 2007).

Although evidence shows variances across cultures, there can also be variances within the same geographical areas and within similar games or forms of play, depending on local and national value systems, among families and their communities. In a survey of cultural influences on parenting in the United States, researchers found that although all of the 1,615 parents lived in the same country, African American parents did not value routines as much as Hispanic parents did and had different expectations about when a child should be expected to take turns or to understand emotions (Spicer, 2010). The differences between cultures in the same country exist independent of the majority culture within a geographical setting. Therefore, parental practices are shaped by both community and cultural influences from within their own family communities, as well as within geographical communities (Bornstein et al., 2008; Göncü et al., 2000).

Environmental Influences

Multiple environmental influences have been identified that impact mother–infant play, including factors such as weather and the close presence of others in the social community (Lancy, 2007). For example, Inuit mothers were noted to play frequently with their infants due to the climate that restricted them to long periods indoors. Elsewhere, the influence of the proximity of the social community was evident in Central Africa, where adult–infant play was evident more than mother–infant play, among the whole of the foraging community, as the childcare was shared among the adults. This included men, which was not common in other cultures. This higher frequency of adult–child play was also evident in other foraging communities in Bengal, New Guinea, and South West Africa (Lancy, 2007). In contrast, in a nearby farming community where there were larger families, children played more together than with adults (Lancy, 2007). Similarly, in a U.S. study, Haight et al. (1999) found that children from Irish-American families sought more peer play than the Taiwanese children, who initiated more play with their caregivers than their peers (Bornstein et al., 2008). This seemed to be an outcome of having more peers to play with on a regular basis via informal playdates with neighbors and cousins who lived nearby. From these diverse studies it appears that children choose play partners based on proximity, availability, and willingness to play, irrespective of whether they are siblings, peers, parents, grandparents, or other adults (see **Figure 15.2**).

Adult Values in Relation to Play

From an international study of significant breadth and depth across 16 different nations, researchers found many similar trends across the four continents of North and South America, Europe, Asia, and Africa (Singer et al., 2009). Irrespective of geography, language, culture, or religious orientation, in this study of 2,400 mothers' perspectives on play, 77% wished they had more time to play with their children, while 87% wished their children had more opportunities for playing with their friends. So, despite the many differences across cultures, there is also a strong similar valuing of play and happiness in childhood.

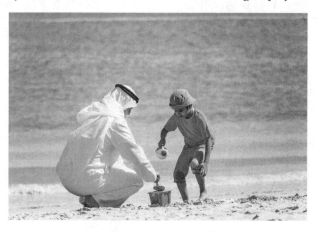

Figure 15.2 In this example of intergenerational play, a boy plays with his grandfather at the beach in Saudi Arabia
© oonal/E+/Getty Images.

Multiple studies have identified similarities across cultures whereby play is valued for supporting a child's learning. For example, in a cross-cultural study between Turkey and Norway, researchers found that although some cultural differences existed, parents of preschoolers in both cultures agreed that play was important for learning and development (Ivrendi et al., 2019). In several studies with parents in the United States, evidence shows that play was prioritized as the preferred route for learning rather than direct teaching in infancy (Bornstein et al., 1999), with parents typically stressing the cognitive values of play most of all (Roopnarine et al., 1993). This was also evident among parents from Ireland in other studies, where play was considered important to support child development (Bornstein et al., 1999; Coughlan & Lynch, 2011). Overall, it appears that cultural groups who are aligned with more advanced technological cultures are most consistent in associating play with its role in child development (Roopnarine, 2011).

With this cultural context in mind, it is not surprising therefore that researchers have found that structured play routines involving the adult and child together have become more prevalent. By striving to enhance their child's play, adults in more advanced technological cultures are increasingly taking part in play unlike in earlier generations. Lancy notes that parents in the United States, Europe, and Asia seem to be "duty bound to carefully orchestrate their child's play curriculum" (Lancy, 2007, p. 279), as evidenced in the high frequency of bedtime reading, structured afterschool activities, and organized sports with an associated commercialization of childhood (Haight & Miller, 1993). In these cultural contexts, which are frequently in countries with a longer history of industrial development, the general consensus is that adult–infant play and, in particular, mother–infant play serves to enhance the child's learning specifically around literacy and intellectual development. So, it is evident that when the purpose of the play occupation in families is play for learning, the play form appears to become more structured.

From the adult–child play research evidence, it is evident that play is valued differently across cultures and is not only associated with learning and development. In one study, parents in Turkey valued play for learning as noted earlier, but they also valued play for the opportunities it provided for keeping children occupied (Ivrendi et al., 2019). In another study in India, researchers found that Indian parents in New Delhi played with their children for enjoyment (Roopnarine et al., 1993). Other studies have found more implicit reasons for mother–child play based on sociocultural values. For example, in studies with Taiwanese mothers, researchers found a particular emphasis on pretend play, whereby the mother used this form of play to influence the child's awareness of social norms (Haight et al., 1999). Similar findings were found in studies among Chinese, Japanese, and Korean cultures, where play was often the medium through which mothers established a strong bond with the child, a task that was considered essential if she was to socialize the child into the community, which was her role culturally (Lancy, 2007). Consequently, it is clear from these studies that it is important to understand the meaning of play among mothers in order to understand the performance patterns of play in families.

Yet studies also show that in some cultures, play is not always considered important. As infants grow into toddlers and children, play appears to diminish in many cultures, especially where children are required to become workers sooner, become involved in childcare of younger siblings, or take on other culturally valued roles. In cultures from South America or Polynesia, this was common. In a cross-cultural study across four cultures, researchers found that play was tolerated but not encouraged by adults in one community in Mexico; play was neither encouraged nor discouraged by adults in India; and play was actively encouraged by adults in Japan and the United States (Whiting & Edwards, 1992). In another study, it was found that some Guatemalan and Mayan cultures did not value play as a family activity[2] and hence did not orchestrate play activities between parent and child (Bazyk et al., 2003; Rogoff, 1993, 2003). In the Mayan study, the origin of this cultural perspective appears to be linked to values on family life, where "the ideal [Mayan] child is hardworking, obedient, and responsible; he does not waste his time in play" (Modiani, 1973, p. 55). Based on this evidence, the consequence is that childhood can be shorter in some cultures than others (Sutton-Smith, 1993).

While children in North American or European contexts, in contrast, may not be viewed as workers at such a young age, they do, however, grow up in cultures that demand academic achievement, which has been a noted factor in changing the shape of adult–child play (Singer et al., 2009). As noted earlier, children in these progress-oriented cultures are more typically scheduled for structured play or learning activities rather than able to access free, unstructured

---

[2] Yet, it is also important to note that, in these studies, the children still played. The child's perspective on play across cultures will be explored in the next section.

play outdoors. This approach to play is deemed to be evidence of hothousing children for society's benefit (Sutton-Smith, 1994), which can equally result in shortening of childhood.

Outdoor play has evolved as a particular aspect of cultural variance at a family and societal level. In some cultures, outdoor play was valued for the opportunity it gave children to use up energy (Ivrendi et al., 2019). However, in cultures such as Australia, Canada, and the United States, outdoor play has become a point of contention. The overriding issue for parents has moved away from valuing active outdoor play, to worrying about hazards in the environment. This has resulted in parents placing restrictions on their children's independent mobility outdoors, with the consequence of restricting licenses to play (Hasluck & Malone, 1999; Hirsch-Pasek et al., 2009; Malone, 2007; Tranter & Pawson, 2001). Given the global nature of media and news reports, there appears to be a heightened awareness of hazards related to road traffic accidents, abductions, and gang violence, for example, that has resulted in an unquestioning acceptance of danger that is over and above the actual risk (Gray, 2011). In response to this significant shift of attitudes toward outdoor play, efforts to examine risk and promote rich-risk play have become more prevalent in research for health promotion to counteract the negative attitudes in society (e.g., Brussoni et al., 2015; Sandseter, 2007). Yet interestingly, risky play was not a recognized play category until recent decades and appears to have emerged as a counterresponse to sociocultural contexts of modern life (Sandseter, 2019). This changing view of outdoor play's risk and benefit is a good example of how play evolves across generations and contexts.

Values and attitudes to play evolve and align with more dominant cultural scripts, which some researchers have explored using concepts relating to views of collectivism or individualism. These concepts refer to both ends of a spectrum of societal values, where an individualistic society values and promotes independence and autonomy, compared to a collectivist society that values social interdependence more (Bornstein et al., 1999). Bornstein et al. identified that U.S. society scores highest for individualism compared to 20 other countries, and this societal difference impacts on play. These findings were characterized in their study of play between U.S. and Argentinean cultures, where Argentinean mothers tended to emphasize socialization in their play compared to U.S. mothers, who focused on functional use of toys and independence. The interpretation of such findings is that cultures that are

deemed more collectivist in nature are seen to use more physical contact and stimulation than individualist cultures that rely more on object play and visual contact (Kärtner et al., 2008). As noted earlier, while such perspectives on culture can be useful to differentiate values and predict behaviors, it needs careful application, as the reality is that cultural differences exist *within* as well as *between* societies (Göncü et al., 2000). It is important that occupational therapy practitioners use this knowledge to inform their practice (see **Box 15.2** for a summary of considerations for addressing family perspectives on play in diverse cultures).

Box 15.2 Considerations for Occupational Therapy in Addressing a Family's Perspective on Play in Diverse Cultures

1. Play appears to be universally accepted by adults as a way that children have fun. However, this does not mean that play is universally valued among adults or for the same reasons.
2. Beyond more industrialized cultures, parent–infant play is quite rare (Lancy, 2007).
3. In many cultures, play belongs in early childhood (0–8 years), and beyond that, children are expected to help with housework, caring for younger siblings, and other valued daily routines.

In more industrialized cultures, adults value play for learning and tend to engage in more frequent structured forms of play with the child in response to this cultural value.

Children's Co-Construction of Culture and Play

Another way play is evident across cultures is within the culture of childhood itself. Children's play generates and forms a culture of childhood, with its own rituals, norms, and values, evident in shared games and rules, rhymes and songs, and favored characters in stories. So, while the study of play in families and among adult–child interactions tells us how children are assimilated into family and community cultures in their play, there is an equal need to explore how children shape and reconstruct culture within childhood among peers (Gosso & Carvalho, 2013). Indeed, some researchers have found that children find their way to play through siblings and peers rather than parents in many cultures (see **Figure 15.3**) (Roopnarine & Krishnakumar, 2006).

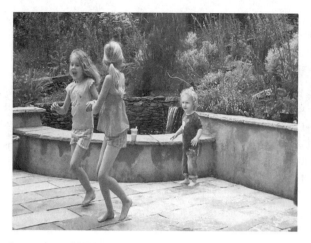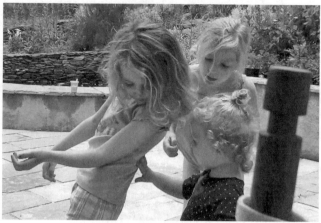

Figure 15.3 Children finding the way to play via peers

Courtesy of Helen Lynch.

Central to the pursuit of understanding a child's view of play is the question: What is play? Is soccer a form of play? Can schoolwork be play? The answer for a child-centered profession like occupational therapy lies within research that seeks to find the answer from the children themselves, as play can only be truly understood from the perspective of the player and is frequently misunderstood by practitioners who overlook this imperative (McInnes, 2019).

Yet to date, evidence from children is harder to locate, and instead, adult voices predominate as proxies for the child, or in lieu of children's perspectives. The result as noted earlier is the heavy focus on the productive value of play, rather than a focus on understanding the occupation of play from the players' experience. This gap is an important one that warrants serious attention. The underrepresentation of children's voices in research is complex but primarily due to the lack of commitment to establishing the child's perspective as an important concern, alongside the challenges in developing child-centered, participatory methods, combined with the ethical barriers of consent and assent. Traditionally, in research, the overreliance on interviews and the spoken word to elicit data is restrictive for many children, who use other forms of communication more effectively (Lynch, 2018; Lynch & Stanley, 2017), and has resulted in excluding, in particular, younger children and children with disabilities (Wickenden & Kembhavi-Tam, 2014). In recent times, researchers have developed more authentic child-centered approaches that include the use of diverse methods to maximize the "voice" of the child, including the following: photovoice, focus groups with arts-based methods and storytelling, behavioral mapping, time-use and play diaries, mosaic methods, and including

child participation in research design and coding (e.g., Berinstein & Magalhaes, 2009; Glenn et al., 2012; King & Howard, 2014; Lynch, 2009; Moore & Lynch, 2018a; Spitzer, 2003). The following section explores play research from the child's perspective, drawing evidence from studies conducted with children in different cultures across five continents (see **Table 15.1**). Guided by Miller and Kuhaneck (2008), the findings are organized into four main areas: (a) the meaning of play for children, (b) play forms, (c) with whom children like to play, and (d) the context of where children like to play. Common to the studies is that all children played, irrespective of whether they had multiple or minimal resources in terms of space, objects, or others with whom to play. Despite many similarities in children's views of play, these perspectives may conflict with adult perspectives. Occupational therapy practitioners can use this knowledge to help identify the play perspectives of children from diverse cultures and to negotiate conflicting views with parents and other adults.

The Meaning of Play for Children

When children were asked what play meant to them or to describe its place in their lives, they reported that it is enjoyable (Brockman Jago & Fox 2011) and fun (Miller & Kuhaneck, 2008; Nicholson et al., 2014), gives them a sense of belonging (Promona et al., 2019), makes them happy (Liu-Yan et al., 2005; Moore & Lynch, 2018a), is planned by children (Ivrendi et al., 2019), is mostly unstructured (Nicholson et al., 2014), and might not have a purpose but is more about the process than the outcome (Glenn et al., 2012). For children with disabilities, similar meanings have been identified,

Table 15.1 Selected Research on the Meaning of Play for Children in Different Cultures

Study Location	Authors	Children's Demographics	Study Aim	Methods	Play Findings
Australia	Howard, Jenvey, & Hill (2006)	92 children 4–6 years	Explore children's categorization of play and learning based on social context	24 cards depicting activities for children to sort	Children associated teacher absence with play in preschool. They chose pictures of play with others predominantly.
Canada	Glenn, Knight, Holt, & Spence (2012)	38 students 7–9 years	Explore what play means to children	Focus groups with multiple methods, including arts-based, group activities, and storytelling	Anything can be a play opportunity, and play can happen anywhere. Play includes four types: active, creative, games, and social activities.
China	Liu-Yan, Yuejuan, & Hongfen (2005)	150 children in 15 kindergartens 5–6 years	Explore children's perceptions of play	Photo classification using 22 photos and interviews	Majority of children (57%) prefer learning knowledge than playing. Play was mostly associated with the presence of toys, the absence of teachers, feelings of happiness, and freedom.
Greece	Prompona, Papoudi, & Papadopoulou (2019)	82 children 6–12 years	Explore the meaning of play during recess	Focus groups	Four main themes emerged: socializing, freedom and choice, personal satisfaction, and intense feelings and struggle.
Iceland	Norðdahl & Einarsdóttir (2015)	200 children 4–9 years	Explore children's preferences about outdoor play and playspaces in school playground	Observations and interviews	Children want diversity in play opportunities; physical challenge; to be secure and to explore; to play with others and find a "nest" (i.e., a secret place out of sight, a hideaway); and to enjoy beautiful things.

(continues)

Table 15.1 Selected Research on the Meaning of Play for Children in Different Cultures   (continued)

Study Location	Authors	Children's Demographics	Study Aim	Methods	Play Findings
India	Oke, Khattear, Pant, & Saraswathi (1999)	240 children 6–12 years	Explore the effect of urban environments on children's play	Observations of 340 episodes of play and interviews	Children played with whomever and whatever was available to them. Children preferred playing with their own age group or similar gender if they had the opportunity.
Ireland	Lynch (2009)	34 children 5–8 years	Explore patterns of occupation among children	Time diaries and observations	Highest preferences were for unstructured social and physical play while playing outside.
	Moore & Lynch (2018)	31 children 6–8 years	Explore fun and happiness as a proxy of well-being	Mosaic methods	Children identified the importance of play, people, and place as contributing to well-being.
Puerto Rico	Trawick-Smith (2010)	49 children 4–5 years	Explore nature of play	Observations in school setting	Prevalence of motor play as a dominant form alongside music and construction play.
Sweden	Prellwitz & Skär (2007)	20 children 7–12 years	Explore how children of diverse abilities use playgrounds for play	Interviews	Playgrounds are valued places for private and group play and a place for friends. Swings are the most important ____. Challenge and risk was valued by children of all abilities.
Turkey and Norway	Ivrendi, Cevher-Kalburan, Sandseter, Storli, & Siversten (2019)	40 children in preschool 4–6 years	Explore how play is defined by children across two cultures; examine differences in play preferences across two cultures	Interviews using a game format	In both countries, children defined play according to what they do (play with toys or in places for play), alongside feelings (fun) and types of play (action, social, imagination).

Study Location	Authors	Children's Demographics	Study Aim	Methods	Play Findings
Uganda	Njelesani, Sedgwick, Davis, & Polatajko (2011)	Approximately 100 children between infancy and prepubescence	Explore outdoor play among a community of children	Naturalistic observation	Children chose to engage in active and creative play with objects and with each other, including imaginative, social, and physical play.
UK (England and Wales)	Brockman, Fox, & Jago (2011)	77 children, 10–11 years	Explore children's perceptions of active play	Focus groups	Play is doing what you want such as running around, hanging out with friends or siblings, and unstructured free play.
	King & Howard (2014)	22 children 6–11 years	Examine children's perception of choice in their free play at home, school and after-school club	Use of a "Play Detective Diary"	Physical activity play with footballs and skipping ropes were the most popular forms of play. In all three environments, play was influenced by policy and license/ permission for play.
United States	Nicholson et al., (2014)	98 children 3–17 years	Examine how children describe play in their lives	Interviews	Children's play preferences favored outdoor play, relationships, and toys.
	Miller & Kuhaneck (2008)	10 children 7–11 years	Explore children's perceptions of play and play preferences	Interviews	Four main categories emerged relating to play: activity, relational, child, and contextual characteristics.
Zanzibar	Berinstein & Magalhaes (2009)	16 children ages 10–12 years	Explore meaning of play	Photovoice using photography and focus groups	Creative, physical, and free-play football were most favored play forms. Social play was most valued with no adult involvement.

where play is considered as something enjoyable and fun, makes them feel positive (Graham et al., 2017), and is self-controlled and related to a lack of stress or worry (Pollock et al., 1997). Glenn et al. found that when Canadian children in their study described an activity as fun, it was consequently considered play. Hence, the critical role of fun in play appears to be a consistent feature across cultures.

Yet play did not always relate to the expression of laughter or high spiritedness. Play was also described by children in the United States as something that requires concentration and was related to challenge and not being too easy or hard (Miller & Kuhaneck, 2008). This balance between easy and hard or challenge and security was also noted in an Icelandic study, where children valued challenge, but mostly when they also were feeling secure in their risk-taking (Norðdahl & Einarsdóttir, 2015). For children with disabilities in Sweden, play in playgrounds was about something being a challenge as well as fun (Prellwitz & Skär, 2007). This characteristic of being a challenge was associated with mastery. For example, in a study from Ireland, play was associated with activities that gave children a sense of achievement such as doing math (Moore & Lynch, 2018a). The link with play and learning was also a factor in Liu-Yan et al.'s study (2005). In their research with kindergarteners in China, the majority of children (57%) valued learning more than playing. The authors noted that this reflects the traditional beliefs about the importance of academic learning within Chinese culture (Liu-Yan et al., 2005). However, it may be that children in certain cultures view learning as part of play and vice versa, or as a totally separate activity and experience. As noted in Chapter 1, due to this variance of what is work or learning versus what is play, many play scholars propose the need to consider play as a continuum that ranges from being most to least playful (Bundy, 1997; Pellegrini, 1991; Wing, 1995).

Other forms of play have particular meaning within cultures due to their historical and cultural significance and are associated with developing valued self-identity within that culture. For example, in a study of older children in Zanzibar (ages 10 to 12 years), children played free-play football, which was highly valued (Berinstein & Magalhaes, 2009). In this culture, football was introduced during British colonization, evolved into an important aspect of Zanzibar society, and remains embedded in Zanzibar culture. In contrast, in another country

where colonization was experienced, an alternative outcome is evident. In studies of children from Ireland, children spoke of playing hurling as a favored play activity (Lynch, 2009). Hurling is a traditional Irish game that has been documented since the Middle Ages and is played in Ireland with a stick and small ball. The game of hurling was banned for many years during British colonization in Ireland but then revived in the 1880s by a sporting and cultural organization who tried to protect Irish cultural traditions. Since then it has become one of the top sports in Ireland and has a valued historical and cultural significance in Irish childhoods (see **Figure 15.4**).

However, for some children the meaning of play is not always associated with happiness and fun. In Prellwitz and Skär's study (2007), a group of Swedish children with disabilities (some with visual impairment and others with developmental disabilities) talked of feeling afraid to try playground equipment if other children were there due to their fear of being teased. Yet for them, the playground was still a special place for play that they valued. Similarly, in one UK study with children with physical disabilities, children said that sometimes play was not fun, that they could be excluded, and they often felt that no one wanted to play with them (Graham et al., 2017). It is apparent that play in childhood therefore has a significant contribution to make for well-being and belonging. Especially in social spaces for play, children need to know they are safe emotionally as well as socially and physically.

Finally, the meaning of play for children is also captured in studies that asked what they considered was "not play." In Glenn's study in Canada, even though almost anything could be a play opportunity, these children also considered what was not play. Similar to Miller and Kuhaneck's U.S. study (2008), this included watching television, which some said was boring. However, others included television as a play activity when it was related to a specific play-related event.

Play Forms

Studies of outdoor play across cultures have shown that play forms appear to be quite universal despite varied levels of socioeconomic advantage or disadvantage. For example, in the study of older children in Zanzibar, key play forms were identified for 16 children living in challenging circumstances due to poverty (Berinstein & Magalhaes, 2009). Imaginative

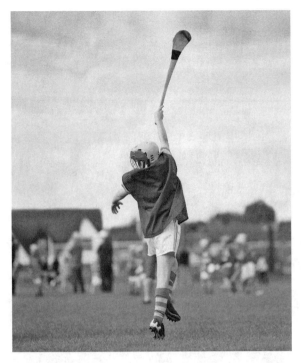

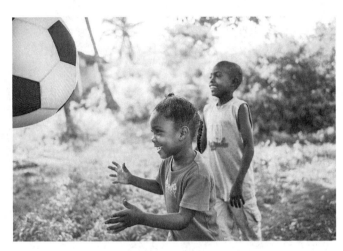

Figure 15.4 Play can have significant historical meaning in communities such as playing hurling in Ireland and soccer in Zanzibar

play, physical play, and games such as free-play football were evident, all using available resources such as sticks and loose parts. Like other studies of children from varied socioeconomic contexts in Ireland (Lynch, 2009), the UK (King & Howard, 2014), and the United States (Miller & Kuhaneck, 2008), all children spoke of playing free-play outdoor sports (like football and hurling) as favored play activities. Having space to play and gather, with a simple ball or stick enabled these forms of play to become universally accessible to diverse socioeconomic communities, in diverse cultures.

From the studies in this review, the forms of outdoor play reported by children were typically free-play unstructured sports taking place with peers and excluding adults (Berinstein & Magalhaes, 2009; King & Howard, 2014; Lynch, 2009; Miller & Kuhaneck, 2008). This is an important issue, as in some studies, sport has been named by children as a form of play but analyzed by researchers as a nonplay activity because it is typically an adult-led occupation involving structured training (Holt et al., 2008). Therefore, when analyzing how children communicate about play, it is important to explore what they mean by the activities they name to ensure that we as adults understand their meaning.

Adults and children differ in how they name play activities and what they mean by them. For example, from the child's perspective, they often described their play as simply "playing outside," which has been noted in studies in the UK, Ireland, and Sweden (Brockman Fox & Jago., 2011; Lynch, 2009; Prellwitz & Skär, 2007; see **Figure 15.5**), while in an observational study in Uganda, the children were observed to be simply "hanging out'" (Njelesani et al., 2011). Although these forms of play can be deemed as passive play by adults, they are more accurately defined as unstructured play, which is noted to be crucial for child health and well-being (Canadian Public Health Association [CPHA], 2019).

Some studies have identified the popularity of play forms rarely included in common play categorizations (e.g., Garvey, 1990; Piaget, 1962). For example, in a study with preschoolers in Puerto Rico, the researcher observed a high level of music play that included chanting, playground singing, and rhymes for use with skipping (Trawick-Smith, 2010). In addition, children in this study played using a high level of teasing and humor to the extent that the researcher categorized it as a form of play in its own right. He argued for more detailed research to be conducted to explore this underexplored play form further across diverse cultures.

Overall, it is clear that more studies of play occupation from a child's perspective are needed. As Sutton-Smith argues, many of the categorizations of play come more from an adult's need to categories rather than

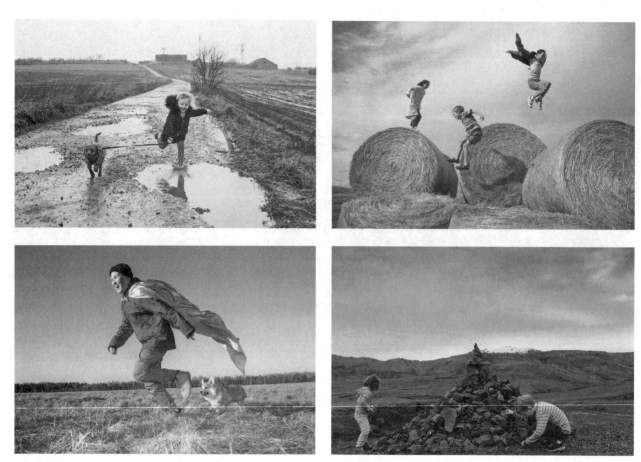

Figure 15.5 "Playing outside" includes "running through puddles" game in the Netherlands, "jumping over bales" game in Montana, "I'm a superhero" game in the Steppes, and "making a stone fort" game in Iceland

Top left: © Sally Anscombe/DigitalVision/Getty Images; Top right: © Zia Soleil/Stone/Getty Images; Bottom left: © Westend61/Getty Images; and Bottom right: © Cavan Images/Cavan/Getty Images.

viewing play from a child's perspective (Sutton-Smith, 1986). While developmental play research has elicited many forms of play such as object play or social play, researching with children illuminates other play forms such as hanging out play or music play that are relatively underexplored to date. Unlike adult activities, play occupations are not always given a name or evident in terms of their form or meaning, and there is a need for more in-depth analysis of childhood play occupations from the child's perspective (Hocking, 2009; Humphry, 2009; Lynch & Moore, 2016). When working with children, occupational therapists must be open to recognize play in diverse and unexpected forms.

Context: Where Children Like to Play

According to Senda (as cited in Drianda & Kinoshita, 2015), the environment provides children with six main forms of play spaces: (1) nature, (2) open spaces, (3) streetscapes, (4) anarchy space, (5) hideout or secret spaces, and (6) structured spaces such as playgrounds. The majority of these relate to outdoor play, which has been identified as the most common preferred space for children to play and influences play in specific ways, suggesting it be assessed and utilized in intervention. Studies with children in North America and Europe have consistently reported that they prefer to play outside where they can play more actively and freely (e.g., Glenn et al., 2012; Kilkelly et al., 2015; Norðdahl & Einarsdóttir, 2015). This preference for outdoor freedom for play has also been noted in a study with children with autism spectrum disorder (ASD) in Ireland, where the freedom to play outside in nature without judgment was also a factor (Blake et al., 2018). Outdoor play is typically more active and consists of a higher level of physical activity play and risky play than that of indoor play (Oke et al., 1999; Stephenson, 2002). It also tends to be less influenced by adult oversight and supervision, thus allowing more freedom. Yet outdoor play is not always about intensive physical activity play. It has also been noted as a place where play can be more flexible, with opportunities to build hideaways and create secret spaces like nests in the middle of a flattened area of tall grass or underneath hedgerows (Norðdahl & Einarsdóttir, 2015).

Some studies have identified that weather influences play more than the places in which play happens. For example, children in Glenn et al.'s (2012) study who live in Canada spoke of their preferences to play outside even when the weather is cold or snowy. In contrast, in a national study of what it is like to be a child in Ireland, 18% of children (*n* = 9,794) voted that bad weather was the second-worst thing for children living in Ireland because the cold, wet weather stopped them from playing outside. Many wished for snow instead of rain (Coyne et al., 2012).

Relational: Who Children Like to Play With

Common also across these studies is the fact that when children talk of playing with others, they do not usually include parents or other adults, but rather talk of play that is planned and executed by children themselves. Play appeared to be linked more closely with social play with other peers, siblings, or cousins but not adults. This was evident in Zanzibar (Berinstein & Magalhaes, 2009), the United States (Miller & Kuhaneck, 2008), Canada (Glenn et al., 2012), and the UK (Brockman Fox & Jago, 2011) and was evident among Australian children as young as 4 in preschool (Howard et al., 2006). The children in the Zanzibar study valued playing together without adult involvement and the freedom of doing what they wanted. In one study in India, peer play was similarly valued, especially if it was with others close in age or of a similar gender; however, these children were seen to play with whomever was available among their group of peers (Oke et al., 1999). In some studies, children included pets as play partners also (Moore & Lynch, 2018a). However, play was not always social, and many children also spoke of valuing playing alone. Certainly, peer play is important to consider if occupational therapists are truly to address play for children of diverse cultures.

"Good Versus Bad" Play: When Children and Adult Play Cultures Clash

Some forms of play are documented by children as important but not valued by adults. According to the children in many play studies, adults have a different view on play than they have, resulting in differences in priorities and play agendas. For example, risky play is highly valued by children, across studies in Ireland, Australia, Sweden, Greece, and Norway (Hinchion et al., 2021; Little & Eager, 2010; Prellwitz & Skär, 2007; Promona et al., 2019; Sandseter, 2010; Yates & Oates, 2019), although children do not use this term themselves. Instead, they talk about play that affords adventure and excitement,

or something that "tickles their tummy!" (Sandseter, 2010). From an adult perspective as noted earlier, parents across many cultures are becoming overly protective toward children's risky play. This has resulted in parents taking a restrictive approach (Oke et al., 1999) and limiting this form of play. Yet an Australian study with 38 4- to 5-year-old children showed that these children had developed an ability to appraise risk and make appropriate judgements regarding their risky play, showing due caution when it was required (Little & Wyver, 2010). Parents restricting outdoor play was viewed by children in Canada as a barrier to participation and was attributed to their parents' fear for safety (Glenn et al., 2012). Therefore, protection is a significant reason why parents can hold opposite views to the child about what form of play is "good" versus "bad."

Overall, studies in Canada and the United States have found that as children mature, their understanding of play becomes increasingly different to the adult's perspective and is often a point of tension between adult and child (Glenn et al., 2012; Nicholson et al., 2014). For example, an area of play that can cause tension between adults and children is around playing video games due to the lack of perceived value among parents. In a Canadian study, this was noted as one of the main differences between adults' and children's perspectives (Glenn et al., 2012), where children valued video games for their excitement in contrast to the adults, who restricted their use based on national guidelines on sedentary behavior (i.e., Tremblay et al., 2011). In this case, it seems that parents restricted video game play due to the developing research that shows how it can negatively impact on health and well-being, which has become an increasing public health concern (CRC, 2013).

Other forms of play have also been contentious. For example, playing with guns and war games in real time and not just on the screen is a common concern in many cultures, yet research has shown that children often use play to make sense of violent events through this type of play, which is important for their mental health (Delaney, 2017). However, it seems that adult carers or parents often lack this play knowledge. The result is that adults place restrictions on the child's license to play certain forms of play. Interestingly, this point of tension became a form of play in itself for children in Greece, where they identified that disputing the adult's authority during recess at school was itself fun and part of their risky play (Promona et al., 2019). Clearly, as children grow, their sense of autonomy and need for freedom to play increases, but often in opposition to adult approval.

Sociocultural perspectives on play also bring insights into how sociocultural values and attitudes are in themselves barriers to play, especially in relation to children with disabilities. In Farrugia's study in Australia, parents spoke of being viewed as bad parents with naughty children and receiving glares and stares in public when their child with ASD behaved inappropriately (Farrugia, 2009). The inappropriate behavior may have involved repetitive patterns of movement or unusual fear reactions to some sensory experiences, which is often how children with ASD respond and express their play. However, these forms of play expression are often deemed inappropriate in many sociocultural settings. Sociocultural contexts by their very nature evolve from shared values and attitudes in communities and include shared understanding about what is acceptable behavior in public settings. Yet, the play expression of children with ASD appears to be unaccepted in some cultures, and many families of children with ASD are left dealing with feelings of exclusion from community play settings. For example, in one study of five families of preschool children with ASD, parents spoke of feeling unwelcome and unsafe in their community playgrounds due to other adult responses to their child's unusual play behaviors (Blake et al., 2018). Like the Australian study (Farrugia, 2009), this sense of being unwelcome resulted in them avoiding public situations and the ensuing pain of stigma. The outcome for many families of children with disabilities is that they experience occupational apartheid based on societal prejudices about their right to share culturally valued occupations together (Wilcock & Hocking, 2015).

Although there is little evidence to date about what play means to children with ASD, there have been some studies with adults who have ASD about their memories of childhood. In Conn's work on adult autobiographies, she found common themes across studies whereby adults with ASD spoke of remembering the intense pleasure and fun they experienced from their childhood play, e.g.: 'the physical thrill from running on the lines of tennis courts … the ecstasy attack of listening to flour-and-water paste being stirred' (Conn, 2015, p. 1197). These play memories differ from the forms of play that children have reported earlier in this chapter. Yet this study informs us that across many autobiographies of people with ASD, a unique play culture is apparent, and Conn argues for the need to respect this play culture in its own right. To date, few studies have examined play forms and subcultures among children with diverse abilities, and it is an emergent area of concern if we are to truly understand play in childhood. As a result, occupational therapists often explore new play forms and negotiate subcultures of children with diverse abilities in the context of practice.

To conclude, play from a child's perspective is a highly valued occupation. While it is associated with fun, it includes a range of important characteristics, including concentration, challenge, mastery, learning, freedom, and autonomy. It is not surprising why some play scholars describe play as being about serious fun because it is about taking fun seriously. See **Box 15.3** for a summary of children's perspectives on play in diverse cultures to inform practice when addressing play.

Box 15.3 Considering Children's Perspectives About Play from Diverse Cultures

- Play occupation is what makes us happy and feel good.
- Play usually happens when there are no adults.
- Play is something we decide for ourselves and is most fun when it is unstructured.
- The opposite of play is boredom.
- Playing outside is highly favored and usually preferred to indoor play when it is free of hazards and there are nearby friends to play with.
- Playing with friends is highly favored but not the only way to play.
- Sometimes we like to play in ways adults do not agree with. We like to take risks, play online, and play in a way that makes us feel good.
- We may name our play differently than adults do.

Policy Perspective: International to National Policy

While the chapter thus far has reviewed evidence of play from adult and child perspectives in the micro system of the home and community context, this next section addresses macro-level issues concerning play policy. As occupational therapists, there is an equal need to consider the child and family not just in relation to their home and community contexts, but also in relation to examining how play and childhood is addressed at a political and government level, as an issue of occupational justice. More specifically, "occupational therapists round the world are obliged to promote occupational rights as an actualization of human rights" (World Federation of Occupational Therapists [WFOT], 2019, p. 1).

International Policy

The study of play as an issue of occupational justice and human rights is informed by the international policy context, which has arisen from the realization that childhood is frequently under threat from humanitarian crises, poverty, disability, and migration among other factors that lead to exclusion and deprivation. Consequently, child human rights are important to protect children and are established internationally primarily from the United Nations Convention on the Rights of the Child ([UNCRC], 1989). Within this UN convention, there are 54 articles, which can be grouped into the following three general areas of concern: protection, participation, and provision (often called the 3-Ps) (Lester & Russell, 2010). Play is included as a human right in article 31 of the UNCRC and is detailed as the right "to engage in play and recreational activities appropriate to the age of the child and to participate freely in cultural life and the arts" (article 31, p. 9). In addition, article 31 states that governments need to provide for play and leisure as an issue of equality because all children have a right to participate in these occupations of childhood on an equal basis. Therefore, article 31 is part of the group of participation rights of children, and the consequences of this right are that governments are required to provide for play.

It is important to note that not all governments across the world have ratified the convention on the rights of the child (the United States being one example). Nonetheless the principles of children's rights are internationally acknowledged, and the UNCRC provides practitioners with guidance for enabling play according to local cultural contexts. Primarily it identifies key areas for consideration, largely related to play advocacy and provision. Some countries such as Belgium, Norway, and Spain have incorporated aspects of the UNCRC into law (Lundy et al., 2012). Others have used it to inform good practice such as Turkey, where the government followed ratification of the UNCRC by supporting national education institutions to work according to play-based learning in early years (Ivrendi et al., 2019).

Yet, despite the almost universal international ratification of the UNCRC in countries around the world, the UN found that the right to play was not being taken seriously, and in 2012–2013 a group came together to draft a General Comment to advance the implementation of this right to play.[3] Consequently, General Comment 17 was developed and published in 2013 to help support the international community to provide for play more effectively (see http://ipaworld.org/ipa-video-this-is-me-the-childs-right-to-play/) (CRC, 2013).

General Comment 17 offers us further insight into potential barriers to participation and solutions

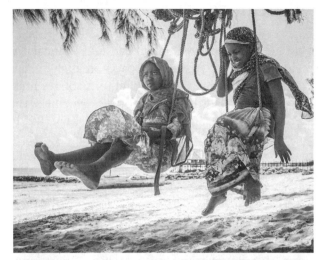

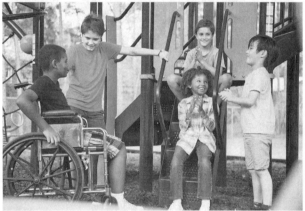

Figure 15.6 Children are at risk of play deprivation in many cultures due to gender or disability
Top: © Jasmin Merdan/Moment/Getty Images; Bottom: © fstop123/E+/Getty Images.

for play. Barriers that are identified in this document include the overemphasis on safety over provision of risk-rich play, the resistance in many urban areas to the presence of children, and lack of access to nature in many contexts. In addition, General Comment 17 identified specific groups of children who are more at risk of play deprivation, based on gender (i.e., girls), ethnicity, migration, disability, or poverty, among other aspects (see **Figure 15.6**). General Comment 17 went on to outline obligations that governments are duty bound to follow relating to nondiscrimination and regulation. This includes the need to ensure, for example, that all play and recreational areas are accessible and that all planning and development of play facilities should be done in collaboration with children themselves. Significantly, universal design was proposed as the approach of choice to address

---

[3] General Comments are typically developed over time in response to the review process that is built into the implementation and review of the UNCRC by the UN. General Comments often seek to clarify the reporting duties of state parties with respect to certain provisions and provide extra guidance by suggesting approaches to their implementation. For details, see https://www.ohchr.org/EN/HRBodies/Pages/TBGlossary.aspx#gc.

design for inclusion in playgrounds. This has led to renewed interest among occupational therapists to examine how universal design can inform inclusive play design and to ensure playspaces are high in play value, which is an underexplored area of research (e.g., Lynch et al., 2019a; Moore & Lynch, 2015; Moore et al., 2020; Prellwitz & Lynch, 2018). Readers are referred to other summary articles for further exploration of children's rights documents and the place of play within them (e.g., Lynch & Moore, 2018; McKendrick et al., 2018).

There have been some critiques of the UNCRC and the assertion of the right to play. This criticism has come from those concerned with the universal assumptions about family life, childrearing, child development, and best practice (Lancy, 2007; Monaghan, 2012). There is a need to ensure that any responses to play provision are culturally relative and not universally applied as one size does not fit all. In these critiques, the pressing issue of concern is the need to include diverse perspectives and variations of sociocultural childhoods to balance the normative development perspective that typically dominates many approaches to service delivery in childhood.

National Policies

Even though the UNCRC is ratified in most countries across the world, it is difficult to determine how play is addressed in policy at national levels. Consequently in 2017–2018, a study was conducted to explore play policy in Europe for children with disabilities. From a play policy review across 28 European countries, the researchers found that European states have progressed policy and the rights of the child to play in different ways. However, few states had developed specific play policies, and few had established guidelines for children's participation in outdoor play design. Only two states had developed play policy at a national level (Ireland and the four nations of the UK), while none had developed any national policy on the inclusion of children in outdoor play design, which was identified in article 31 as a key aspect of children's participation in matters that affect them (Lynch et al., 2018). While it is likely there may be some gaps in this review due to the diverse languages across Europe, data were collected from representatives of 28 countries who were best placed to identify and locate their own national policies for the review (https://www.ludi-network .eu/). Further exploration is needed internationally across continents to determine the full breadth of play policy throughout the world, especially in countries where play is valued among adults as an important part of childhood.

International Initiatives

The importance of play has become more evident in international initiatives to address social inclusion and well-being. For example, with the growing evidence of play deprivation and the increase in psychopathology in childhood (Gray, 2011), there is a growing countermovement to try to redress the balance and increase outdoor play through the development of position papers and research, in particular on physical activity and risky play (Brussoni et al., 2015; Niehues et al., 2013; Tremblay et al., 2015; Tremblay et al., 2011). Other strategies evident across continents are seen in efforts to mobilize governments and municipalities to develop playful cities or national playdays (e.g., Toscano, 2019; UNICEF, 2018). So, from a societal level, policymakers are using evidence to develop guidelines to help redress the knowledge gap among adults who care for children, on the value of providing high play value and risk-rich opportunities for children for their health and well-being.

Policy Implications

To conclude, while play has been recognized as the right of the child, there is a significant lack of policy at national levels to operationalize a whole government response to providing for play. Yet, there are many examples internationally of play initiatives showing that play is valued at the heart of many communities (see **Appendix 15.1**). As occupational therapists, we are committed to enabling occupation and defending the rights of the child to play as an issue of occupational justice, consistent with their family and community culture and beliefs (WFOT, 2019), irrespective of whether national governments have progressed to developing policy or not. See **Box 15.4** for a summary of considerations and possibilities for addressing play in diverse cultures from a policy perspective. The remainder of this chapter explores the place of play in occupational therapy practices internationally to determine how to progress the agenda for play for all.

Play in Occupational Therapy: An International Perspective

A primary focus of this chapter has been on understanding play occupation from the child, family, and sociocultural perspective, in order to strengthen our insights into play first as an occupation. Many key themes have been highlighted that serve to inform occupational therapy practice. First, there is a need to acknowledge

Box 15.4 Policy Considerations for Addressing Play in Diverse Cultures

- Article 31 of the UNCRC states that all children have a right to play, including those with disabilities.
- Although the UNCRC is ratified by most countries across the world, few countries have developed national play policies.
- Despite the lack of national play policies, occupational therapists who work within countries that have ratified the UNCRC have a duty to protect and to promote the rights of the child to play, as an issue of occupational justice and human rights (WFOT, 2019).
- General Comment 17 guides occupational therapists to address play rights of children, and identifies key areas of concern, including the need to provide inclusive play facilities, to apply a universal design approach, to include children in designing for play, and to work collaboratively to build inclusive societies.

Data from World Federation of Occupational Therapists. (2019). *Position statement: Occupational therapy and human rights* (revised). https://www.wfot.org/resources/occupational-therapy-and-human-rights

cultural variability regarding play and the subsequent implications for occupational therapy practice. Play can mean many different things to different cultures from both adults' perspectives and children's perspectives. Parent–child play differs across cultures depending on cultural values and attitudes toward play and childhood. In fact, as noted by Lancy's review (2007), parent–child play is relatively rare in many cultures. Second, whether adults value play or simply tolerate it, nevertheless, children in every culture play. And third, across studies to date, children generally agree with what play is—it happens when they have freedom to do what they choose, typically without adults present. Collectively this evidence suggests specific strategies that can be implemented to strengthen occupational therapy practice when implementing a play-based perspective with children and families (see **Box 15.5**).

In order to address the sociocultural embeddedness of play occupation, it is important to consider the specific as well as universal aspects of play as a phenomenon (Roopnarine et al., 1994). One of the ways that this can be done is by considering the concept of parental reasoning, which was an outcome of an occupational science study of play in home settings (Lynch et al., 2016). Different types of parental reasoning are based on decision making during parenting and childrearing (see **Table 15.2**). Although these modalities are similar to professional reasoning from occupational therapy literature, personal and

Box 15.5 Strategies for Culturally Relevant Practice for Play Occupation

Is your play intervention based on cultural values of the child and family? In order to answer this, ask essential questions as part of your assessment, for example:

- Parent/caregiver:
  - What does play mean to you as a family?
  - What does play look like in your home?
  - How do you like to play? Do you value playing together with your child, or organizing playdates or both?
  - What do you remember about play in your family growing up?
  - Are there any particular routines or plans around play that you organize in your family?
  - What do you think of toys, and how do they find their way to your home? (e.g., Is it mostly through gifts, or at special events like birthdays; do you like to buy toys or to make them; do you agree or disagree with the current level of commercialization?)
  - Is there any kind of play you don't like/don't agree with/don't allow your child to play? Tell me more …
  - What, if any, is your biggest play challenge at home/with your child?
- Child:
  - What do you think about play?
  - What is your favorite and least favorite thing to play or do? Why?
  - Is there anything you would like to be able to play but find it too hard?
  - Where do you like to play, and where is your favorite place to play? Why?
  - What do you like to play when you have friends to play with?
  - What do you like to play when you are alone?
  - What are you not allowed to play? Why?
  - What would you really like to play if you were allowed?
- Once you have a clearer idea of play in this family culture, then consider:
  - Is adult–child play part of this family culture? If not, then what does this mean for the intervention you are choosing to do?
  - What are the play preferences of the child, and do these differ from those of the adult caregivers? If so, how will you establish a play goal that works for both child and family?
  - Can you consider adding a play goal that is based on play occupation—not to teach skills but to solve a play challenge for this child and family—e.g., to educate adults on benefits of risky play, advocate for more time to play and have fun in free-play, advocate for inclusive playgrounds, or get involved in other community play initiatives?

Data from Lancy, D. (2007). Accounting for variability in mother-child play. *American Anthropologist, 109*, 273–284. https://10.1525/AA.2007.109.2.273

Table 15.2 Forms of Parental Reasoning

Form of Reasoning	Description	Relationship to Professional Reasoning in Occupational Therapy
Personal reasoning	Characteristic-based and draws from the parents' own disposition or personality traits, which determine their emotional responses, among other things.	Draws from a transactional model (Bronfenbrenner & Morris, 2007), which emphasizes the role of parent characteristics as a force that shapes development in the child.
Knowledge-based reasoning (factual)	Draws from theoretical or scientific knowledge about parenting and child development.	Comparable to procedural reasoning in occupational therapy studies (Fleming, 1994b).
Future-based reasoning	Relates to the ideas that parents hold of the "future" child.	Relates to *conditional* reasoning, which focuses on a future narrative for the person (Fleming, 1994a).
Practical-based reasoning	Relates to the availability and access to resources, which influences choices about what is feasible or possible.	Matches *pragmatic* reasoning in the occupational therapy literature (Schell & Schell, 2007).
Sociocultural reasoning	Draws from the social and cultural attitudes and values of the parents and therefore is strongly linked to the communities in which they live.	Significantly shaped by the parents' own experiences of parenting and therefore has a strong historical connection. Along with personal reasoning, it is not so evident in professional reasoning.
Narrative reasoning	Evident in parenting practices when participating in social networks through storytelling, sharing of puzzling stories to make sense of what is happening or establishing ideas about how to deal with childrearing issues.	Similar to the meaning-making that therapists also do (Hamilton, 2008).

sociocultural reasoning are specific to parental reasoning and reflect the embedded nature of the developmental niche of families and communities (Super & Harkness, 1986). From this perspective, parental reasoning incorporates a focus on the social setting, including the cultural customs of childcare and childrearing and the psychology of the caretakers. These key considerations were identified as essential by Super and Harkness (1986) when exploring the interface between an individual child and family and their cultural context. Consideration of parental reasoning can help occupational therapists consider the cultural specificity of play within a family.

Now we also need to consider how to strengthen play in occupational therapy intervention as an alternative to relying on the developmental perspective. As noted in this and earlier chapters, occupational therapy practice has been dominated by developmental discourses of play. If we apply Sutton-Smith's (1997) analysis (see **Box 15.6**), occupational therapists typically prioritize a "play as progress" rhetoric, i.e., that we most value the psychological evidence of play for

learning and use this approach to inform our practices and to guide the development of effective intervention. This perspective is often identified as a focus on the future child rather than the child in the present.

While there is indeed an imperative to enable play among children with special needs, developmental approaches are not the only means to do so. From an

Box 15.6 The Origins of the Concept of Play Rhetorics

Brian Sutton-Smith was a Professor of Education and influential play theorist from New Zealand who led the field in advancing play in the late 20th century. In his text, *The Ambiguity of Play* (1997), he proposed that there are seven rhetorics of play: (1) play as self, (2) the imaginary, (3) competition or power, (4) community, (5) identity, (6) fate, frivolity, or foolishness, and (7) play as progress. These seven rhetorics represent multiple perspectives from diverse disciplines, with 'play as progress' being the most common rhetoric in child development and rehabilitation (Sutton-Smith, 1997).

occupational science perspective, where doing, being, becoming, and belonging is explored (Wilcock & Hocking, 2015), the concept of the child as *being in the present* helps us to shift away from the developmental perspective. From this standpoint, the occupation of play (in terms of form and function) can be understood from the child's subjective experience (meaning) in the "now" of childhood. This occupational science perspective is informed by the new social studies of childhood (James & Prout, 2015), which argue for the need to respect the "being" rather than the "becoming" aspect of children's lives. In addition, a rights-based approach is a central concern, whereby there is a recognized right of the child to have a childhood. Furthermore, for children with disabilities, there is a further issue of the pathologizing of play, whereby children with special needs are often viewed as nonplaying and in need of intervention (Goodley & Runswick-Cole, 2010). The outcome for children with disabilities is that play is often hijacked for rehabilitation purposes and relegated to training and skills development, with the priority on "becoming," where the product is more important than the process of play. The combination of each of these perspectives leads to the argument for the need to unshackle play from more traditional developmental approaches (Fahy et al., 2020; Goodley & Runswick-Cole, 2010). By integrating these perspectives within occupational science and occupational therapy, we can consider new directions and possibilities for addressing occupational injustices in enabling play occupation (Prellwitz & Skär, 2016).

Toward an Integration of Play Occupation in Occupational Therapy

Play has long been valued by the profession of occupational therapy. Play was established from the outset as a core aspect of occupational therapy in the early 1900s but quickly receded. Play did not come to the fore again until the 1970s when research emerged on occupational behavior from Mary Reilly (1974) and sensory integration from Jean Ayres (1972, 2005), which was further expanded with the emergence of the new science of occupation in the 1980s and 1990s (Hocking, 2009). Since then, play scholarship in occupational therapy and occupational science has continued to evolve with the result that there are now tools to assess play alongside play programs that are evidence based (e.g., Bundy, 2004; Bundy et al., 2009; Knox, 2008; Stagnitti, 2007; Stagnitti et al., 2011; Wilkes-Gillan, Bundy, Cordier, & Lincoln, 2016, Wilkes-Gillan, Bundy, Cordier, Lincoln, & Chen,

2016). Helped also by the evolution of ideas of participation, occupational therapy has moved from impairment-focused practice toward occupational engagement in life situations more specifically (AOTA, 2020; World Health Organization [WHO], 2001).

Yet in some studies from the United States, Ireland, Sweden, and Switzerland, researchers have consistently noted that play as an occupation is rarely the focus in occupational therapy practice (Bundy, 1991; Couch et al., 1998; Lynch et al., 2017; Miller Kuhaneck et al., 2013; Moore & Lynch, 2018b). From these studies that span almost 30 years, therapists agreed that they used play in practice and that it was an important occupation in childhood. Yet most therapists reported that they used play as a means to an end and rarely selected play as a goal in therapy. Similar results have been identified in other studies in Canada and the UK, where it was identified that few addressed participation in play or measured outcomes for play, and instead worked more on client impairments (Dunford et al., 2013; Saleh et al., 2008). This means that play in occupational therapy *may not be play at all* if it is often utilizing a playful approach to target other skills. Consequently, it is evident that there is a tension between what occupational therapists value (play occupation) and practice (play activity as a means to an end).

From this analysis, it is important to acknowledge that there is a difference between play activity and play occupation. Occupation denotes the clients' personalized experience of meaningful engagement in an occupation such as play, whereas activity denotes action that is nonspecific to a client and their context (AOTA, 2020). The evidence from the multiple studies reviewed in this chapter show that when children are asked about play, it is very important to them, it is about fun and happiness, it is something they do mostly without adults and involves contexts where they can set challenges for themselves and take risks together or alone. Therefore, it becomes clear that when we talk of play in occupational therapy, we need a way to consider two separate aspects of play, play as an activity or play as an occupation. And furthermore, how do we work more to protect the child's right to play, to ensure play as an occupation is embedded as an important part of child-centered occupational therapy practice, and how do we work to enable play occupation? We need to develop a clearer articulation of play occupation alongside play activity.

A Continuum of Play in Practice

From the review of occupational therapy practice and play, it is possible to propose a continuum of play in practice. This model aims to enable play in occupational therapy by clarifying the relationship of play occupation with play activity. The continuum of play intervention moves from extrinsic to intrinsic motivation, from external to internal control as follows: from a teaching approach, to directed play, to guided play, and to play occupation (see **Figure 15.7**) (Lynch, 2016; Ray-Kaeser & Lynch, 2017).

The continuum starts on the left with the least amount of play in intervention. In this form of intervention, therapists teach a child the skills for play directly. This approach has a focus on "work," without a playful approach, and thus is labeled *work/nonplay*. A developmental approach typically underpins these work practices, with the application of acquisitional frame of reference, motor learning, or cognitive approaches to teach skills related to play activity (Miller Kuhaneck, Spitzer, & Miller, 2010). However, there is little evidence as yet that working on play skills results in improvements in engagement in play itself (Bundy, 2010). This approach to play was not very evident in the surveys of occupational therapy practice to date.

The next type of intervention is where therapists use play primarily as a tool (as a means to an end), which can be described as *playful work* (Henricks, 2015). In these reviews of play in occupational therapy to date, play activity was a central aspect of therapy intervention when used to motivate the child to behave or develop skills identified as deficits and associated with intervention goals (Lynch et al., 2017; Miller Kuhaneck et al., 2013). Like nonplay work, therapists direct the intervention and are informed by developmental approaches primarily. There is evidence that using playful activities generates better results compared with repeated exercises (Melchert-McKearnan et al., 2000). However, the main focus is not on play itself but on functional skills development.

Therefore, when the goal is to improve function using a playful approach, this use of play in practice can be described as playful work, whereby play is utilized to make learning fun.

Moving along the continuum, the next form of play in therapy is *worklike play*. This is where therapists use a child-initiated, play-based approach in their therapy interventions. There is evidence that a child-directed play approach can be more useful than a therapist-directed approach for enabling fine-motor skills, for example (DeGangi et al., 1993). One example of a renowned play-based approach in occupational therapy is Ayres sensory integration, which is done in the context of play and establishes play as one of the 10 process elements within the fidelity to treatment (Parham et al., 2011); indeed, Ayres described play as a hallmark of this approach (Smith-Roley et al., 2007). When a play-based approach is adopted, this means that the child initiates the play activity, and the therapist scaffolds by providing a positive emotional atmosphere and the just-right challenge within the therapy context (Bundy, 1991). While a developmental approach is a core feature, it is tempered by features of mastery motivation and play theory. Although the child chooses what to play, the therapist guides the play, negotiates activities that are not preplanned, and alters the task or the environment based on the child's responses. Therefore, a play-based approach conforms with key features of play whereby it is selected by the child, who is motivated to play and has internal control and inner drive to play. However, it is not fully play centered as the child is not free to play in an unstructured way and has no control of choice of playmate. Similar to playful work discussed earlier, the goal of therapy may not be about improvements in play per se, but on improving performance skills, client factors, or nonplay areas of occupational performance.

Therapist-initiated and directed	Therapist-initiated/child responsive	Child-initiated/therapist scaffolded and guided	Child-initiated, child led and child directed
Activities are taught and practiced	Activities are playful or play-based	Activities are playful, play-based, self-chosen and voluntary	Activities are intrinsically motivated, self-chosen, voluntary
Therapist may apply a technique to the child e.g., brushing, massage	*Therapist works on play skills with child, e.g., teaching turn-taking in a game*	*Therapist follows child's lead, e.g., AYRES SENSORY INTEGRATION*	*Therapist works to enable PLAY, PARTICIPATION AND PLAYFULNESS, e.g., ensure local playgrounds are Universally Designed*
Play type: Work/non-play	Play type: Directed play i.e., playful work	Play type: Guided play i.e., work-like play	Play type: PLAY OCCUPATION

←←←←moving from extrinsic motivation.................... to intrinsic motivation→→→→
External control to internal control

Figure 15.7 Continuum from therapist-directed to child-directed play

Reproduced from Ray-Kaeser, S., & Lynch, H. (2017). Occupational therapy perspective on play for the sake of play. In S. Besio, D. Bulgarelli, & V. Stancheva-Popkostadinova (Eds.), *Play development in children with disabilities* (pp. 155–165). De Gruyter. https://doi.org/10.1515/9783110522143-014

At the end of the continuum is the fourth form of play in therapy, *play occupation*, where the child initiates and directs play activities fully. This form is the most closely associated with a play-centered approach. To develop practice that supports play occupation, the therapist must set goals that relate to the playing child in the now of childhood. Therefore, a developmental approach is not aligned with this approach as much as a child-rights-based approach. Here the focus for the therapist must be on play itself and not just making therapy playful. The assessments, goals, and intervention are play centered, and the intended outcome is that the child has fun and is provided with licenses to play according to their play needs and preferences (Ray-Kaeser et al., 2018; Ray-Kaeser & Lynch, 2017). Central to this approach is that play is not about the product but the process of play itself. Given the evidence we have reviewed from children, that play often happens when there are no adults there, it is clear that to enable play occupation is to attend primarily to the context for play. Furthermore, given the diverse nature of play across cultures, the social and physical contexts need to be considered according to the values and attitudes of the family and community, and within that context, play may not be important to the adult, or may differ in its form and meaning compared to other families.

Although play occupation and play-centered interventions are not well developed to date in occupational therapy, there are some examples of research and practice that is moving in this direction. For example, interventions guided by a context-focused approach can be considered in relation to play occupation where the goal is to address environmental changes rather than working on the child's abilities (e.g., Darrah et al., 2011; Law et al., 2011). Context-focused interventions have already been explored in relation to playgrounds and the use of loose parts to increase playfulness (Bundy et al., 2011), to increase physical activity (Engelen et al., 2013), and to explore the impact on risk-taking for children with disabilities (Niehues et al., 2013). Designing inclusive play environments has also begun to be part of occupational therapy practice to promote occupational justice at a community level (Lynch et al., 2019b; Moore & Lynch, 2015). Context-focused play interventions also can provide an opportunity for addressing various crises across the globe (see **Practice Opportunity 15.2**).

Designing toys with high play value to match the child's motivation for play (Ríos-Rincón et al., 2016) and working with peers and parents to support play (Wilkes-Gillan, Bundy, Cordier, & Lincoln, 2016, Wilkes-Gillan, Bundy, Cordier, Lincoln, & Chen, 2016) have been shown to be effective in impacting play occupation. In each case, the child's play preferences and playfulness are at the center, and the goal is

Practice Opportunity 15.2 Strategies for Play in Crisis Situations

Although, to date, we do not have much research about occupational therapy practices in relation to play and populations of children living in crises, there is a lot we can learn from projects such as those carried out in collaboration with the International Play Association: Play in Crisis project (Chatterjee, 2017). They included research on natural disasters (Great East Japan Earthquake, 2011; Nepal Earthquake, 2015), humanitarian crises (Roma community living in Turkey; Syrian refugees since 2011), and everyday crises (slums of India; migrants in Thailand). For example, in the natural disaster situation of the earthquake in Japan, researchers found that communities were destroyed, and despite a commitment to supporting play for children, significant challenges ensued:

> Irrespective of where children were staying, evacuation centers, at a relative's house, or public temporary housing, or even when children returned to their original house directly from the evacuation shelter, children had no adequate space or opportunity to play. In the atmosphere of great sadness, loss and despair, many children refrained from playing and they were told not to play by adults in many of the temporary living spaces. The disaster destroyed spaces where children used to play. Parks and schoolyards became dominated by construction work for temporary houses and left-over spaces around them were covered in tarmac and used for parking cars. Friends got separated while moving to temporary and other housing options in different locations. (Chatterjee, 2017, p. 24)

In response, community organizations established local volunteer groups to develop pop-up temporary playgrounds and to provide play opportunities through mobilizing "play cars" to bring materials to different locations. Significantly, successful interventions across all of these crisis situations were usually embedded in programs related to providing *Child Friendly Spaces (CFSs)*. The effectiveness of CFS interventions seems to rest on three core ingredients: (1) they serve to provide a protection for children from further risk of abuse and violence, (2) they provide a means to strengthen the child's own resilience and well-being, and (3) they focus on mobilizing the community around the child.

Data from Chatterjee, S. (2017). Access to play for children in situations of crisis synthesis of research in six countries. *International Play Association.* http://ipaworld.org/wp-content/uploads/2020/04/IPA-APC-Research-Synthesis-Reportsinglepg-1.pdf

enabling play occupation through addressing changes in the physical and social environments. The intervention is contextual, emphasizes participation, and takes place in home and community settings. It is hoped that such studies help establish a clearer perspective on how to centralize play occupation in occupational therapy intervention and support the development of intervention protocols to guide practice. Culturally relevant practices need to underpin these evolving practices, to ensure cultural sensitivity is embedded, and to maximize the goodness of fit with the values and meaning of play within a specific community (Gerlach et al., 2014).

Barriers to Strengthening Occupational Therapy Practice and Play Occupation

In order to strengthen play in practice, it is also important to identify current barriers. Across these studies, therapists in Canada, the United States, the UK, Ireland, Switzerland, and Sweden reported many similar barriers to prioritizing play. Therapists reported that they were constrained by policy and service expectations (e.g., related to how the service was funded); that their priorities needed to be placed on remediation of daily living skills; that occupational therapy departments were cautious about including play interventions; and that they lacked knowledge about play theory, occupation-centered practice, and play interventions (Lynch et al., 2017; Miller Kuhaneck et al., 2013; Page et al., 2015). Inadvertently, a professional concern for prioritizing skill development over play risks creating barriers to play occupation and eroding opportunities in childhood for free play. This is a critical issue, as we know that children in general are experiencing a decline in free play (Singer et al., 2009), while children with disability are at a higher risk for play deprivation (CRC, 2013). While most therapists reported learning about play primarily in their professional education, it has been noted in a study comparing occupational therapy curricula across Australia, Canada, and New Zealand that no specific play interventions were taught (Rodger et al., 2006). Perhaps by strengthening the understanding of occupational science and play, alongside knowledge and skills for applying a play-centered approach in practice, these barriers can be overcome (for an example of such a program, see www.p4play.eu). Please see Appendix 15.1 for resources to promote participation in play.

While there is much play knowledge available for therapists to learn and apply in practice

as evidenced by this book, more specific research is needed. To date, few studies have examined the different approaches to play intervention in occupational therapy. We need research to compare the outcomes of adult-directed play, child-initiated guided play, or child-directed play in enabling play occupation. A more specific analysis of how play is used in occupational therapy practice is needed to help identify the different approaches to play and methods for overcoming barriers to engaging in more play-occupation-centered interventions. Furthermore, more studies are needed in relation to culturally sensitive ways of enabling play in cultures and families where play is not valued, in order to protect the rights of the child to play.

Conclusion

With a call to embed the f-words of function, family, fitness, fun, friends, and future in our work with children with disabilities (Rosenbaum & Gorter, 2011), it is timely that, as experts in occupation, we analyze our practice. Where is fun for the children we serve? Where is play as occupation? To move our practice toward play, this chapter has reviewed sociocultural, individual, international, and policy perspectives on play that can inform practice. We can translate this evidence to provide play for children in general and for children with disabilities, creating opportunities for inclusive environments and providing culturally sensitive education on play for promoting health, well-being, and a playful life. Specifically, a continuum of play in practice is proposed that includes contextual intervention as a way to embed play occupation. Contextual approaches not only can be employed to address play needs at the individual level but also at community and policy levels through engagement in social or political action (Moore & Lynch, 2015). By considering the continuum from playful work to guided play and play occupation, we can take a more critical analytical perspective on play and advance our thinking about how to enable and adopt a more play-occupation approach. This continuum acknowledges that children learn in different ways, that instruction is not the only form of learning, that play occupation is also a means of learning in itself, especially in young children (Wood, 2007).

As occupational therapists, we need to rethink our role in play in two critical respects. First, without a focus on child-initiated and child-directed play in occupational therapy, play occupations may not be enhanced. Both therapists and adults do not always value or view play in the same way as children. Second, we have a role in enabling play participation and need to ensure we become part of the play solution. If play is the serious work of the child, then we must ensure that play occupation is evident in our work, as part of our role in enabling play. Although play is viewed as relating to fun, it should not be confused with being frivolous; it is the means through which the child learns and develops, the source of well-being, and consequently an aspect of childhood that requires serious consideration.

References

Adolph, K. E., Karasik, L. B., & Tamis-LeMonda, C. S. (2010). Moving between cultures: Cross-cultural research on motor development. In M. Bornstein (Ed.), *Handbook of cultural developmental science* (pp. 61–88). New York: Taylor and Francis Group.

American Occupational Therapy Association (AOTA). (2020). Occupational therapy practice framework: Domain and process (4th ed.). *American Journal of Occupational Therapy, 74.*

Ayres, A. J. (1972). *Sensory integration and learning disorders.* Los Angeles, CA: Western Psychological Services.

Ayres, A. J. (2005). *Sensory integration and the child: Understanding hidden sensory challenges.* Los Angeles, CA: Western Psychological Services.

Bazyk, S., Stalnaker, D., Llerena, M., Ekelman, B., & Bazyk, J. (2003). Play in Mayan children. *American Journal of Occupational Therapy, 57*(3), 273–283. https://doi.org/10.5014/ajot.57.3.273

Berinstein, S., & Magalhaes, L. (2009). A study of the essence of play experience to children living in Zanzibar, *Tanzania. Occupational Therapy International, 16*(2), 89–106. https://doi.org/10.1002/oti.270

Blake, A., Sexton, J., Lynch, H., Moore, A., & Coughlan, M. (2018). An exploration of the outdoor play experiences of preschool children with autism spectrum disorder in an Irish preschool setting. *Todays' Children Tomorrow's Parents: An Interdisciplinary Journal, 47–48*, 100–116.

Bonder, B., Martin, L., & Miracle, A. (2004). Culture emergent in occupation. *American Journal of Occupational Therapy, 58*, 159–168. https://doi.org/10.5014/ajot.58.2.159

Bornstein, M., Haynes, O., Pascual, L., Painter, K., & Galperin, C. (1999). Play in two societies: Pervasiveness of process, specificity of structure. *Child Development, 70*(2), 317–331. https://www.jstor.org/stable/i247432

Bornstein, M., Putnick, D., Heslington, M., Gini, M., Suwalsky, J., Venuti, P.,... de Galperin, C. (2008). Mother–child emotional availability in ecological perspective: Three countries, two regions, two genders. *Developmental Psychology, 44*(3), 666–680. https://doi.org/10.1037%2F0012-1649.44.3.666

Brockman, R., Fox, K., & Jago, R. (2011). What is the meaning and nature of active play for today's children in the UK? *International Journal of Behavioural Nutrition and Physical Activity, 8*(15). http://www.ijbnpa.org/content/8/1/15

Brockman, R., Jago, R., & Fox, K. (2011). Children's active play: Self-reported motivators, barriers and facilitators. *BMC Public Health, 11*(461). http://www.biomedcentral.com/1471-2458/11/461

Bronfenbrenner, U., & Morris, P. (2007). The bioecological model of human development. In R. Lerner (Ed.), *Handbook of child psychology: Theoretical models of human development* (6th ed., Vol. 1, pp. 793–828). New York: Wiley and Sons.

Brussoni, M., Gibbons, R., Gray, C., Ishikawa, T., Sandseter, E. B. H., Beinenstock, A., & Tremblay, M. (2015). What is the relationship between risky outdoor play and health in children? A systematic review. *International Journal of Environmental Research and Public Health, 12*(6), 6423–6454. https://doi.org/10.3390/ijerph120606423

Bundy, A. (1991). Play theory and sensory integration. In A. Fisher, E. Murray, & A. Bundy (Eds.), *Sensory integration: Theory and practice* (pp. 46–68). Philadelphia: F. A. Davis.

Bundy, A. (1997). Play and playfulness: What to look for. In L. D. Parham & L. Fazio (Eds.), *Play in occupational therapy for children* (pp. 52–66). St. Louis, MO: Mosby.

Bundy, A. (2004). *Test of playfulness (ToP) (Version 4.0).* Sydney, Australia: The University of Sydney.

Bundy, A. (2010). Evidence to practice commentary: Beware the traps of play assessment. *Physical & Occupational Therapy in Pediatrics, 30*(2), 98–100. https://doi.org/10.3109/01942631003622723

Bundy, A., Luckett, T., Tranter, P., Naughton, G., Wyver, S., Ragen, J., & Spies, G. (2009). The risk that there is "no risk": A simple, innovative intervention to increase children's activity levels. *International Journal of Early Years Education, 17*(1), 33–45. https://doi.org/10.1080/09669760802699878

Bundy, A., Naughton, G., Tranter, P., Wyver, S., Baur, L., Schiller, W.,... Brentnall, J. (2011). The Sydney playground project: Popping the bubblewrap—unleashing the power of play: A cluster randomised controlled trial of a primary school playground-based intervention aiming to increase children's physical activity and social skills. *BMC Public Health, 11*(680), 1–9. https://10.1186/1471-2458-11-680

Burghardt, G. (2014). A brief glimpse at the long evolutionary history of play. *Animal behavior and cognition, 1*(2), 90–98. https://doi.org/10.12966/abc.05.01.2014

Canadian Public Health Association (CPHA). (2019). *Children's unstructured play position statement: March 2019.* https://www.cpha.ca/childrens-unstructured-play

Chatterjee, S. (2017). *Access to play for children in situations of crisis synthesis of research in six countries.* Cardiff, UK: International Play Association. http://ipaworld.org/wp-content/uploads/2018/02/IPA-APC-Research-Synthesis-Report-A4.pdf

Chick, G. (2015). Anthropology and the study of play. In J. Johnson, S. Eberle, T. Henricks, & D. Kuschner (Eds.), *The handbook of the study of play* (pp. 71–84). London: Rowman & Littlefield, and the Strong.

Committee on the Rights of the Child (CRC). (2013). *General comment No.17 (2013) on the right of the child to rest, leisure, play, recreational activities, cultural life and the arts (art.31)*. Geneva: United Nations.

Conn, C. (2015). "Sensory highs," "vivid rememberings" and "interactive stimming": Children's play cultures and experiences of friendship in autistic autobiographies. *Disability & Society*, 30(8), 1192–1206. http://dx.doi.org/10.1080/09687599.2015.1081094

Couch, K., Deitz, J., & Kanny, E. (1998). The role of play in pediatric occupational therapy. *American Journal of Occupational Therapy*, 52(2), 111–117. https://doi.org/10.5014/ajot.52.2.111

Coughlan, M., & Lynch, H. (2011). Parents as environmental managers: The Irish home as a play space for toddlers. *Irish Journal of Occupational Therapy*, 39(1), 34–41.

Coyne, I., Dempsey, O., & Comiskey, C. (2012). *Life as a child and young person in Ireland: Report of a national consultation*. Dublin: Government Publications. https://assets.gov.ie/34614/e4ac092807aa4317b79bad218b1e3b1d.pdf

Darrah, J., Law, M., Pollock, N., Wilson, B., Russell, D., Walter, S.,... Galupp, B. (2011). Context therapy: A new intervention approach for children with cerebral palsy. *Developmental Medicine & Child Neurology*, 53(7), 615–620. https://doi.org/10.1111/j.1469-8749.2011.03959.x

DeGangi, G., Wietlisbach, S., Goodin, M., & Scheiner, N. (1993). A comparison of structured sensorimotor therapy and child-centered activity in the treatment of preschool children with sensorimotor problems. *American Journal of Occupational Therapy*, 47, 777–786. http://dx.doi.org/10.5014/ajot.47.9.777

Delaney, K. (2017). Playing at violence: Lock-down drills, "bad guys" and the construction of "acceptable play" in early childhood. *Early Child Development and Care*, 187(5–6), 878–895. https://doi.org/10.1080/03004430.2016.1219853

Dickie, V. (2004). Culture is tricky: A commentary on culture emergent in occupation. *The American Journal of Occupational Therapy*, 58, 169–173. https://doi.org/10.5014/ajot.58.2.169

Drianda, R., & Kinoshita, I. (2015). The safe and fun children's play spaces: Evidence from Tokyo, Japan and Bandung, Indonesia. *Journal of Urban Design*, 20(4), 437–460. https://doi.org/10.1080/13574809.2015.1044507

Dunford, C., Bannigan, K., & Wales, L. (2013). Measuring activity and participation outcomes for children and youth with acquired brain injury: An occupational therapy perspective. *British Journal of Occupational Therapy*, 76(2), 67–76. https://doi.org/10.4276/030802213X13603244419158

Edwards, C. (2000). Children's play in cross-cultural perspective: A new look at the six cultures study. *Cross-Cultural Research*, 34, 318–338. https://doi.org/10.1177%2F106939710003400402

Engelen, L., Bundy, A., Naughton, G., Simpson, J., Bauman, A., Ragen, J.,... van der Ploeg, H. (2013). Increasing physical activity in young primary school children—it's child's play: A cluster randomised controlled trial. *Preventative Medicine* (56), 319–325. https://doi.org/10.1016/j.ypmed.2013.02.007

Fahy, S., Delicate, N., & Lynch, H. (2020). Now, being, occupational: Outdoor play and children with autism. *Journal of Occupational Science*. 1–19 https://doi.org/10.1080/14427591.2020.1816207

Farrugia, D. (2009). Exploring stigma: medical knowledge and the stigmatisation of parents of children diagnosed with autism spectrum disorder. *Sociology of Health &*

Illness, 31(7), 1011–1027. https://doi.org/10.1111/j.1467-9566.2009.01174.x

Fernald, A., & O'Neill, D. (1993). Peekaboo across cultures: How mothers and infants play with voices, faces, and expectations. In K. MacDonald (Ed.), *Parent–child play: Descriptions and implications* (pp. 259–287). New York: SUNY Press.

Fleming, M. (1994a). Conditional reasoning: Creating meaningful experiences. In C. Mattingly & M. Fleming (Eds.), *Clinical reasoning: Forms of inquiry in a therapeutic practice* (pp. 197–235). Philadelphia, PA: F. A. Davis.

Fleming, M. (1994b). Procedural reasoning: Addressing functional limitations. In C. Mattingly & M. Fleming (Eds.), *Clinical reasoning: Forms of inquiry in a therapeutic practice* (pp. 137–177). Philadelphia, PA: F. A. Davis.

Garvey, C. (1990). *Play: The developing child*. Cambridge, MA: Harvard University Press.

Gaskins, S., Haight, W., & Lancy, D. (2007). The cultural construction of play. In A. Goncu & S. Gaskins (Eds.), *Play and development: Evolutionary, sociocultural, and functional perspectives* (pp. 179–202). Mahwah, NJ: Erlbaum.

Gerlach, A., Browne, A., & Suto, M. (2014). A critical reframing of play in relation to indigenous children in Canada. *Journal of Occupational Science*, 21(3), 243–258. http://dx.doi.org/10.1080/14427591.2014.908818

Glenn, N., Knight, C., Holt, N., & Spence, J. (2012). Meanings of play among children. *Childhood*, 20, 185–199. https://doi.org/10.1177%2F0907568212454751

Göncü, A., Mistry, J., & Mosier, C. (2000). Cultural variations in the play of toddlers. *International Journal of Behavioral Development*, 24(3), 321–329. https://doi.org/10.1080/01650250050118303

Goodley, D., & Runswick-Cole, K. (2010). Emancipating play: Dis/abled children, development and deconstruction. *Disability & Society*, 25(4), 499–512. https://doi.org/10.1080/09687591003755914

Gosso, Y., & Carvalho, A. (2013). *Play and cultural context*. http://www.child-encyclopedia.com/play/according-experts/play-and-cultural-context. Encyclopedia of Early Childhood Development.

Gosso, Y. (2010). Play in different cultures. In P. Smith (Ed.), *Children and play: Understanding children's worlds* (pp. 80–98). West Sussex, UK: Wiley-Blackwell.

Graham, N., Nye, C., Mandy, A., Clarke, C., & Morriss-Roberts, C. (2017). The meaning of play for children and young people with physical disabilities: A systematic thematic synthesis. *Child Care Health and Development*, 44, 173–182. https://doi-org.ucc.idm.oclc.org/10.1111/cch.12509

Gray, P. (2011). The decline of play and the rise of psychopathology in children and adolescents. *American Journal of Play*, 3, 443–463.

Haight, W., & Miller, P. (1993). *Pretending at home: Early development in a sociocultural context*. New York: State University of New York Press.

Haight, W., Wang, X., Han-tih Fung, H., Williams, K., & Mintz, J. (1999). Universal, developmental, and variable aspects of young children's play: A cross cultural comparison of pretending at home. *Child Development*, 70(6), 1477–1488. https://www.jstor.org/stable/1132319

Hamilton, T. B. (2008). Narrative reasoning. In B. Schell & J. Schell (Eds.), *Clinical and professional reasoning in occupational therapy* (pp. 125–168). Baltimore, MD: Lippincott Williams & Wilkins.

Hammell, K. W. (2013). Occupation, well-being, and culture: Theory and cultural humility. *Canadian Journal of Occupational Therapy*, *80*(4), 224–234. https://doi .org/10.1177/0008417413500465

Hasluck, L., & Malone, K. (1999). Location, leisure and lifestyle: young people's retreat to home environments. In F. Berardo & C. Shehan (Eds.), *Contemporary perspectives on family research* (pp. 177–196). Bingley, UK: JAI Press.

Hasselkus, B. R. (2002). Occupation as a source of well-being and development. In *The meaning of everyday occupation* (pp. 59–69). Thorofare, NJ: Slack.

Heider, K. (1997). *Grand Valley Dani: Peaceful warriors*. Fort Worth, TX: Harcourt Brace College Publishers.

Henricks, T. (2015). *Play and the human condition*. Chicago: University of Illinois Press.

Hinchion, S., McAuliffe, E., & Lynch, H. (in press). Fraught with frights or full of fun: Perspectives of risky play among six-to-eight-year-olds. European Early Childhood Education Research Journal. https://doi.org/10.1080/1350293X.2021.1968460

Hirsch-Pasek, K., Golinkoff, R., Berk, L., & Singer, D. (2009). *A mandate for playful learning in preschool: Presenting the evidence*. Thousand Oaks, CA: Sage.

Hocking, C. (2009). The challenge of occupation: Describing the things people do. *Journal of Occupational Science*, *16*(3), 140–150. https://doi.org/10.1080/14427591.2009.9686655

Holmes, R. (2013). Children's play and culture. *Scholarpedia*, *8*(6), 31016. https://doi.org/10.4249/scholarpedia.31016

Holt, N., Spence, J., Sehn, Z., & Cutumisu, N. (2008). Neighborhood and developmental differences in children's perceptions of opportunities for play and physical activity. *Health & Place*, *14*(1), 2–14. https://doi.org/10.1016/j .healthplace.2007.03.002

Howard, J., Jenvey, V., & Hill, C. (2006). Children's categorisation of play and learning based on social context. *Early Child Development and Care*, *176*(3–4), 379–393. https://doi .org/10.1080/03004430500063804

Humphry, R. (2009). Occupation and development: A contextual perspective. In E. Crepeau, E. Cohn, & B. Schell (Eds.), *Willard and Spackman's occupational therapy* (11th ed., pp. 22–32). London: Wolters Kluwer/Lippincott Williams & Wilkins.

Ivrendi, A., Cevher-Kalburan, N., Sandseter, E. B. H., Storli, R., & Siversten, H. (2019). Children, mothers, and preschool teachers' perceptions of play: Findings from Turkey and Norway. *Journal of Early Childhood Studies*, *3*(1), 32–54. https:// doi.org/10.24130/eccd-jecs.196720193119

James, A., & Prout, A. (2015). *Constructing and reconstructing childhood: Contemporary issues in the sociological study of childhood* (3rd. ed.). London: Routledge/Falmer.

Kärtner, J., Keller, H., Lamm, B., Abels, M., Yovsi, R. D., Chaudhary, N., & Su, Y. (2008). Similarities and differences in contingency experiences of 3-month-olds across sociocultural contexts. *Infant Behaviour & Development*, *31*, 488–500. https://doi.org/10.1016/j.infbeh.2008.01.00

Kilkelly, U., Lynch, H., Moore, A., O'Connell, A., & Field, S. (2015). Children and the outdoors: Contact with the outdoors and natural heritage among children aged 5 to 12: Current trends, benefits, barriers and research requirements. http://

www.heritagecouncil.ie/fileadmin/user_upload/Publications /Corporate/Chiuldren_full_report_web.pdf

King, P., & Howard, J. (2014). Children's perceptions of choice in relation to their play at home, in the school playground and at the Out-of-School club. *Children & Society*, *28*, 116–127. https://doi.org/10.1111/j.1099-0860.2012.00455.x

Knox, S. (2008). Development and current use of the Revised Knox Preschool Play Scale. In L. D. Parham & L. Fazio (Eds.), *Play in occupational therapy for children* (2nd ed., pp. 55–70). St. Louis, MO: Mosby Elsevier.

Lancy, D. (2007). Accounting for variability in mother–child play. *American Anthropologist*, *109*, 273–284. https://10.1525 /AA.2007.109.2.273

Law, M., Darrah, J., Pollock, N., Wilson, B., Russell, D., Walter, S.,... Galuppi, B. (2011). Focus on function: A cluster, randomized controlled trial comparing child-versus context-focused intervention for young children with cerebral palsy. *Developmental Medicine & Child Neurology*, *53*, 621–629. https://doi.org/10.1111/j.1469-8749.2011.03962.x

Lester, S., & Russell, W. (2010). *Children's right to play: An examination of the importance of play in the lives of children worldwide*. https://issuu.com/bernardvanleerfoundation/docs /childrens_right_to_play_an_examination_of_the_impo/66

Lindsay, S., Tétrault, S., Desmaris, C., King, G. A., & Piérart, G. (2014). Le travail de médiation culturelle effectué par des ergothérapeutes offrant des soins adaptés à la culture [The cultural brokerage work of occupational therapists in providing culturally sensitive care]. *Canadian Journal of Occupational Therapy*, *81*(2), 114–123. https://doi.org /10.1177/0008417413520441

Little, H., & Eager, D. (2010). Risk, challenge and safety: Implications for play quality and playground design. *European Early Childhood Education Research Journal*, *18*(4), 497–513. https://doi.org/10.1080/1350293X.2010.525949

Little, H., & Wyver, S. (2010). Individual differences in children's risk perception and appraisals in indoor play environments. *International Journal of Early Years Education*, *18*(4), 297–313. https://doi.org/10.1080/09669760.2010.531600

Liu-Yan, Yuejuan, P., & Hongfen, S. (2005). Comparative research on young children's perceptions of play—an approach to observing the effects of kindergarten educational reform. *International Journal of Early Years Education*, *13*(2), 101–112. https://doi.org/10.1080/09669760500170982

Lundy, L., Kilkelly, U., Byrne, B., & Kang, J. (2012). *The UN Convention on the Rights of the Child: A study of legal implementation in 12 countries*. UK: UNICEF.org.uk http://www .ipjj.org/fileadmin/data/documents/reports_monitoring _evaluation/UNICEF-UK-QUB_ConventionImplementation 12Countries_2012_EN.pdf

Lynch, H. (2009). Patterns of activity of Irish children aged five to eight years: City living in Ireland today. *Journal of Occupational Science*, *16*(1), 44–49. https://doi.org/10.1080/14427591.200 9.9686641

Lynch, H. (2016). *From play research to practice*. Paper presented at the Fifth European Sensory Integration Conference, Vienna, Austria.

Lynch, H. (2018). Beyond voice: An occupational science perspective on researching through doing. In M. Twomey & C. Carroll (Eds.), *Seen and heard: Exploring participation, engagement and voice for children with disabilities* (pp. 243–266). Oxford, UK: Peter Lang.

Lynch, H., Hayes, N., & Ryan, S. (2016). Exploring socio-cultural influences that impact on infant play occupations in Irish home environments. *Journal of Occupational Science, 23*(3), 352–369. https://doi.org/10.1080/14427591.2015.1080181

Lynch, H., & Moore, A. (2016). Play as an occupation in occupational therapy. *British Journal of Occupational Therapy.* https://doi.org/10.1177/0308022616664540

Lynch, H., & Moore, A. (2018). What barriers to play do children with disabilities face? In P. Encarnação, S. Ray-Kaeser, & N. Bianquin (Eds.), *Guidelines for supporting children with disabilities' play. Methodologies, tools, and contexts* (pp. 27–40). Berlin: De Gruyter. https://content.sciendo.com/view/book/9783110613445/10.1515/9783110613445-007.xml?language=de&result=2&rskey=7IAMdc

Lynch, H., Moore, A., Edwards, C., & Horgan, L. (2019a). Advancing play participation for all: The challenge of addressing play diversity and inclusion in community parks and playgrounds. *British Journal of Occupational Therapy, 38*(2), 107–117. https://doi.org/10.1177/0308022619881936

Lynch, H., Moore, A., Edwards, C., & Horgan, L. (2019b). *Community parks and playgrounds: Intergenerational participation through universal design.* http://nda.ie/Publications/Others/Research-Promotion-Scheme/Community-Parks-and-Playgrounds-Intergenerational-Participation-through-Universal-Design1.pdf

Lynch, H., Moore, A., & Prellwitz, M. (2018). From policy to play provision: Universal design and the challenge of inclusive play. *Children, Youth and Environment, 28*(2), 12–34. https://www.jstor.org/stable/10.7721/chilyoutenvi.28.2.0012

Lynch, H., Prellwitz, M., Schulze, C., & Moore, A. (2017). The state of play in children's occupational therapy: A comparison between Ireland, Sweden and Switzerland. *British Journal of Occupational Therapy,* 1–9. https://doi.org/10.1177/0308022617733256

Lynch, H., & Stanley, M. (2017). Beyond words: Using qualitative video methods for researching occupation with young children. *OTJR: Occupation, Participation and Health, 38*(1), 56–66. https://doi.org/10.1177/1539449217718504

Malone, K. (2007). The bubble-wrap generation: Children growing up in walled gardens. *Environmental Education Research, 13*(4), 513–527. https://doi.org/10.1080/13504620701581612

McInnes, K. (2019). Playful learning in the early years—through the eyes of children. *Education 3–13, 47*(7), 796–805. https://doi.org/10.1080/03004279.2019.1622495

McKendrick, J., Loebach, J., & Casey, T. (2018). Realising article 31 through General Comment No. 17: Overcoming challenges and the quest for an optimum play environment. *Children, Youth and Environment, 28*(2), 1–11. https://www.jstor.org/stable/10.7721/chilyoutenvi.28.2.0001

Melchert-McKearnan, K., Deitz, J., Engel, J., & White, O. (2000). Children with burn injuries: Purposeful activity versus rote exercise. *American Journal of Occupational Therapy, 54*(4), 381–390. https://doi.org/10.5014/ajot.54.4.381

Miller, E., & Kuhaneck, H. (2008). Children's perceptions of play experiences and play preferences: A qualitative study. *American Journal of Occupational Therapy, 62*(4), 407–415. https://doi.org/10.5014/ajot.62.4.407

Miller Kuhaneck, H., Spitzer, S., & Miller, E. (2010). *Activity analysis, creativity, and playfulness in pediatric occupational therapy.* Sudbury, MA: Jones and Bartlett Publishers.

Miller Kuhaneck, H., Tanta, K., Coombs, A., & Pannone, H. (2013). A survey of pediatric occupational therapists' use of play. *Journal of Occupational Therapy, Schools and Early Intervention, 6,* 213–227. https://doi.org/10.1080/19411243.2013.850940

Modiani, N. (1973). *Indian education in the Chiapas highlands.* New York: Holt, Rinehart and Winston.

Monaghan, K. (2012). Early childhood development policy: The colonisation of the world's childrearing practices? In A. Twum-Danso Imoh & R. Ame (Eds.), *Childhoods at the intersection of the local and the global* (pp. 56–74). London: Palgrave Macmillan. https://doi.org/10.1057/9781137283344_4

Moore, A., & Lynch, H. (2015). Accessibility and usability of playground environments for children under 12: A scoping review. *Scandinavian Journal of Occupational Therapy, 22*(5), 331–344. https://doi.org/10.3109/11038128.2015.1049549

Moore, A., & Lynch, H. (2018a). Understanding a child's conceptualisation of well-being through an exploration of happiness: The centrality of play, people and place. *Journal of Occupational Science, 25*(1), 124–141. https://doi.org/10.1080/14427591.2017.1377105

Moore, A., & Lynch, H. (2018b). Play and play occupation: A survey of paediatric occupational therapy practice in Ireland. *Irish Journal of Occupational Therapy, 46*(1), 59–72. https://doi.org/10.1108/IJOT-08-2017-0022

Moore, A., Lynch, H., & Boye, B. (2020). Can universal design support outdoor play, social participation, and inclusion in public playgrounds? *A scoping review. Disability and Rehabilitation,* 1–22. https://doi.org/10.1080/09638288.2020.1858353

Nicholson, J., Shimpi, P., Kurnik, J., Carducci, C., & Jevgjovikj. (2014). Listening to children's perspectives on play across the lifespan: Children's right to inform adults' discussions of contemporary play. *International Journal of Play, 3*(2), 136–156. https://doi.org/10.1080/21594937.2014.937963

Niehues, A., Bundy, A., Broom, A., Tranter, P., Ragen, J., & Engelen, L. (2013). Everyday uncertainties: Reframing perceptions of risk in outdoor free play. *Journal of Adventure Education and Outdoor Learning, 13*(3), 223–237. https://doi.org/10.1080/14729679.2013.798588

Njelesani, J., Sedgwick, A., Davis, J., & Polatajko, H. (2011). The influence of context: A naturalistic study of Ugandan children's doings in outdoor spaces. *Occupational Therapy International, 18,* 124–132. https://doi.org/10.1002/oti.310

Norðdahl, K., & Einarsdóttir, J. (2015). Children's views and preferences regarding their outdoor environment. *Journal of Adventure Education & Outdoor Learning, 15*(2), 152–167. https://doi.org/10.1080/14729679.2014.896746

Oke, M., Khattear, A., Pant, P., & Swarawathi, T. (1999). A profile of children's play in urban India. *Childhood, 6*(2), 207–219.

Opie, I., & Opie, P. (1969). *Children's play in streets and playgrounds.* London: Clarendon Press.

Page, J., Roos, K., Banziger, A., Margot-Cattin, I., Agustoni, S., Rossini, E.,... Meyer, S. (2015). Formulating goals in occupational therapy: State of the art in Switzerland. *Scandinavian Journal of Occupational Therapy, 22*(6), 403–415. https://doi.org/10.3109/11038128.2015.1049548

Parham, L. D., Roley, S. S., May-Benson, T. A., Koomar, J., Brett-Green, B., Burke, J. P., et al. (2011). Development of a fidelity measure for research on the effectiveness of the Ayres Sensory Integration Intervention. *American Journal of Occupational Therapy*, 65(2), 133–142. https://doi.org/10.5014/ajot.2011.000745

Parten, M. (1932). Social participation among preschool children. *Journal of Abnormal Child Psychology*, 27, 243–269. https://psycnet.apa.org/doi/10.1037/h0074524

Pellegrini, A. (1991). *Applied child study: A developmental approach.* Hillsdale, NJ: Erlbaum.

Piaget, J. (1962). *Play, dreams and imitation in childhood.* New York: W. W. Norton.

Pierce, D. (2003). *Occupation by design: Building therapeutic power.* Philadelphia: F. A. Davis.

Pollock, N., Stewart, D., Law, M., Sahagian-Whalen, S., Harvey, S., & Toal, C. (1997). The meaning of play for young people with physical disabilities. *Canadian Journal of Occupational Therapy*, 64, 25–31. https://doi.org/10.1177%2F000841749706400105

Prellwitz, M., & Lynch, H. (2018). Universal design for social inclusion: Playgrounds for all. In M. Twomey & C. Carroll (Eds.), *Seen and heard: Exploring participation, engagement and voice for children with disabilities* (pp. 267–296). Oxford, UK: Peter Lang.

Prellwitz, M., & Skär, L. (2007). Usability of playgrounds for children with different abilities. *Occupational Therapy International*, 14(3), 144–155. https://doi.org/10.1002/oti.230

Prellwitz, M., & Skär, L. (2016). Are playgrounds a case of occupational injustice? Experiences of parents of children with disabilities. *Children, Youth and Environment*, 26(2), 28–42. https://doi.org/10.7721/chilyoutenvi.26.2.0028

Primeau, L. (1998). Orchestration of work and play within families. *American Journal of Occupational Therapy*, 52, 188–195. https://doi.org/10.5014/ajot.52.3.188

Promona, S., Papoudi, D., & Papadopoulou, K. (2019). Play during recess: Primary school children's perspectives and agency. *Education 3–13*. https://doi.org/10.1080/03004279.2019.1648534

Ramugondo, E. (2012). Intergenerational play within family: The case for occupational consciousness. *Journal of Occupational Science*, 19(4), 326–340. https://doi.org/10.1080/14427591.2012.710166

Ray-Kaeser, S., Chatelain, S., Kindler, V., & Schneider, E. (2018). The evaluation of play from occupational therapy and psychology perspectives. In S. Besio, D. Bulgarelli, & V. Stancheva-Popkostadinova (Eds.), *Evaluation of children's play: Tools and methods* (pp. 19–57). Berlin: De Gruyter. https://doi.org/10.1515/9783110610604-004

Ray-Kaeser, S., & Lynch, H. (2017). Occupational therapy perspective on play for the sake of play. In S. Besio, D. Bulgarelli, & V. Stancheva-Popkostadinova (Eds.), *Play development in children with disabilities* (pp. 155–165). Berlin: De Gruyter. https://doi.org/10.1515/9783110522143-014

Reilly, M. (1974). *Play as exploratory learning.* Beverly Hills, CA: Sage Publications.

Ríos-Rincón, A., Adams, K., Magill-Evans, J., & Cook, A. (2016). Playfulness in children with limited motor abilities when using a robot. *Physical & Occupational Therapy in Pediatrics*, 36(3), 232–246. http://doi.org/10.3109/01942638.2015.1076559

Rodger, S., Brown, T., Brown, A., & Roever, C. (2006). A comparison of paediatric occupational therapy university program curricula in New Zealand, Australia and Canada. *Physical & Occupational Therapy in Pediatrics*, 26(1/2), 153–180. https://doi.org/10.1080/J006v26n01_10

Rogoff, B. (1993). Children's guided participation and participatory appropriation in sociocultural activity. In R. Wozniak & K. Fischer (Eds.), *Development in context: Acting, thinking in specific environments* (pp. 121–153). London: Erlbaum.

Rogoff, B. (2003). *The cultural nature of human development.* Oxford, UK: Oxford University Press.

Roopnarine, J. (2011). Cultural variations in beliefs about play, parent–child play, and children's play: Meaning for childhood development. In A. Pellegrini (Ed.), *The Oxford handbook of the development of play* (pp. 19–40). New York: Oxford University Press.

Roopnarine, J., Hooper, F., Ahdmeduzzaman, M., & Pollack, B. (1993). Gentle play partners: other–child and father–child play in New Delhi, India. In K. MacDonald (Ed.), *Parent–child play: Descriptions and implications* (pp. 287–304). Albany: State University of New York Press.

Roopnarine, J., Johnson, J., & Hooper, F. (1994). *Children's play in diverse cultures.* Albany: State University of New York Press.

Roopnarine, J., & Krishnakumar, A. (2006). Parent–child and child–child play in diverse cultural contexts. In D. Fromberg & D. Bergen (Eds.), *Play from birth to twelve: Contexts, perspectives and meanings* (2nd ed., pp. 275–288). New York: Routledge.

Rosenbaum, P., & Gorter, J. (2011). The "F-words" in childhood disability: I swear this is how we should think? *Child Care Health and Development*, 36, 457–463. http://doi.org/10.1111/j.1365-2214.2011.01338.x

Ruckenstein, M. (2010). Toying with the world: Children, virtual pets and the value of mobility. *Childhood*, 17(4), 500–513. https://doi.org/10.1177%2F0907568209352812

Saleh, M., Korner-Bitensky, N., Snider, L., Malouin, F., Mazer, B., Kennedy, D., & Roy, M. (2008). Actual vs. best practices for young children with cerebral palsy: A survey of paediatric occupational therapists and physical therapists in Quebec, Canada. *Developmental Neurorehabilitation*, 11(1), 60–80. https://doi.org/10.1080/17518420701544230

Sandseter, E. (2007). Categorising risky play—How can we identify risk-taking in children's play? *European Early Childhood Education Research Journal*, 15(2), 237–252. https://doi.org/10.1080/13502930701321733

Sandseter, E. (2010). "It tickles my tummy!" Understanding children's risk-taking in play through reversal theory. *Journal of Early Childhood Research*, 8(1), 67–88. https://doi.org/10.1177/1476718x09345393

Sandseter, E. (2019). Outdoor play: Outdoor risky play. *In Encyclopedia on Early Childhood Development*. http://www.child-encyclopedia.com/outdoor-play/according-experts/outdoor-risky-play

Schell, B., & Schell, J. (2007). *Clinical and professional reasoning in occupational therapy.* Baltimore, MD: Lippincott, Williams & Wilkins.

Schwartzman, H. (1979). The sociocultural context of play. In B. Sutton-Smith (Ed.), *Play and learning* (pp. 239–255). New York: Gardner Press.

Shonkoff, J., & Phillips, D. (2000). *From neurons to neighbourhoods: The science of early childhood development.* Washington, DC: National Academy Press.

Singer, D., Singer, J., D'Agnostino, H., & DeLong, R. (2009). Children's pastimes and play in sixteen nations: Is free-play declining? *American Journal of Play*, 2(3), 283–312.

Smilansky, S. (1968). *The effects of sociodramatic play on disadvantaged preschool children*. New York: Wiley.

Smith-Roley, S., Mailloux, Z., Miller-Kuhaneck, H., & Glennon, T. (2007). Understanding Ayres sensory integration. *OT Practice*, 12(17), CEA007. https://digitalcommons.sacredheart.edu/cgi/viewcontent.cgi?article=1017&context=ot_fac

Spicer, P. (2010). Cultural influences on parenting. *Zero to Three*, 30(4), 28–32.

Spitzer, S. (2003). Using participant observation to study the meaning of occupations of young children with autism and other developmental disabilities. *American Journal of Occupational Therapy*, 57(1), 66–76. https://doi.org/10.5014/ajot.57.1.66

Stagnitti, K. (2007). *Child-initiated pretend play assessment (ChIPPA) manual and kit*. Melbourne, Vic: Coordinates Publications. http://hdl.handle.net/10536/DRO/DU:30010526

Stagnitti, K., Malakellis, M., Kenna, R., Kershaw, B., Hoare, M., & de Silva-Sanigorski, A. (2011). Evaluating the feasibility, effectiveness and acceptability of an active play intervention for disadvantaged preschool children: A pilot study. *Australian Journal of Early Childhood*, 36(3), 66–72. https://doi.org/10.1177%2F183693911103600309

Stephenson, A. (2002). Opening up the outdoors: Exploring the relationship between the indoor and outdoor environments of a centre. *European Early Childhood Education Research Journal*, 10(1), 29–38. https://doi.org/10.1080/13502930285208821

Super, C., & Harkness, S. (1986). The developmental niche: A conceptualisation of the interface of child and culture. *International Journal of Behavioral Development*, 9(4), 545–569. https://doi.org/10.1177/016502548600900409

Sutton-Smith, B. (1986). *Toys as culture*. New York: Gardner.

Sutton-Smith, B. (1993). Dilemmas in adult play with children. In K. MacDonald (Ed.), *Parent child play: Descriptions and implications* (pp. 15–40). New York: SUNY Press.

Sutton-Smith, B. (1994). Paradigms of intervention. In J. Hellendoorn, R. van der Kooij, & B. Sutton-Smith (Eds.), *Play and intervention* (pp. 3–22). New York: State University of New York Press.

Sutton-Smith, B. (1997). *The ambiguity of play*. Cambridge, MA: Harvard University Press.

Toscano, I. (2019). Welcome to the European playful cities! *URBACT*. https://urbact.eu/welcome-european-playful-cities.

Tranter, P., & Pawson, E. (2001). Children's access to local environments: A case-study of Christchurch, *New Zealand*. *Local Environment*, 6(1), 27–48. https://doi.org/10.1080/13549830120024233

Trawick-Smith, J. (2010). Drawing back the lens on play: A frame analysis of young children's play in Puerto Rico. *Early Education and Development*, 21(4), 536–567. https://doi.org/10.1080/10409280903118432

Tremblay, M., Gray, C., Babcock, S., Barnes, J., Bradsheet, C., Carr, D.,... Brussoni, M. (2015). Position statement on active outdoor play. *Environmental Research and Public Health*, 12, 6475–6505. https://doi.org/10.3390/ijerph120606475

Tremblay, M., LeBlanc, A., Janssen, I., Kho, M., Hicks, A., Murumets, K.,... Duggan, M. (2011). Canadian sedentary behaviour guidelines for children and youth. *Applied Physiology, Nutrition, and Metabolism*, 36(1), 219–235. https://doi.org/10.1139/h11-012

UNICEF. (2018). *Child-friendly cities and communities handbook*. https://s25924.pcdn.co/wp-content/uploads/2018/05/CFCI-handbook-NewDigital-May-2018.pdf

United Nations Convention on the Rights of the Child (UNCRC). (1989). *Convention on the rights of the child*. Geneva: United Nations.

Wachs, T. (1987). Specificity of environmental action as manifest in environmental correlates of infants' mastery motivation. *Developmental Psychology*, 23(6), 782–790. https://doi/10.1037/0012-1649.23.6.782

Whiting, B., & Edwards, C. (1992). *Children of different worlds: The formation of social behavior*. Cambridge, MA: Harvard University Press.

Wickenden, M., & Kembhavi-Tam, G. (2014). Ask us too! Doing participatory research with disabled children in the global south. *Childhood*, 21(3), 400–417. https://doi.org/10.1177/0907568214525426

Wilcock, A., & Hocking, C. (2015). *An occupational perspective of health* (3rd ed.). Thorofare, NJ: Slack.

Wilkes-Gillan, S., Bundy, A., Cordier, R., & Lincoln, M. (2016). Child outcomes of a pilot parent-delivered intervention for improving the social play skills of children with ADHD and their playmates. *Developmental Neurorehabilitation*, 19, 238–245. https://doi.org/10.3109/17518423.2014.948639

Wilkes-Gillan, S., Bundy, A., Cordier, R., Lincoln, M., & Chen, Y. (2016). A randomised controlled trial of a play-based intervention to improve the social play skills of children with attention deficit hyperactivity disorder (ADHD). *PLoS One*, 11(8), 1–22. https://doi.org/10.1371/journal.pone.0160558

Wing, L. (1995). Play is not the work of the child: Young children's perceptions of work and play. *Early Childhood Research Quarterly*, 10(2), 223–247. https://doi.org/10.1016/0885-2006(95)90005-5

Wood, E. (2007). New directions in play: Consensus or collision? *Education 3–13*, 35(4), 309–320. https://doi.org/10.1080/03004270701602426

World Federation of Occupational Therapists (WFOT). (2019). *Position statement: Occupational therapy and human rights (revised)*. https://www.wfot.org/resources/occupational-therapy-and-human-rights

World Health Organization. (2001). *The international classification of functioning, disability and health (ICF)*. Geneva: WHO. https://apps.who.int/iris/handle/10665/42407

Yates, E., & Oates, R. (2019). Young children's views on play provision in two local parks: A research project by early childhood studies students and staff. *Childhood*, 26(4), 491–508. https://doi.org/10.1177/0907568219839115

APPENDIX 15.1 Resources to Promote Play

Two Play Policy Examples
Ireland: https://www.gov.ie/en/publication/5e246d-ready-steady-play-a-national-play-policy/
Scotland: https://www.playscotland.org/resources/?category=play-strategy

International Play Resources
LUDI

LUDI was a COST Action Network funded by the European Union from 2014 to 2018, devoted to supporting the play of children with disabilities in Europe. The network involved 32 countries and more than 100 practitioners and researchers.

See LUDI's website, where many free resources are located, including information on the development of a play training school, focused on children with disabilities and play for the sake of play:
https://www.ludi-network.eu/

Toys and Games Usability Evaluation Tool (TUET)

The TUET questionnaire was designed to assess usability of toys for children with a disability. Research showed that it provides reliable and valid measures for assessing the accessibility and usability of toys and games for children with hearing, visual, and upper-limb motor impairments. The instrument is available at:
http://www.tuet.eu/.

Learning About Play Across Cultures

Free online course for exploring the importance of play across cultures, from Sheffield University, UK:
https://www.futurelearn.com/courses/play/6

Brussoni and Risky Play

Dr. Mariana Brussoni is a leading researcher in the area of outdoor physical activity play with a special focus on risky play. She is a developmental child psychologist who has specialized in child injury prevention and has come to promote risky play as a key aspect in child health and well-being. See her website for resources and project information to see what initiatives she has developed that might trigger ideas for a project in your work:
https://brussonilab.ca/projects/

Playing Out Initiative for Safe Streets

Playing Out is a not-for-profit organization set up by parents in the UK to promote safer streets for play in their communities.
https://www.childinthecity.org/2017/11/28/bbc-video-on-playing-out-receives-8-million-views/
https://playingout.net/play-streets/faqs/

Other International Initiatives and Resources

International Play Association: https://ipaworld.org/resources/
Toy Industries Europe Resources: https://www.toyindustries.eu/resource-category/play/

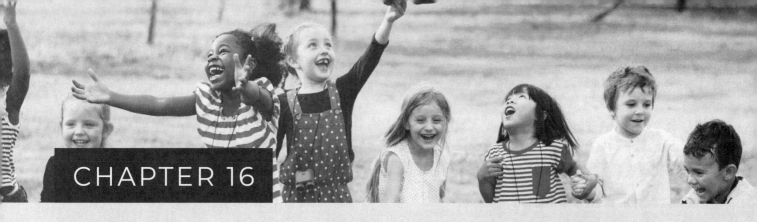

CHAPTER 16

Creatively Negotiating Play Dilemmas

Susan L. Spitzer, PhD, OTR/L

After reading this chapter, the reader will:

- Extend client interests for play despite oppositionality.
- Build pretend play in the face of limited ideas, resistance, and strong emotions.
- Identify and manage challenges when presented with problematic or underground play themes.
- Describe strategies for promoting humor and joking as play.
- Promote healthy video gaming.
- Grade and modify challenge, risk, and competition in play.
- Implement structure and limit setting while maintaining flexibility in play.
- Use play for children with serious health conditions.
- Identify dilemmas and possibilities for using telehealth to promote play in occupational therapy.

The creation of something new is not accomplished by the intellect but by the play instinct.

—Carl Jung

When occupational therapy practitioners firmly commit to play in their practice, a number of particular dilemmas inevitably arise. Some common dilemmas are tied directly to play difficulties of children such as absent or narrow play interests, problematic play themes, resistance to pretend play, ineffective use of humor, unhealthy video gaming, and derailment with challenge and competition. Other dilemmas exist within the therapeutic play space and are rooted in the conflicting nature of play and the role of therapeutic intervention such as the balance between structure and flexibility, trying to promote play in medical contexts, and adapting strategies for telehealth. Many difficulties emerge as therapists balance the value of true play with therapeutic goals and client needs.

Given their frequency and complexity, these predicaments and their management merit individual review. The most common dilemmas have been addressed in previous chapters. This chapter recognizes additional important challenges and illustrates how the professional reasoning presented in earlier chapters applies to these complex issues. This is not a comprehensive listing of problems and solutions because all challenges cannot be anticipated for the variety of clients and contexts encountered in occupational therapy. Therefore, the specifics here are designed to illustrate how to plan for and adjust therapy plans to contend with the real difficulties of play in particular situations. By having multiple exemplars of how to analyze and manage play dilemmas, you will be better able to anticipate and adapt to similar and novel challenges as both arise in your own practice.

Child-Related Play Dilemmas

Narrow Play Focus

Many of the children receiving occupational therapy begin therapy with limited play interests and resistance to change. Therefore, expanding play interests can be an important focus of therapy. Although the fundamentals for incorporating play interests were covered in Chapter 8, this process becomes more complicated in practice when children have limited interests with which to begin. For some children, restricted interest is associated with constrained self-initiated attempts to engage in activities. They may not be interested in the toys or other objects available, and they may show no interest in other children's play. They may not have the skills to engage, or they may not have had a positive experience with a number of activities. They may not object to the therapist's ideas, but it can be very difficult to find play or other activities in which they genuinely enjoy participating. For other children, their specific interests are so strong and compelling that they resist anything outside of those narrow interests. Either way, the occupational therapy practitioner is challenged to help pediatric clients extend their interests and increase play participation in a diversity of activities, places, and social settings. While the bulk of the research on play interests has been conducted with children with autism spectrum disorder (ASD), it clearly has implications for children with other diagnoses who have limited interests.

Using Current Play Interests in Social Play

Play and interests often go hand in hand. Research shows that including a child's interests can be effective for promoting play participation, especially for children with ASD (i.e., Baker, 2000; DiCarlo, Schepis, & Flynn, 2009; Jung & Sainato, 2013, 2015; Koegel et al., 2012; Kryzak et al., 2013; Owens et al., 2008; Porter, 2012; Reinhartsen, Garfinkle, & Wolery, 2002; Vismara & Lyons, 2007; Wimpory, Hobson, & Nash, 2007). In a review of 20 published studies, all found gains in engagement/motivation from incorporating personal interests for children with ASD (Gunn & Delafield-Butt, 2015). Incorporating children's interests is best practice in occupational therapy and person-centered planning (Didden et al., 2008; Tomchek

& Koenig, 2016). Access to special interests has also been associated with quality of life for children with ASD (Tavernor et al., 2013).

Strong play interests can hinder or support social play, however. Children who have intense play interests often have an interest different from that of their potential playmates. If a client is not interested in playing what the other children are playing, and the other children lack the knowledge or interest to play what the client is playing, socially interactive play that is truly playful does not occur. But such hindrances can be transformed into opportunities. Embracing a child's play interest, however unconventional it may be, is to appreciate diversity (Mitchell & Lashewicz, 2018). The use of special interests has been highly effective in increasing social engagement of children and adolescents with ASD in play and leisure activities (Boyd et al., 2007; Dunst et al., 2012; Kaboski et al., 2014; Koegel et al., 2012; Koegel, Kim, Koegel, & Schwartzman, 2013; Kryzak, Bauer, Jones, & Sturmey, 2013; Kryzak & Jones, 2014; Lindsay et al., 2017; Vismara & Lyons, 2007; Watkins, O'Reilly, Kuhn, & Ledbetter-Cho, 2019; Wimpory, Hobson, & Nash, 2007; Winters-Messiers, 2007). Because of the social nature of such play, the interests and skills of both child and peer are valued and considered for adaptation.

One way to use special interests in social play is to have preferred items available or create an environment where those play themes are valued (Kabooski et al., 2014; Kryzak & Jones, 2014; Lindsay et al., 2017; Watkins et al., 2019). Specific toys, play objects, or lunch clubs can be the conduit for both to share a play interest. If a child cannot access their interests, then they are unlikely to engage in any play. Individuals with disabilities can feel that their different strengths and interests are devalued and unimportant if the focus is just on others' conventional interests. When their interests are used as strengths in social play, children are more likely to want to participate. If the environment has opportunities for a child to use their interests in play, then social play is also more likely (Reszka, Odom, & Hume, 2012), and social anxiety may be lessened (Kaboski et al., 2014). However, this is not necessarily the case for items with very high motivation such as highly preferred sensory stimulating items for children with ASD (Sautter et al., 2008; White, 1959), which must be assessed individually. Children tend to be motivated to engage with others in and around their special interest. The other child(ren) are exposed to new interests or to interests in a more intense manner, potentially expanding their knowledge and interest in less-familiar play. The limit to this approach is that these unique interests may not always be of adequate or lasting interest to other children.

Current play interests can also be adapted into shared interests. Transforming limited play interest in ways that encompass what other children can and will want to play creates additional opportunities for social play to emerge. Elements of two children's different play preferences can be fused together to create a new activity, such as combining ponies and *Star Wars* characters to make up a new story that both children can play together. Tag games, follow-the-leader, ball games, and new pretend games are social games that have been successfully modified to accommodate children's unique interests (Baker, 2000; Baker, Koegel, & Koegel, 1998; Koegel, Dyer, & Bell, 1987; Koegel et al., 2012; Koegel et al., 2013; Kuhaneck et al., 2010; Owens et al., 2008). Interests such as geography, airplanes, dinosaurs, and presidents can be incorporated easily into such play forms by using terms about these topics while maintaining the standard form of the game. For example, a game of catch looks similar even when a different object is used or when the players say *president* before throwing the ball. A cognitive approach may use a visual reminder card of how to incorporate a child's interests into social interaction (Spencer, Simpson, Day, & Buster, 2008). For adolescents, it is often possible to find interests that overlap even if all interests do not (Cho et al., 2017). It is not necessary that all elements are of equal value or meaning to both parties, simply that there are elements that are meaningful to each as depicted in **Practice Example 16.1**. Including the interests of both the child and others shows that both are valued and respected. Involving children in the process of modifying social activities can also help them learn to negotiate and appropriately assert their own needs and preferences to build social interaction skills.

As children age, it often becomes increasingly easier to find or create groups of peers who innately share similar passions such as chess clubs, science camps, and robotics programs. Bringing together children who truly share each other's passions can be very rewarding intellectually and socially. Such children can be a good match for friendships that occur with less effort and outside support. Shared interests have been identified as critical to maintaining friendships for boys with ASD (Daniel & Billingsley, 2010).

Expanding Play Interests

The professional reasoning process for expanding interests is informed by the evaluation and activity analysis. The occupational therapy practitioner compares how the activity is done currently with the child's interests and needs. This analysis allows the therapist to identify possible modifications based on interests, strengths, skills, or needs to expand engagement (see worksheet in **Appendix 16.1** to assist with this process).

Cultivating Seeds of Interest. At times, it can be hard to find anything that interests a child. In these cases, the occupational therapy practitioner must create occupational appeal (Munier, Myers, & Pierce, 2008) and focus on the precursors of play (Holloway, 2008). Even limited interests can be identified by the evaluation and used to support active engagement by the child. For example, children with Angelman syndrome tend to have stronger preferences for water-related items (Didden et al., 2008), or a child may like a particular character, or something as simple as the color red or shiny objects. These materials can be used in therapy as objects toward which the child will move or reach. Or, the child may show a relative strength with

---

PRACTICE EXAMPLE 16.1 Tommy, Interests, and Social Play

Contributed by Heather M. Kuhaneck, PhD, OTR/L, FAOTA

Tommy was a bright and smiling 7-year-old who loved maps. He had a library of atlases at home and was particularly fond of Antarctica and any stories of the explorers who traveled with Sir Ernest Shackleton. Tommy's peers were less than interested in this topic, and Tommy generally had few friends to play with at recess.

His occupational therapist was able to create a game for Tommy that allowed him to engage with his peers in a way that was fun and developmentally appropriate for them but that also engaged him in an area in which he was quite interested. The occupational therapist created a "tag"-like game that provided rough-and-tumble play and recreated the adventures of Shackleton in the exploration of the Arctic. The occupational therapist set the situation so that each child got to add a rule to the game; Tommy got to tell the children if the rule matched the real story of the adventure (so he got to share his knowledge), and the children got to make up a fun game with the rules they wanted for the game. The game included some sharing and working together (the explorers had to work together to survive), some rough-and-tumble climbing and racing (who could make it to the top of the mountain first), and lots of sensory motor activity on the playground (pulling, pushing, hauling) as the children acted out the explorer's adventures.

visual perception and thus be more inclined to find constructional activities or object relationships intrinsically satisfying. Or a parent or other caregiver may be able to share what makes the child smile. Any of these small interests can be the opening for the therapist to "get into" the play of a child with limited interests.

The occupational therapy practitioner does not stop here. Extending such a narrow interest into broader engagement in play and other functional daily activities requires a continuously graded approach. As the child consistently shows interest in actively participating, the therapist upgrades the challenge so that there is a delay in reaching/obtaining the object or more complex ways of using the object. For example, if a child likes shiny red objects, the therapist may place a string of shiny red beads easily within the child's reach and gradually move some farther away to sustain engagement while working on trunk rotation. The occupational therapist may place an object of interest in a tunnel, at the top of a structure, or behind another object to encourage a child to crawl, climb, or negotiate obstacles. Later, that preferred object might be included in a reciprocal modified game of catch or in pretending it is treasure. To promote play, the occupational therapy practitioner grades the challenge so that the child is continually able to *obtain* the object of interest and experience the pleasure of doing so. When meaning is created for a child, occupation then emerges (Price & Miner, 2007). Momentum is generated, encouraging further repetition and perseverance (Carlson, 1996). Once the child is willing to participate in a broader range of activities, the therapist can create greater opportunities for practice and skill development. As occupational therapy practitioners balance out the child's limited interests and the goals desired for the child's future, they reflect

on this question: Is this a step that helps the child move forward in making therapeutic gains toward his or her goals? If the answer is in the affirmative, therapists can know that their reasoning is sound.

Broadening Interests Despite Opposition.

Some children get so focused on their own particular interests or ways of doing things that anything else is met with great opposition and resistance. A child may insist on exclusively playing cars, monsters, horses, or a particular character. The problem with a constricted passion is when the child is so involved in this one play activity that he or she cannot adjust to play with other peers or tolerate changes that promote therapeutic goals. Research indicates that narrow interests in children with ASD can greatly interfere with participation and limit enjoyment in activities not related to their specific interest (Eversole et al., 2016; Klin et al., 2007). The client often reacts as if all the therapist's ideas are work and can be extremely resistant to adult direction. In these situations, the occupational therapy practitioner must balance two initially competing commitments—the personal meaning of the interest and the need for functional participation.

To bridge the chasm between what the child wants to do and what the child needs to do, the occupational therapy practitioner adapts the child's play in a manner that simultaneously is consistent both with play and intervention goals. The activity can still be play if the modifications are consistent with the child's personal meaning. For example, a boy who insists he only wants to play with his toy helicopter might be enticed to roll small balls of white playdough to cover a helicopter's propellers in a pretend blizzard to work on play expansion and fine-motor development (see **Figure 16.1**). The

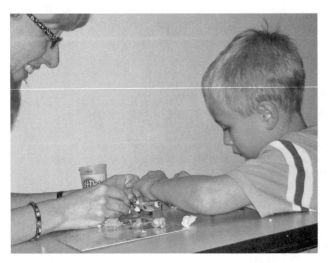 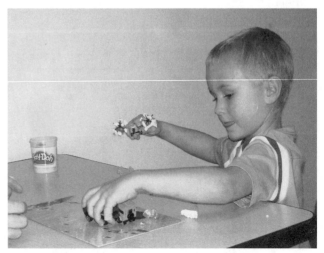

Figure 16.1 An occupational therapist demonstrates respect for and valuing of a child's play interests in toy vehicles by incorporating these toys in a new play activity of rolling small playdough snowballs to cover a plane's propellers in a pretend blizzard

therapist is challenged to find as many ways as possible to combine the child's obsessive play focus with therapeutic goals. The occupational therapist uses activity analysis to identify multiple ways to play the child's specific interest. It is extremely important that these ideas are presented in a playful manner to minimize resistance and ease transitions to modified play. Adaptations can close the gap between wants and needs by combining elements of both through modifications or grading.

Modifying Structure and Choice to Expand Interests. The occupational therapy practitioner may opt to give the client choices or turns in selecting activities with clear elements of both the child's interests and therapeutic properties. The therapist plans creative activities that are both playful and therapeutic so that clients will try to actively participate, as the case of Javier illustrates (see **Practice Example 16.2**). An older child can be

---

PRACTICE EXAMPLE 16.2 Javier, Interests, and Resistance

Javier was a 7-year-old with obsessive compulsive disorder and attention-deficit/hyperactivity disorder (ADHD). He was being seen for poor motor planning and postural control because his parents wanted him to be able to imitate others' movements to adjust to new play activities with peers and to be able to move safely around the environment (without bumping into stable objects) for unsupervised independent play.

Javier was not very interested in doing anything in the clinic. Instead, he loved to talk perseveratively about his various interests or things that were on his mind. When he talked, he was unable to initiate or continue a therapeutic activity because he had to stop to talk. Thus, his talking about his interests was a barrier to engagement in therapeutic activities. It was very difficult to interrupt or stop this narrative. One of these interests was the *Miss Nelson* book series (Allard, 1985, 1988).

To physically engage Javier, his occupational therapist suggested enacting some of these stories. Javier liked to pretend to transform into the character Coach Swamp and have the therapist "athlete" do "exercises" (run around). Although this activity helped engage Javier in pretend play and build therapeutic rapport, the motor demands were primarily talk without addressing his therapeutic need. The therapist wanted to adapt this activity to provide additional therapeutic gains and increase variety in play. The occupational therapist analyzed Javier's repetitive play in light of his other abilities, strengths, and needs in order to identify possible modifications (see **Table 16.1**).

Table 16.1 Analysis of Javier's Repetitive Play to Determine Modification Opportunities

Activity Components	Child's Performance (Occupational Analysis)	Other Child Interests, Abilities, Strengths	Areas of Need	Analysis: Possible Modifications
Materials (toys, objects, shape, color, size, etc.)	None	Books	Increased variety	Exercise cards
Sensory features (visual, auditory, tactile, vestibular, proprioceptive)	Minimal demands for his abilities	Good visual processing and reading	Body awareness	Have him determine adequate space for himself to do exercises. Ask him where therapist should perform as well.
Motor/action features (eyes, posture, hand use, movements, motor skill/ coordination/ control, etc.)	Repetitive talking is primary Minimal other demands	Simple motor actions intact	Postural control; bilateral coordination	Have him demonstrate exercises involving postural and bilateral coordination demands.
Cognitive features (sequencing, problem solving, construction, imagination, etc.)	Remember exercises, terms	Excellent memory	Flexibility	Allow him to determine and select the order.
Social features (interaction with another)	Talking quickly to people to give information	Likes other people and peers	Reciprocal social interaction (allowing and waiting for other person's response)	Ask him about how to do the exercise, is this right, etc., to build more dynamic interaction.

(continues)

PRACTICE EXAMPLE 16.2 Javier, Interests, and Resistance *(continued)*

Because "exercises" could be therapeutic, the occupational therapist decided to develop "Coach Swamp" exercises. She made cards with pictures and labels of different exercises that would help Javier build kinesthetic awareness, postural control, and bilateral coordination, which would address his other goals. She presented these "Coach Swamp" exercise cards to Javier, telling him he could pick which ones to do. As the therapist played the role of the lazy student athlete, she explained how she did not know how to do each exercise and would need the coach to show and teach her. Thus, "coach" Javier demonstrated each exercise and did them alongside the occupational therapist "athlete." The exercises were transformed from work into a specific preferred play activity as Javier adjusted to novelty in his play.

---

involved directly in the explicit process of combining elements of what he or she wants and needs to do (Kuhaneck et al., 2010; Spitzer, 2008, 2017). Clients can be informed that a particular area needs to be addressed and why (e.g., "better balance will help you play on the playground without getting hurt"), and the therapist then gathers the child's ideas for how to do this. For other children, it can be framed as a social interaction dilemma of needing to find a way for both ideas to be included and played together. One way to explicate this process and make it seem fair is to have both therapist and child write their top ideas for the session on different index cards and then pair index cards from each one into a single activity. In one case, one client came up with an idea of playing space travel (his index card) to visit aliens and return to earth, and then writing (the therapist's index card) a letter to the aliens about the visit to thank them for the interesting food and so on. In another case, when a child saw the cards of his choices, he stated, "Wow, I can't wait! There is so much fun stuff to do!" Having concrete reminders of all the personal meaning can help counter the demands of expanding into previously less preferred areas.

Grading to Expand Interests. For children who cannot make choices or tolerate structural modifications to their preferred activities, downgrading demands and introducing very small changes can be effective to start expanding interests. In such cases, the occupational therapy practitioner starts where the child is and builds a bridge through a series of very carefully graded activities. Each activity adaptation is a small step toward the goal, as the case of Paul illustrates (see **Practice Example 16.3**). The process of expanding a strong, particular play focus can take time and occurs gradually (Paley, 1990).

When a child's interests cause resistance to nonplay therapeutic goals, honoring the child's play interests can be extraordinarily challenging. Yet, using these special interests can be especially effective in educational programs for students with ASD (Kluth & Schwarz, 2008; Koegel, Singh, & Koegel, 2010). The occupational therapy practitioner

---

PRACTICE EXAMPLE 16.3 Paul, Interests, and Opposition

Paul was a 3-year-old with ASD, who demonstrated extreme anger with any adult attempts at intervention. His tantrums were frequent and extreme in volume, aggression, and duration. Even when someone tried to help him do what he wanted, he would tantrum. His language was severely limited, and despite explanations and demonstrations, he may not have understood that the adult was trying to help him.

The occupational therapy evaluation found restricted play interests. Paul preferred rough physical play and novel nontoy items (such as a flashlight or pencil sharpener), but he also liked to watch cartoons; hold, throw, and mouth balls; roll cars on different surfaces; and dump, kick, throw, or step on most other toys. He appreciated positive emotional reactions from adults such as smiling with praise, "yay's," and clapping. His gross-motor skills were well developed for his age, and he seemed to rely on visual learning. Given the nature of his interests, he could be very destructive and had to be monitored closely and continuously by adults.

Because any involvement in what Paul was doing would be met with tantrums, the occupational therapist opted to let Paul engage in what he selected, monitor him for safety, and model play with selected other materials in strategic locations so that he would notice her. The occupational therapist selected one item at a time that she determined Paul was likely to be successful and enjoy based on his other interests. For example, the therapist selected a number of sensory-motor materials that gave sensory feedback. Given his visual strengths, she also determined that constructional play would be a likely category of play that Paul could perform and might want to perform once he realized that construction provides opportunities for destruction. Therefore, she used blocks that she stacked up and then knocked down. She used long blocks laid out like a road with a car to drive on the "road." She gradually modeled other constructional activities as well such as building a garage for the car to "bust" out of.

With the occupational therapist's modeling of play, Paul began to come over and imitate what she had done. He began indicating that he wanted the occupational therapist to get an item for him, which gave the occupational therapist another dimension to her role in his expanding play repertoire. Gradually, over the course of these first 2 months, she had established a small role in his play. Initially, he took over each activity and would not allow the occupational therapist to be involved. Then, over the course of the next 4 months, the occupational therapist began to establish "turns," first in parallel by repeating the activity Paul had done with extra materials and emphasizing "my turn" and "your turn" with gestures. Later, the occupational therapist was able to bring out a construction/demolition game, Don't Break the Ice®. She very quickly took her turn between each of his turns at hitting the blocks. Eventually, she was able to get Paul to wait for her to take a turn. In this way, Paul learned to tolerate adult interaction, laying the groundwork for further intervention, and he broadened his play repertoire to participate in social play and play with constructional toys in a safe and independent manner (see **Figure 16.2A and B**).

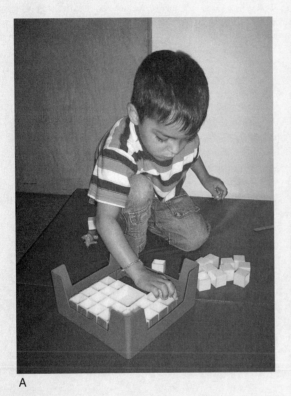 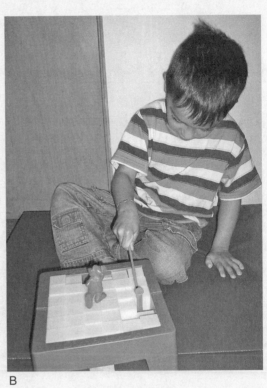

A   B

Figure 16.2 Strengths and interest in construction (A) and destruction (B) play themes may be blended with a cooperative turn-taking game to build tolerance for social play with a game of Don't Break the Ice®

Courtesy of Susan L. Spitzer.

may help create a new play activity that combines the child's interest with therapeutic, skill-building activities, as illustrated in **Practice Example 16.4**.

Relinquishing Preferred Objects

When a child's focused interest involves an object that impedes participation in other needed activities, adults often want to remove the object. Based on the information presented earlier, it should not surprise you to learn that great caution is urged in weighing such a move. If a child is very attached to an object, having to

let go of that object even briefly can be very upsetting, which in itself can create further challenges for participation. Furthermore, the child may become very angry and distrustful with you for having taken the object, jeopardizing the therapeutic relationship and play.

Instead, it is often advisable to consider whether the object needs to be removed. Perhaps there are ways to incorporate it in new ways or to work around the object. Often a duplicate or similar object can be used to model a different way to use the object. Once trust is established, the therapist may be able to take a brief turn with the object or establish a resting place

---

PRACTICE EXAMPLE 16.4 Isabella, Presidents, and Geography

Isabella was a bright kindergartner with an anxiety disorder who had developed a strong interest in information related to American presidents and world geography. She loved to talk about recent knowledge she had gained in these areas and was inattentive and unengaged with other activities. Occupational therapy was focused on building self-confidence, balance, bilateral coordination, and timing for greater participation at recess, and increased visual-spatial constructional skills for improved ability to draw, write, and make class projects. She was being seen in a school therapy room using a sensory integration approach.

Isabella's occupational therapist suggested that they play world traveling. Isabella asked if they could play American presidents traveling the world; and her occupational therapist agreed. To work on gross-motor skills, they used different equipment to represent different countries or modes of traveling to each location. Isabella was quick to identify countries to start at and where to travel to, but despite her studied knowledge of the world, she was unable to identify their relative locations and distances. Her occupational therapist borrowed a world map from a teacher so that Isabella could look at the location of each country before making the trip on suspended equipment. In this way, the occupational therapist helped Isabella to work on spatial orientation through determining direction and estimating relative spatial distance to determine long, medium, and short trips.

PRACTICE EXAMPLE 16.5 Mark and His Car

Contributed by Heather M. Kuhaneck, PhD, OTR/L, FAOTA

Mark came to therapy each visit holding a small toy car that he refused to relinquish. Attempts to remove it led to tantrums and sessions that were less than productive. His occupational therapist quickly made the decision to allow Mark to keep the car and eventually to use it in activities to motivate him.

The therapist brought in another toy car for herself and modeled placing the car in her pocket so she could use her hands to play with playdough. Then she modeled rolling the car in the playdough and then putting it back in her pocket. She repeatedly placed and removed the car and then handed Mark her car. Mark was able to imitate the therapist with her car and return it to her. Over time, he was able to put his toy car in his pocket briefly as long as he was able to pull it out as he chose. Eventually, as Mark was able to trust that his therapist would not take his car away, he allowed the therapist to pick up his toy car and place it in his pocket.

The occupational therapist determined that Mark was beginning to enjoy climbing, and she created activities and obstacles to climb that required him to let go of his car briefly. The therapist would then quickly take the car and place it up just slightly higher so that Mark could see it, climb up to it, and retrieve it. As long as he could quickly get it back and could see it, he was not upset by this. They continued to play this type of game until over time, Mark could give up the car for greater distances as long as he could see it up ahead. They were eventually able to create a similar game using a scooter board as a car he was riding on, to chase and try to catch his toy car that the therapist kept pushing slightly further away. Over time, this grew into a hide-and-seek game with his toy car. He was not only able to handle having the toy car out of his sight, but this also became an enjoyable game that transferred over time to his home and his family.

---

for the object so that the child becomes accustomed to gradually letting it go without having to worry about getting it back. See **Practice Example 16.5**.

Difficulties Pretending

Although pretend play can be a very powerful way to engage children in therapeutic activities (Parham, 1992), some children need help to participate in pretend play. Even when they have the foundational cognitive skills of at least 18 months developmentally (Stagnitti & Unsworth, 2000), pretend play can still be difficult. Some children do not know what to pretend or how to pretend. Other children pretend in ways that peers or adults dislike. Others resist pretend play. And yet other children get so engrossed in the emotional aspects, that they cannot regulate their emotions to sustain pretend play.

Building Pretend Play

Strong research supports the effectiveness of interventions targeting functional play with pretense and symbolic play for children with disabilities, especially ASD (Barton, 2015; Barton, Choi, & Mauldin, 2019; Barton, Ledford, Zimmerman, & Pokorski, 2018; Barton, Murray, O'Flaherty, Sweeney, & Gossett, 2020; Barton & Wolery, 2008; Chang, Shih, Landa, Kaiser, & Kasari, 2018; Lang et al., 2009). Interventions were delivered directly to the child and/or via a parent or teacher and consisted primarily of modeling, prompting (usually graded to use the least intrusive and most natural visual and verbal prompts needed), using the child's interest or self-direction, imitating the child, narrating actions (i.e., "the boy is eating") and specific descriptive reinforcement (i.e., "wow, how creative that you added a garage for your house"). One study found that while providing role-play material increases the frequency of pretend play, adult support increases the frequency and quality of pretend play in preschoolers (Kalkusch et al., 2020).

Few studies have examined more advanced imaginative play for children and adolescents with disabilities, but their findings are positive (Dimitropoulos, Zyga, Doernberg, & Russ, 2021; Doernberg, Russ, & Dimitropoulos, 2020; Goldingay et al., 2020; Porter, 2012). Goldingay and colleagues found that a play-based approach positively impacted a wider range of social abilities for adolescents than a cognitive behavior approach to social skills. These interventions for imaginative and dramatic play typically involve modeling and very general prompts to make up or act out a story or create a movie about a topic, question "what's next?" or ask what could happen differently. The studies also involved strategies designed to increase the child's knowledge and understanding about physical, social, and emotional factors whether through modeling, embedded explanations, or supplemental learning activities (such as a field trip to a train museum to learn about the history and role of trains in society).

Expanding Pretend Play Ideas

Ideas for pretend play involve different aspects of cognitive processing, which are linked both to creativity and action. Specifically, creativity has been closely linked with pretend play because both involve openness, spontaneous associations, and generation of new ideas, which is also frequently referred to as divergent thinking (Chylińska & Gut, 2020; Russ, 2018, 2020). Play involves creative action, and increased pretend play has been associated with increased creativity (Chylińska & Gut, 2020; Russ, 2018, 2020). But play and creativity are not the same. Some children with disabilities struggle with creating conceptual play ideas such as themes and stories (Dos Santos, Lucisano, & Pfeifer, 2019). On the other hand, children may have creative imaginations but, as in the case of those with dyspraxia, have difficulties with ideation for what they can enact motorically with their bodies or the environment, including in relation to other children (Bodison, 2015; Serrada-Tejeda, Santos-del-Riego, May-Benson, & Pérez-de-Heredia-Torres, 2021). Sensory processing factors such as body awareness, balance, and touch have also been associated with pretend play (Roberts, Stagnitti, Brown, & Bhopti, 2018). Children with weaknesses in motor planning, motor skills, and process skills may struggle with creative problem solving and planning to organize their play ideas into an integrated pattern or story; to identify which objects, space, and environmental features to

use; and to determine how to use them to implement various creative play ideas. Notably, pretend play is not just the thinking of ideas but also selecting and enacting those ideas in relation to the physical and social environment in a meaningful way (Chylińska & Gut, 2020).

Occupational therapy practitioners can support children with general ideas for pretend play, ideation for physical action, and pragmatic enactment of ideas. General ideas for pretend play can be stimulated with storybooks, movies or videos, and common daily life activities in the home and community (feeding a baby or pet, delivering mail, getting groceries, etc.). The therapist may be able to suggest the child think of something from one of these categories or downgrade the demands by providing more specific ideas. The therapist can model ideas for creative changes such as including a super power, an injury, a need for help, a "found" item, or other plot twist. The therapist can upgrade by asking, "What happens next?" or "What about a different ending?" Even for a child with a specific narrow interest, such as dinosaurs, the therapist can help the child generate other related ideas such as feeding them, taking care of baby dinosaurs, making them a home, and fighting off other dinosaurs, which later can be expanded further such as to being a paleontologist or having a dinosaur pet. The therapist can provide indirect cues for ideation of how to enact the play using objects and the physical space. The therapist can provide structure for ideas of what objects to use such as, "What could be the treasure?" or may need to downgrade to suggest looking in an area, helping the child to identify the important criteria of the object (such as color or size) and find something that has that criteria, giving options, or even suggesting a specific item if necessary. The therapist can support the child in ideas of where to set up for play and the arrangement of that space to support play (such as the castle here, the jail over there, and the forest between them).

Improving Engagement in Pretend Play

Superhero play, a common form of pretend play for children (Singer & Singer, 1990) and a commonly used theme in imaginative pretend play interventions, supports child engagement in play (Goldstein, 2018; Hoffmann & Russ, 2016). A superhero may be anyone the child sees as having great "power," anyone whom the child respects, or anyone the child wants to be. Thus, the exact type of superhero may vary. Young children may admire and want to be a mother, father, firefighter, Dora the Explorer, or Diego the Adventurer. Older children may pretend to be conventional superheroes like Spider-Man, Superman, or Luke Skywalker, or more everyday superheroes like an astronaut, a pilot, or a doctor. In play, superhero titles may be invented in relation to the other aspects of play. For example, a child suddenly may be acknowledged by self or the therapist as "super jumper," "the amazing frog boy," or "the incredible flying girl." Whom the child might experience as being a hero depends on the child's cognitive functioning, experience, and social context.

By playing a superhero, the child takes on these superhero qualities. The child becomes powerful and a helper to others. The child gets to imagine and experience the possibilities of what might be and what could be. This is very beneficial for children in general, who often inhabit a role of being helped and of being told what to do, and when to do things (Kelly-Byrne, 1989). For children with disabilities, who often experience greater loss of power over their own lives and who may suffer from low self-esteem, superhero play can be transformative (Parham, 1992). Through superhero play, the child is empowered to perform great feats or to help others. This can be a healing, coping strategy (Singer & Singer, 1990). Superhero play can be a beneficial alternative to destructive play in children who are angry (Livesay, 2007). Superhero play is consistent with our profession's valuing of intrinsic motivation, empowerment, and active engagement in occupation.

Managing Underground Play Themes

Some pretend play themes can be disturbing to adults. For example, many adults feel uncomfortable when they see children playing common play themes related to aggression and violence (such as guns, jail, fighting, and war; see **Figure 16.3**), death and dying, abuse and trauma, and bodily parts and functions. Therapists, parents, caregivers, teachers, or other adults often prefer other types of play. Yet research indicates this type of play can be very important for children to understand the world and feel empowered (Delaney, 2016). Even if this play is prohibited, children still may play these underground themes and may even enjoy breaking the rules to do so (Hinchion, McAuliffe, & Lynch, 2021). This conflict creates a therapeutic dilemma for the occupational therapy practitioner who wants to honor the child's play interests but also must contend with adult reservations about allowing such play. Additionally, therapists must beware of underground play themes that signal true

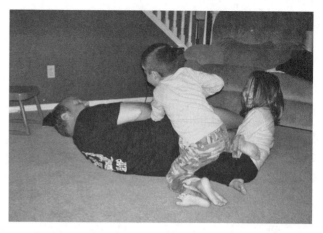

Figure 16.3 In some families, rough-and-tumble play is acceptable for all children, whereas other families may discourage or not allow aggressive-themed pretend play for some or all children. Play that is discouraged or prohibited may continue underground, outside the view or presence of adult authority figures
Courtesy of David A. Morales.

problems necessitating adult intervention. Professional reasoning must be relied on heavily when confronted with underground play ideas.

Therapists need to reflect on their own values and knowledge of play, as well as the values, needs, and interests of the child and other relevant adults (**Box 16.1**). The therapist must be careful not to push his or her own values onto the child. The therapist may consider information about the common presence of such themes in typical children's play and the potential function of this play for the child's understanding of these difficult concepts. The occupational therapy practitioner must determine whether and how underground play themes can be incorporated into therapeutic activities, as seen in **Practice Example 16.6**. Therapists can share their knowledge with parents/caregivers, schools, or other relevant parties to help them make informed decisions about tolerating and sanctioning play. Even with this knowledge, a parent/caregiver or institution may set rules against a certain type of play, thus setting the social-cultural boundaries for therapy. If a therapist feels strongly that such a type of play is important for a child, the therapist may advocate for changes to these rules on behalf of the client.

Many children need help with the limits of underground play, as it is often only sanctioned until a certain point or under certain circumstances. Typically, children learn to control and limit these play themes to fit their sociocultural parameters. They play a variety of play themes beyond "potty talk" in their games when out of earshot of adults. Children begin to recognize which objects can be thrown and hit, and which objects break. They learn to regulate force so as not to really hurt someone when play fighting. Often, it is adult feedback and rules that help them control and shape this form of play. When a child with a disability is learning to play, the therapist and adults in his or her life may have to play both roles of supporting and limiting or guiding this play. For example, therapists may shape destructive forms of play away from "killing" and toward things that are socially acceptable to be destroyed or disciplined (such as litter, weeds, monsters, bad guys), or they may help the child enact a sequence of events related to aggression (such as rebuilding a building or giving "first aid" for "injuries"). In some cases, the therapist may also have to set explicit limits/rules, especially where there is undue risk of injury to self or others or damage to property. Or, the occupational therapy practitioner may suggest alternative forms of play such as cooperative games that are inconsistent with aggression and allow the child to develop alternative social skills (Bay-Hinitz & Wilson, 2005).

Another professional reasoning factor in underground play is assessing whether such play is within the range of typical play or whether it may be a sign that the child is struggling with an unusually strong emotional experience and needs adult help and perhaps

underground play. They begin to understand when and with whom they can play such types of play—for example, 7- and 8-year-old boys learn to use

PRACTICE EXAMPLE 16.6 Joey and the Dying Game

Joey was a 10-year-old with ASD and intellectual disabilities. He demonstrated difficulties with self-regulation of emotions and behavior. He was easily frustrated and upset, which usually resulted in aggression (hitting or grabbing others) and destruction of nearby physical property. Even when calm, he had significant difficulties with motor planning and grading force; he often accidentally hurt other people, broke objects, or ruined projects. He was being seen in the school occupational therapy room with a focus on play and sensory integration. He was easily frustrated and would try to stop or get out of most therapeutic and daily life activities.

During one session, he dropped to the ground and announced, "I died." Not sure he completely understood death and wondering if this was escape behavior, the occupational therapist focused on the immediate priorities to keep play going and emphasize the social emotional themes, commenting, "Oh no, I'm going to miss you! Should I give you some medicine to help you feel better?" "No!" replied Joey. "What should I do?" asked the therapist. "Bury me," said Joey. "Okay," said the therapist, "will this big pillow work?" "Yea," he replied. And she placed a large pillow on top of him and commented how she wished he would come back to play. After a moment, he pushed the pillow back and said, "I'm alive." "Yay!" the therapist said. Joey then wanted the therapist to take a turn, and she did, with Joey carefully placing the pillow on top of her as she directed "gentle, just pretend."

This became the basis for a more elaborate "dying game." First, they selected equipment that they could use together (determining adequate physical space for their two bodies). He would ask her, "Do you want to dance?" and hold out his hand. She put her hand in his and together they would get on moving equipment, being very attentive to maintain body space and be careful "like a gentleman." They would move the swing around in a "dance" and fall off together into a pillow, where he would say who was dead. The "alive" person would bury the "dead" one, carefully grading force. Then the "dead" person would come back to life, and the game was repeated. In the "dying game," Joey experienced sustained participation and learned to regulate his muscle force and emotions in social interactions.

additional mental health intervention. Children at play regardless of disability may express their traumatic experiences from various adverse events such as abuse; neglect; violence; painful medical care; a suddenly departed family member (death, abandonment, divorce); or a close family member who has a substance abuse disorder, has a mental illness, is incarcerated, or is the victim of domestic violence (Hoover, 2015; Lynch, Ashcroft, & March Tekell, 2017; Stenman et al., 2019). For example, sometimes children begin to play with themes of death and dying when a pet or someone they know has died. If this theme comes up frequently or with unusually strong real emotions shown, it may indicate that the child needs assistance with the grieving process, and the team psychologist or social worker should be consulted. A child who demonstrates real anger and aggression in play fighting may also need psychological intervention to express and understand the source of their anger in addition to a focus on cooperative play. Occupational therapy practitioners can use trauma-informed approaches such as building regulation through play (Fette, Lambdin-Pattavina, & Weaver, 2019). However, for children and adolescents who need help to express their feelings about and heal from trauma through play activities, additional expertise and training in play therapy is necessary as well as additional research (Blunden, 2001; Humble et al., 2019; Parker, Hergenrather, Smelser, & Kelly, 2021).

Play with sexual themes is a form of underground play that requires careful professional reasoning. Sexual development in children is normal but often uncomfortable for adults. Typically, children with a normal interest in their bodies may start to talk about these factual discoveries, ask questions about body functions, engage in touching of or looking at their genitalia, and show interest in and curiosity about other aspects of sexuality (Cacciatore, Ingman-Friberg, Lainiala, & Apter, 2020; Larsson & Svedin, 2002; Sandnabba, Santtila, Wannas, & Krook, 2003; Sciaraffa & Randolph, 2011). These behaviors are commonly observed in children, peaking at 3 to 5 years of development, but the behaviors at this age do not have the same cognitive and erotic meaning as adult sexuality (Counterman & Kirkwood, 2013; Pluhar, 2007; Sciaraffa & Randolph, 2011). Limited research indicates that similar behaviors related to sexual development also occur in children with disabilities (Chan & John, 2012; Wilkinson, Theodore, Raczka, 2015). Typically, children learn to differentiate aspects of sexuality that are public and private; however, this may be more difficult for some children with disabilities, especially those with ASD (Chan & John, 2012). Practitioners can promote healthy sexuality by responding with developmentally appropriate

honesty as well as role modeling and education about modesty, privacy, and safety in alignment with family values (Counterman & Kirkwood, 2013; Wilkinson et al., 2015). Nonetheless, clinicians must be alert and report suspicious incidences or descriptions of sexual behavior to the authorities as required by law. After all, children with disabilities are at increased risk of sexual abuse (Chan & John, 2012). Increasing sexuality and the rare occurrence of child sexual behaviors that imitate adult sexual behavior (oral–genital contact and insertion of object or body part into another child), and sexual preoccupation in a young child who does not demonstrate other preoccupations indicate that the child is unlikely to have invented this behavior on his or her own and is more likely to have been exposed to sexual activity or to have been sexually abused, which is truly concerning when observed in children's play (Davies, Glaser, & Kossoff, 2000).

Reducing Resistance to Pretending

Shifting to pretend play can be met with resistance by some children. Children may find unreal ideas confusing and uncomfortable and even feel it is wrong to spend time on ideas that are untrue. This is very common in children with ASD (Moor, 2002), who tend to do better with concrete rather than abstract thinking. When you suggest pretending, the child may tell you, "I'm not Superman, I'm Peter," or "That's not a phone, it's a block." In such cases, the occupational therapy practitioner may have to grade activities carefully, slowly introducing pretend components into the child's current play, and may need to address the child's cognitive and emotional processing (see **Box 16.2** for a list of strategies).

Grading Pretend Play. It is often best to start pretend play with objects related to the child's own body and behavior because this tends to occur first in typical development (Hellendoorn, 1994). The development of pretend play and related age expectations as described in Chapter 1 can provide a basis for this process. For example, functional or presymbolic play involves the use of real or real-looking objects or props in conventional ways. Pretending to drink from a cup, eat from a spoon, sleep with a pillow, and talk on a phone are examples of the most basic form of pretending. Because the pretending is very concrete and closely related to the real use of objects, it can be easier for a child to understand and enjoy doing (Moor, 2002). Gradually expanding the type of objects and the way they are used allows the child to gain foundational pretend play skills. For example, real objects can also be used in relation to someone else (such as pretending to feed a parent/

Box 16.2 Strategies for Adapting Concrete Play to Pretend Play

---

- Grade developmentally to gradually:
  - Expand pretending with toys and objects
    - Utilize toys and objects in different ways such as:
      - Constructing different kinds of buildings
      - Making other things from blocks such as statues
    - Use real or realistic objects (such as kitchen items) and actions related to child's body (e.g., pretend to drink from a cup)
    - Use real or realistic objects and actions related to another's body (e.g., parent/caregiver) or doll/toy figure (e.g., feed the toy dog)
      - Objects to consider starting with include: baby, vehicles, animal and people figures
    - Employ realistic props (e.g., firefighter's hat, superhero cape)
    - Substitute open-ended objects with a resemblance to the real represented object (e.g., rectangular block as a "candy bar")
      - Pieces of cloth, boxes, sponges, paper, and pipe cleaners work well, but anything can do
    - Substitute open-ended objects without a clear resemblance to the real represented object (e.g., a pink ball as a "candy bar")
    - Remove real objects and props (completely imagine the objects)
  - Assume roles:
    - Reality-based role (e.g., mother, police officer, doctor)
    - Fantasy roles (e.g., superhero, an animal)
    - Switch and play different characters (be the "helper" instead of the "hero")
    - Include feelings
  - Organize the elements
    - Use a familiar sequence such as eat–drink–sleep, get ready for school or bed, go to store, have a party, visit a doctor or vet
    - Include narrative plots
      - Beginning, middle, end
      - A familiar plot from a favorite book or video
      - Novel plots or combining plots from two or more stories (e.g., Superman in Star Wars; live on the moon; super powers)
      - Make unexpected plot twists, dilemmas (such as loss of a toy or an injury), silly sequences (such as suddenly growing antennae), alternate endings ("what if ...")
- Use favorite interests
- Model pretend play
- Emphasize difference between "pretend" and "real"
- Use a prop to signify changes in role from "real" to "pretend"
- Explore how an object or action is "like" something else
- Discuss or develop a story to explicitly explain the pretend play activity and/or its value

---

caregiver or sibling), a doll, or other toy character. Expanding symbolic play next involves the use of "real" props such as a fireman's hat, pretend dishes, or pretend lawn mower. Then the occupational therapy practitioner may introduce using objects that merely resemble a real object. For example, a plastic banana may be a "phone," a rectangular block may be a "car," a red ball may be an "apple," and so on. The more closely the object resembles the true item in size, color, and shape, the more easily it may be accepted by the child. A small red ball looks more like a strawberry than a big purple block does, but eventually even a big purple block may become a strawberry during pretend play.

At higher developmental levels, the occupational therapy practitioner may want to encourage themes and narrative plots because this tends to become the more dominant form of pretend play. Usually, this involves the child becoming someone else, such as a superhero, pirate, firefighter, ballerina, Olympic star, mother, pilot, or animal. Pretending to be someone else can present significant difficulty for some children who resist this notion. It can be helpful to start with "real people" roles, such as a firefighter or mother, because the child has seen these roles and knows that people really can be mothers or firefighters. Pretending to ride a horse is closer to real life than pretending to be a horse. Other children may be more receptive to characters and story lines with which they are familiar in favorite books, movies, and television shows. Later, the child may become more open to pretending something unreal, such as a unicorn or alien.

As with most play skills, the occupational therapy practitioner balances the opportunity to repeat, practice, and master each new pretend play skill with encouraging further expansion of these themes. As pretend play is learned, each child needs different amounts of time to practice this new skill by repeating the pretend play. Just like learning to use stairs, some children want to repeat the same pretend sequence extensively before they are ready to expand it. As these are repeated, the therapist may grade the introduction of other pretend play into these repetitions. A child who has difficulty understanding the value and reasoning for pretend play may benefit from additional strategies for pretend play to be meaningful.

Processing Strategies for Pretend Play.

A child may be more open to pretend play when real areas of interest are included, even if it is a narrow interest (Porter, 2012; see **Practice Example 16.7**). Most successful pretend play interventions have included toys in which the child is most interested (Chang et al., 2018; Lang et al., 2009). In this way, the occupational therapy practitioner helps children connect pretend play to their interests and dreams. The familiarity of an interest can be a strength such as the joy of pretending favorite story lines from books or films whose stories are well-known without having to come up with unique pretend ideas. When paired with intrinsic meaning, pretend play becomes more than just a skill, but a truly enjoyable occupation.

The child may need to observe first before feeling comfortable to try pretend play. The occupational therapy practitioner may model pretend play so that the child can observe this phenomenon before asking the child to think of him- or herself differently. A prop that signifies the role change, such as a firefighter hat or cape, may also help the child to differentiate or mark between the world of make-believe and the everyday real world.

The occupational therapy practitioner may initially emphasize use of the words *pretend* and *not real* to help the child understand and accept the imaginative play ideas: "We are doing *pretend* eating, *not real* eating." This strategy is also helpful when the therapist has concerns about the child's ability to manage and separate reality from make-believe. This cognitive strategy can help the child differentiate pretend stealing from a bad guy from actually stealing from a classmate, even a "bad" classmate. A physical prop (such as a hat) or even a sign or label (masking tape with the words *pretend robber* put on a shirt) can help clarify this difference between real and pretend for children who struggle with these concepts.

To start, the occupational therapy practitioner may simply comment on how what the child is doing is "like" something else; for example, "You are flying through the air (on a swing) like birds fly in the air." The therapist may need to clarify, "You are *not* a bird, but you are doing what birds do, so you are *like* a bird, you are *pretending* to be a bird." The occupational therapist may even encourage the child to think of other things that are "like" this, for example, other things that fly. Again, emphasizing the use of the words *pretend* and *not real* can help the child understand and accept the imaginative play ideas. A paper or digital therapeutic story with pictures to explain how and why pretend play is done can be read multiple times and may also help the child to understand and build interest for this form of play (Barry & Burlew, 2004; Smith, Constantin, Johnson, & Brosnan, 2021; see **Appendix 16.2** for sources to assist in writing therapeutic stories.)

For children who understand pretend play but dislike playing untrue ideas, they may appreciate an explanation of how pretend play can connect to another value they have. For example, children may be fascinated to learn that pretend play can enable them to play *with* other children and help their brain learn creative problem solving for becoming a scientist like Albert Einstein.

Managing Strong Emotions in Pretend Play

Affect and emotional experience have been identified as integral to pretend play as cognitive processing (Russ,

---

PRACTICE EXAMPLE 16.7 Olivia and Pretend Play

Olivia was 8 years old and diagnosed with a learning disability and post-traumatic stress disorder. She loved board games but resisted pretend play. Whenever the occupational therapist suggested a pretend theme, Olivia repeatedly asked, "What are you doing?" and "Why?" Despite encouragement, modeling, and explanations, Olivia would comply with a direction to do a particular action but never initiated or responded spontaneously to various pretend play themes. Instead, Olivia repeatedly asked to play her current favorite games of Perfection® and Mouse Trap®. To combine Olivia's interests in board games with therapeutic goals to increase variation and flexibility in play, the occupational therapist suggested that they create large pretend versions of the games in the form of obstacle courses. Olivia was delighted with this idea and actively participated with designing and going through the game "boards" as she actively pretended to be the game "pieces." From this base, as the occupational therapist explained how other pretend themes were similar to pretending board games. Olivia then happily accepted more pretend play themes offered by her therapist and then other children.

2018). Research has found that pretend play interventions can improve emotional control (Dimitropoulos et al., 2021; Goldstein, 2018; Goldstein & Lerner, 2018). In fact, Russ, Fehr, and Hoffman (2013) found that pretend play interventions that emphasized emotional expression were more effective in building play skills than those focused on imagination and organization. Typically, intervention includes modeling of emotional understanding ("I'm feeling __ because__") and how to regulate emotions ("I'm going to talk to my mom to feel better"); encouraging the character/toy talk about emotions; and prompting or asking how the child/character is feeling (Hoffmann & Russ, 2016; Russ et al., 2013).

Story lines that involve strong emotions tend to include more drama, suspense, or tragedy such as the threat of danger, fear, and fighting. Many children like these themes because it can be exciting to watch out for dangerous animals (such as sharks, crocodiles, alligators, bears, lions, or spiders), make-believe creatures (such as ghosts, monsters, pirates, and villains), and other threats (such as storms). This fear and the threat of danger add an element of excitement and potential risk if the child makes a mistake, falls, or goes too close to where the danger is. Playing with fears is thought to help children feel more in control of their fears if they successfully express and manage them in play (Goetze, 1994; Mook, 1994; Singer & Singer, 1990). The use of such potential dangers can be a playful technique for directing a child to do an activity in a certain way: "Stay on the path so the crocodiles don't get you!" It can also be used to help children persevere through an extra challenge or error when they slip: "Oh no, it's quicksand, use all your muscles, and you can get out." Overcoming danger or risk is what superheroes do, too.

These otherwise playful threats can also be the source of much fear and anxiety in some children. Young children are especially vulnerable because they may have difficulty recognizing and remembering that the danger is only pretend and not real (Singer & Singer, 1990). Other children do not have the emotional strength to handle such potential threats, which seem too real. Significant fear is associated with less willingness to take a risk and more protective behaviors in typical children of various ages (Cook et al., 1999; Morrongiello & Matheis, 2007b). Even if the child suggests it, he or she may have difficulty playing with this theme. Also, novelty itself can evoke some element of real fear and anxiety in children and impact the child's tolerance for pretend fear and danger. Therefore, the occupational therapist must carefully monitor the child when playing with themes of danger and fear, grade the activity carefully to ensure that the child is mostly successfully overcoming or escaping the "danger," and be

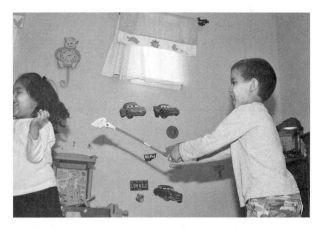

Figure 16.4 Playing with themes of pretend danger and fear with a toy shark can be very enjoyable for many children. However, the occupational therapy practitioner must be ready to adapt or intervene if the play is too scary and threatening for a child

Courtesy of David A. Morales.

ready to alter the activity and offer emotional support if needed (see **Figure 16.4**).

Limited Understanding of Humor

Children with ASD, language impairments, and intellectual disabilities often have difficulty with humorous play, especially in later childhood and adolescence (Agius & Levey, 2019; Chadwick & Platt, 2018; Samson, 2013). They typically do best with explicit and non-social content (Silva, Da Fonseca, Esteves, & Deruelle, 2017). They may have difficulty comprehending and recognizing another's humor, especially sarcasm and irony, which can be misunderstood as real or misinterpreted as lies (Chadwick & Platt, 2018; Samson, 2013). They may mistakenly think others are laughing *at* them. Indeed, they may be the target of hurtful and stigmatizing humor (Chadwick & Platt, 2018). The amount, duration, and timing of their laughter may be interpreted as inappropriate at times (Chadwick & Platt, 2018). Attempts at humor may cross the line into maladaptive humor, such as teasing and mocking, which can have negative effects on social relationships when others are hurt or offended (Martin, Puhlik-Doris, Larsen, Gray, & Weir, 2003). Some may use self-defeating humor to make others laugh at their own expense, which can negatively impact well-being and self-esteem (Martin et al., 2003). However, pediatric clients who struggle with humor often do value humor and are motivated to develop their humor (Silva et al., 2017).

Humor is used commonly as a tool for playful therapeutic use of self in occupational therapy (Leber & Vanoli, 2001; see also Chapter 6); but it also may be the targeted play outcome. Research indicates that humor is trainable in general (Ruch & McGhee, 2014). Developmentally young children can benefit from activities that scaffold and encourage absurdity in play as well as unexpected silly faces, sounds, and words (Loizou & Loizou, 2019). Modeling adaptive humor such as incongruities and silliness can also help youth learn adaptive humor (Chiang, Lee, & Wang, 2016). Therapists also may need to explicitly state or draw attention to humor by marking it as "I'm joking" or "I'm just being silly." Children as young as 5 years developmentally can be taught to understand sarcasm and double meanings (Jackson, Nuñez, Maraach, Wilhite, & Moschella, 2021; Lee, Sidhu, & Pexman, 2020). Adaptive forms of humor, termed self-enhancing and affiliative, can be beneficial for mental health when directed internally and for building social relationships and friendships when directed toward others (Chadwick & Platt, 2018; Jones, James, Fox, & Blunn, 2021; Martin et al, 2003; Paine, Karajian, Hashmi, Persram, & Howe, 2020).

The research on intervention efficacy for children and adolescents with disabilities is limited but positive. Adolescents with ASD can benefit from humor training to increase understanding and use of humor, especially for nonsense jokes and to facilitate interactions with others (Wu, Liu, Kuo, Chen, & Chang, 2016). In this study, intervention focused on training the adolescents to analyze jokes to better understand them as well as sharing and practicing jokes with each other. Humor training is sometimes included within effective social skills training programs for youth with ASD (e.g., Laugeson, Frankel, Gantman, Dillon, & Mogil, 2012).

In order to help children develop humor, therapists must understand its typical development, a topic not always a focus of occupational therapy education. Humor is developed with a child's language and cognition, especially a deeper understanding of how other people think (Paine et al., 2020; Purser, Van Herwegen, & Thomas, 2020). Infants laugh at others' bodily displays of incongruities as well as silly faces and sounds (Paine et al., 2020). Toddlers and young children also display a variety of incongruities with actions (such as putting a toy on one's head) and language (making up words, intentionally using incorrect words), exaggerated sounds, and humorous acts (clowning around), as well as share their humor by smiling, laughing, and looking for a reaction (Hoicka & Akhtar, 2012). In middle childhood, children's humor tends to focus on play with language such as riddles and multiple meanings of words (Paine et al., 2020). At 8 years of age developmentally, laughter becomes reliably connected with comprehension of humor (Purser et al., 2020). In adolescence, sarcasm, irony, and metaphor are

used more frequently (Chang et al., 2014). Humor can be an effective strategy to engage in social play for children with a high level of physical disability (Graham, Mandy, Clarke, & Morriss-Roberts, 2019). Humor is commonly associated with playfulness into adulthood (Barnett, 2007; Bergen & Rousta, 2019; Guitard, Ferland, & Dutil, 2005).

Due to the increasing subtlety of humor as children mature, a cognitive approach is often indicated to assist with judgment in both producing and appreciating humorous incidents. Older children and adolescents often may humorously entertain extreme ideas despite the impossibility and consequences of reality. For example, a child might think, "Wouldn't it be cool if I could jump off the building with my bike and land without getting hurt?" or wish "I dare you to throw the tests out the window" and so on. Likewise, a child may want to escalate a prank of a plastic bug at the family dinner table to a real dead bug in the food at a restaurant. Therapeutically, it is important to make sure clients understand the reality that such ideas cannot be acted on because they may not recognize their own mortality and may minimize the long-term real consequences of their actions.

Some older children and adolescents may need help to analyze the difference between adaptive and maladaptive humor such as the difference between teasing and joking and the difference between witty and hostile sarcasm. Some may need help with the social interaction skills of conveying their own intentionality as sender of humor, monitoring the response of how their humor attempts are received, recognizing cues of the intentionality of someone else sending possible humorous messages, and conveying their responses to humor clearly. Some individuals may need help to consider the other person's thinking and feeling to determine what may be sensitive, offensive, or inappropriate despite its apparent humor in other contexts such as in a movie or online material. For older children and adolescents, a clinician may need to consider the client's vocabulary, world knowledge, metalinguistic knowledge, and figurative language to support understanding of jokes, sarcasm, puns, funny stories, and irony (Agius & Levey, 2019).

Unhealthy Video Gaming

Video games are a common leisure and play interest across ages when electronic devices are available. Video games can be socially appealing because they allow youth the opportunity to engage in competitive play even if they do not excel at sports, offer a means for companionship when playing in a group, provide social capital for discussion topics and relating to peers, and can promote prosocial outcomes (Greitemeyer & Mügge, 2014; Raney, Smith, & Baker, 2006; See **Figure 16.5**). Some parents of children with disabilities support video game play as having a positive impact on their children (Finke, Hickerson, & McLaughlin, 2015). However, inequality in high-speed Internet and device access can limit these opportunities for low-income and minority children (Katz, Gonzalez, & Clark, 2017).

Video play and screen use can also be problematic. Although moderate use of video games appears to be generally safe for children 2 years of age or older and poses no long-term health problems (Griffiths, 2005; American Academy of Pediatrics [AAP] Council on Communications and Media, 2016), excessive or unbalanced video gaming has been linked with a number of negative outcomes. High use of media in general (including video games) has been associated with negative health outcomes, including obesity, sleep disruption, and adolescent smoking (AAP Council on Communications and Media, 2016; Common Sense Media, 2008; Hale & Guan, 2015). From childhood through adulthood, high rates of screen time have been associated with decreased attention, memory, and learning; increased mental health issues

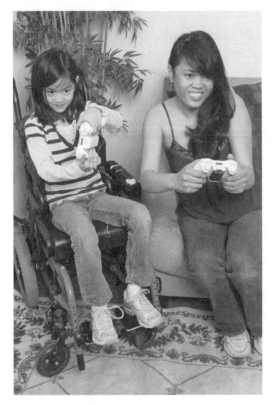

Figure 16.5 As a common play interest for youth, video games may be used as an intervention tool or may be targeted as play outcomes in occupational therapy

© ktaylorg/E+/Getty Images.

and addictions; and an increased risk of premature cognitive decline (Neophytou et al., 2019). High screen time in young children also has been associated with decreased fine-motor, visual-motor, bilateral coordination skills, and posture (Dadson, Brown, & Stagnitti, 2020; Howie, Coenen, Campbell, Ranellli, & Straker, 2017; Kipling Webster, Martin, & Staiano, 2019). Excessive use and checking of smartphones have been associated with increased time spent on gaming and social networking in children and adolescents (Fischer-Grote, Kothgassner, & Felnhofer, 2019). Video game use may conflict with the family's values (Erdogan, Johnson, Dong, & Qiu, 2019). Video games can also expose children to violent images, unsafe behavior, sexual content, negative stereotypes, substance use, cyberbullies and predators, advertising, misleading or inaccurate information, and gambling (American Academy of Child & Adolescent Psychiatry, 2020). Violent video games tend to increase aggression and aggression-related variables and decrease prosocial outcomes (Greitemeyer & Mügge, 2014). Video gaming can create strong habits for ongoing use, so it is important that its negative risks be weighed carefully in determining its use in occupational therapy either as an intervention or targeted outcome.

Evidence does support using video and computer games within occupational therapy as an intervention tool to improve attention, mental health, positive behavior, social participation, visual perception, and occupational performance for children and teens with a range of different disabilities (Egan, 2019; García-Redondo, García, Areces, Núñez, & Rodríguez, 2019; James, Ziviani, Ware, & Boyd, 2015; Lee, Grey, Gurfinkel, Leb, Stern, & Sytner, 2013; Schuurmans, Nijhof, Engels & Granic, 2018; Vasquez et al., 2015). For older children and adolescents, they can be age appropriate, normalizing, and culturally appropriate (Gooch & Living, 2004). Many devices are portable and allow a range of accessibility modifications that help create just right play as both ends and means (American Occupational Therapy Association [AOTA], 2016; Proffitt, 2016). Manufacturers are increasingly adopting game controllers often in collaboration with occupational therapists to increase accessibility for diverse abilities. Factors linked to the success of computer play as an intervention include graded challenges for targeted skills, feedback for self-efficacy, and positive reinforcement for progress toward therapy goals, as well as the therapist's interactions as coach or player (Biddiss, Chan-Viquez, Cheung, & King, 2021). The use of peers with video games may also increase the play experience (Jozkowski & Cermak, 2019). Video games also can be useful tools for increasing therapy frequency without the physical presence of a therapist (James, Ziviani, King, & Boyd, 2016).

Occupational therapy practitioners also help children achieve a healthy balanced use of electronic media (AOTA, 2020; Garfinkel & Minard, 2021). A healthy balance is based on the amount of time a child spends playing video games, the type of video games, and how they fit within the youth's overall daily play routines. The American Academy of Pediatrics (AAP Council on Communications and Media, 2016) recommends setting daily limits of total screen use (including video games and television) and offers a free online program that can be used to guide families to plan daily media time use for different-aged children (www.healthychildren.org/MediaUsePlan). Therapists can help with establishing routines and habits to support implementing daily limits. Another critical factor in achieving a healthy balance is ensuring that children also have physical hands-on play that they can and want to do that does not involve screen use, which may even counteract negative effects on motor skill development (American Academy of Child & Adolescent Psychiatry, 2020; AAP Council on Communications and Media, 2016; Dadson et al., 2020). Occupational therapists can help families match video games to a child's developmental abilities, learn online privacy and safety practices, and recognize and mitigate risks (Garfinkel & Minard, 2021). For example, they may examine how violence is presented and how negative issues are resolved and whether this fits a specific client's understanding, especially in how it relates to reality. A variety of computerized parental controls can be used to assist parents and other caregivers in ensuring positive play experiences (for example, see the guide provided by Common Sense Media at https://www.commonsensemedia.org/blog/parents-ultimate-guide-to-parental-controls?utm_source=021014_Parent+Default&utm_medium=email&utm_campaign=weekly).

Difficulties Playing with Challenge, Risk, and Competition

Challenge and competition emerge as prominent aspects of play in middle childhood in the forms of games with rules, sports, and computer/video games (Florey & Greene, 2008). As a common form of play, pediatric clients may want to engage in challenging and competitive play and/or may need to develop skills in this form of play. Clients may not have been allowed to engage in nominal risk, may resist challenge, or be unable to tolerate losing. Although it may be appropriate to include these elements in occupational therapy sessions, the use of these features is not always play. For such children, occupational therapy must carefully grade and modify challenge, risk, and competition.

Assuring Manageable Challenge and Risk

Many children enjoy the playful thrill and possibility that challenge offers in the face of some risk of defeat or failure. Even young children seek out and enjoy physical risk taking despite its "scariness" (Stephenson, 2003). Children enjoy its uncertainty and thrill (Hinchion, McAuliffe, & Lynch, 2021). Through limited risk experiences, children have described how they learn from their own mistakes (Christensen & Mikkelsen, 2008). A systematic review found overall positive effects of risky outdoor play on various aspects of healthy child development with usually minor injuries at a similar level to sports (Brussoni et al., 2015). Factors influencing a child's willingness to take risks versus avoidance of risk taking include various child attributes (i.e., age, sex, experience, values, temperament), parent–family characteristics (i.e., socialization and teaching practices; parent modeling, style, and attributes; older sibling behavior and encouragement), and social-situational factors (peer risk taking and persuasion, media exposure, and convenience), as well as socioeconomics, culture, and neighborhoods (Jelleyman, McPhee, Brussoni, Bundy, & Duncan, 2019; Morrongiello & Lasenby-Lessard, 2007; Niehues & Bundy, 2019). Additionally, adults concerned for safety and injury prevention often limit opportunities for risky play (Brussoni et al., 2015, 2018).

Sometimes children with disabilities do not experience the same enjoyment of challenge in play (Messier, Ferland, & Majnemer, 2008). Clients with anxiety, low self-esteem, or high awareness of their limitations may avoid the mere attempt at a challenging task and prefer very easy tasks that they have mastered, where there is no risk of failure. In these cases, the occupational therapy practitioner must adapt challenge so the client can play. Many children enjoy having challenges framed in pretend play, where challenge is intrinsic to the theme, such as advancing levels in a video game, Olympics, circus/magic tricks, rodeo, television game show, and so on.

Grading can help a child to build tolerance for challenge. First the occupational therapy practitioner suggests an easy challenge, a very simple action that the child can meet with ease. Before increasing the demands, the therapist may have the child repeat the success a few times to increase sense of mastery. Then the therapist keeps gradually increasing the activity demands slightly, including the child's ideas for increased challenges when possible. The therapist also may notify the child of the increasing challenge so the child can prepare emotionally. The therapist may comment playfully about how hard it is in general and elicit or offer positive comments about the child's potential for doing it—"This is pretty hard, but do you think you can do it? I think you can do it." If the activity has been carefully graded, by the time the child reaches the point of true challenge to his or her abilities, the child should have experienced repeated success in previous "challenge" attempts. This momentum increases the likelihood that the child will now attempt a true challenge and be willing to try again, even if he or she fails. The occupational therapist has created a game where the challenge is fun because it is met successfully, where children experience satisfaction in meeting a challenge and begin to see themselves as successful conquerors of challenges. The child has taken a risk and succeeded.

Children with disabilities often have fewer opportunities to engage in risky play such as incorporating greater heights, speed, dangerous objects (such as sharp, hard, rough), and play fighting/wrestling. Well-intentioned adults striving to protect children with disabilities, often limit risk-taking opportunities common for other children (Spencer et al., 2016). This lack of opportunity can increase risk aversion and disrupt the developmental process for gradually assuming more complex responsibilities in life (Bundy et al., 2015). Preliminary research suggests that adults' barriers to risky play may be reduced by learning to reframe their thinking to (1) locate the risk within the play activity as opposed to the child with disabilities and (2) recognize the value in risk taking to increase tolerance of risk as well as learn strategies to make everyday risks manageable (Brussoni et al., 2018; Bundy et al., 2015; Spencer et al., 2016; Sterman, Villeneuve, et al, 2020).

A note of caution is warranted here. The goal is *manageable* risk-taking that, motivates the child to go further but can be met successfully (Burke, 1977; White, 1959). Risk taking should be balanced with understanding and self-control to avoid truly dangerous, risky play that can injure the child (Little & Wyver, 2010; Morrongiello & Matheis, 2007b). Children must have an accurate understanding of the challenge in relation to their abilities and their vulnerability for injury (Little & Wyver, 2010; Morrongiello & Mathesis, 2007a, 2007b). The child should have some sense of fear of real dangers to be cautious and must be able to find excitement in safe activities too (Cook, Peterson, & DiLillo, 1999; Morrongiello & Matheis, 2007b). Research indicates that typical 4- and 5-year-olds are able to identify injury risk behavior and use these judgments in their play to inform their decisions about risk-taking (Little & Wyver, 2010). They selected activities that offered challenge and excitement and were cautious about engaging in activities beyond their current capacities. Occupational therapy practitioners can use a cognitive approach to help children learn calculated risk taking to play safely by assisting them in developing insight into their own abilities and an understanding of physical properties in the environment.

Promoting Healthy Competition

Competition involves a striving for performance that is compared and evaluated. This may be a challenge between the client and the therapist, family members, and/or peers. Competitive play such as team sports are common in Western society, especially as children age. Typically, children become developmentally ready for competitive play from 7–12 years of age based on individual and contextual factors (Kochanek et al., 2019). Developmentally appropriate competition may help children develop emotional and social skills; however, hypercompetition can inhibit performance, promote negative social behavior, increase maladaptive self-perceptions, and decrease inclusion of people with diverse backgrounds and abilities such as those with disabilities (Bay-Hintz & Wilson, 2005; Kochanek et al., 2019; Spaaij et al., 2019).

Maintaining a healthy, balanced level of competition requires careful adapting on the part of the occupational therapy practitioner (see **Figure 16.6**).

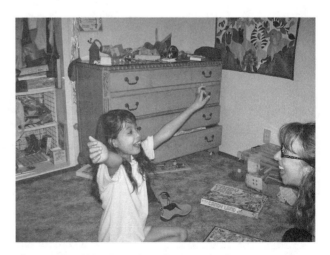

Figure 16.6 Winning a board game can be very exciting for a child, but the occupational therapy practitioner may need to grade competition to help the child learn to manage competition and tolerate losing as well

Clients may have difficulty tolerating losing or even the possibility of losing and may gloat excessively with winning. These features make them unattractive playmates for competitive games, and without a playmate, children lose out on opportunities to play. Some children are so afraid of losing that they avoid this large category of play altogether. Issues of competition commonly arise when children are seen in group therapy sessions, which provide natural opportunities to address competition.

Interventions that emphasize the experiential process of the activity itself as well as personal improvement over winning are likely to yield an environment where competition truly can be play (see **Table 16.2**). Mastery and improvement can be highlighted over performance comparisons with others (Kochanek et al., 2019). Games may be modified to avoid having

Table 16.2 Interventions for Addressing Competitive Play

Intervention	Description and Examples
Select and modify competitive play activities for participation	■ Use games of personal challenge where the child focuses on mastery and improving performance rather than winning (Kochanek et al., 2019). ■ Focus attention on the play process more than the outcome. • Include elements that are exciting, fun, and interesting besides winning (Kochanek et al., 2019). • Play games where no one wins or loses despite the game structure. • Play typically competitive games without computing or discussing points, winning, losing, or being ahead to focus on the process of playing. • Play games of pure chance—as long as the child can cognitively understand the explanation that it is just chance as to who wins or loses. • Establish rules where points are awarded (only) for good sportsmanship, such as saying "good job" to teammates regardless of whether he or she is winning or losing. • Restructure competitive games into cooperative games where players work together to reach a common goal (Bay-Hinitz & Wilson, 2005). ■ Partner or team up children to support each other through loss (Murphy, 2019).
Grade competitiveness demands	■ Gradually increase turn-taking in noncompetitive activities so that the child learns to tolerate the challenges of sharing an activity with another person. ■ Gradually alter the relative amount/frequency of winning/losing to gradually stretch the child's ability to handle loss (Murphy, 2019): • Alternate between winning and losing so that therapist and client essentially "take turns" with winning and losing. • Have therapist get close to winning (creating a threat of loss for the client) but then lose. • Have "a tie," where no one wins or loses. ■ Gradually decrease number and directness of preparations for losing such as • Warnings about the possibility of losing. • Structured choices/reminders to either continue playing a fun game the child might lose or stop/miss out on this fun game.
Educate and train skills	■ Make a story or have discussions about the process of playing games. Important points include: • One person loses and one wins. • Everybody loses sometime (reviewing game statistics from a favorite team easily proves this). • How to handle both winning and losing (good sportsmanship). • How it is more fun to play, regardless of winning or losing, than not to play at all. ■ Model coping skills for losing and good sportsmanship. ■ Track dates and outcomes in a journal or other concrete means so that children can remember and reflect on the times they did win (Murphy, 2019).

a winner or loser or may be graded to focus on the role of winner or loser, depending on the child's needs. This may be games of personal challenge, where one competes against oneself. The occupational therapist can emphasize how the client beat his or her last record, setting a new record. Even when the client does not beat his or her last record, that client still holds "the record" and may do better next time.

Dilemmas Related to Using Play Therapeutically

Another set of dilemmas arises as occupational therapy practitioners attempt to reconcile their value of true play in itself with various other demands of providing therapy. Therapists can find that the dynamic, flexible nature of play can be at odds with their need to be structured and organized to enable progress. Objects, space, and the physical interactions of play can be at odds with telehealth, especially given the lack of research and development of play interventions. Play for its own sake is not just at odds with but can be disrupted in medical contexts, at a time when many children are in great need of play.

Adapting Structure to Balance Flexibility

Occupational therapy intervention usually involves some amount of structure, whether indirectly through environmental modifications and consultation or directly through grading, modeling, and targeting goals. Most play interventions also utilize structure for play. Yet, play is characterized more heavily by spontaneity and self-direction. Therefore, to encourage play, pediatric occupational therapy practitioners try to limit externally imposed structure and share as much control as possible with the child, allowing for flexibility and novelty within limited structure.

The difficulty here is that children's needs and ability to tolerate structure vary dramatically. Some children prefer high levels of structure and routine and have trouble tolerating the uncertainty of novelty and flexibility inherent in play. Some children get so disorganized with unstructured free play that they cannot implement their own ideas for play. In both cases, play novelty and spontaneity must be graded for what the child can tolerate and needs. Balancing between structure and flexibility involves ongoing clinical reasoning based on sound occupational analysis to create an enjoyable just right challenge (Ayres, 1972). Providing choices and developing routines are two ways of adapting flexibility and structure in play (see **Table 16.3**).

Providing Choices

Choice has been found to be critical for play and play intervention for children with disabilities who often have fewer choices (Barnett, 2018; Graham et al., 2019; Hui & Dimitropoulou, 2020; Sterman, Naughton, Bundy, Froude, & Villeneuve, 2020; Sterman, Villeneuve, et al., 2020). Giving children as much choice as possible is

Table 16.3 Strategies for Adapting Structure with Flexibility in Play

General Strategy	Examples
Providing choices	■ Ask children which activity or material they want to use (grading the range available from which to select). ■ Show two or more play objects. ■ Show pictures of two or more play objects or actions. ■ Give the child a cognitive framework for identifying possible play choices (such as "look," "remember"). ■ Offer an activity consistent with child's identified preferences, movements (e.g., jumping), eye gaze, sounds, etc.
Developing routines	■ Use a similar structure/organization (sequence of steps, materials, time, etc.). ■ Provide an explicit schedule (see Figure 16.7). ■ Use visual supports (pictures or words). ■ Give reminders about upcoming transitions. ■ Use key phrases and gestures to indicate and reinforce the order (e.g., first, next, last). ■ Develop explicit rules for an activity to clarify setup, steps, or ending. ■ Use a timer (visual and/or auditory). ■ Provide an object to use in the next activity as a transition object.

one way of valuing their input in occupational therapy. Choice is important in selecting what to play and how to play it. Providing choices can be especially effective for engaging a child who is resistant or oppositional.

Some children have trouble making a choice, initiating an activity, or identifying potential choices to play. For these children, choices must be adapted in accordance with the individual child's needs, abilities, and therapeutic goals. The number and type of items offered or the field from which to select should be graded to provide structure. For example, a child may be overwhelmed by a large number of options available in a space. This child may need to start with a limited number of options, which are gradually increased over time. The therapist may show the child two toys or two pictures of activities and see which one the child selects, reaches/leans toward, or gazes at (Van Tubbergen, Warschausky, Birnholz, & Baker, 2008). A child with ideation problems may have difficulty identifying potential choices that are present and be unable to find anything to do during unstructured play time. This child may require a modified structure to identify the realm of possible choices such as "let's pick something your friends are doing [at recess]" or "let's see what games there are [on the playground]." For those children who do not initiate a selection in the presence of clear options, the therapist may guide them toward an option that is similar to the movement the child is doing or another preference. For example, if the child is jumping around, the occupational therapy practitioner might suggest a structured jumping game, such as jumping from one spot to another, jumping over something, or jumping on a trampoline.

Developing Routines

Play routines are established sequences that provide a structure that can promote play (AOTA, 2020). Many children find reassurance in a basic routine so they know what to expect next and how to prepare for it. Routines can structure individual play activities or multiple play activities within a session. Notably, some clients have trouble understanding a general implicit flow of a therapy session, and the uncertainty can cause emotional distress or disorganization. For example, some children may repeatedly ask about what is next, when will _____ happen, will they be doing _____ today. Others may act out with a transition to another activity because it was unexpected, or they thought they were going to follow the same series of activities as last time.

In such situations, the occupational therapy practitioner makes the implicit flow more explicit and structured to help the child participate. The challenge is to modify routines while still maintaining flexibility and opportunities for the child's internal organization of play. Children who thrive on structure can easily become dependent on a schedule or following steps and lose out on opportunities for spontaneous play because they view it as "not time" for a particular play activity. They may focus predominantly on the routine, missing the play experience. The more open the routine is, the more the therapist can take advantage of opportunities or new information that may arise within a treatment session. The occupational therapist provides just enough structure to help the child participate, grading it over time as needed (Baron, 1991; Moor, 2002; see **Practice Example 16.8**).

PRACTICE EXAMPLE 16.8 Christopher and Structure

Christopher was a 4-year-old with cerebral palsy (CP) and an anxiety disorder. Because his occupational therapist was committed to promoting play and his intrinsic motivation, she consistently asked Christopher what he wanted to do. In the first few sessions, he was unable to offer any ideas, so the occupational therapist suggested some activities. Then Christopher began telling the therapist what he wanted to do (an activity from a previous session). Eventually, he wanted to do the same series of activities in the same order.

Christopher's occupational therapist wanted to encourage more variation in play and other skills, so she began to suggest different activities or changes in the activity. Each time he screamed and cried "no" and said the activity he wanted. At this point, it became very difficult to get him to calm and try the alternate activity. The occupational therapist recognized that this level of change and flexibility was too disorganizing for Christopher. At the same time, the occupational therapist also recognized that with this inflexible preference for predictable structure, Christopher could become dependent on a rigid structure. Therefore, the occupational therapist introduced a simple structure of alternating between the child's choice and the occupational therapist's choice for an activity. Initially, she provided warnings and reminders about these changes with emotional assurances that he would get to do fun things. She first used Christopher's ideas during her choice times and Christopher's tantrums subsided immediately. Next, she asked his help in picking her choice from 1 of 2 of his preferred activity options. Gradually, the therapist graded increasing novelty in her selections over time. Eventually, with preparing Christopher, she also alternated whose choice was first each session and the number of choices per session.

Example 1	Example 2
My choice/turn Your choice/turn My choice/turn Your choice/turn	Body/gym activities Snack Get my things Go home/Go to class
Example 3	**Example 4**
Use ball Play game at table Write Walk to class	Take shoes off Swing Write Obstacle course Craft Put shoes on Wait for mommy and _____ to talk Walk to car Drive to park

Figure 16.7 Examples of schedules with differing levels of structure for pediatric occupational therapy sessions

The amount and type of structure are graded to match the child's needs and therapeutic goals. Some children need a general routine for a session and daily activities, and others need a detailed schedule or list (see **Figure 16.7** for examples in therapy sessions). A general category or time may be enough, or exact details may be needed. For example, it may be enough to "play a board game," or it may be necessary to list all the steps to playing a board game in general or a specific board game. Visual supports (pictures or written words) may be a necessary modification for a child who has difficulty with language processing, memory, or attention. Many children simply need to know what they are transitioning toward in order to end the activity they are doing. Other children require reminders throughout the session to help the child prepare for transitions and get ready for the next activity. Understanding and anticipating the end of play can seem very arbitrary and unfair from a child's perspective, so modifications such as establishing time limits or other clear end points or making an activity into a game with rules can help. Several websites have freely available games and game board templates that can be downloaded and customized for a particular child's needs.

Maintaining Therapeutic Goals and Structuring for Too Much Playing Around

A particular dilemma in practice is when children focus exclusively on fun. Some children seem to find ways to be silly, make jokes, or play games all the time. Others find something fun and want to continue to play this same activity endlessly. Although

this fun-seeking sounds like a trait the authors of this book might support, it may be problematic at certain times and places. When therapy is addressing activities that require a child's serious focus, such as accuracy in writing or cutting, a client's playful approach can detour therapeutic efforts, with cuts and lines all over the paper. This playful behavior also can be disruptive during certain family and cultural events and in classrooms, which require quiet attention or diligent work. For example, a second-grader deciding to make a pencil into a puppet that makes silly sounds when the class is writing quietly in their journals can be very aggravating for a school-based therapist as well as others in the class. Children with attention-deficit disorders often have difficulty attending to activities that are less than highly interesting. Other children may seek strong play experiences to avoid even the smallest challenge. These can be very stressful moments for the therapist, who may wonder if this momentary detour from therapy may turn into total derailment. Although the entire goal of this book is facilitating play, we also advocate facilitating play in therapy sessions for the *purpose* of therapeutic gains. When the child's engagement in play seems to be a roadblock for therapy, the occupational therapist's professional reasoning is challenged. How can the therapist maintain play when it seems incompatible with therapy?

It takes creative thinking to adapt these play activities based on sound activity analysis. At these times, the occupational therapist must make clinical judgments about the relative valuation of play, the setting, the work at hand, and the possibilities for creating activity adaptations. When the activity can be modified to meet the child's interests and the environmental demands, as discussed in Chapter 8, this is often the preferred route. If no effective adaptations can be found, then sometimes the therapist will have to set more explicit structure that allows for some play and some "work." Permitting some of this playfulness at first may be necessary to allow the child mastery over a new ability and encourage willingness to "buy in" to work, as the two cases of Sophia and Eddie illustrate (see **Practice Examples 16.9** and **16.10**).

Playing in the Context of Medical Care

Various medical conditions can create a number of challenges for play. Medical interventions can create pain, anxiety, depression, and trauma for children (Jones, Kirkendall, Grissim, Daniels, & Boles, 2021; Kyriakidis, Tsamagou, & Magos, 2021; Potaszi, Varela,

PRACTICE EXAMPLE 16.9 Sophia and Play Limits

Sophia was a 2½-year-old with developmental delays and sensory processing disorder. Although she was socially interactive, she generally wandered around without engagement in play activities and became easily fearful during a range of therapy activities. The occupational therapist was using a sensory integration approach to optimize her arousal level, encouraging her to actively reach and throw various balls and toys into a bin. Sophia had played with these toys before and always recoiled when she saw the spider balls in the bin. She appeared genuinely scared and commented, "Ick." The occupational therapist always put them aside with an exaggerated "Ick" followed by a smile.

During one session, Sophia asked for the spiders. Each time, she took the spider and waved it in the therapist's face, laughing as the therapist feigned exaggerated fear. At first, the occupational therapist was delighted with Sophia's management of her own discomfort and her interest in playing a new game. But as it became clear that Sophia wanted to continue this game indefinitely, the occupational therapist realized that something would have to change to continue along the therapeutic path—to extend complexity of play. So the occupational therapist set a limit, allowing Sophia to briefly scare the therapist and then, more seriously, having her let the spider go into a barrel because "Now it is time for the spider to go to bed." Although Sophia did not want to alter her play in this way, the therapist successfully encouraged her with an offer of getting another spider with which to do the same. It took some direction from the therapist, but Sophia did allow her spider game to be adapted by the therapist for improved therapeutic outcomes.

PRACTICE EXAMPLE 16.10 Eddie and His Strong Play Drive

Eddie was a 4-year-old who had delayed fine-motor skills as a result of sustaining a traumatic brain injury earlier that year. He avoided manipulating small toys, scissors, crayons, and other materials that would build his fine-motor skills. He had a good sense of playfulness and especially enjoyed a range of transportation vehicles such as cars, trucks, trains, motorcycles, and airplanes. He quickly resisted all activities with even mild fine-motor demands.

The occupational therapist suggested a small wind-up train with open cart and round track that she knew could be upgraded. Eddie was immediately interested in watching the train go around and picking it up to look at it more closely. Once Eddie was playing, the occupational therapist upgraded the demands by bringing out some small pegs as cargo to fill up the empty cart. Again, Eddie willingly helped fill up the cart. Although the occupational therapist was getting Eddie's playful engagement, she knew the activity still needed to be upgraded further for it to be therapeutic for Eddie. She brought out some tongs, whose correct use would be therapeutic for Eddie's fine-motor needs. She suggested that the tongs were a crane to load and unload the train. Eddie accepted this and began using the tongs with his whole hand in a more gross form than the finger precision the occupational therapist had envisioned. Nonetheless, she opted to let Eddie continue in this manner for a few minutes to build his comfort, acceptance, and interest in the activity before upgrading the demand of precise use of the tongs. If she pushed the increased precision demand too fast, Eddie would stop the activity because he would no longer experience it as play. Because the occupational therapist waited and allowed Eddie to continue to engage in the playing that she had shaped, he was willing to tolerate her upgraded demands just a few minutes later.

Carvalho, Prado, & Prado, 2013). Health conditions can also create direct challenges to play in daily life (Bambrick, Dennis, & Wilkinson, 2018; Jasem, Darlington, Lambrick, Grisbrooke, & Randall, 2020; Jones, 2018; Riso, Cambrisi, Bertini, & Miscioscia, 2020). Children's play can be disrupted when not able to attend school, when hospitalized, when undergoing medical treatments, and when experiencing condition-dependent limitations (Jasem et al., 2020). Play deprivation is even more striking here in contrast with the unique benefits of play participation for children with health conditions.

Play can be very therapeutic for children undergoing medical procedures or dealing with life-threatening and life-limiting conditions. Evidence consistently shows that play-based techniques can help reduce pain, anxiety, and other negative reactions in children undergoing needle-related medical procedures, chemotherapy, hospitalization, peripheral catheterization, cast removal, and routine medical visits (Kyriakidis et al., 2021; Mohammadi et al., 2021; Orhan & Yildiz, 2017; Potaszi et al., 2013; Rashid, Cheong, Hisham, Shamsuddin, & Roslan, 2021; Stein Duker, Schmidt, Pham, Ringold, & Nager, 2021; William Li, Lopez, & Lee, 2007; Wong et al., 2018; Zengin, Yayan, & Düken, 2021). In many cases, the interventions involve providing information about the procedure via play (Orhan & Yildiz, 2017; William Li, Lopez, & Lee, 2007; Wong et al., 2018). The child is prepared by having the procedures demonstrated and explained and by getting to touch the items or simulated items used in the procedure. Some studies also use role-playing where the child plays the parent to a "sick" toy (Rashid et al., 2021). Some studies also used play as a distraction from the medical procedure (Wong et al., 2018). Recent research suggests that such methods can be provided effectively in a group setting as well as individually (Jones et al., 2021). This use of play as an intervention tool is employed by occupational therapy practitioners as well as other healthcare providers such as child life specialists, play specialists, play therapists, and nurses.

In occupational therapy, play as a tool also is incorporated through the use of preferred play activities, play objects, and a playful approach to goals (Bambrick et al., 2018; Mohammadi et al., 2021). Mohammadi and colleagues (2021) found that a play-based approach can increase the effectiveness of occupational therapy on symptoms and participation in daily activities for children undergoing chemotherapy. Potaszi and colleagues (2013) found that hospitalized children who participated in play activities supervised by occupational therapists demonstrated greater stress reduction than those who did not.

Occupational therapy practitioners also directly target play as an outcome for children with various health conditions. Typically, this involves addressing limited play opportunities in terms of play objects, spaces, and peers (Jasem et al., 2020). Adaptations, education, and advocacy are common intervention approaches. Play for the sake of play can be especially important in occupational therapy at the end of a child's life to have meaning in the remaining life and death (Bambrick et al., 2018; Jasem et al., 2020).

Promoting Play via Telehealth

Telehealth, the use of information and communication technology to deliver occupational therapy (AOTA, 2018), is increasingly being used in pediatrics. Typically, its use has been to increase client access across the distances of rural or underserved areas and pandemic health precautions (AOTA, 2018; Dinesen et al., 2016; Little, Pope, Wallisch, & Dunn, 2018a, 2018b; Robinson et al., 2021). Telehealth can be very convenient for families who have access to devices and quality Internet service (Dinesen et al., 2016; Little et al., 2018b; Wallisch, Little, Pope, & Dunn, 2019). Overall, telehealth has been shown to have positive effects; however, the studies are weak (Dinesen et al., 2016; Parsons, Cordier, Vaz, & Lee, 2017). This state of early research in addition to the need to create new ways to adapt telehealth for play are key dilemmas for occupational therapy practitioners.

Limited research supports telehealth parent/caregiver training, consultation, and coaching as effective for promoting play, especially for children with ASD.

In one study, teleconferencing was used to provide occupation-based coaching with caregivers, where therapists ask reflective questions and make reflective comments regarding the caregiver-identified goals for their children with ASD (Little et al., 2018a). This intervention was effective in increasing parent efficacy and child participation, including a significant increase in play activity frequency. In another study, videoconferencing was used to provide parent training and coaching effectively to promote parent understanding and use of play for skill development in children with ASD (Vismara, Young, & Rogers, 2012). A similar play-based program for building skills in children with Prader-Willi syndrome was found to be a feasible intervention for research (Zyga, Russ, & Dimitropoulos, 2018). Recorded web-based parent training and parent coaching via videoconferencing for imitation training, which may be used in and for play, has been effective for increasing spontaneous imitation in children with ASD (Wainer & Ingersoll, 2015). While not focused on play, it is interesting to note that one study found that adding coaching and live feedback to a web-based educational program was more effective in building social skills and positive parent perceptions of their children with ASD (Ingersoll, Wainer, Berger, Pickard, & Bonter, 2016).

Very limited research has explored direct play-based telehealth interventions with children. In one case, an occupational therapist used videoconferencing to observe computer game play and provide consultation to increase the motor skills of a 5-year-old with CP (Reifenberg et al., 2017). In a feasibility study, researchers were able to develop an intervention where children were given the same set of toys as the interventionist who modeled play and encouraged the child with Prader-Willi syndrome to "make up a story about___," except that the children did not always want to play with these toys (Dimitropoulos, Zyga, & Russ, 2017).

A second dilemma in play and telehealth is the need to adapt interventions specifically for telehealth (Dinesen et al., 2016; Ekberg, Danby, Theobald, Fisher, & Wyeth, 2019). This is likely to require the efforts of both researchers and practicing therapists. This is especially needed in direct work with children through telehealth for parent/caregiver–child play and therapist–child play. To successfully meet a child's needs in telehealth, an occupational therapy practitioner relies on activity and occupational analyses specific to this virtual context in order to select and adapt play activities specific to telehealth.

Direct therapy with children and parents via telehealth has different affordances and challenges of in-person direct therapy (Ekberg et al., 2019). A key benefit is to access the child's natural play environment at home or in the community (AOTA, 2018). One practical challenge is that it does not allow physical engagement between therapist and client through shared manipulable space (Ekberg et al., 2019). This constrains both play and the therapist's ability to provide physical assistance and visual cues and to adapt physical elements in the middle of sessions. Furthermore, given that families may struggle to adjust the camera in a way that enables adequate visual observation and the compromised ability of a camera to focus on a detail in a broad view (Dimitropoulos, Zyga, & Russ, 2017; Reifenberg et al., 2017), the therapist must work with far less information on the physical environment than if physically present in that environment. In a study of how play-based speech therapy was delivered through telehealth, Ekberg et al. (2019) described how a therapist can still facilitate a child's active and playful engagement with an object even if the child cannot physically access it. For example, in one session, a therapist blew bubbles and encouraged the child to blow and pop the bubbles. Other examples of therapist–child play may include covering and uncovering the camera for drama especially with a drumroll, turning the camera sideways or upside down, creating small paper "snowballs" to flick at each other for a snowball fight, and getting inside a "fort" with the camera. A cognitive approach to play is especially well-suited for telehealth. For example, a child can be coached to problem-solve how to build a road to help his car get from location to location. A parent or other caregiver may also be engaged to facilitate play interaction by encouraging the child, commenting playfully, cuing the child to look at something specific on the screen or on their side of the screen, or physically assisting the child.

Clinicians also are using telehealth to train parents directly in play with their children (CLASI, 2020). In this approach, therapists may first ask to be shown around the home to see toys, common play areas, and environmental affordances. The parent/caregiver, therapist, or child may suggest an activity to play. The therapist observes, comments on these observations, and makes suggestions while the parent or other caregiver plays with the child.

Conclusion

A number of common dilemmas in using play in occupational therapy were presented here. You will certainly encounter your own practice dilemmas with similarities and differences to those here because play presents novel challenges. There will be things you have never seen before, and you will be required to adapt in ways you never have before. This book provides occupational therapy practitioners with tools to contend with these dilemmas in order to manage the dilemmas in play without managing play itself so that children can play. Future research is likely to assist further in clinical reasoning. It is my hope that you will find your dilemmas to be just right challenges so that there may be play despite the dilemmas.

References

Agius, J., & Levey, S. (2019). Humor intervention approaches for children, adolescents, and adults. *Israeli Journal for Humor Research*, 8(1), 8–28. http://www.israeli-humor-studies.org /media/02-humanintervention_approaches_for_children.pdf

Allard, H. (1985). *Miss Nelson is missing!* New York: Houghton Mifflin.

Allard, H. (1988). *Miss Nelson has a field day.* New York: Houghton Mifflin.

American Academy of Child & Adolescent Psychiatry. (2020, February). Screen time and children. https://www.aacap.org /AACAP/Families_and_Youth/Facts_for_Families/FFF-Guide /Children-And-Watching-TV-054.aspx

American Academy of Pediatrics (AAP) Council on Communications and Media. (2016). Media and young minds. *Pediatrics*, 138(5), e20162591. https://doi.org/10.1542/peds .2016-2591

American Occupational Therapy Association (AOTA). (2016). Assistive technology and occupational performance. *American Journal of Occupational Therapy, 70*, 7012410030. http:// dx.doi.org/10.5014/ajot.2016.706S02

American Occupational Therapy Association (AOTA). (2018). Telehealth in occupational therapy. *American Journal of Occupational Therapy*, 72(Supplement_2). https://doi .org/10.5014/ajot.2018.72s219

American Occupational Therapy Association (AOTA). (2020). Occupational therapy practice framework: Domain and process (4th ed.). *American Journal of Occupational Therapy*, 74(Suppl. 2), 7412410010. https://doi.org/10.5014 /ajot.2020.74S2001

Ayres, A. J. (1972). *Sensory integration and learning disorders*. Los Angeles, CA: Western Psychological Services.

Baker, M. J. (2000). Incorporating the thematic ritualistic behaviors of children with autism into games: Increasing social play interactions with siblings. *Journal of Positive Behavior Interventions*, 2(2), 66–84. https://doi .org/10.1177/109830070000200201

Baker, M. J., Koegel, R. L., & Koegel, L. K. (1998). Increasing the social behavior of young children with autism using their obsessive behaviors. *Journal of the Association for Persons with Severe Handicaps, 23*(4), 300–308.

Bambrick, R. L., Dennis, C. W., & Wilkinson, K. (2018). Understanding therapists' use of play with children with life-threatening conditions: A qualitative study. *The Open Journal of Occupational Therapy, 6*(2), 4. http://dx.doi .org/10.15453/2168-6408.1283

Barnett, J. H. (2018). Three evidence-based strategies that support social skills and play among young children with autism spectrum disorders. *Early Childhood Education Journal, 46*(6), 665–672. https://doi.org/10.1007/s10643-018-0911-0

Barnett, L. A. (2007). The nature of playfulness in young adults. *Personality and Individual Differences, 43*, 949–958.

Baron, K. B. (1991). The use of play in child psychiatry: Reframing the therapeutic environment. *Occupational Therapy in Mental Health, 11*(2/3), 37–56.

Barry, L. M., & Burlew, S. B. (2004). Using social stories to teach choice and play skills to children with autism. *Focus on Autism and Other Developmental Disabilities, 19*(1), 45–51. https://doi.org /10.1177/10883576040190010601

Barton, E. E. (2015). Teaching generalized pretend play and related behaviors to young children with disabilities. *Exceptional Children, 81*, 489–506. https://doi.org /10.1177/0014402914563694

Barton, E. E., Choi, G., & Mauldin, E. G. (2019). Teaching sequences of pretend play to children with disabilities. *Journal of Early Intervention, 41*(1), 13–29. https://doi.org /i10.177/105381511879466

Barton, E. E., Ledford, J. R., Zimmerman, K. N., & Pokorski, E. A. (2018). Increasing the engagement and complexity of block play in young children. *Education and Treatment of Children, 41*(2), 169–196. DOI: https://doi.org/10.1353/etc.2018.0007

Barton, E. E., Murray, R., O'Flaherty, C., Sweeney, E. M., & Gossett, S. (2020). Teaching object play to young children with disabilities: A systematic review of methods and rigor. *American Journal on Intellectual and Developmental Disabilities, 125*(1), 14–36. https://doi.org/10.1352/1944-7558-125.1.14

Barton, E. E., & Wolery, M. (2008). Teaching pretend play to children with disabilities: A review of the literature. *Topics in Early Childhood Special Education, 28*(2), 109–125. https://doi.org/10.1177/0271121408318799

Bay-Hinitz, A. K., & Wilson, G. R. (2005).A cooperative games intervention for aggressive preschool children. In L. A. Reddy, T. M. Files-Hall, & C. E. Schaefer (Eds.), *Empirically based play interventions for children* (pp. 191–211). Washington, DC: American Psychological Association.

Bergen, D., & Rousta, M. M. (2019).Developing creativity and humor: The role of the playful mind. In S. R. Luria, J. Baer, & J. C. Kaufman (Eds.), *Explorations in creativity research. Creativity and humor* (pp. 61–81). Cambridge, MA: Elsevier Academic Press. https://doi.org/10.1016/B978-0-12-813802 -1.00003-X

Biddiss, E., Chan-Viquez, D., Cheung, S. T., & King, G. (2021). Engaging children with cerebral palsy in interactive computer play-based motor therapies: Theoretical perspectives. *Disability and Rehabilitation, 43*(1), 133–147. https://doi.org /10.1080/09638288.2019.1613681

Blunden, P. (2001).The therapeutic use of play. In L. Lougher (Ed.), *Occupational therapy for child and adolescent mental health* (pp. 67–86). Edinburgh, Scotland: Churchill Livingstone.

Bodison, S. C. (2015). Developmental dyspraxia and the play skills of children with autism. *American Journal of Occupational Therapy, 69*(5), 6905185060. https://doi.org/10.5014/ajot .2015.017954

Boyd, B. A., Conroy, M. A., Mancil, G. R., Nakao, T., & Alter, P. J. (2007). Effects of circumscribed interests on the social behaviors of children with autism spectrum disorders. *Journal of Autism and Developmental Disorders, 37*, 1550–1561. https:// doi.org/10.1007/s10803-006-0286-8

Brussoni, M., Gibbons, R., Gray, C., Ishikawa, T., Sandseter , E. B. H., Bienenstock, A., . . . Tremblay, M. S. (2015). What is the relationship between risky outdoor play and health in children? A systematic review. *International Journal of Environmental Research and Public Health, 12*(6), 6423–6454. https://doi.org/10.3390/ijerph120606423

Brussoni, M., Ishikawa, T., Han, C., Pike, I., Bundy, A., Faulkner, G., & Mâsse, L. C. (2018). Go play outside! Effects of a risk-reframing tool on mothers' tolerance for, and parenting practices associated with, children's risky play: Study protocol for a randomized controlled trial. *Trials, 19*(1), 173. http://dx.doi.org/10.1186/s13063-018 -2552-4

Bundy, A. C., Wyver, S., Beetham, K. S., Ragen, J., Naughton, G., Tranter, P., . . . Sterman, J. (2015). The Sydney playground project-levelling the playing field: A cluster trial of a primary school-based intervention aiming to promote manageable risk-taking in children with disability. *BMC Public Health, 15*(1), 1–6. https://doi.org/10.1186/s12889-015-2452-4

Burke, J. P. (1977). A clinical perspective on motivation: Pawn versus origin. *American Journal of Occupational Therapy, 31*(4), 254–258.

Cacciatore, R. S., Ingman-Friberg, S., Lainiala, L. P., & Apter, D. L. (2020). Verbal and behavioral expressions of child sexuality among 1–6-year-olds as observed by daycare professionals in Finland. *Archives of Sexual Behavior, 49*(7), 2725–2734. http:// dx.doi.org/10.1007/s10508-020-01694-y

Carlson, M. (1996). The self-perpetuation of occupations. In R. Zemke & F. Clark (Eds.), *Occupational science: The evolving discipline* (pp. 143–157). Philadelphia: F. A. Davis.

Chadwick, D. D., & Platt, T. (2018). Investigating humor in social interaction in people with intellectual disabilities: A systematic review of the literature. *Frontiers in Psychology, 9*, 1745. https:// doi.org/10.3389/fpsyg.2018.01745

Chan, J., & John, R. M. (2012). Sexuality and sexual health in children and adolescents with autism. *The Journal for Nurse Practitioners, 8*(4), 306–315. https://doi.org/10.1016/j.nurpra .2012.01.020

Chang, H. J., Wang, C. Y., Chen, H. C., & Chang, K. E. (2014). The analysis of elementary and high school students' natural and humorous responses patterns in coping with embarrassing situations. *Humor, 27*(2), 325–347. https://doi.org/10.1515 /humor-2013-0059

Chang, Y. C., Shih, W., Landa, R., Kaiser, A., & Kasari, C. (2018). Symbolic play in school-aged minimally verbal children with autism spectrum disorder. *Journal of Autism and Developmental Disorders, 48*(5), 1436–1445. https://doi.org/10.1007/s10803 -017-3388-6

Chiang, Y., Lee, C., & Wang, H. (2016). Effects of classroom humor climate and acceptance of humor messages on adolescents' expressions of humor. *Child & Youth Care Forum, 45*(4), 543–569. http://dx.doi.org/10.1007/s10566-015 -9345-7

Cho, I. Y. K., Jelinkova, K., Schuetze, M., Vinette, S. A., Rahman S., McCrimmon, A., . . . Bray, S. (2017). Circumscribed interests in adolescents with autism spectrum disorder: A look beyond trains, planes, and clocks. *PLoS One, 12*(11), e0187414. https://doi.org/10.1371/journal.pone.0187414.

Christensen, P., & Mikkelsen, M. R. (2008). Jumping off and being careful: Children's strategies of risk management in everyday life. *Sociology of Health & Illness, 30*(1), 112–130.

Chylińska, M., & Gut, A. (2020). Pretend play as a creative action: On the exploratory and evaluative features of children's pretense. *Theory & Psychology, 30*(4), 548–566. https://doi.org/10.1177/0959354320931594

CLASI. (2020). *Ayres sensory integration and telehealth.* [Video]. YouTube. https://www.youtube.com/watch?v=exOp49GPLq0

Common Sense Media. (2008). *Media + child and adolescent health: A systematic review.* http://www.commonsensemedia.org/sites/default/files/CSM_media+health_v2c%20110708.pdf

Cook, S., Peterson, L., & DiLillo, D. (1999). Fear and exhilaration in response to risk: An extension of a model of injury risk in a real-world context. *Behavior Therapy, 30*(1), 5–15.

Counterman, L., & Kirkwood, D. (2013). Understanding healthy sexuality development in young children. *Voices of Practitioners, 8*(2), 1–13.

Dadson, P., Brown, T., & Stagnitti, K. (2020). Relationship between screen-time and hand function, play and sensory processing in children without disabilities aged 4–7 years: A exploratory study. *Australian Occupational Therapy Journal, 67*(4), 297–308. https://doi.org/10.1111/1440-1630.12650

Daniel, L. S., & Billingsley, B. S. (2010). What boys with an autism spectrum disorder say about establishing and maintaining friendships. *Focus on Autism and Other Developmental Disabilities, 25*(4), 220–229. https://doi.org/10.1177/1088357610378290

Davies, S. L., Glaser, D., & Kossoff, R. (2000). Children's sexual play and behavior in pre-school settings: Staff perceptions, reports, and responses. *Child Abuse & Neglect, 24*, 1329–1343.

Delaney, K. K. (2016). Playing at violence: Lock-down drills, "bad guys" and the construction of "acceptable" play in early childhood. *Early Child Development and Care, 187*(5–6), 878–895. https://doi.org/10.1080/03004430.2016.1219853

DiCarlo, C. F., Schepis, M. M., & Flynn, L. (2009). Embedding sensory preference into toys to enhance toy play in toddlers with disabilities. *Infants & Young Children, 22*(3), 188–200. doi: 10.1097/IYC.0b013e3181abe1a1

Didden, R., Korzilius, H., Sturmey, P., Lancioni, G. E., & Curfs, L. M. G. (2008). Preference for water-related items in Angelman syndrome, Down syndrome and non-specific intellectual disability. *Journal of Intellectual & Developmental Disability, 33*(1), 59–64. doi:http://dx.doi.org/10.1080/13668250701872126

Dimitropoulos, A., Zyga, O., Doernberg, E., & Russ, S. W. (2021). Preliminary efficacy of a remote play-based intervention for children with Prader-Willi syndrome. *Research in Developmental Disabilities, 108*, 103820. https://doi.org/10.1016/j.ridd.2020.103820

Dimitropoulos, A., Zyga, O., & Russ, S. (2017). Evaluating the feasibility of a play-based telehealth intervention program for children with Prader–Willi syndrome. *Journal of Autism and Developmental Disorders, 47*(9), 2814–2825. https://doi.org/10.1007/s10803-017-3196-z

Dinesen, B., Nonnecke, B., Lindeman, D., Toft, E., Kidholm, K., Jethwani, K.. . . . Nesbitt, T. (2016). Personalized telehealth in the future: A global research agenda. *Journal of Medical Internet Research, 18*(3), e53. https://doi.org/10.2196/jmir.5257

Doernberg, E. A., Russ, S. W., & Dimitropoulos, A. (2020). Believing in make-believe: Efficacy of a pretend play intervention for school-aged children with high-functioning autism spectrum disorder. *Journal of Autism and Developmental Disorders*, 1–13. https://doi.org/10.1007/s10803-020-04547-8

Dos Santos, D. M., Lucisano, R. V., & Pfeifer, L. (2019). An investigation of the quality of pretend play ability in children with cerebral palsy. *Australian Occupational Therapy Journal, 66*, 210–218.

Stein Duker, L. I., Schmidt, A. R., Pham, P. K., Ringold, S. M., & Nager, A. L. (2021). Use of Audiobooks as an Environmental Distractor to Decrease State Anxiety in Children Waiting in the Pediatric Emergency Department: A Pilot and Feasibility Study. *Frontiers in Pediatrics, 8*, 556805. https://doi.org/10.3389/fped.2020.556805

Dunst, C. J., Trivette, C. M., & Hamby, D. W. (2012). Effect of interest-based interventions on the social-communicative behavior of young children with autism spectrum disorders. *Center for Early Literacy Learning, 5*(6), 1–10.

Egan, B. (2019). *Video and computer game interventions for children 5–21 years. Systematic review of related literature from 2010 to 2017* [Critically Appraised Topic]. Bethesda, MD: American Occupational Therapy Association.

Ekberg, S., Danby, S., Theobald, M., Fisher, B., & Wyeth, P. (2019). Using physical objects with young children in "face-to-face" and telehealth speech and language therapy. *Disability and Rehabilitation, 41*(14), 1664–1675. http://dx.doi.org/10.1080/09638288.2018.1448464

Erdogan, N. I., Johnson, J. E., Dong, P. I., & Qiu, Z. (2019). Do parents prefer digital play? Examination of parental preferences and beliefs in four nations. *Early Childhood Education Journal, 47*(2), 131–142. https://doi.org/10.1007/s10643-018-0901-2

Eversole, M., Collins, D. M., Karmarkar, A. Colton, L., Quinn, J. P., Karsbaek, R., . . . Hilton, C. L. (2016). Leisure activity enjoyment of children with autism spectrum disorders. *Journal of Autism and Developmental Disorders, 46*(1), 10–20.

Fette, C., Lambdin-Pattavina, C., & Weaver, L. L. (2019). Understanding and applying trauma-informed approaches across occupational therapy settings. *OT Practice.* https://www.aota.org/-/media/Corporate/Files/Publications/CE-Articles/CE-Article-May-2019-Trauma.pdf

Finke, E. H., Hickerson, B., & McLaughlin, E. (2015). Parental intention to support video game play by children with autism spectrum disorder: An application of the theory of planned behavior. *Language, speech, and hearing services in schools, 46*(2), 154-165. https://doi.org/10.1044/2015_LSHSS-13-0080

Fischer-Grote, L., Kothgassner, O. D., & Felnhofer, A. (2019). Risk factors for problematic smartphone use in children and adolescents: A review of existing literature. *Neuropsychiatrie, 33*, 179–190. https://doi.org/10.1007/s40211-019-00319-8

Florey, L. L., & Greene, S. (2008).Play in middle childhood. In L. D. Parham & L. S. Fazio (Eds.), *Play in occupational therapy for children* (2nd ed., pp. 279–299). St. Louis, MO: Mosby Elsevier.

García-Redondo, P., García, T., Areces, D., Núñez, J. C., & Rodríguez, C. (2019). Serious games and their effect improving attention in students with learning disabilities. *International Journal of Environmental Research and Public Health, 16*(14), 2480. https://doi.org/10.3390/ijerph16142480

Garfinkel, M., & Minard, C. (2021). Supporting occupational balance in children using everyday technologies: The distinct value of occupational therapy. *SIS Quarterly Practice Connections, 6*(1), 5–7.

Goetze, H. (1994).Processes in person-centered play therapy. In J. Hellendoorn, R. van der Kooij, & B. Sutton-Smith (Eds.), *Play and intervention* (pp. 63–76). Albany: State University of New York Press.

Goldingay, S., Stagnitti, K., Robertson, N., Pepin, G., Sheppard, L., & Dean, B. (2020). Implicit play or explicit cognitive behaviour therapy: The impact of intervention approaches to facilitate social skills development in adolescents. *Australian Occupational Therapy Journal, 67*(4), 360–372. https://doi.org/10.1111/1440-1630.12673

Goldstein, T. R. (2018). Developing a dramatic pretend play game intervention. *American Journal of Play, 10*(3), 290–308.

Goldstein, T. R., & Lerner, M. D. (2018). Dramatic pretend play games uniquely improve emotional control in young children. *Developmental Science, 21*(4), e12603. https://doi.org/10.1111/desc.12603

Gooch, P., & Living, R. (2004). The therapeutic use of videogames within secure forensic settings: A review of the literature and application to practice. *British Journal of Occupational Therapy, 67*, 332–341.

Graham, N., Mandy, A., Clarke, C., & Morriss-Roberts, C. (2019). Play experiences of children with a high level of physical disability. *American Journal of Occupational Therapy, 73*(6), 7306205010p1-7306205010p10. https://doi.org/10.5014/ajot.2019.032516. PMID: 31891340.

Greitemeyer, T., & Mügge, D.O. (2014). Video Games Do Affect Social Outcomes: A Meta-Analytic Review of the Effects of Violent and Prosocial Video Game Play. *Personality and Social Psychology Bulletin, 40*(5), 578–589. https://doi.org/10.1177/0146167213520459

Griffiths, M. (2005). Video games and health: Video gaming is safe for most players and can be useful in health care. *British Medical Journal, 331*, 122–123. http://www.bmj.com/cgi/reprint/331/7509/122

Guitard, P., Ferland, F., & Dutil, E. (2005). Toward a better understanding of playfulness in adults. *OTJR: Occupation, Participation and Health, 25*, 9–22.

Gunn, K. C., & Delafield-Butt, J. T. (2015). Teaching children with autism spectrum disorder with restricted interests. *Review of Educational Research, 86*(2), 408–430. https://doi.org/10.3102/0034654315604027

Hale, L., & Guan, S. (2015). Screen time and sleep among school-aged children and adolescents: A systematic literature review. *Sleep Medicine Reviews, 21*, 50–58. https://doi.org/10.1016/j.smrv.2014.07.007

Hellendoorn, J. (1994).Imaginative play training for severely retarded children. In J. Hellendoorn, R. van der Kooij, & B. Sutton-Smith (Eds.), *Play and intervention* (pp. 113–122). Albany: State University of New York Press.

Hinchion, S., McAuliffe, E., & Lynch, H. (2021). Fraught with frights or full of fun: Perspectives of risky play among six- to eight-year-olds. *European Early Childhood Education Research Journal, 29*(5), 696–714. https://doi.org/10.1080/1350293X.2021.1968460

Hoffmann, J. D., & Russ, S. W. (2016). Fostering pretend play skills and creativity in elementary school girls: A group play intervention. *Psychology of Aesthetics, Creativity, and the Arts, 10*(1), 114. http://dx.doi.org/10.1037/aca0000039

Hoicka, E., & Akhtar, N. (2012). Early humour production. *British Journal of Developmental Psychology, 30*(4), 586–603. https://doi.org/10.1111/j.2044-835X.2011.02075.x

Holloway, E. (2008).Fostering early parent-infant playfulness in the neonatal intensive care unit. In L.D. Parham & L.S. Fazio (Eds.), *Play in occupational therapy for children* (2nd ed., pp. 335–350). St. Louis, MO: Mosby Elsevier.

Hoover, D. W. (2015). The effects of psychological trauma on children with autism spectrum disorders: A research review. *Review Journal of Autism and Developmental Disorders, 2*(3), 287–299. https://doi.org/10.1007/s40489-015-0052-y

Howie, E. K., Coenen, P., Campbell, A. C., Ranelli, S., & Straker, L .M. (2017). Head, trunk and arm posture amplitude and variation, muscle activity, sedentariness and physical activity of 3 to 5 year-old children during tablet computer use compared to television watching and toy play. *Applied Ergonomics, 65*, 41–50. https://doi.org/10.1016/j.apergo.2017.05.011.

Hui, S., & Dimitropoulou, K. (2020). iCan-Play: A practice guideline for assessment and intervention of play for children with severe multiple disabilities. *The Open Journal of Occupational Therapy, 8*(3), 1–14. https://doi.org/10.15453/2168-6408.1696

Humble, J. J., Summers, N. L., Villarreal, V., Styck, K. M., Sullivan, J. R., Hechler, J. M., & Warren, B. S. (2019). Child-centered play therapy for youths who have experienced trauma: A systematic literature review. *Journal of Child & Adolescent Trauma, 12*(3), 365–375. https://doi.org/10.1007/s40653-018-0235-7

Ingersoll, B., Wainer, A. L., Berger, N. I., Pickard, K. E., & Bonter, N. (2016). Comparison of a self-directed and therapist-assisted telehealth parent-mediated intervention for children with ASD: A pilot RCT. *Journal of Autism and Developmental Disorders, 46*(7), 2275–2284. https://doi.org/10.1007/s10803-016-2755-z

Jackson, M. L., Nuñez, R. M., Maraach, D., Wilhite, C. J., & Moschella, J. D. (2021). Teaching comprehension of double-meaning jokes to young children. *Journal of Applied Behavior Analysis, 54*(3), 1095–1110. http://dx.doi.org/10.1002/jaba.838

James, S., Ziviani, J., King, G., & Boyd, R. N. (2016). Understanding engagement in home-based interactive computer play: Perspectives of children with unilateral cerebral palsy and their caregivers. *Physical & Occupational Therapy in Pediatrics, 36*(4), 343–358. DOI: 10.3109/01942638.2015.1076560

James, S., Ziviani, J., Ware, R. S., & Boyd, R. N. (2015). Randomized controlled trial of web-based multimodal therapy for unilateral cerebral palsy to improve occupational performance. *Developmental Medicine & Child Neurology, 57*(6), 530–538. https://doi.org/10.1111/dmcn.12705

Jasem, Z. A., Darlington, A., Lambrick, D., Grisbrooke, J., & Randall, D. C. (2020). Play in children with life-threatening and life-limiting conditions: A scoping review. *American Journal of Occupational Therapy, 74*(1), 7401205040. https://doi.org/10.5014/ajot.2020.033456

Jelleyman, C., McPhee, J., Brussoni, M., Bundy, A., & Duncan, S. (2019). A cross-sectional description of parental perceptions and practices related to risky play and independent mobility in children: The New Zealand state of play survey. *International Journal of Environmental Research and Public Health, 16*(2). doi: http://dx.doi.org/10.3390/ijerph16020262

Jones, M. (2018). The necessity of play for children in health care. *Pediatric Nursing, 44*(6), 303.

Jones, M. T., Kirkendall, M., Grissim, L., Daniels, S., & Boles, J. C. (2021). Exploration of the relationship between a group medical play intervention and children's preoperative fear and anxiety. *Journal of Pediatric Health Care: Official Publication of National Association of Pediatric Nurse Associates & Practitioners, 35*(1), 74–83. http://dx.doi.org/10.1016/j.pedhc.2020.08.001

Jones, S., James, L., Fox, C., & Blunn, L. (2021).Laughing together: The relationships between humor and friendship in childhood through to adulthood. In T. Altmann (Ed.), *Friendship in cultural and personality psychology: International perspectives*. New York: Nova.

Jozkowski, A. C., & Cermak, S. A. (2019). Moderating effect of social interaction on enjoyment and perception of physical activity in young adults with autism spectrum disorders. *International Journal of Developmental Disabilities, 66*(3), 222–234. https://doi.org/10.1080/20473869.2019.1567091

Jung, S., & Sainato, D. M. (2013). Teaching play skills to young children with autism. *Journal of Intellectual & Developmental Disability, 38*(1), 74–90. https://doi.org/10.3109/13668250.2012.732220

Jung, S., & Sainato, D. M. (2015). Teaching games to young children with autism spectrum disorder using special interests and video modeling. *Journal of Intellectual & Developmental Disability, 40*(2), 198. http://dx.doi.org/10.3109/13668250.2015.1027674

Kaboski, J. R., Diehl, J. J., Beriont, J., Crowell, C. R., Villano, M., Wier, K., & Tang, K. (2014). Brief report: A pilot summer robotics camp to reduce social anxiety and improve social/vocational skills in adolescents with ASD. *Journal of Autism and Developmental Disorders, 45*, 3862–3869. https://doi.org/10.1007/s10803-014-2153-3

Kalkusch, I., Jaggy, A. , Bossi, C. B., Weiss, B., Sticca, F., & Perren, S. (2020). Promoting social pretend play in preschool age: Is providing roleplay material enough? *Early Education and Development*, 1–17. https://doi.org/10.1080/10409289.2020.1830248

Katz, V. S., Gonzalez, C., & Clark, K. (2017). Digital inequality and developmental trajectories of low-income, immigrant, and minority children. *Pediatrics, 140*(Supplement 2), S132–S136. DOI: https://doi.org/10.1542/peds.2016-1758R

Kelly-Byrne, D. (1989). *A child's play life: An ethnographic study*. New York: Teachers College.

Kipling Webster, E., Martin, C. K., & Staiano, A. E. (2019). Fundamental motor skills, screen-time, and physical activity in preschoolers. *Journal of Sport and Health Science, 8*(2), 114–121. https://doi.org/10.1016/j.jshs.2018.11.006

Klin, A., Danovitch, J. H., Merz, A. B., & Volkmar, F. R. (2007). Circumscribed interests in higher functioning individuals with autism spectrum disorders: An exploratory study. *Research and Practice for Persons with Severe Disabilities, 32*, 89–100.

Kluth, P., & Schwarz, P. (2008). *"Just give him the whale!": 20 ways to use fascinations, areas of expertise, and strengths to support students with autism*. Baltimore, MD: Paul H. Brookes.

Kochanek, J., Matthews, A., Wright, E., DiSanti, J., Neff, M., & Erickson, K. (2019). Competitive readiness: Developmental considerations to promote positive youth development in competitive activities. *Journal of Youth Development, 14*(1), 48–69. http://dx.doi.org/10.5195/jyd.2019.671

Koegel, R. L., Dyer, K., & Bell, L. K. (1987). The influence of child-preferred activities on autistic children's social behavior. *Journal of Applied Behavior Analysis, 20*, 243–252.

Koegel, R., Fredeen, R., Kim, S., Danial, J., Rubinstein, D., & Koegel, L. (2012). Using perseverative interests to improve interactions between adolescents with autism and their typical peers in school settings. *Journal of Positive Behavior Interventions, 14*(3), 133–141. http://doi.org/10.1177/1098300712437043

Koegel, R., Kim, S., Koegel, L., & Schwartzman, B. (2013). Improving socialization for high school students with ASD by using their preferred interests. *Journal of Autism and Developmental Disorders, 43*(9), 2121–2134.

Koegel, L. K., Singh, A. K., & Koegel, R. L. (2010). Improving motivation for academics in children with autism. *Journal of Autism and Developmental Disorders, 40*(9), 1057–1066.

Kryzak, L. A., Bauer, S., Jones, E. A., & Sturmey, P. (2013). Increasing responding to others' joint attention directives using circumscribed interests. *Journal of Applied Behavior Analysis, 46*(3), 674–679. https://doi.org/10.1002/jaba.73

Kryzak, L. A., & Jones, E. A. (2014). The effect of prompts within embedded circumscribed interests to teach initiating joint attention in children with autism spectrum disorders. *Journal of Developmental and Physical Disabilities, 27*, 265–284. https://doi.org/10.1007/s10882-014-9414-0

Kuhaneck, H., Spitzer, S., & Miller, E. (2010). *Activity analysis, creativity and playfulness in pediatric occupational therapy: Making play just right*. Sudbury, MA: Jones & Bartlett Learning.

Kyriakidis, I., Tsamagou, E., & Magos, K. (2021). Play and medical play in teaching pre-school children to cope with medical procedures involving needles: A systematic review. *Journal of Paediatrics and Child Health, 57*(4), 491–499. http://dx.doi.org/10.1111/jpc.15442

Lang, R., O'Reilly, M., Rispoli, M., Shogren, K., Machalicek, W., Sigafoos, J., & Regester, A. (2009). Review of interventions to increase functional and symbolic play in children with autism. *Education and Training in Developmental Disabilities, 44*(4), 481–492.

Larsson, I., & Svedin, C. G. (2002). Teachers' and parents' reports on 3- to 6-year-old children's sexual behavior—A comparison. *Child Abuse & Neglect, 26*, 247–266.

Laugeson, E. A., Frankel, F., Gantman, A., Dillon, A. R., & Mogil, C. (2012). Evidence-based social skills training for adolescents with autism spectrum disorders: The UCLA PEERS program. *Journal of Autism and Developmental Disorders, 42*(6), 1025–1036. https://doi.org/10.1007/s10803-011-1339-1

Leber, D., & Vanoli, E. (2001). Therapeutic use of humor: Occupational therapy clinicians' perceptions and practices. *American Journal of Occupational Therapy, 55*(2), 221–226.

Lee, K., Sidhu, D. M., & Pexman, P. M. (2020). Teaching sarcasm: Evaluating metapragmatic training for typically developing children. *Canadian Journal of Experimental Psychology = Revue Canadienne De Psychologie Experimentale, 75*(2), 139–145. http://dx.doi.org/10.1037/cep0000228

Lee, S. C., Grey, C., Gurfinkel, M., Leb, O., Stern, V., & Sytner, G., (2013). The effect of computer-based intervention on enhancing visual perception of preschool children with autism: A single-subject design study. *Journal of Occupational Therapy, Schools, and Early Intervention, 6*, 31–43. http://dx.org/10.1080/19411243.2013.776425

Lindsay, S., Hounsell, K. G., & Cassiani, C. (2017). A scoping review of the role of LEGO® therapy for improving inclusion and social skills among children and youth with autism. *Disability Health Journal, 10*(2), 173–182. https://doi.org/10.1016/j.dhjo.2016.10.010.

Little, H., & Wyver, S. (2010). Individual differences in children's risk perception and appraisals in outdoor play environments. *International Journal of Early Years Education, 18*(4), 297.

Little, L. M., Pope, E., Wallisch, A., & Dunn, W. (2018a). Occupation-based coaching by means of telehealth for families of young children with autism spectrum disorder. *American Journal of Occupational Therapy, 72*, 7202205020. https://doi .org/10.5014/ajot.2018.024786

Little, L. M., Wallisch, A., Pope, E., & Dunn, W. (2018b). Acceptability and cost comparison of a telehealth intervention for families of children with autism. *Infants & Young Children, 31*, 275–286. https://doi.org/10.1097/IYC.0000000000000126.

Livesay, H. (2007). Making a place for the angry hero on the team. In R. C. Lawrence (Ed.), *Using superheroes in counseling and play therapy* (pp. 121–142). New York: Springer.

Loizou, E., & Loizou, E. K. (2019). Visual and verbal humor productions after a series of creative structured activities: A case study of two pre-schoolers, *Early Years*, 1–17. https://doi .org/10.1080/09575146.2019.1683721

Lynch, A., Ashcraft, R., & March Tekell, L. (2017). Understanding children who have experienced early adversity: Implications for practitioners practicing sensory integration. *SIS Quarterly Practice Connections, 2*(3), 5–7.

Martin, R. A., Puhlik-Doris, P., Larsen, G., Gray, J., & Weir, K. (2003). Individual differences in uses of humor and their relation to psychological well-being: Development of the Humor Styles Questionnaire. *Journal of Research in Personality, 37*, 48–75. https://doi.org/10.1016/S0092-6566(02)00534-2

Messier, J., Ferland, F., & Majnemer, A. (2008). Play behavior of school age children with intellectual disability: Their capacities, interests and attitude. *Journal of Developmental and Physical Disabilities, 20*, 193–207.

Mitchell, J., & Lashewicz, B. (2018). Quirky kids: Fathers' stories of embracing diversity and dismantling expectations for normative play with their children with autism spectrum disorder. *Disability & Society, 33*(7), 1120–1137. http://dx.doi .org/10.1080/09687599.2018.1474087

Mohammadi, A., Mehraban, A. H., Damavandi, S. A., Zarei, M. A., & Haghani, H. (2021). The effect of play-based occupational therapy on symptoms and participation in daily life activities in children with cancer: A randomized controlled trial. *British Journal of Occupational Therapy*, 0308022620987125. https:// doi.org/10.1177/0308022620987125

Mook, B. (1994). Therapeutic play: From interpretation to intervention. In J. Hellendoorn, R. van der Kooij, & B. Sutton-Smith (Eds.), *Play and intervention* (pp. 39–52). Albany: State University of New York Press.

Moor, J. (2002). *Playing, laughing and learning with children on the autism spectrum: A practical resource of play ideas for parents and carers*. Philadelphia, PA: Jessica Kingsley.

Morrongiello, B. A., & Lasenby-Lessard, J. (2007). Psychological determinants of risk-taking by children: An integrative model and implications for interventions. *Injury Prevention, 13*, 20–25.

Morrongiello, B. A., & Matheis, S. (2007a). Addressing the issue of falls off playground equipment: An empirically-based intervention to reduce fall-risk behavior on playgrounds. *Journal of Pediatric Psychology, 32*, 819–830.

Morrongiello, B. A., & Matheis, S. (2007b). Understanding children's injury-risk behaviors: The independent contributions of cognitions and emotions. *Journal of Pediatric Psychology, 32*(8), 926–937.

Munier, V., Myers, C. T., & Pierce, D. (2008). Power of object play for infants and toddlers. In *Play in occupational therapy for children* (pp. 219–249). St. Louis, MO: Mosby.

Murphy, L. (2019). Approaching competitive games with care: Five tips to help kids become better at losing. *Autism Asperger's Sensory Digest*, 28–30.

Neophytou, E., Manwell, L. A., & Eikelboom, R. (2019). Effects of excessive screen time on neurodevelopment, learning, memory, mental health, and neurodegeneration: A scoping review. *International Journal of Mental Health and Addiction*, 1–21. https://doi.org/10.1007/s11469-019-00182-2

Niehues, A., & Bundy, A. (2019). Parents' perceptions of risk and the influence on children's everyday occupations. *American Journal of Occupational Therapy, 73*(4_Supplement_1), 7311505150. https://doi.org/10.5014/ajot.2019.73S1-PO5013

Orhan, E., & Yildiz, S. (2017). The effects of pre-intervention training provided through therapeutic play on the anxiety of pediatric oncology patients during peripheral catheterization. *International Journal of Caring Sciences, 10*(3), 1533–1544.

Owens, G., Granader, Y., Humphrey, A., & Baron-Cohen, S. (2008). LEGO therapy and the social use of language programme: An evaluation of two social skills interventions for children with high functioning autism and Asperger syndrome. *Journal of Autism and Developmental Disorders, 38*, 1944–1957. https:// doi.org/10.1007/s10803-008-0590-6

Paine, A. L., Karajian, G., Hashmi, S., Persram, R. J., & Howe, N. (2020). "Where's your bum brain?" Humor, social understanding, and sibling relationship quality in early childhood. *Social Development*, 1–20. https://doi.org/10.1111 /sode.12488

Paley, V. G. (1990). *The boy who would be a helicopter: The uses of storytelling in the classroom*. Cambridge, MA: Harvard University Press.

Parham, L. D. (1992). Strategies for maintaining a playful atmosphere during therapy. *Sensory Integration Special Interest Section Newsletter, 15*(1), 2–3.

Parker, M. M., Hergenrather, K., Smelser, Q., & Kelly, C. T. (2021). Exploring child-centered play therapy and trauma: A systematic review of literature. *International Journal of Play Therapy, 30*(1), 2–13. https://doi.org/10.1037/pla0000136

Parsons, D., Cordier, R., Vaz, S., & Lee, H. C. (2017). Parent-mediated intervention training delivered remotely for children with autism spectrum disorder living outside of urban areas: Systematic review. *Journal of Medical Internet research, 19*(8), e198.

Pluhar, E. (2007). Childhood sexuality. In M. S. Tepper & A. F. Owens (Eds.), *Sexual health: Vol. 1. Psychological foundations* (pp. 155–181). Westport, CT: Praeger.

Porter, N. (2012). Promotion of pretend play for children with high-functioning autism through the use of circumscribed interests. *Early Childhood Education Journal, 40*, 161–167. https://doi.org/10.1007/s10643-012-0505-1

Potaszi, C., Varela, M. J. V. D., Carvalho, L. C. D., Prado, L. F. D., & Prado, G. F. D. (2013). Effect of play activities on hospitalized children's stress: A randomized clinical trial. *Scandinavian Journal of Occupational Therapy, 20*(1), 71–79. http://dx.doi .org/10.3109/11038128.2012.729087

Price, P., & Miner, S. (2007). Occupation emerges in the process of therapy. *American Journal of Occupational Therapy, 61*(4), 441–450.

Proffitt, R. (2016). Gamification in rehabilitation: Finding the "just-right-challenge." In D. Novák, B. Tulu, & H. Brendryen (Eds.), *Handbook of Research on Holistic Perspectives in Gamification for Clinical Practice* (pp. 132–157). Hershey, PA: IGI Global. http://doi:10.4018/978-1-4666-9522-1.ch007

Purser, H. R., Van Herwegen, J., & Thomas, M. S. (2020). The development of children's comprehension and appreciation of riddles. *Journal of Experimental Child Psychology, 189*, 104709. https://doi.org/10.1016/j.jecp.2019.104709.

Raney, A. A., Smith, J. K., & Baker, K. (2006).Adolescents and the appeal of video games. In P. Vorderer & J. Bryant (Eds.), *Playing video games: Motives, responses, and consequences* (pp. 165–179). Mahwah, NJ: Erlbaum.

Rashid, A. A., Cheong, A. T., Hisham, R., Shamsuddin, N. H., & Roslan, D. (2021). Effectiveness of pretend medical play in improving children's health outcomes and well-being: A systematic review. *BMJ Open, 11*(1). http://dx.doi.org/10.1136/bmjopen-2020-041506

Reifenberg, G., Gabrosek, G., Tanner, K., Harpster, K., Proffitt, R., & Persch, A. (2017). Feasibility of pediatric game-based neurorehabilitation using telehealth technologies: A case report. *American Journal of Occupational Therapy, 71*, 7103190040. https://doi.org/10.5014/ajot.2017.024976

Reinhartsen, D. B., Garfinkle, A. N., & Wolery, M. (2002). Engagement with toys in two-year-old children with autism: Teacher selection versus child choice. *Research and Practice for Persons with Severe Disabilities, 27*(3), 175–187.

Reszka, S. S., Odom, S. L., & Hume, K. A. (2012). Ecological features of preschools and the social engagement of children with autism. *Journal of Early Intervention, 34*(1), 40–56. https://doi.org/10.1177/1053815112452596

Riso, D. D., Cambrisi, E., Bertini, S., & Miscioscia, M. (2020). Associations between pretend play, psychological functioning and coping strategies in pediatric chronic diseases: A cross-illness study. *International Journal of Environmental Research and Public Health, 17*(12), 4364. doi:http://dx.doi.org/10.3390/ijerph17124364

Roberts, T., Stagnitti, K., Brown, T., & Bhopti, A. (2018). Relationship between sensory processing and pretend play in typically developing children. *American Journal of Occupational Therapy, 72*(1).

Robinson, M. R., Koverman, B., Becker, C., Ciancio, K. E., Fisher, G., & Saake, S. (2021). Lessons learned from the COVID-19 pandemic: Occupational therapy on the front line. *American Journal of Occupational Therapy, 75*(2), 7502090010p1-7502090010p7. https://doi.org/10.5014/ajot.2021.047654

Ruch, W., & McGhee, P. E. (2014).Humor intervention programs. In A. C. Parks & S. M. Schueller (Eds.), *The Wiley Blackwell handbook of positive psychological interventions* (pp. 179–193). Malden, MA: Wiley Blackwell. https://doi.org/10.1002/9781118315927.ch10

Russ, S. W. (2018).Pretend play and creativity: Two templates for the future. In R. J. Sternberg & J. C. Kaufman (Eds.), *The nature of human creativity* (pp. 264–279). Cambridge, UK: Cambridge University Press.

Russ, S. W. (2020). Mind wandering, fantasy, and pretend play: A natural combination. In D. D. Preiss, D. Cosmelli, & J. C. Kaufman (Eds.), *Creativity and the wandering mind: Spontaneous and controlled cognition* (pp. 231–248). San Diego, CA: Academic Press. https://doi.org/10.1016/B978-0-12-816400-6.00010-9

Russ, S. W., Fehr, K., & Hoffmann, J. (2013). Helping children develop pretend play skills: Implications for giftedness and talented programs. In K. H. Kim, J. Kaufman, J. Baer, & B. Sriraman (Eds.), *Advances in creativity and giftedness: Vol. 2. Creatively gifted students are not like other gifted students: Research, theory, and practice* (pp. 73–91). Rotterdam, Netherland: Sense Publishers.

Samson, A. C. (2013). Humor(lessness) elucidated—Sense of humor in individuals with autism spectrum disorders: Review and Introduction. *Humor, 26*(3), 393–409.

Sandnabba, N. K., Santtila, P., Wannas, M., & Krook, K. (2003). Age and gender specific sexual behaviors in children. *Child Abuse & Neglect, 27*, 579–605.

Sautter, R. A., LeBlanc, L. A., & Gillett, J. N. (2008). Using free operant preference assessments to select toys for free play between children with autism and siblings. *Research in Autism Spectrum Disorders, 2*(1), 17–27.

Schuurmans, A. A., Nijhof, K. S., Engels, R. C., & Granic, I. (2018). Using a videogame intervention to reduce anxiety and externalizing problems among youths in residential care: An initial randomized controlled trial. *Journal of Psychopathology and Behavioral Assessment, 40*(2), 344–354. https://doi.org/10.1007/s10862-017-9638-2

Sciaraffa, M., & Randolph, T. (2011). You want me to talk to children about what? Responding to the subject of sexuality development in young children. *Young Children 66*(4), 32–38.

Serrada-Tejeda, S., Santos-del-Riego, S., May-Benson, T. A., & Pérez-de-Heredia-Torres, M. (2021). Influence of ideational praxis on the development of play and adaptive behavior of children with autism spectrum disorder: A comparative analysis. *International Journal of Environmental Research and Public Health, 18*(11), 5704. https://doi.org/10.3390/ijerph18115704

Silva, C., Da Fonseca, D., Esteves, F., & Deruelle, C. (2017). Seeing the funny side of things: Humour processing in autism spectrum disorders. *Research in Autism Spectrum Disorders, 43–44C*, 8–17. https://doi.org/10.1016/j.rasd.2017.09.001

Singer, D. G., & Singer, J. L. (1990). *The house of make believe: Children's play and the developing imagination.* Cambridge, MA: Harvard University Press.

Smith, E., Constantin, A., Johnson, H., & Brosnan, M. (2021). Digitally-mediated social stories support children on the autism spectrum adapting to a change in a "real-world" context. *Journal of Autism and Developmental Disorders, 51*, 514–526. https://doi.org/10.1007/s10803-020-04558-5

Spaaij, R., Lusher, D., Jeanes, R., Farquharson, K., Gorman, S., & Magee, J. (2019). Participation-performance tension and gender affect recreational sports clubs' engagement with children and young people with diverse backgrounds and abilities. *PLoS One, 14*(4). http://dx.doi.org/10.1371/journal.pone.0214537

Spencer, G., Bundy, A., Wyver, S., Villeneuve, M., Tranter, P., Beetham, K., . . . Naughton, G. (2016). Uncertainty in the school playground: Shifting rationalities and teachers' sense-making in the management of risks for children with disabilities. *Health, Risk & Society, 18*(5–6), 301–317. http://dx.doi.org/10.1080/13698575.2016.1238447

Spencer, V. G., Simpson, C. G., Day, M., & Buster, E. (2008). Using the power card strategy to teach social skills to a child with autism. *TEACHING Exceptional Children Plus, 5*(1), n1, Article 2. http://escholarship.bc.edu/education/tecplus/vol5/iss1/art2

Spitzer, S. L. (2008).Play in children with autism: Structure and experience. In L. D. Parham & L. S. Fazio (Eds.), *Play in occupational therapy for children* (2nd ed., pp. 351–374). St. Louis, MO: Mosby Elsevier.

Spitzer, S. (2017). *How to make therapeutic work fun for pediatric clients.* MedBridge Blog. https://www.medbridgeeducation.com/blog/2017/07/make-therapeutic-work-fun-pediatric-clients/?a_aid=1655&a_cid=29b49843

Stagnitti, K., & Unsworth, C. (2000). The importance of pretend play in child development: An occupational therapy perspective. *British Journal of Occupational Therapy, 63,* 121–127.

Stenman, K., Christofferson, J., Alderfer, M. A., Pierce, J., Kelly, C., Schifano, E., . . . Kazak, A. E. (2019). Integrating play in trauma-informed care: Multidisciplinary pediatric healthcare provider perspectives. *Psychological Services, 16*(1), 7–15. https://doi.org/10.1037/ser0000294

Stephenson, A. (2003). Physical risk-taking: Dangerous or endangered? *Early Years: An International Journal of Research and Development, 23,* 35–43.

Sterman, J. J., Naughton, G. A., Bundy, A. C., Froude, E., & Villeneuve, M. A. (2020). Mothers supporting play as a choice for children with disabilities within a culturally and linguistically diverse community. *Scandinavian Journal of Occupational Therapy, 27*(5), 373–384. https://doi.org/10.1080/11038128.2019.1684556

Sterman, J., Villeneuve, M., Spencer, G., Wyver, S., Beetham, K. S., Naughton, G., . . . Bundy, A. (2020). Creating play opportunities on the school playground: Educator experiences of the Sydney playground project. *Australian Occupational Therapy Journal, 67*(1), 62–73. https://doi.org/10.1111/1440-1630.12624

Tavernor, L., Barron, E., Rodgers, J., & McConachie, H. (2013). Finding out what matters: Validity of quality of life measurement in young people with ASD. *Child: Care, Health and Development, 39*(4), 592–601.

Tomchek, S. D., & Koenig, K. P. (2016). *Occupational therapy practice guidelines for individuals with autism spectrum disorder.* Bethesda, MD: AOTA Press.

Van Tubbergen, M., Warschausky, S., Birnholz, J., & Baker, S. (2008). Choice beyond preference: Conceptualization and assessment of choice-making skills in children with significant impairments. *Rehabilitation Psychology, 53*(1), 93–100.

Vasquez, E., Nagendran, A., Welch, G. F., Marino, M. T., Hughes, D. E., Koch, A., & Delisio, L. (2015). Virtual learning environments for students with disabilities: A review and analysis of the empirical literature and two case studies. *Rural Special Education Quarterly, 34*(3), 26–32. https://doi.org/10.1177/875687051503400306

Vismara, L. A., & Lyons, G. L. (2007). Using perseverative interests to elicit joint attention behaviors in young children with autism: Theoretical and clinical implications for understanding motivation. *Journal of Positive Behavior Interventions, 9*(4), 214–228.

Vismara, L. A., Young, G. S., & Rogers, S. J. (2012). Telehealth for expanding the reach of early autism training to parents. *Autism Research and Treatment,* 121878. https://doi.org/10.1155/2012/121878

Wainer, A. L., & Ingersoll, B. R. (2015). Increasing access to an ASD imitation intervention via a telehealth parent training program. *Journal of Autism and Developmental Disorders, 45*(12), 3877–3890. https://doi.org/10.1007/s10803-014-2186-7

Wallisch, A., Little, L., Pope, E., & Dunn, W. (2019). Parent perspectives of an occupational therapy telehealth intervention. *International Journal of Telerehabilitation, 11*(1), 15–22. https://doi.org/10.5195/ijt.2019.6274

Watkins, L., O'Reilly, M., Kuhn, M., & Ledbetter-Cho, K. (2019). An interest-based intervention package to increase peer social interaction in young children with autism spectrum disorder. *Journal of Applied Behavior Analysis, 52*(1), 132–149. https://doi.org/10.1002/jaba.514.

White, R. W. (1959). Motivation reconsidered: The concept of competence. *Psychological Review, 66*(5), 297–333.

Wilkinson, V. J., Theodore, K., & Raczka, R. (2015). "As normal as possible": Sexual identity development in people with intellectual disabilities transitioning to adulthood. *Sexuality and Disability, 33*(1), 93–105. https://doi.org/10.1007/s11195-014-9356-6

William Li, H. C., Lopez, V., & Lee, T. L. I. (2007). Effects of preoperative therapeutic play on outcomes of school-age children undergoing day surgery. *Research in Nursing & Health, 30*(3), 320–332.

Wimpory, D., Hobson, R. P., & Nash, S. (2007). What facilitates social engagement in preschool children with autism? *Journal of Autism and Developmental Disorders, 37,* 564–573.

Winter-Messiers, M. A. (2007). From tarantulas to toilet brushes: Understanding the special interest areas of children and youth with Asperger syndrome. *Remedial and Special Education, 28*(3), 140–152.

Wong, C. L., Ip, W. Y., Kwok, B. M. C., Choi, K. C., Ng, B. K. W., & Chan, C. W. H. (2018). Effects of therapeutic play on children undergoing cast-removal procedures: A randomised controlled trial. *BMJ Open, 8,* e021071. https://doi.org/10.1136/bmjopen-2017-021071

Wu, C., Liu, Y., Kuo, C., Chen, H., & Chang, Y. (2016). Effectiveness of humor training among adolescents with autism. *Psychiatry Research, 246,* 25–31. https://doi.org/10.1016/j.psychres.2016.09.016

Zengin, M., Yayan, E. H., & Düken, M. E. (2021). The effects of a therapeutic play/play therapy program on the fear and anxiety levels of hospitalized children after liver transplantation. *Journal of PeriAnesthesia Nursing: Official Journal of the American Society of PeriAnesthesia Nurses, 36*(1), 81–85. http://dx.doi.org/10.1016/j.jopan.2020.07.006

Zyga, O., Russ, S. W., & Dimitropoulos, A. (2018). The PRETEND program: Evaluating the feasibility of a remote parent-training intervention for children with Prader-Willi syndrome. *American Journal on Intellectual and Developmental Disabilities, 123*(6), 574–584. https://doi.org/10.1352/1944-7558-123.6.574

APPENDIX 16.1 Worksheet for Identifying Opportunities to Expand Limited Play Interests

Child's Name:	
Activity Child Likes:	
What factors seem to be most meaningful to the child?	

<u>Directions</u>: Note core elements of the way the child does this activity; the child's general preferences, abilities, and strengths; and the child's areas of need. Then consider the relationship of elements of strengths or needs that might be introduced into the current activity, in ways that are most consistent with its current form and meaning. Try one modification at a time to determine child's level of acceptance, resistance, or interest.

Activity Components	Child's Performance (Occupational Analysis)	Other Child Interests, Abilities, Strengths	Areas of Need	Analysis: Possible Modifications
Materials (toys, objects, shape, color, size, etc.)				
Sensory features (visual, auditory, tactile, vestibular, proprioceptive)				
Motor/action features (eyes, posture, hand use, movements, motor skill/ coordination/control, etc.)				
Cognitive features (sequencing, problem solving, construction, imagination, etc.)				
Social features (interaction with another)				
Location & space				

APPENDIX 16.2 Suggested Resources on Creating Therapeutic Stories

Baltazar, A., & Bax, B. E. (2004). Writing social stories for the child with sensory integration dysfunction: An introductory resource and guide for therapists, teachers, and parents. *Sensory Integration Special Interest Section Quarterly, 27*(1), 1–3.

Fazio, L. S. (2008).Storytelling, storymaking, and fantasy play. In L. D. Parham & L.S. Fazio (Eds.), *Play in occupational therapy for children* (2nd ed., pp. 427–443). St. Louis, MO: Mosby Elsevier.

Gray, C. (2000). *The new social story book.* Arlington, TX: Future Horizons.

Levine, K., & Chedd, N. (2007). *Replays: Using play to enhance emotional and behavioral development for children with autism spectrum disorders.* London: Jessica Kingsley.

Marr, D., & Nackley, V. (2007). Writing your own sensory stories. *OT Practice, 12*(11), 15–19.

The Gray Center for Social Learning and Understanding (www.thegraycenter.org) provides information on social stories.

Index

Note: Figures, tables and boxes are indicated by f, t and b following the page number